P9-CCR-678

ALSO BY MARISA ACOCELLA MARCHETTO

JUST WHO THE HELL IS SHE, ANYWAY?

CANCER VIXEN

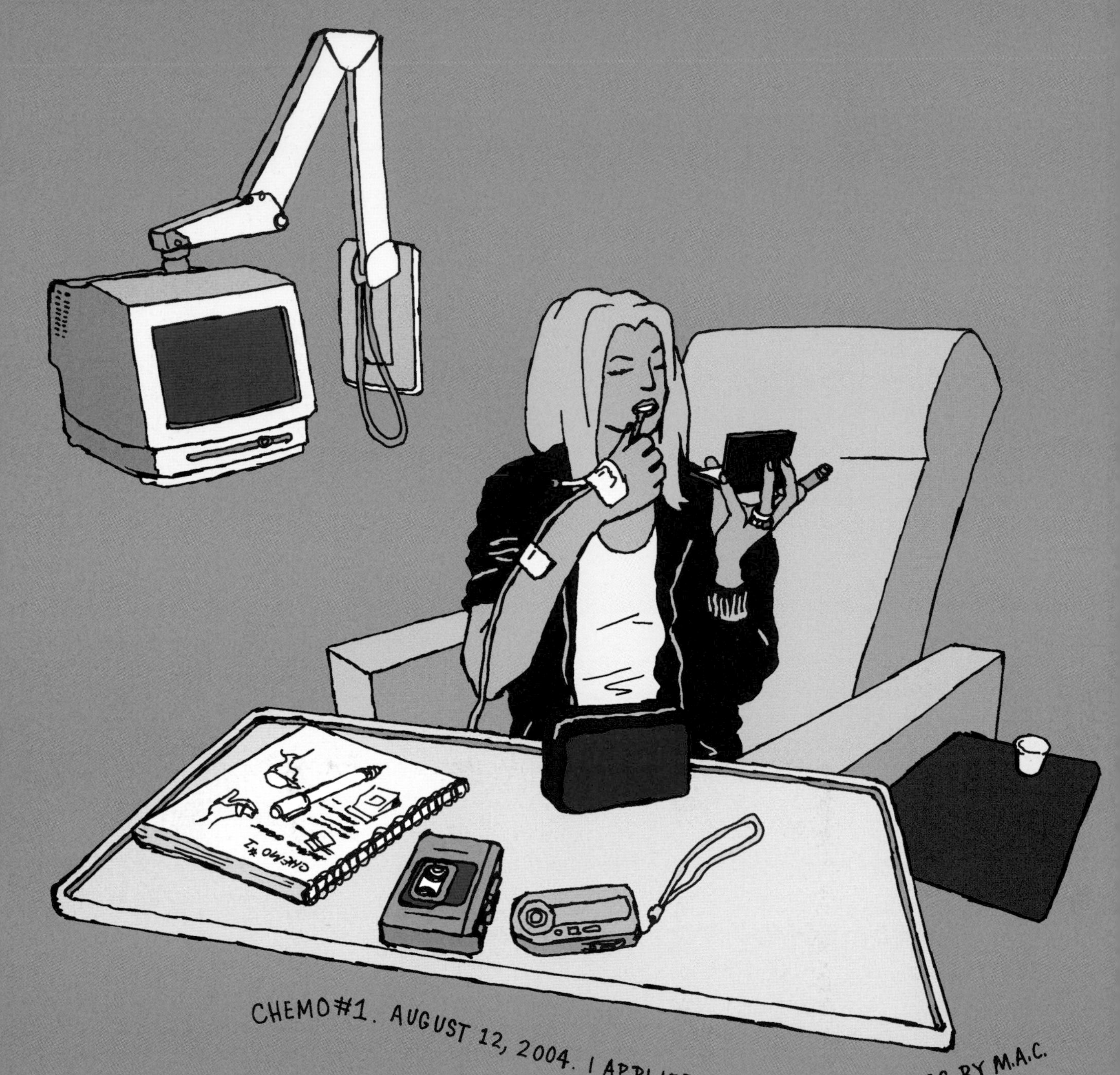

CHEMO #1. AUGUST 12, 2004. I APPLIED *VIVA GLAM* LIPGLASS BY M.A.C.

CANCER VIXEN

A TRUE STORY

MARISA ACOCELLA MARCHETTO

ALFRED A. KNOPF

NEW YORK · TORONTO
2006

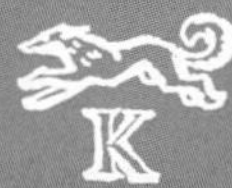

THIS IS A BORZOI BOOK
PUBLISHED BY ALFRED A. KNOPF AND ALFRED A. KNOPF CANADA

PUBLISHED SIMULTANEOUSLY IN CANADA BY ALFRED A. KNOPF CANADA, A DIVISION OF RANDOM HOUSE OF CANADA LIMITED, TORONTO.
www.aaknopf.com
www.randomhouse.ca

LIBRARY OF CONGRESS CATALOGING-IN-PUBLICATION DATA.
MARCHETTO, MARISA ACOCELLA.
CANCER VIXEN: A TRUE STORY/ MARISA ACOCELLA MARCHETTO.—1ST ED.
p. cm.
ISBN-10: 0-307-26357-6 (alk. paper)
1. MARCHETTO, MARISA ACOCELLA—HEALTH—COMIC BOOKS, STRIPS, ETC.
2. BREAST-CANCER—PATIENTS—NEW YORK (STATE)—NEW YORK—BIOGRAPHY—COMIC BOOKS, STRIPS, ETC. I. TITLE.
RC280.B8M343 2006
362.196'994490092—dc22 2006040967

LIBRARY AND ARCHIVES CANADA CATALOGUING IN PUBLICATION
MARCHETTO, MARISA ACOCELLA
CANCER VIXEN: A TRUE STORY/ MARISA ACOCELLA MARCHETTO.
ISBN-13: 978-0-676-97824-7
ISBN-10: 0-676-97824-X
1. MARCHETTO, MARISA ACOCELLA-HEALTH. 2. BREAST-CANCER-PATIENTS-NEW YORK (STATE)-NEW YORK-BIOGRAPHY. 3. CARTOONISTS-NEW YORK (STATE)-NEW YORK-BIOGRAPHY. I. TITLE.
RC280.B8M36 2006
362.196'99449'0092 C2005-907018-8

OUT OF CONCERN FOR THE PRIVACY OF INDIVIDUALS DEPICTED HERE, THE AUTHOR HAS CHANGED THE NAMES OF CERTAIN INDIVIDUALS, AS WELL AS POTENTIALLY IDENTIFYING DESCRIPTIVE DETAILS CONCERNING THEM.

MANUFACTURED IN SINGAPORE
FIRST EDITION

FOR SILVANO

WHAT HAPPENS WHEN A SHOE-CRAZY, LIPSTICK-OBSESSED, WINE-SWILLING, PASTA-SLURPING, FASHION-FANATIC, SINGLE-FOREVER, ABOUT-TO-GET-MARRIED BIG-CITY GIRL CARTOONIST (ME, MARISA ACOCELLA) WITH A FABULOUS LIFE FINDS...

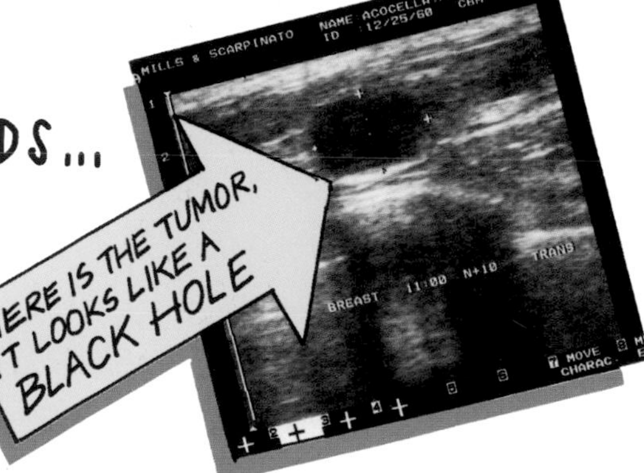

A LUMP IN HER BREAST?!?

I NOTICED SOMETHING FISHY WHILE SWIMMING IN APRIL.
WHY DOES MY ARM HURT?

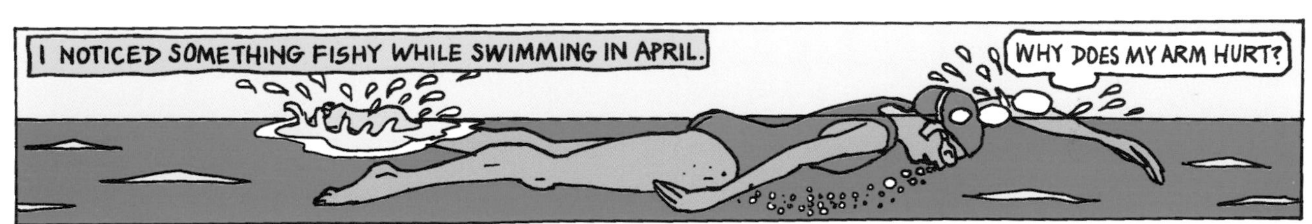

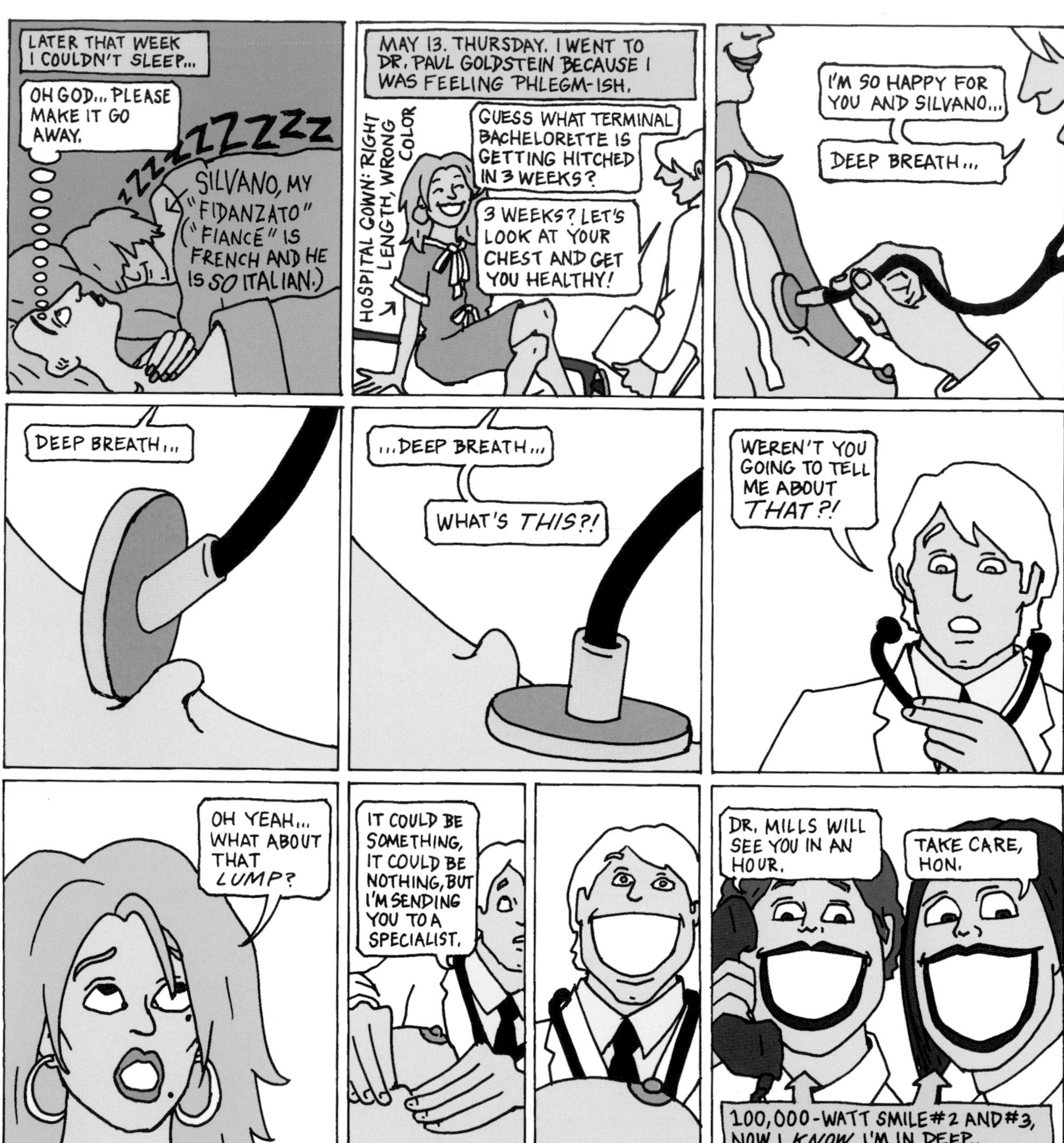

LATER THAT WEEK I COULDN'T SLEEP...
OH GOD... PLEASE MAKE IT GO AWAY.
ZZZZZZZZZZZz
SILVANO, MY "FIDANZATO" ("FIANCÉ" IS FRENCH AND HE IS *SO* ITALIAN.)
MAY 13. THURSDAY. I WENT TO DR. PAUL GOLDSTEIN BECAUSE I WAS FEELING PHLEGM-ISH.
HOSPITAL GOWN: RIGHT LENGTH, WRONG COLOR
GUESS WHAT TERMINAL BACHELORETTE IS GETTING HITCHED IN 3 WEEKS?
3 WEEKS? LET'S LOOK AT YOUR CHEST AND GET YOU HEALTHY!
I'M SO HAPPY FOR YOU AND SILVANO...
DEEP BREATH...
DEEP BREATH...
...DEEP BREATH...
WHAT'S *THIS?!*
WEREN'T YOU GOING TO TELL ME ABOUT *THAT?!*
OH YEAH... WHAT ABOUT THAT *LUMP?*
IT COULD BE SOMETHING, IT COULD BE NOTHING, BUT I'M SENDING YOU TO A SPECIALIST.
DR. MILLS WILL SEE YOU IN AN HOUR.
TAKE CARE, HON.
100,000-WATT SMILE #2 AND #3, NOW I *KNOW* I'M IN DEEP...

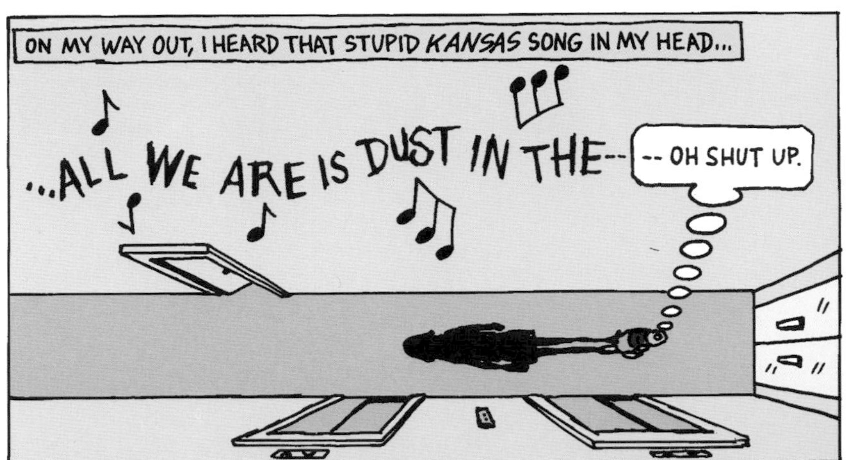
ON MY WAY OUT, I HEARD THAT STUPID *KANSAS* SONG IN MY HEAD...
...ALL WE ARE IS DUST IN THE--
-- OH SHUT UP.

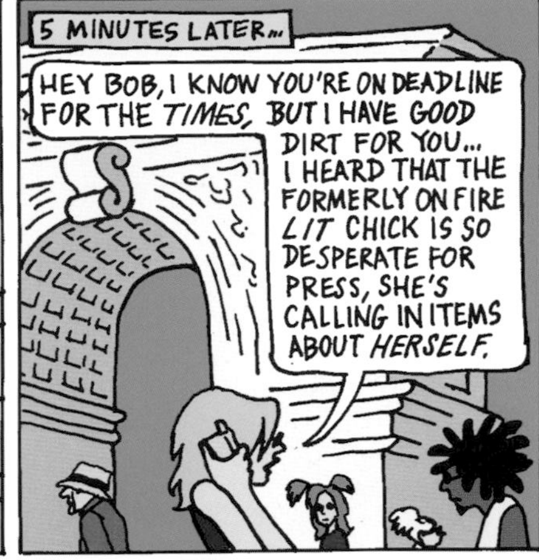
5 MINUTES LATER...
HEY BOB, I KNOW YOU'RE ON DEADLINE FOR THE *TIMES*, BUT I HAVE GOOD DIRT FOR YOU... I HEARD THAT THE FORMERLY ON FIRE *LIT* CHICK IS SO DESPERATE FOR PRESS, SHE'S CALLING IN ITEMS ABOUT *HERSELF*.

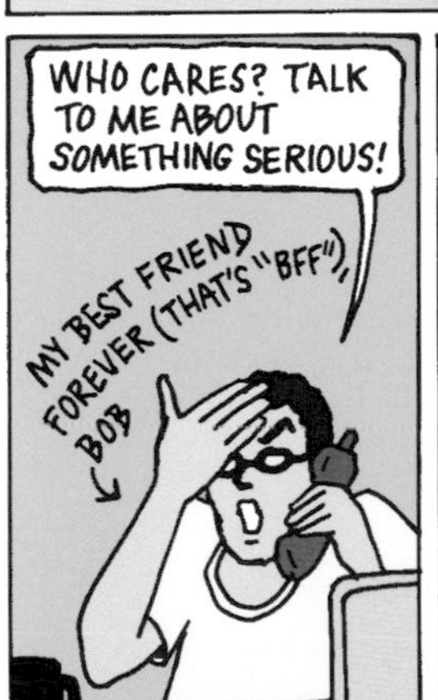
WHO CARES? TALK TO ME ABOUT SOMETHING SERIOUS!
MY BEST FRIEND FOREVER (THAT'S "BFF") BOB

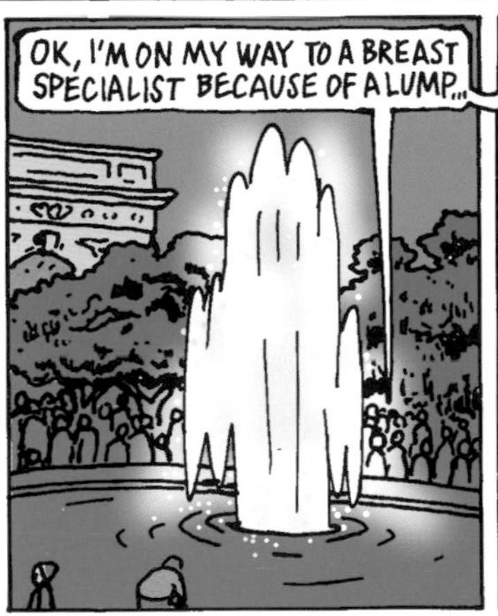
OK, I'M ON MY WAY TO A BREAST SPECIALIST BECAUSE OF A LUMP...

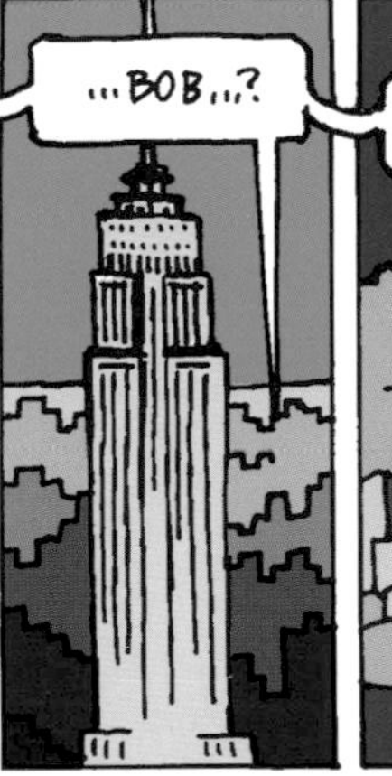
...BOB...?

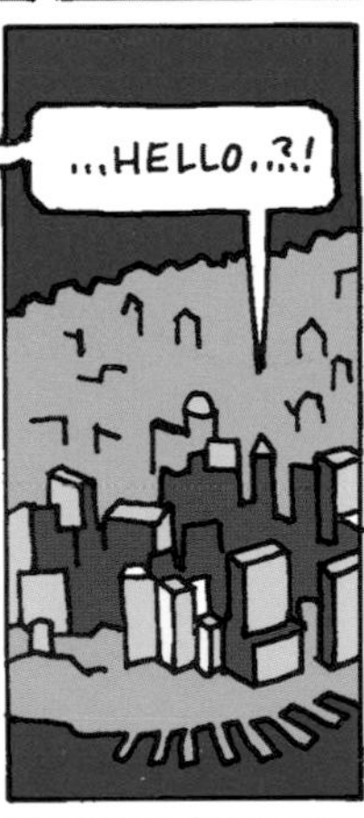
...HELLO...?!

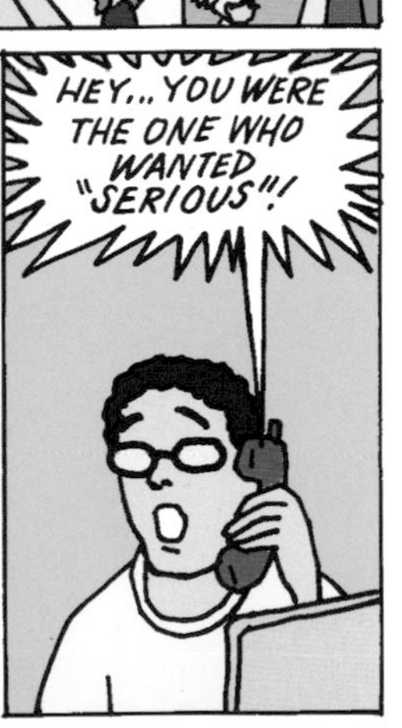
HEY... YOU WERE THE ONE WHO WANTED "SERIOUS"!

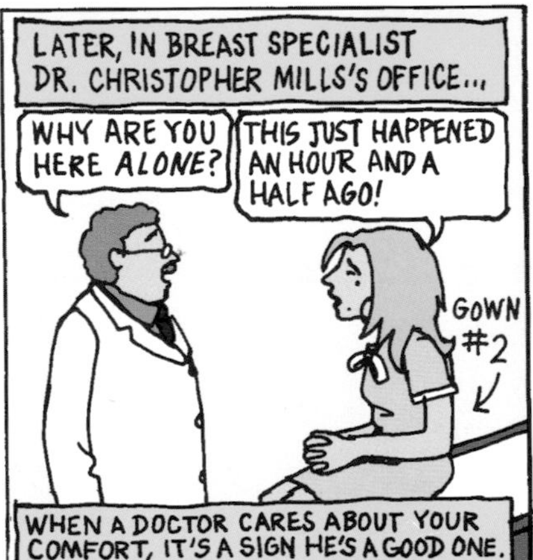
LATER, IN BREAST SPECIALIST DR. CHRISTOPHER MILLS'S OFFICE...
WHY ARE YOU HERE *ALONE*?
THIS JUST HAPPENED AN HOUR AND A HALF AGO!
GOWN #2
WHEN A DOCTOR CARES ABOUT YOUR COMFORT, IT'S A SIGN HE'S A GOOD ONE.

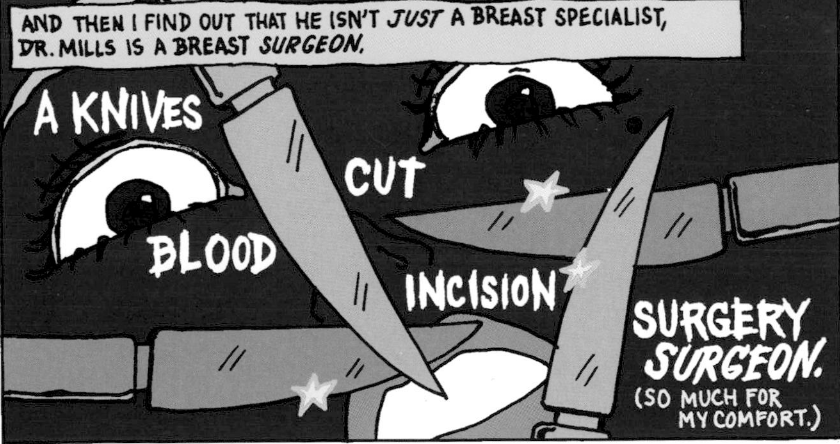
AND THEN I FIND OUT THAT HE ISN'T *JUST* A BREAST SPECIALIST, DR. MILLS IS A BREAST *SURGEON*.
A KNIVES
CUT
BLOOD
INCISION
SURGERY
SURGEON.
(SO MUCH FOR MY COMFORT.)

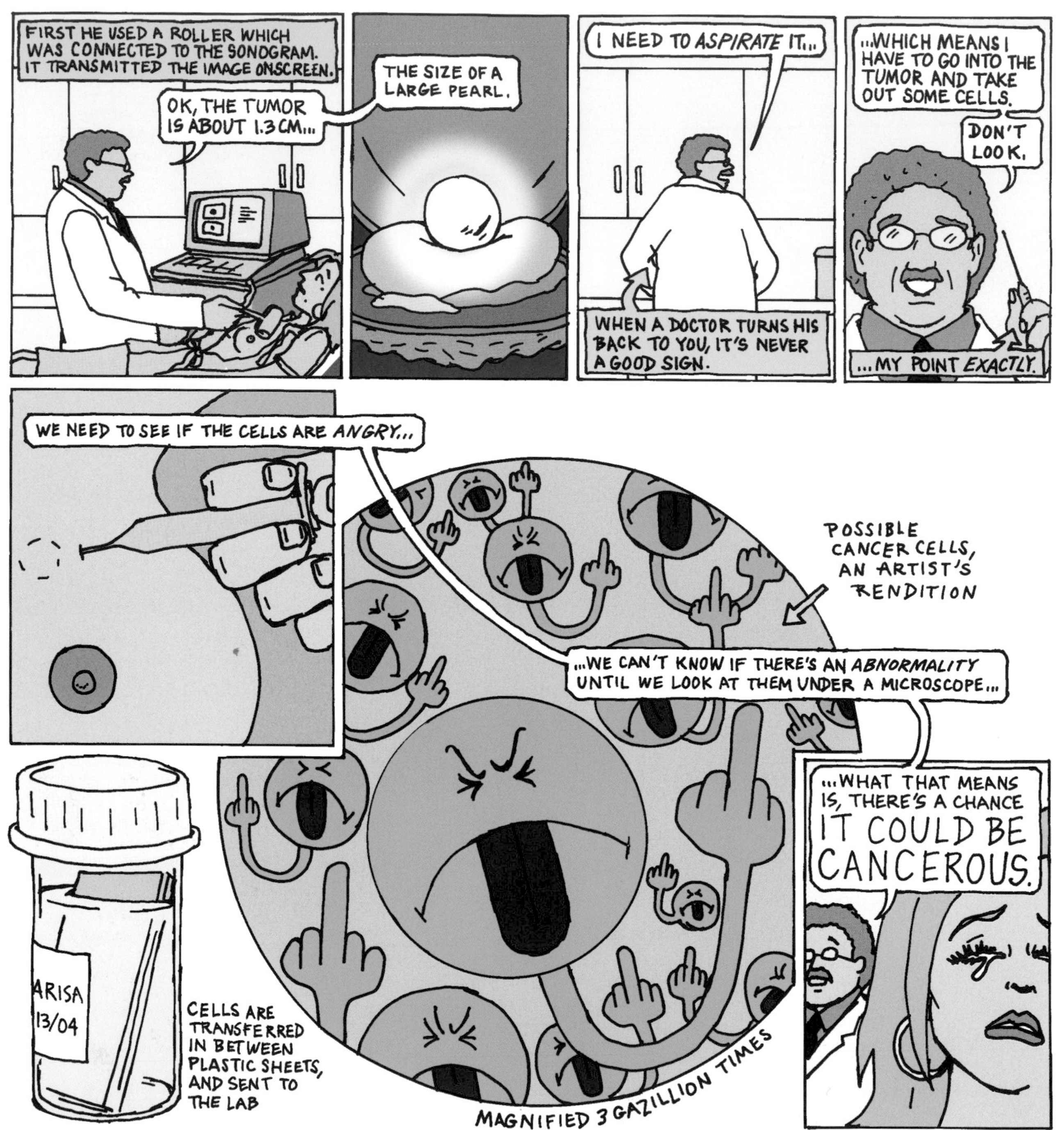
FIRST HE USED A ROLLER WHICH WAS CONNECTED TO THE SONOGRAM. IT TRANSMITTED THE IMAGE ONSCREEN.
OK, THE TUMOR IS ABOUT 1.3 CM...
THE SIZE OF A LARGE PEARL.
I NEED TO ASPIRATE IT...
WHEN A DOCTOR TURNS HIS BACK TO YOU, IT'S NEVER A GOOD SIGN.
...WHICH MEANS I HAVE TO GO INTO THE TUMOR AND TAKE OUT SOME CELLS.
DON'T LOOK.
...MY POINT EXACTLY.
WE NEED TO SEE IF THE CELLS ARE ANGRY...
POSSIBLE CANCER CELLS, AN ARTIST'S RENDITION
...WE CAN'T KNOW IF THERE'S AN ABNORMALITY UNTIL WE LOOK AT THEM UNDER A MICROSCOPE...
...WHAT THAT MEANS IS, THERE'S A CHANCE IT COULD BE CANCEROUS.
ARISA 13/04
CELLS ARE TRANSFERRED IN BETWEEN PLASTIC SHEETS, AND SENT TO THE LAB
MAGNIFIED 3 GAZILLION TIMES

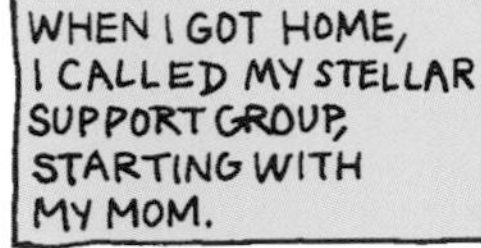
WHEN I GOT HOME, I CALLED MY STELLAR SUPPORT GROUP, STARTING WITH MY MOM.

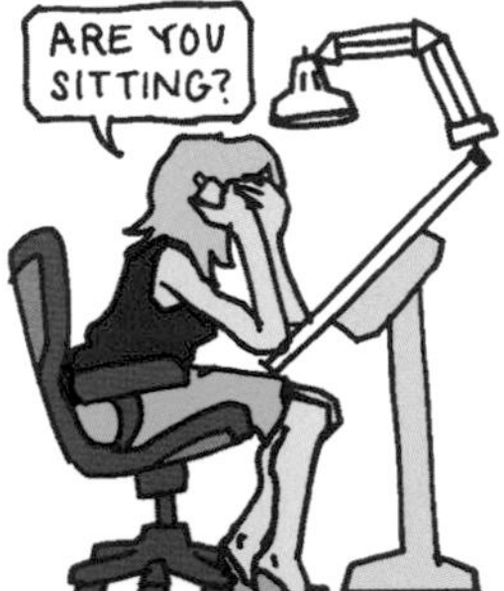
ARE YOU SITTING?

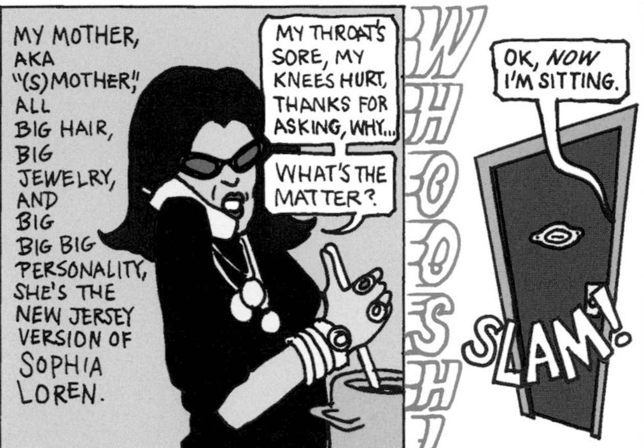
MY MOTHER, AKA "(S)MOTHER," ALL BIG HAIR, BIG JEWELRY, AND BIG BIG BIG PERSONALITY, SHE'S THE NEW JERSEY VERSION OF SOPHIA LOREN.
MY THROAT'S SORE, MY KNEES HURT, THANKS FOR ASKING, WHY...
WHAT'S THE MATTER?
WHOOSH!
OK, NOW I'M SITTING.
SLAM!

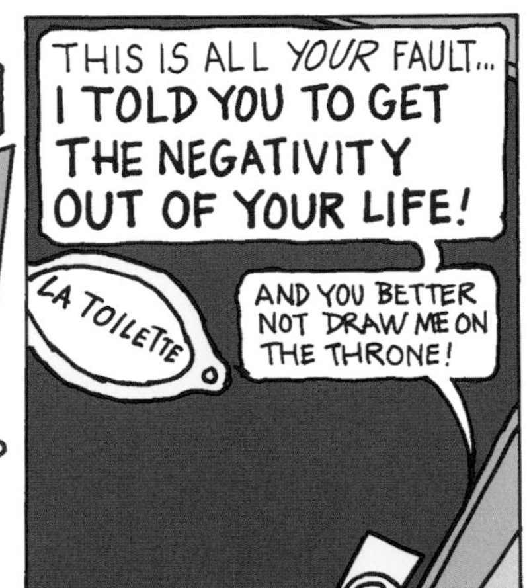
THIS IS ALL YOUR FAULT... I TOLD YOU TO GET THE NEGATIVITY OUT OF YOUR LIFE!
LA TOILETTE
AND YOU BETTER NOT DRAW ME ON THE THRONE!

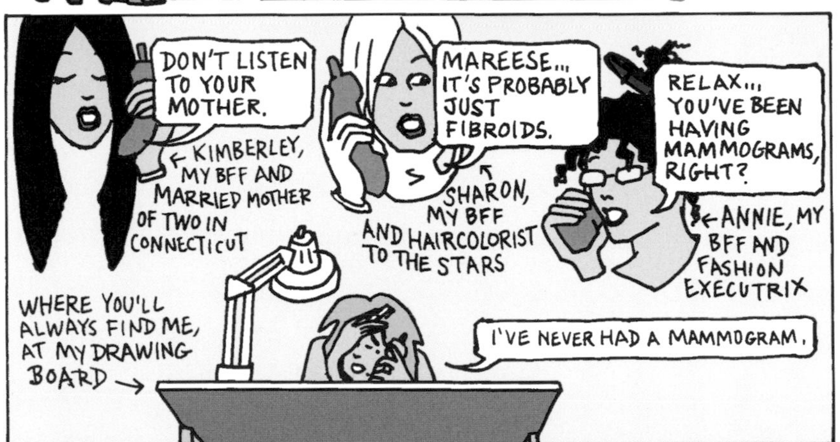
DON'T LISTEN TO YOUR MOTHER.
← KIMBERLEY, MY BFF AND MARRIED MOTHER OF TWO IN CONNECTICUT
MAREESE... IT'S PROBABLY JUST FIBROIDS.
↑ SHARON, MY BFF AND HAIRCOLORIST TO THE STARS
RELAX... YOU'VE BEEN HAVING MAMMOGRAMS, RIGHT?
← ANNIE, MY BFF AND FASHION EXECUTRIX
WHERE YOU'LL ALWAYS FIND ME, AT MY DRAWING BOARD →
I'VE NEVER HAD A MAMMOGRAM.

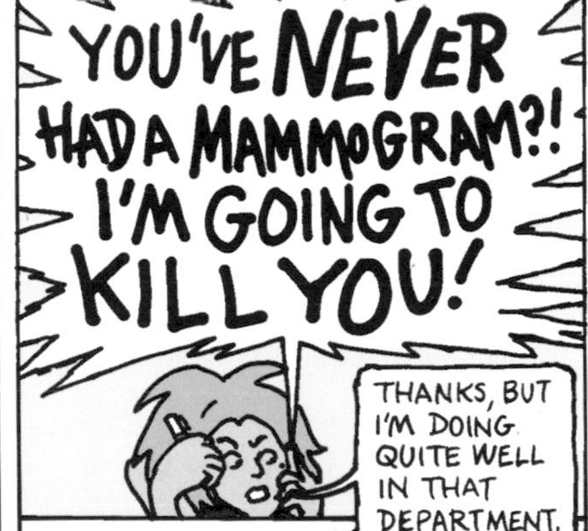
YOU'VE NEVER HAD A MAMMOGRAM?! I'M GOING TO KILL YOU!
THANKS, BUT I'M DOING QUITE WELL IN THAT DEPARTMENT.

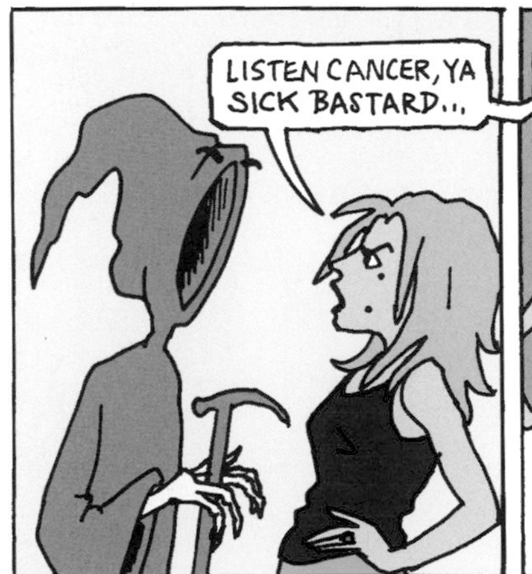
LISTEN CANCER, YA SICK BASTARD...

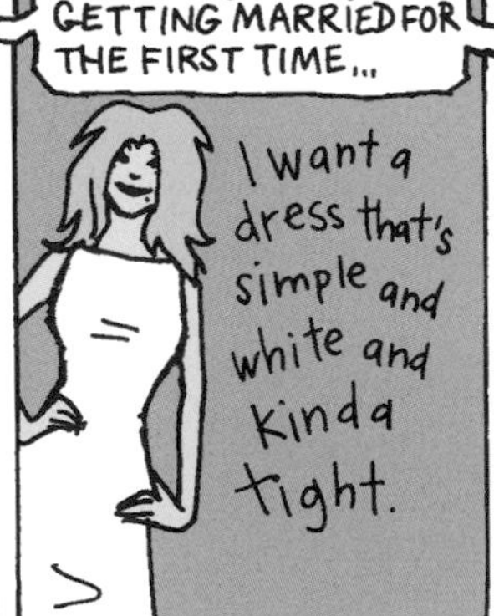
...FINALLY, AT 43, I'M GETTING MARRIED FOR THE FIRST TIME...
I want a dress that's simple and white and kinda tight.

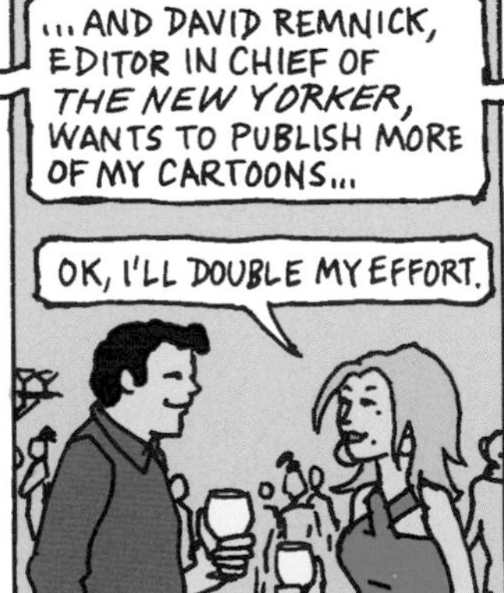
...AND DAVID REMNICK, EDITOR IN CHIEF OF THE NEW YORKER, WANTS TO PUBLISH MORE OF MY CARTOONS...
OK, I'LL DOUBLE MY EFFORT.

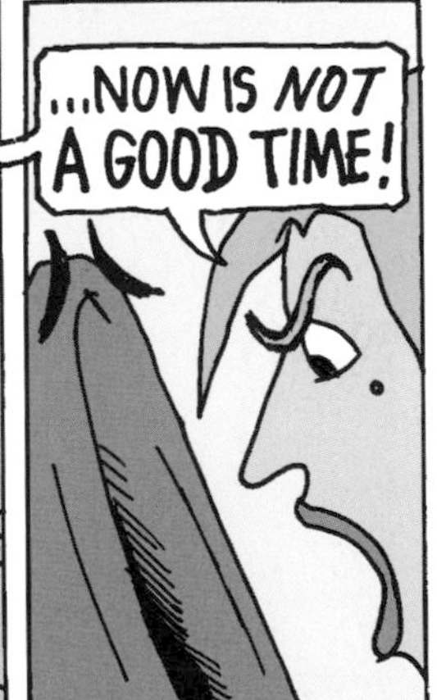
...NOW IS NOT A GOOD TIME!

THAT NIGHT, SILVANO RANG ME FROM THE SPECTACULAR RESTAURANT HE OWNS.
Da Silvano
ALEC BALDWIN LOVED THE SHOVEL-NOSE LOBSTER. I SAVED YOU ONE. COME OVER, I'M HUNGRY!

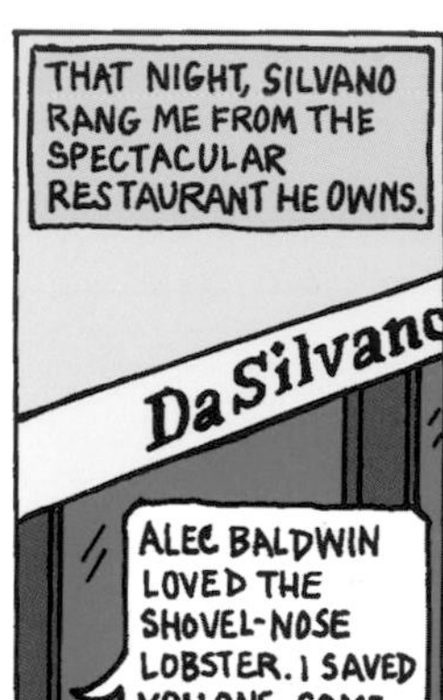

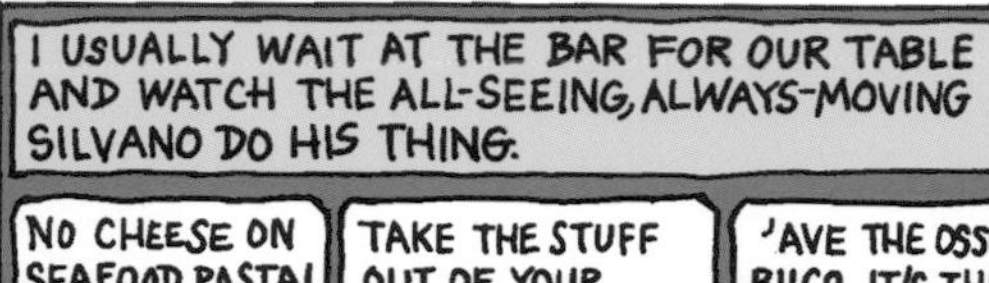

NO CHEESE ON SEAFOOD PASTA! IT'S A SACRILEGE!
TAKE THE STUFF OUT OF YOUR APRON, YOU LOOK LIKE A KANGAROO!
'AVE THE OSSO BUCO. IT'S THE END OF THE WORLD!
THIS ALL HAPPENED IN THE SAME MINUTE, I SWEAR.

THE MOST ENERGETIC MAN ON THE PLANET FINALLY SITS DOWN, AND I TELL HIM ABOUT MY WONDERFUL DAY.
SILVANO, THE DOCTOR ASPIRATED A LUMP IN MY BREAST AND I GET THE RESULTS TOMORROW, BUT DON'T WORRY...

...THERE'S A CHANCE IT MAY *NOT* BE CANCEROUS.

THE NEXT DAY, FRIDAY, MAY 14, I WAS SUPPOSED TO GET THE RESULTS. SO WHENEVER I HEARD...
RING! RING!
WAAA-AHH!
WHOOSH!
THUD!
OUCH.
REPEAT 57 TIMES

IT'S YOUR MOMMA, ANYONE CALL?..
...ABOUT CANCER?
CONVERSATION #4, 5, 6, 9, 10, 11, 12, 13, 14, 16, 17, 18, 19, 20, 21, 23, 24, 25, 26, 27, 29, 35, 44, 45, 46, 47, 48, 51, 52, 55&56

MARISA, GIRL... ANY WORD...
...ABOUT CANCER?
SHARON WORE LATEX GLOVES AND A MASK WHILE COLORING HAIR
CONVERSATION #15, 43

ANYTING NEW...
...ABOUT CANCER?
CONVERSATION #1, 3, 8, 22, 38, 39, 41, 49, 57

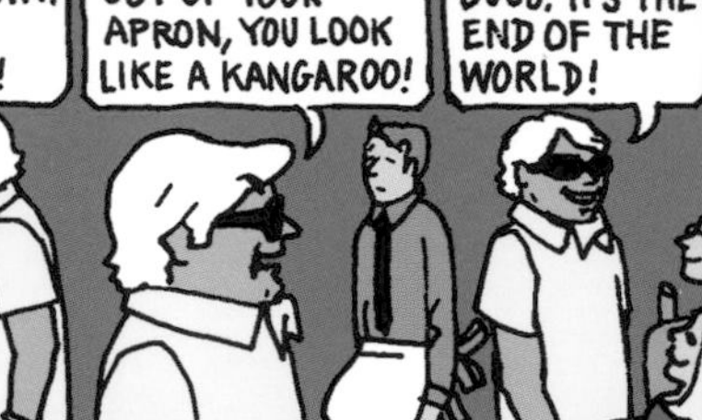

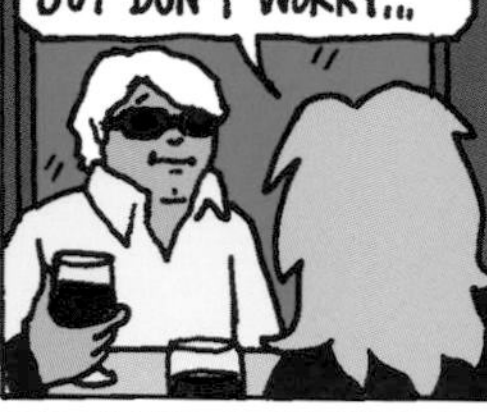

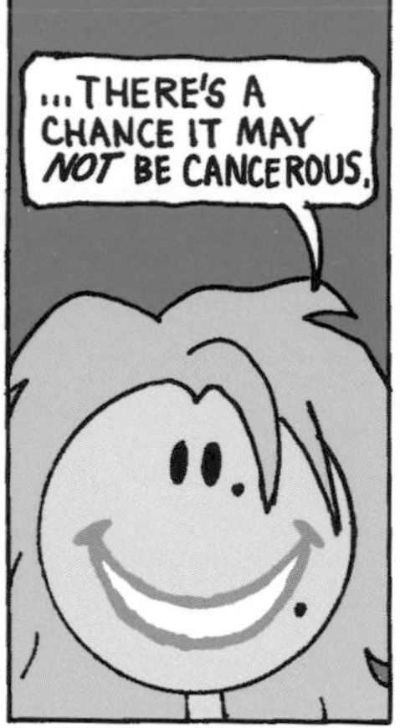

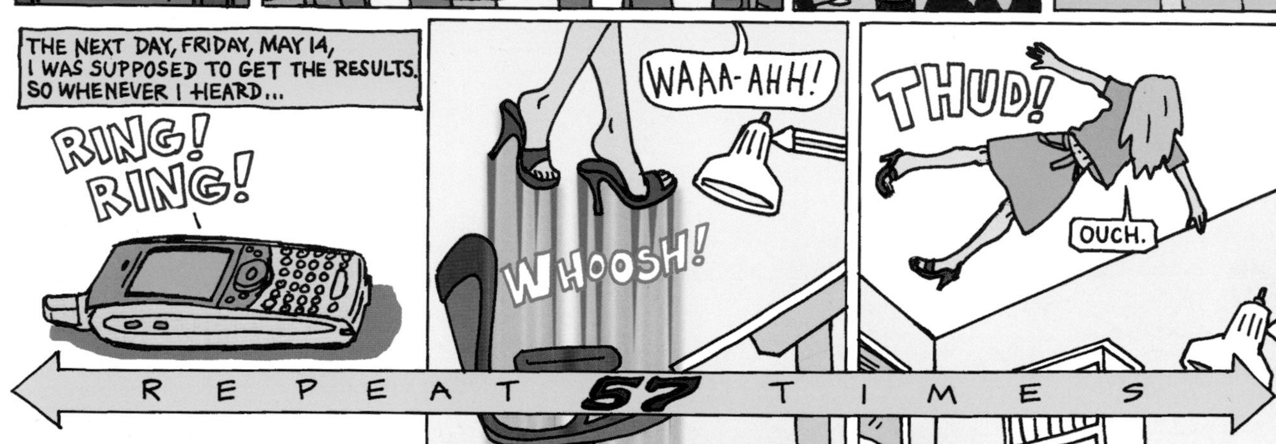

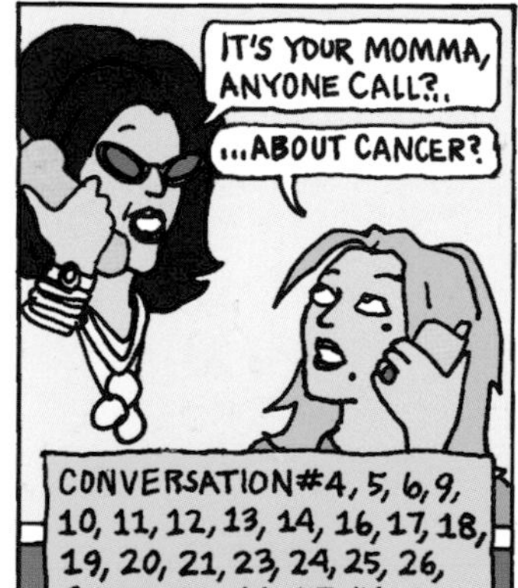

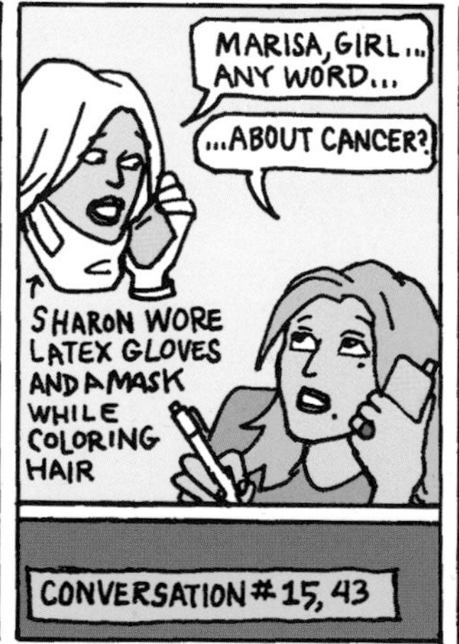

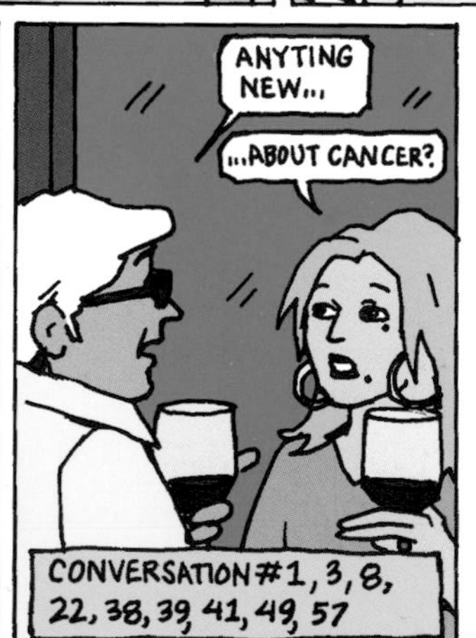

MAY 14 PHONE LOG:

TOTAL # OF INCOMING CALLS: 57

TOTAL # OF CALLS FROM SILVANO: 9

TOTAL # OF CALLS FROM MY BFFs: 17

TOTAL # OF CALLS FROM MY (S)MOTHER: 31

TOTAL # OF CALLS FROM DOCTORS: 0

MAY 15, THE DAY AFTER THE DAY I WAS SUPPOSED TO GET THE RESULTS...

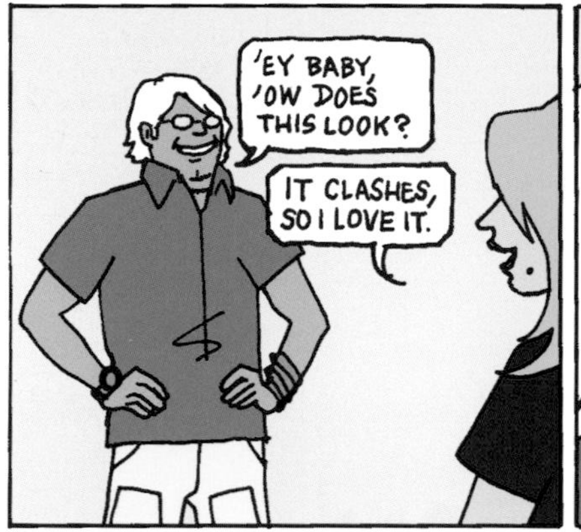

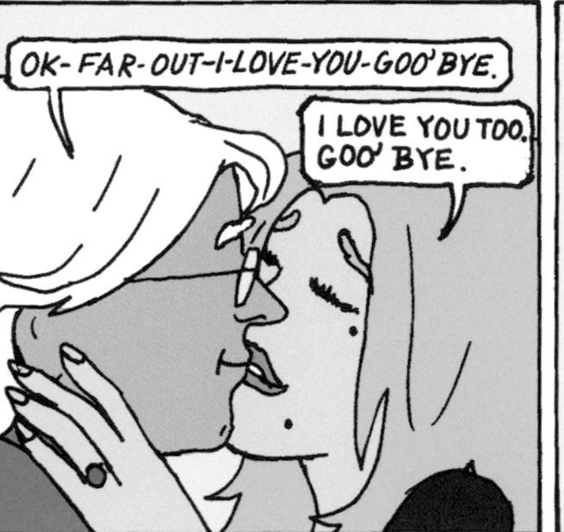

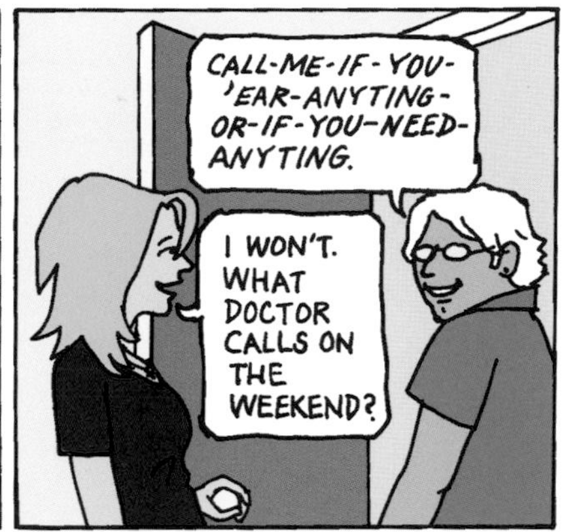

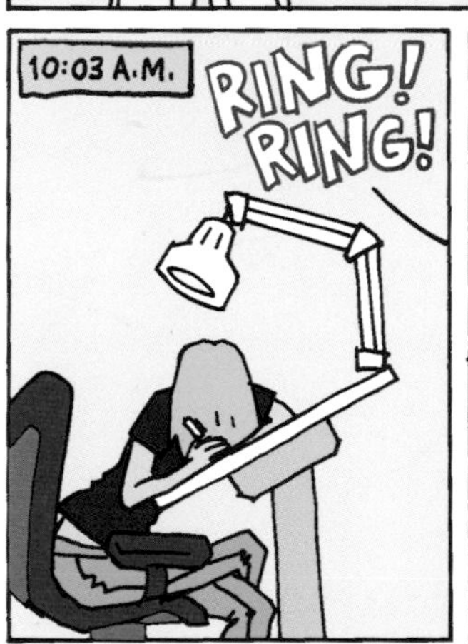

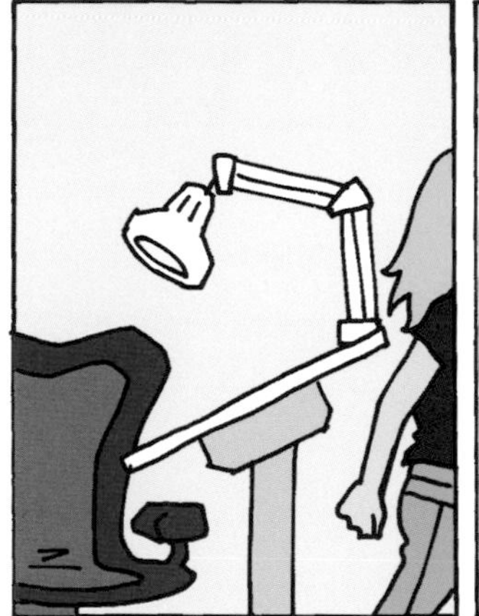

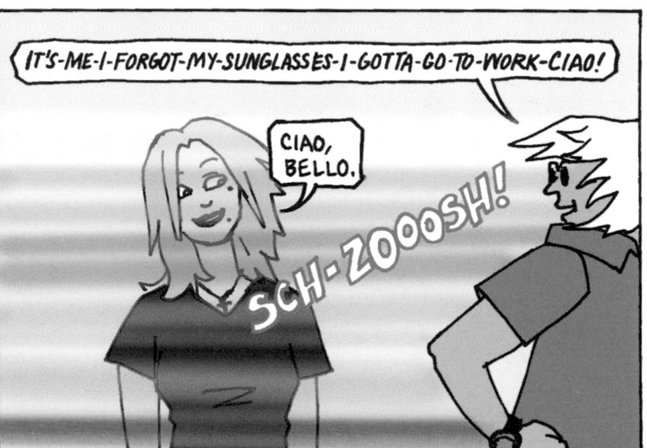

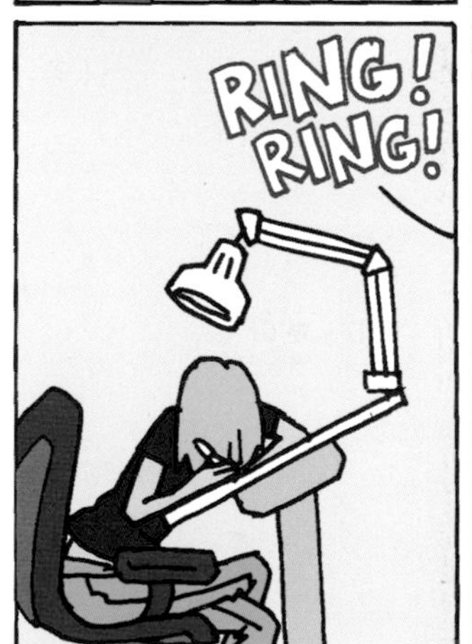

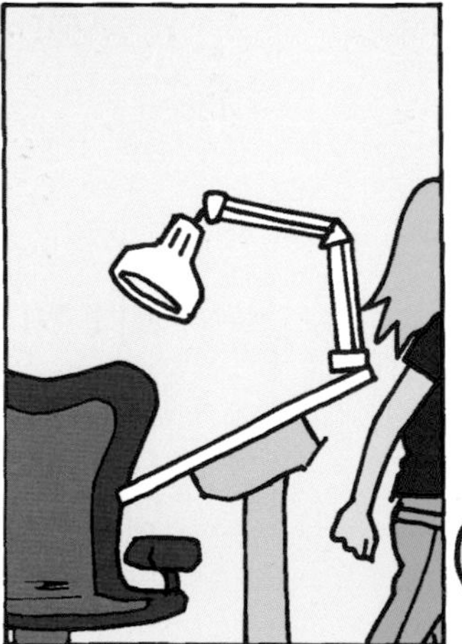

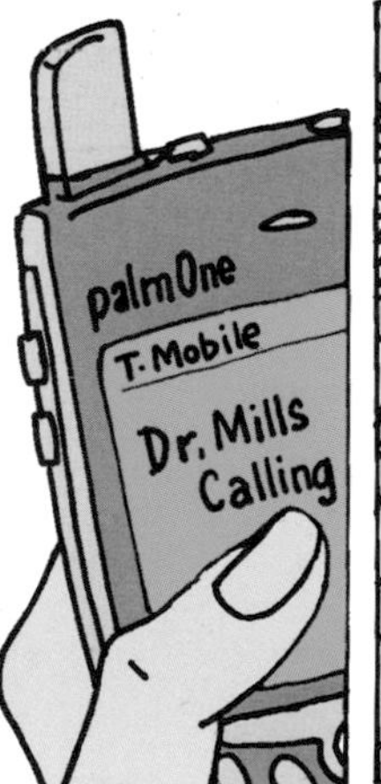

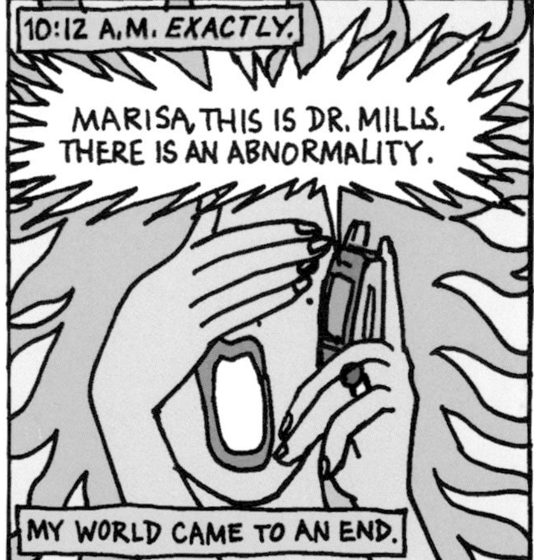

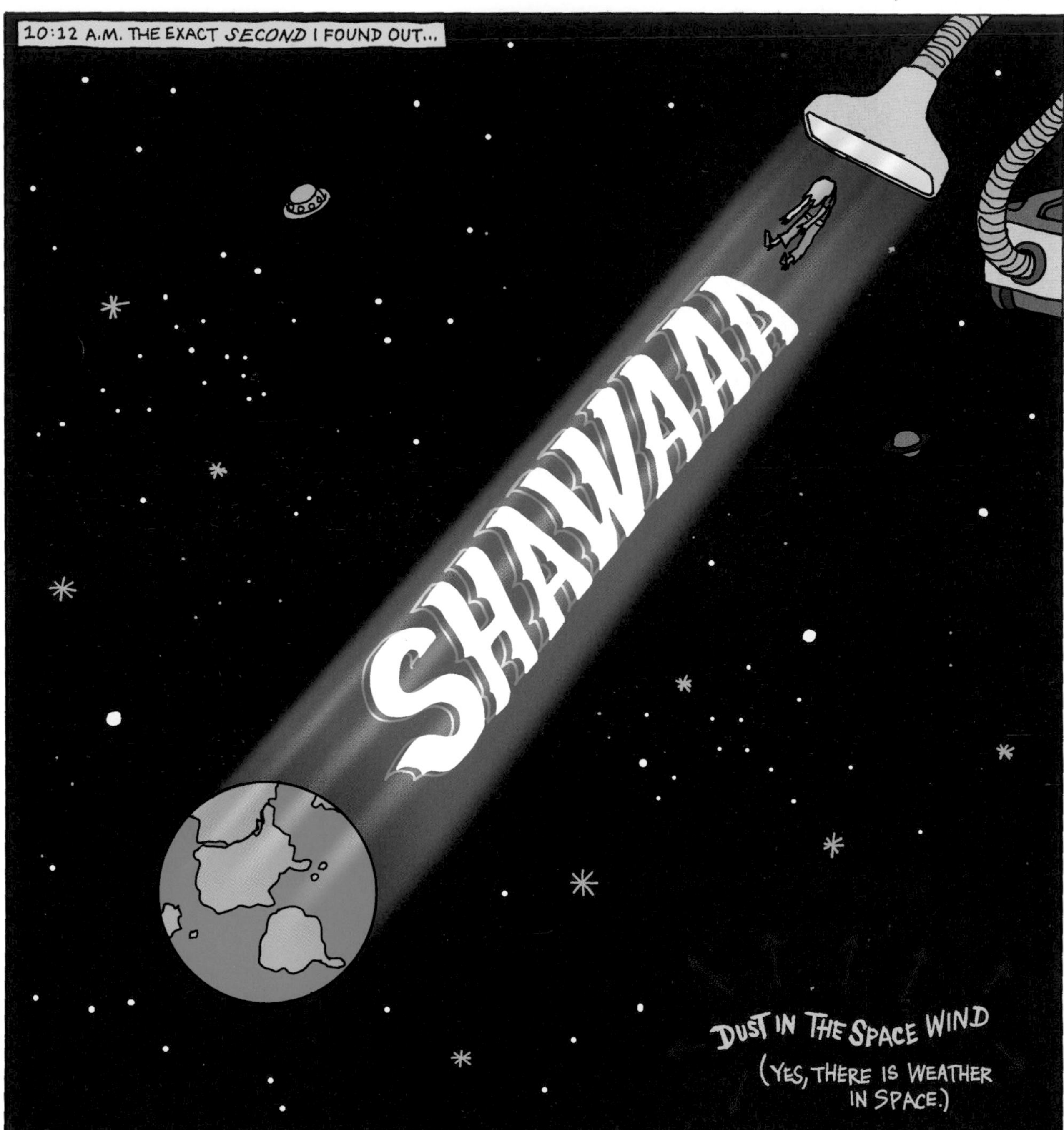
10:12 A.M. THE EXACT SECOND I FOUND OUT...
SHAWAAA
DUST IN THE SPACE WIND
(YES, THERE IS WEATHER IN SPACE.)

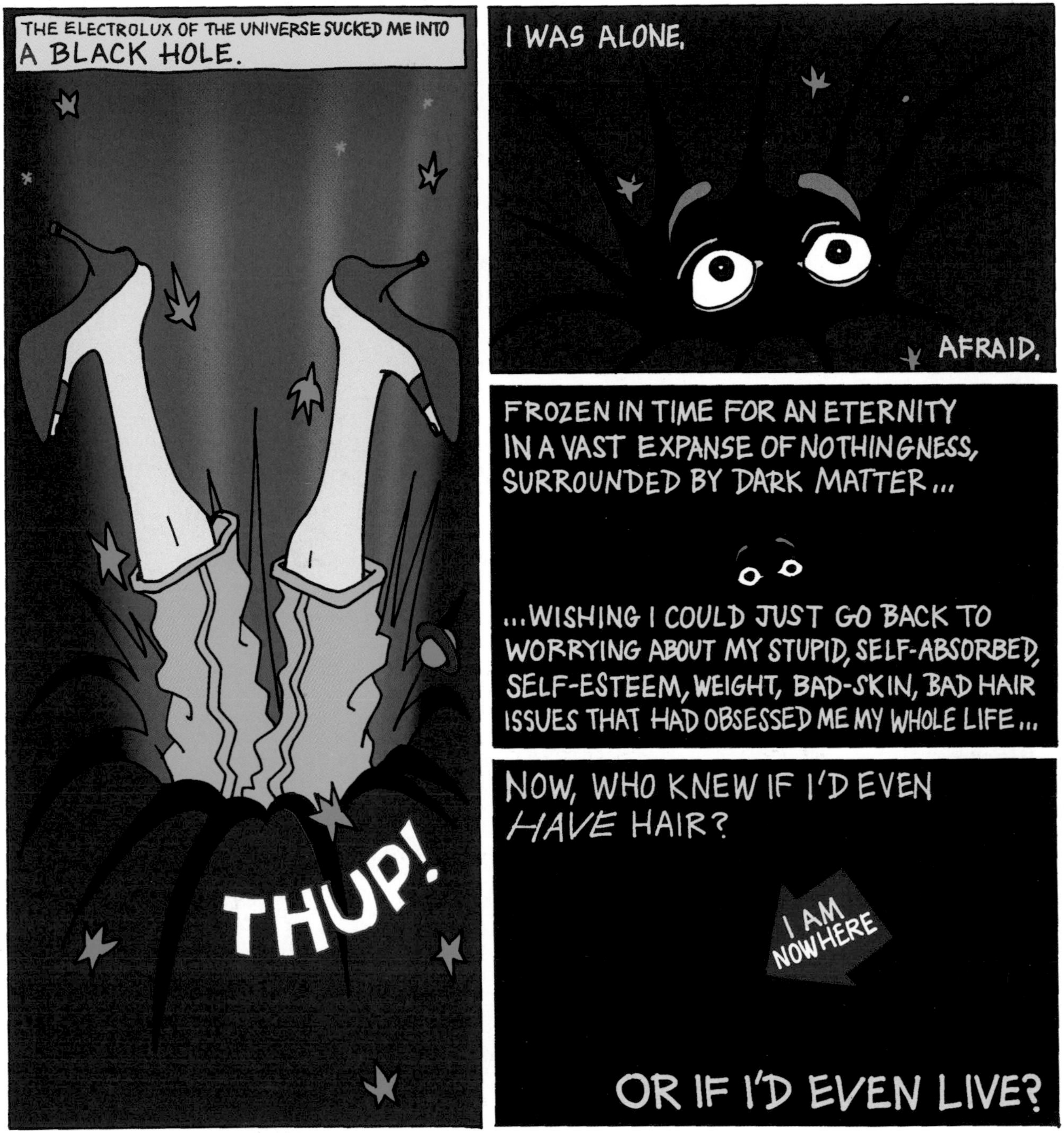

THE ELECTROLUX OF THE UNIVERSE SUCKED ME INTO A BLACK HOLE.

THUP!

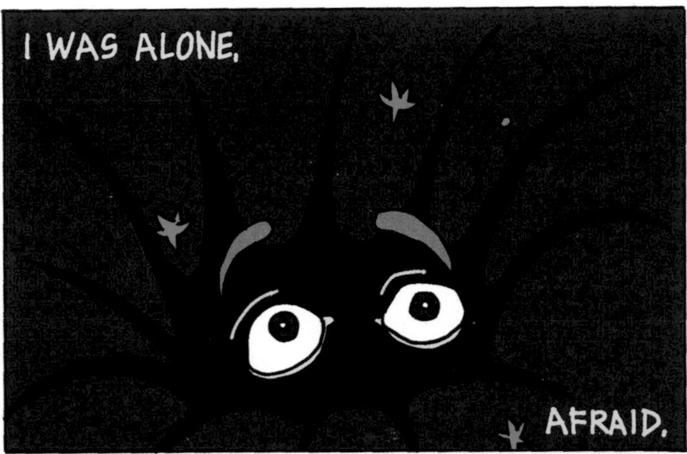

FROZEN IN TIME FOR AN ETERNITY IN A VAST EXPANSE OF NOTHINGNESS, SURROUNDED BY DARK MATTER...

...WISHING I COULD JUST GO BACK TO WORRYING ABOUT MY STUPID, SELF-ABSORBED, SELF-ESTEEM, WEIGHT, BAD-SKIN, BAD HAIR ISSUES THAT HAD OBSESSED ME MY WHOLE LIFE...

NOW, WHO KNEW IF I'D EVEN *HAVE* HAIR?

I AM NOWHERE

OR IF I'D EVEN LIVE?

10:12:03 A.M. THE NEXT MILLISECOND. I HAD TO CALL MY PARENTS...

OF COURSE MY (S)MOTHER PICKED UP THE PHONE FIRST.
OHMYGOD, I'M SICK!
THE JERSEY SHORE

IF MY DAD HATED THE PHONE BEFORE...
MOM JUST RAN INTO THE TUSH.
MARISA, DON'T TELL ME!

OHGOD OHGOD OHGOD OHGOD PLEASE GOD NO!
LA TOILETTE

WHY DO I HAVE CANCER NOW? WHY DO I NEED A LUMPECTOMY NOW? WHY IS THIS HAPPENING NOW? NOW WHEN I'VE NEVER BEEN HAPPIER!

YOU HAVE TO TELL SILVANO RIGHT NOW. HE'S GOING TO BE YOUR HUSBAND.
HON, GET ME THE EXTENSION!

I'M AFRAID TO TELL SILVANO...

MARISA, IT'S MOM. SILVANO IS A MAN OF GREAT CHARACTER.
THIS IS DAD, HON. HE'S NOT JUST ANY MAN, AND THAT'S WHY YOU WAITED 43 YEARS TO GET MARRIED.

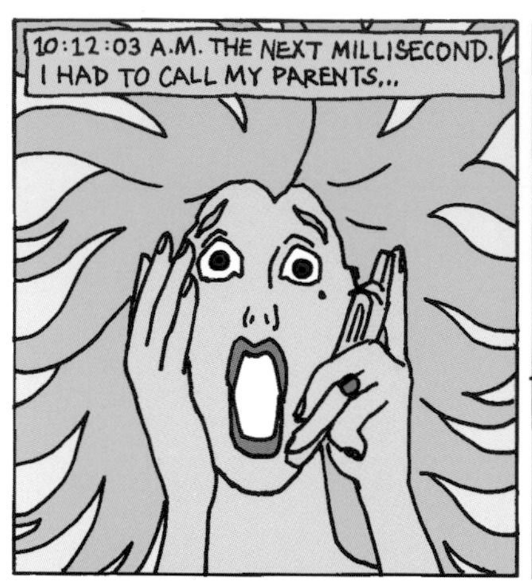

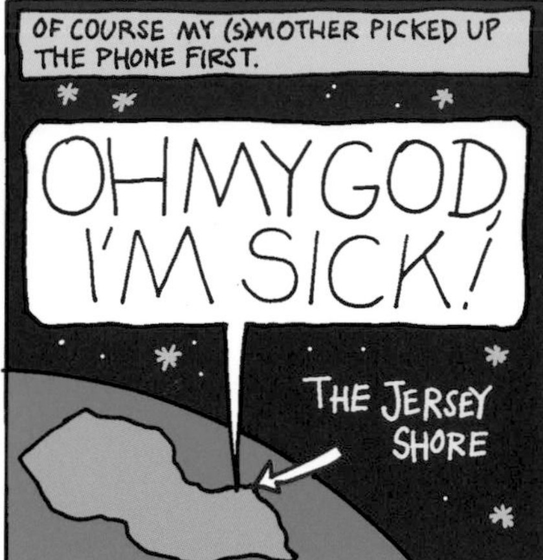

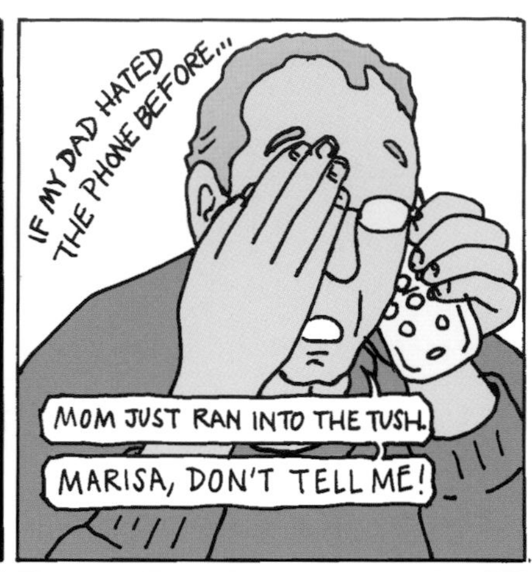

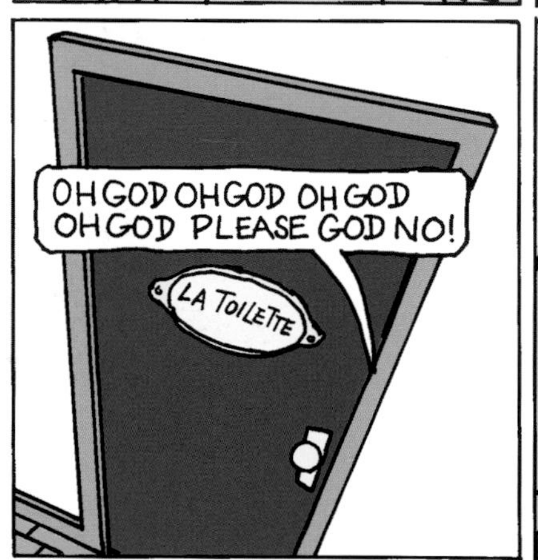

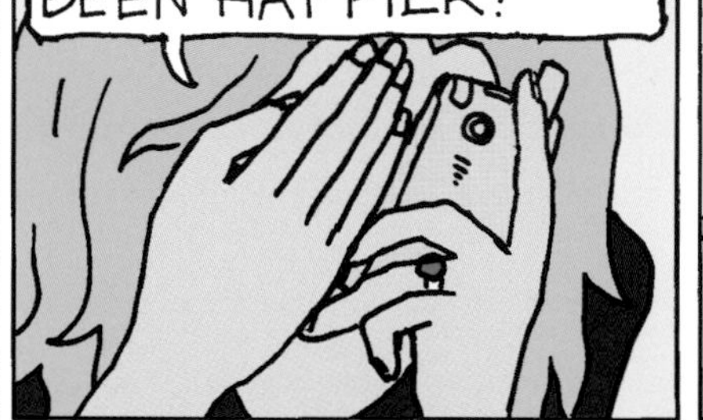

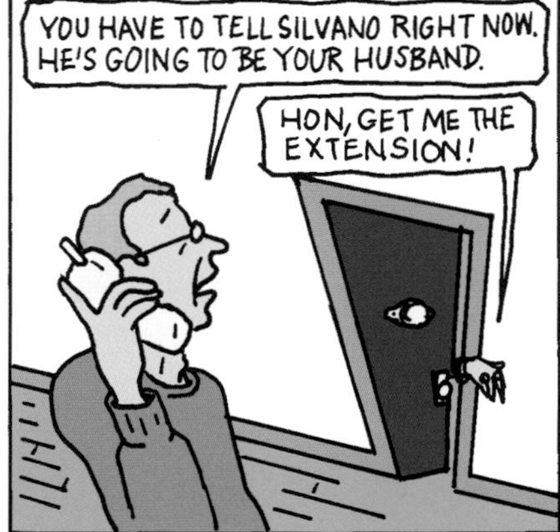

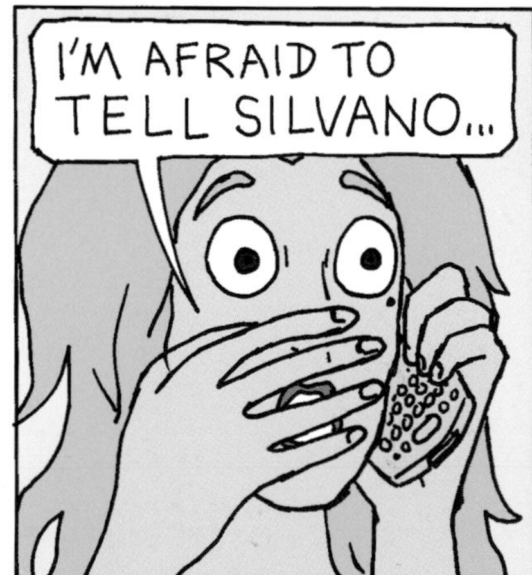

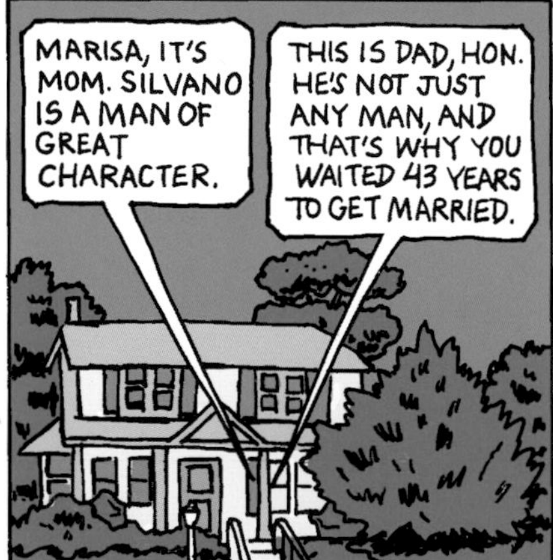

BUT WHEN WOMEN GET SICK MEN LEAVE. HUSBANDS LEAVE THEIR WIVES... AND WE'RE NOT EVEN MARRIED!

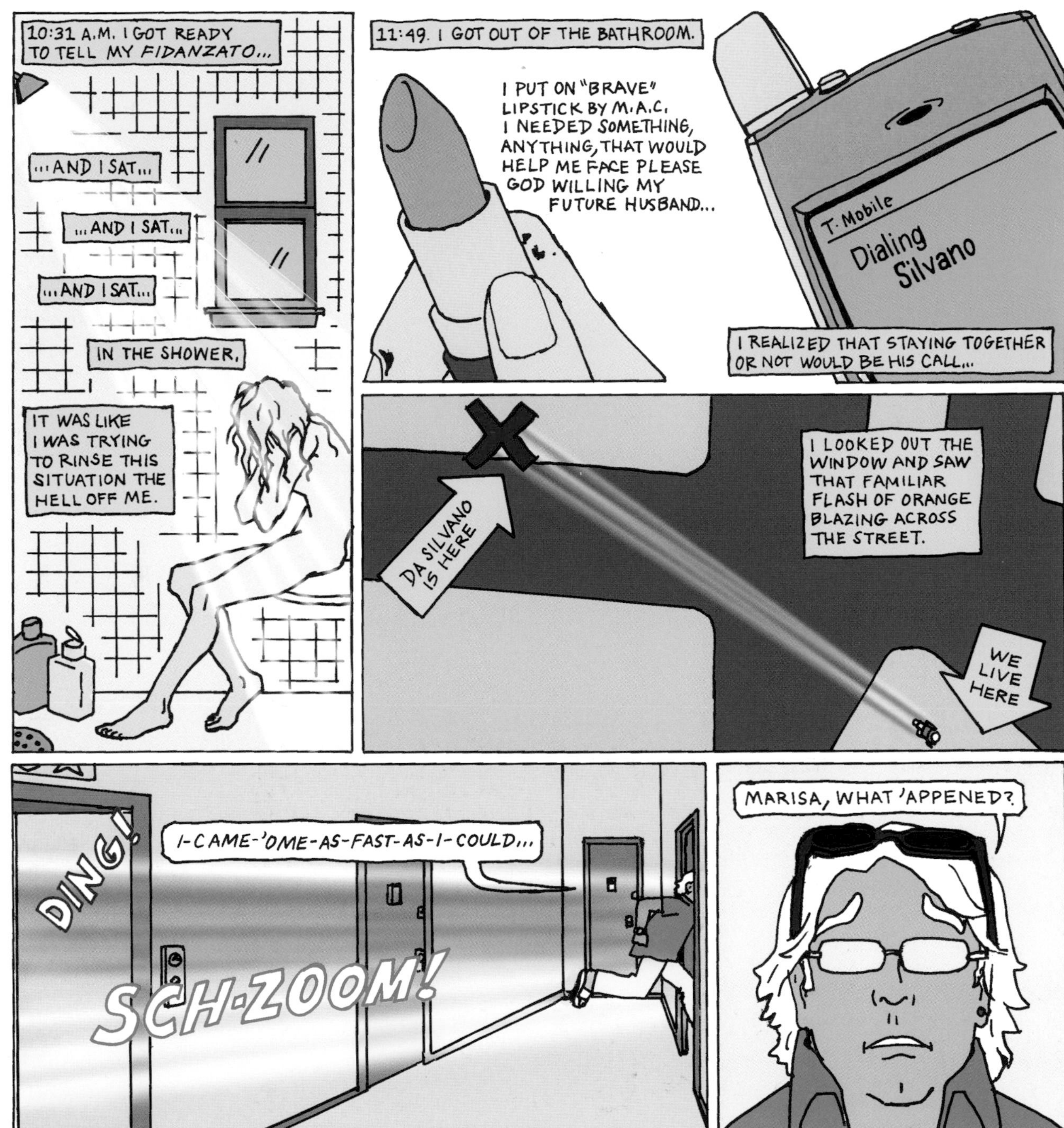

10:31 A.M. I GOT READY TO TELL MY *FIDANZATO*...
...AND I SAT...
...AND I SAT...
...AND I SAT...
IN THE SHOWER.
IT WAS LIKE I WAS TRYING TO RINSE THIS SITUATION THE HELL OFF ME.
11:49. I GOT OUT OF THE BATHROOM.
I PUT ON "BRAVE" LIPSTICK BY M.A.C. I NEEDED SOMETHING, ANYTHING, THAT WOULD HELP ME FACE PLEASE GOD WILLING MY FUTURE HUSBAND...
T-Mobile
Dialing Silvano
I REALIZED THAT STAYING TOGETHER OR NOT WOULD BE HIS CALL...
DA SILVANO IS HERE
I LOOKED OUT THE WINDOW AND SAW THAT FAMILIAR FLASH OF ORANGE BLAZING ACROSS THE STREET.
WE LIVE HERE
DING!
SCH-ZOOM!
I-CAME-'OME-AS-FAST-AS-I-COULD...
MARISA, WHAT 'APPENED?

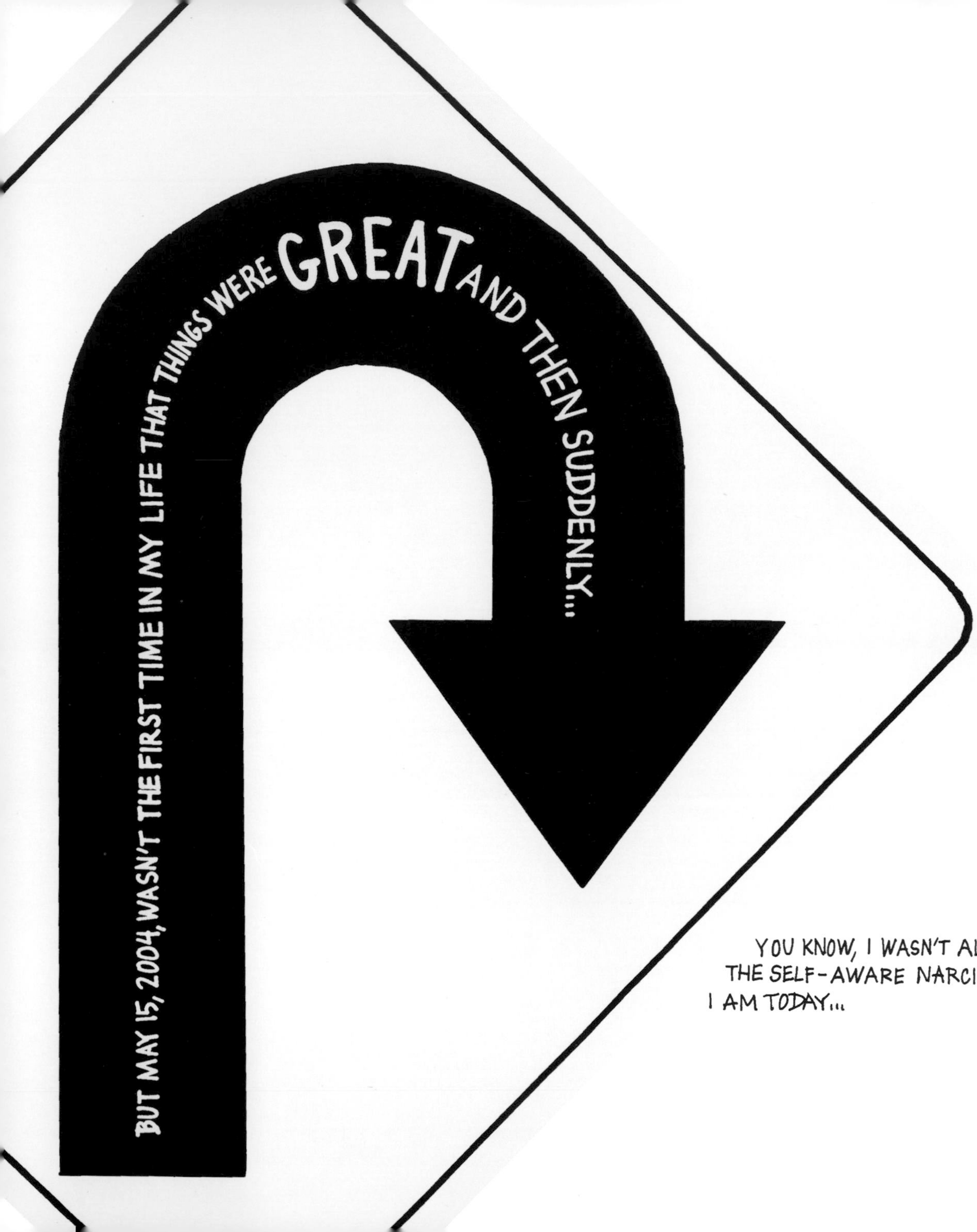

BUT MAY 15, 2004, WASN'T THE FIRST TIME IN MY LIFE THAT THINGS WERE **GREAT** AND THEN SUDDENLY...

YOU KNOW, I WASN'T ALWAYS
THE SELF-AWARE NARCISSIST
I AM TODAY...

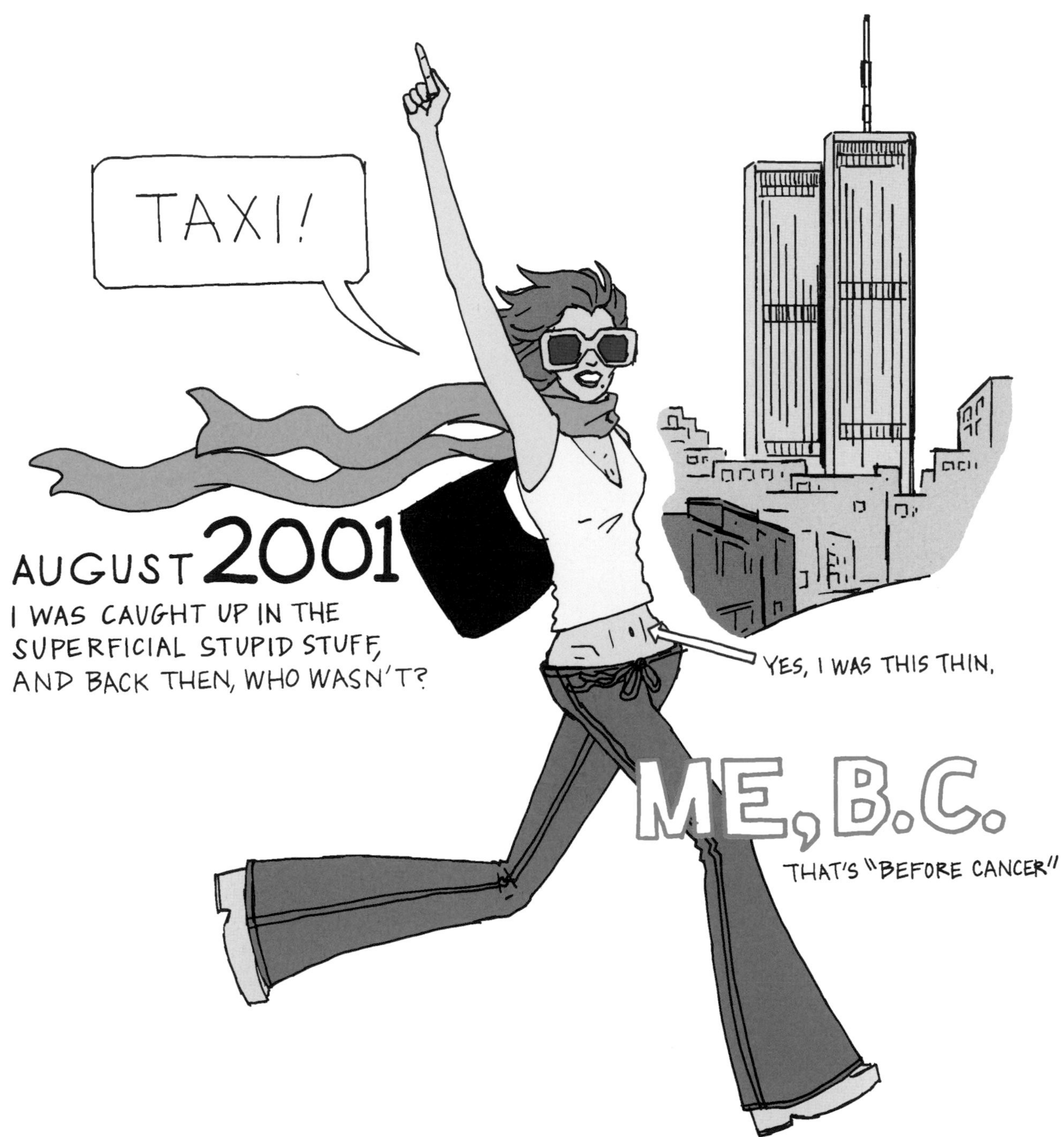
TAXI!
AUGUST 2001
I WAS CAUGHT UP IN THE SUPERFICIAL STUPID STUFF, AND BACK THEN, WHO WASN'T?
YES, I WAS THIS THIN.
ME, B.C.
THAT'S "BEFORE CANCER"

I'M NOT SAYING THE *FABULISTA* LIFE WASN'T FUN. IT WAS. MY BFF BOB AND I WENT TO ALL THE "IT" EVENTS.
FABULOUS. FABULOUS.
WHO WOULDN'T LOVE THE FRONT ROW OF A FASHION SHOW?
PEOPLE WHO AREN'T IN THEM.

...AND WE WENT TO ALL THE "IT" PARTIES.
THERE'S SARAH JESSICA... PHEW! FOR A MOMENT I THOUGHT THERE WAS *NOBODY* HERE!

AFTER 1 OR 10 DIRTY MARTINIS, FASHION COMMENTATOR BOB TURNED HIS ATTENTION TO YOURS TRULY...
LOOK AT YOU... TOO MUCH BLUE EYESHADOW AND TOO MUCH GLITTER IN THAT BLUE EYESHADOW...

...LOUD SILVER PLATFORMS WITH *LOUDER* ORANGE PANTS...
...AND I WON'T EVEN COMMENT ON THE AQUA FROST TOENAIL COLOR.

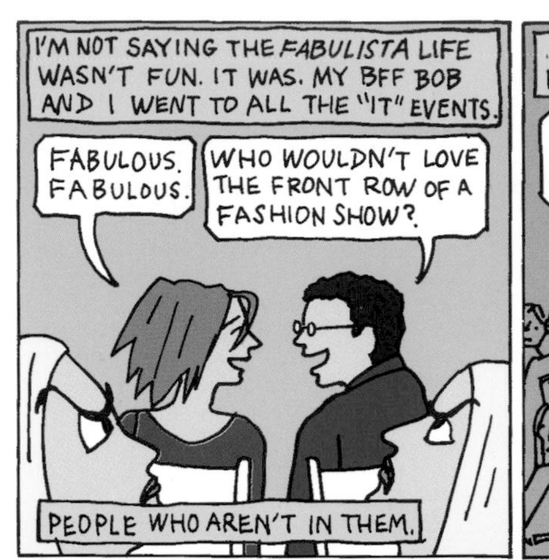

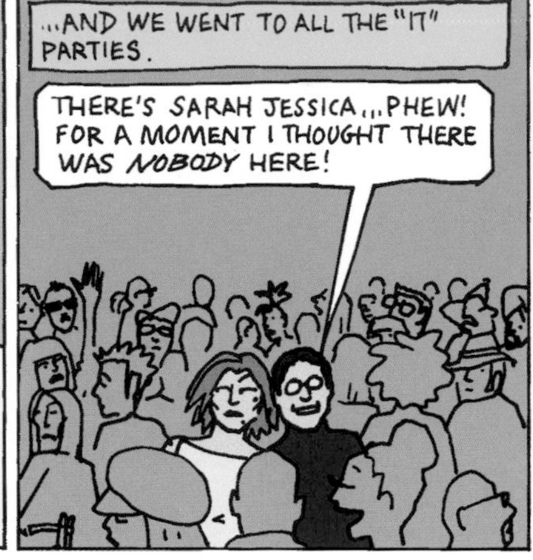

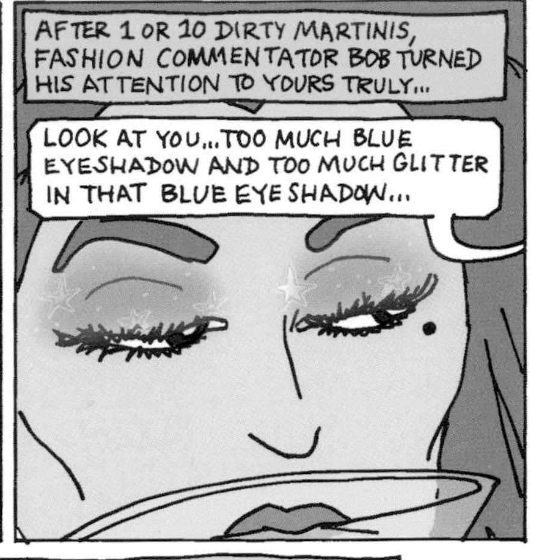

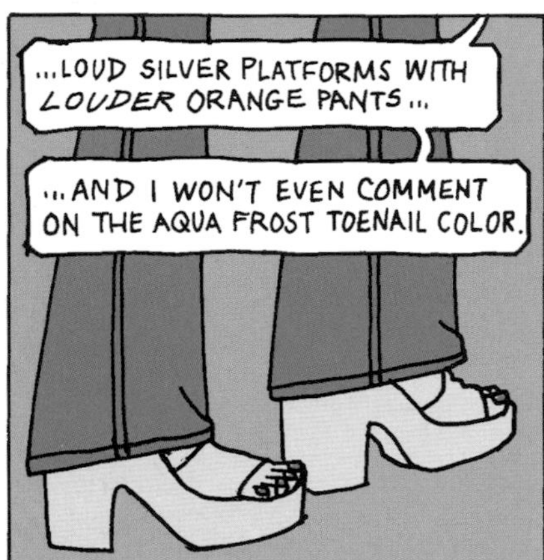

ALL THIS FROM A MAN IN AN IRIDESCENT PURPLE PRADA SUIT!

IT'S A *BLUE* VIOLET. TO BE OF *FASHION* IS TO BE COLD. YOU TRY TOO HARD.

THIS IS THE NEXT THING BOB SAID:

I WOULD HAVE BEEN ANNOYED HAD I NOT GOTTEN A CARTOON OUT OF IT.

THAT'S BASED ON ME
THAT IS BOB
MARISA ACOCELLA

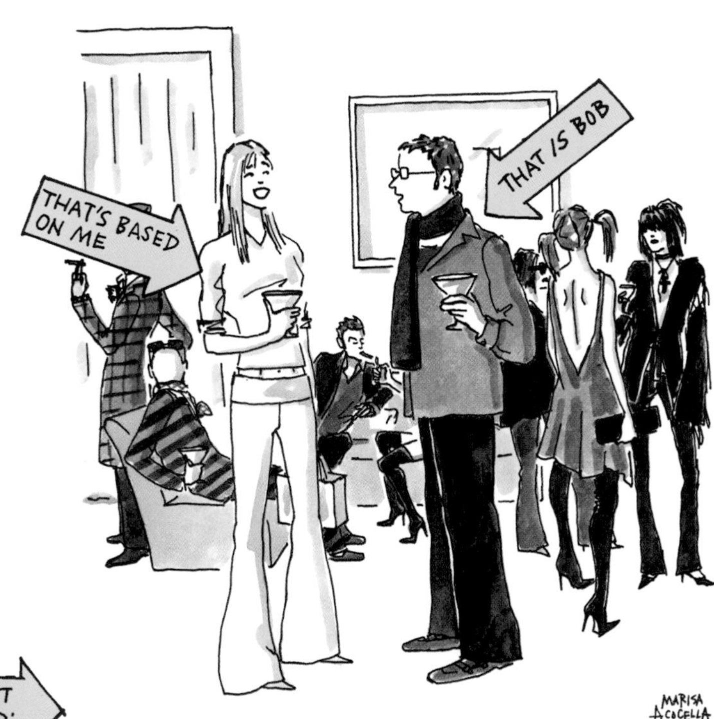

"Stop smiling. You're downtown."

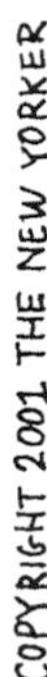

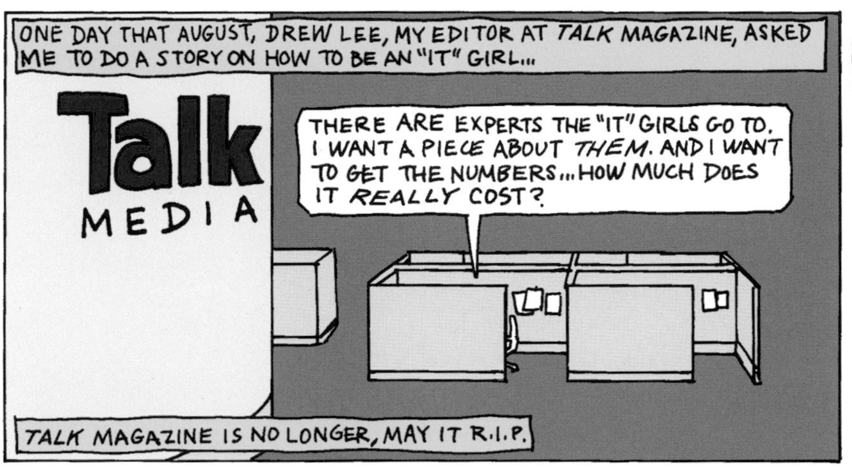
ONE DAY THAT AUGUST, DREW LEE, MY EDITOR AT *TALK* MAGAZINE, ASKED ME TO DO A STORY ON HOW TO BE AN "IT" GIRL...
Talk MEDIA
THERE ARE EXPERTS THE "IT" GIRLS GO TO. I WANT A PIECE ABOUT *THEM*. AND I WANT TO GET THE NUMBERS... HOW MUCH DOES IT *REALLY* COST?
TALK MAGAZINE IS NO LONGER, MAY IT R.I.P.

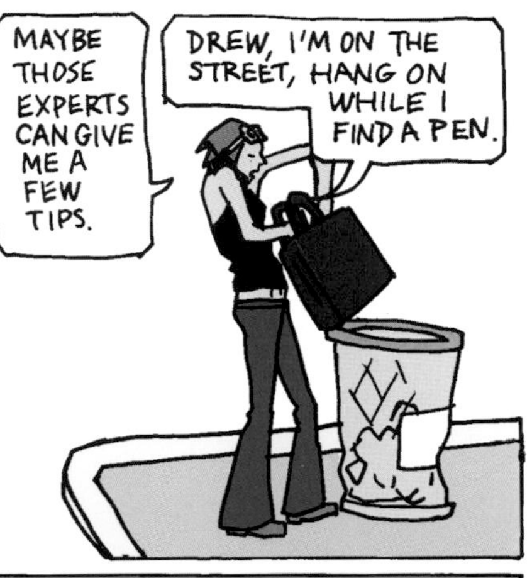
MAYBE THOSE EXPERTS CAN GIVE ME A FEW TIPS.
DREW, I'M ON THE STREET, HANG ON WHILE I FIND A PEN.

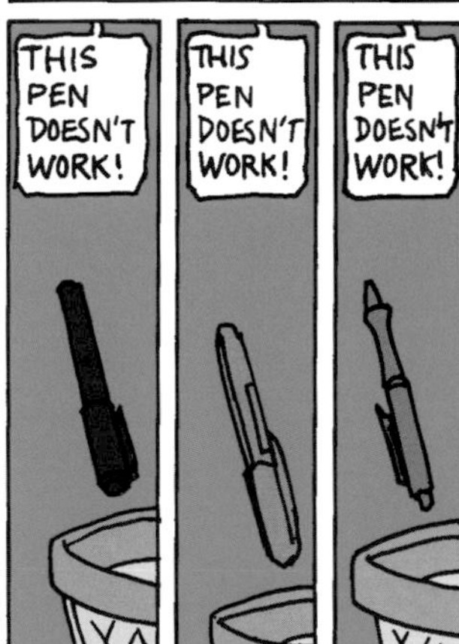
THIS PEN DOESN'T WORK!
THIS PEN DOESN'T WORK!
THIS PEN DOESN'T WORK!

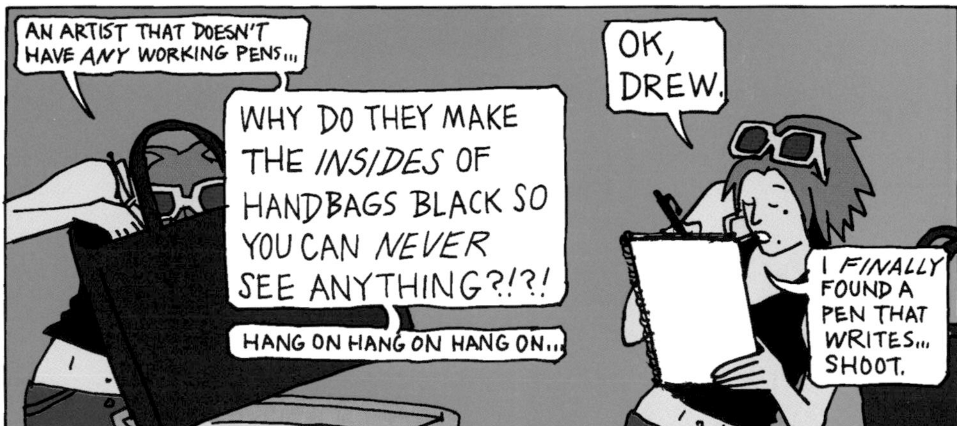
AN ARTIST THAT DOESN'T HAVE *ANY* WORKING PENS...
WHY DO THEY MAKE THE *INSIDES* OF HANDBAGS BLACK SO YOU CAN *NEVER* SEE ANYTHING?!?!
HANG ON HANG ON HANG ON...
OK, DREW.
I *FINALLY* FOUND A PEN THAT WRITES... SHOOT.

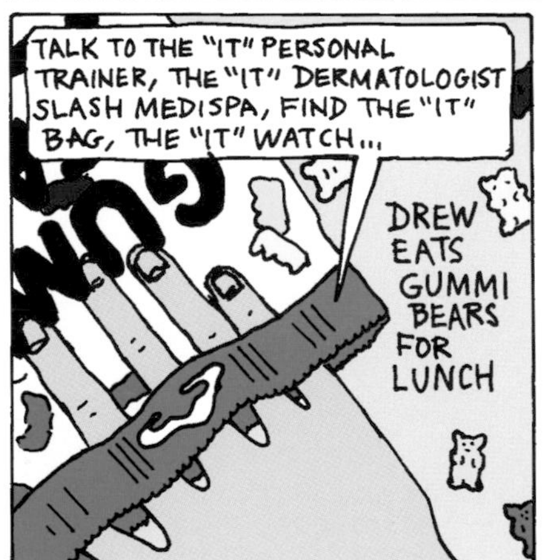
TALK TO THE "IT" PERSONAL TRAINER, THE "IT" DERMATOLOGIST SLASH MEDISPA, FIND THE "IT" BAG, THE "IT" WATCH...
DREW EATS GUMMI BEARS FOR LUNCH

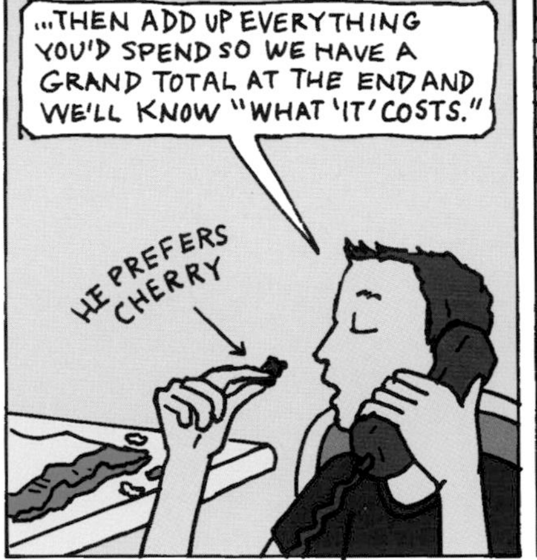
...THEN ADD UP EVERYTHING YOU'D SPEND SO WE HAVE A GRAND TOTAL AT THE END AND WE'LL KNOW "WHAT 'IT' COSTS."
HE PREFERS CHERRY

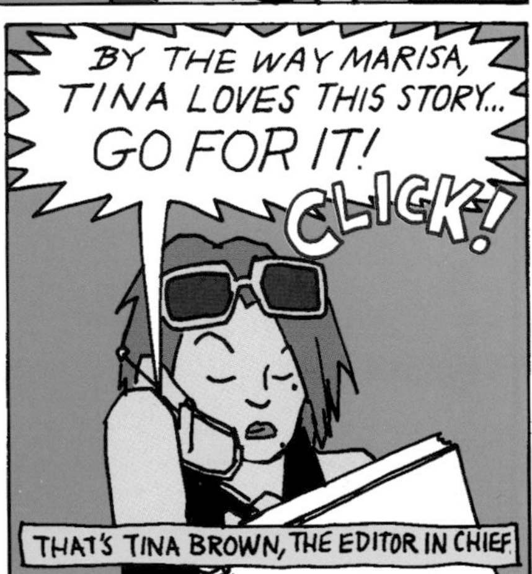
BY THE WAY MARISA, TINA LOVES THIS STORY... GO FOR IT!
CLICK!
THAT'S TINA BROWN, THE EDITOR IN CHIEF.

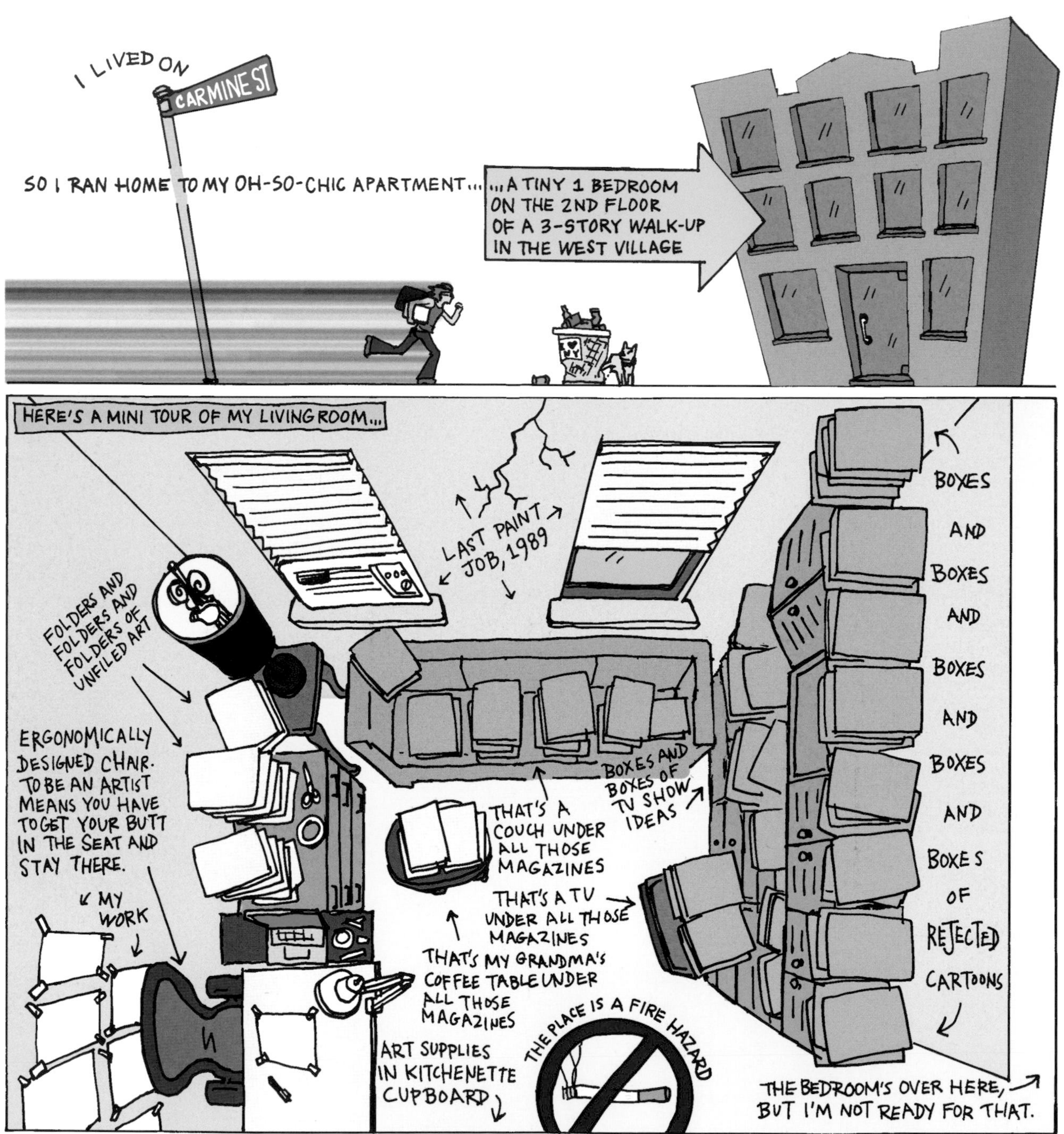

I LIVED ON
CARMINE ST
SO I RAN HOME TO MY OH-SO-CHIC APARTMENT...
...A TINY 1 BEDROOM ON THE 2ND FLOOR OF A 3-STORY WALK-UP IN THE WEST VILLAGE
HERE'S A MINI TOUR OF MY LIVINGROOM...
LAST PAINT JOB, 1989
BOXES AND BOXES AND BOXES AND BOXES AND BOXES AND BOXES OF REJECTED CARTOONS
FOLDERS AND FOLDERS AND FOLDERS OF UNFILED ART
ERGONOMICALLY DESIGNED CHAIR. TO BE AN ARTIST MEANS YOU HAVE TO GET YOUR BUTT IN THE SEAT AND STAY THERE.
MY WORK
BOXES AND BOXES OF TV SHOW IDEAS
THAT'S A COUCH UNDER ALL THOSE MAGAZINES
THAT'S A TV UNDER ALL THOSE MAGAZINES
THAT'S MY GRANDMA'S COFFEE TABLE UNDER ALL THOSE MAGAZINES
ART SUPPLIES IN KITCHENETTE CUPBOARD
THE PLACE IS A FIRE HAZARD
THE BEDROOM'S OVER HERE, BUT I'M NOT READY FOR THAT.

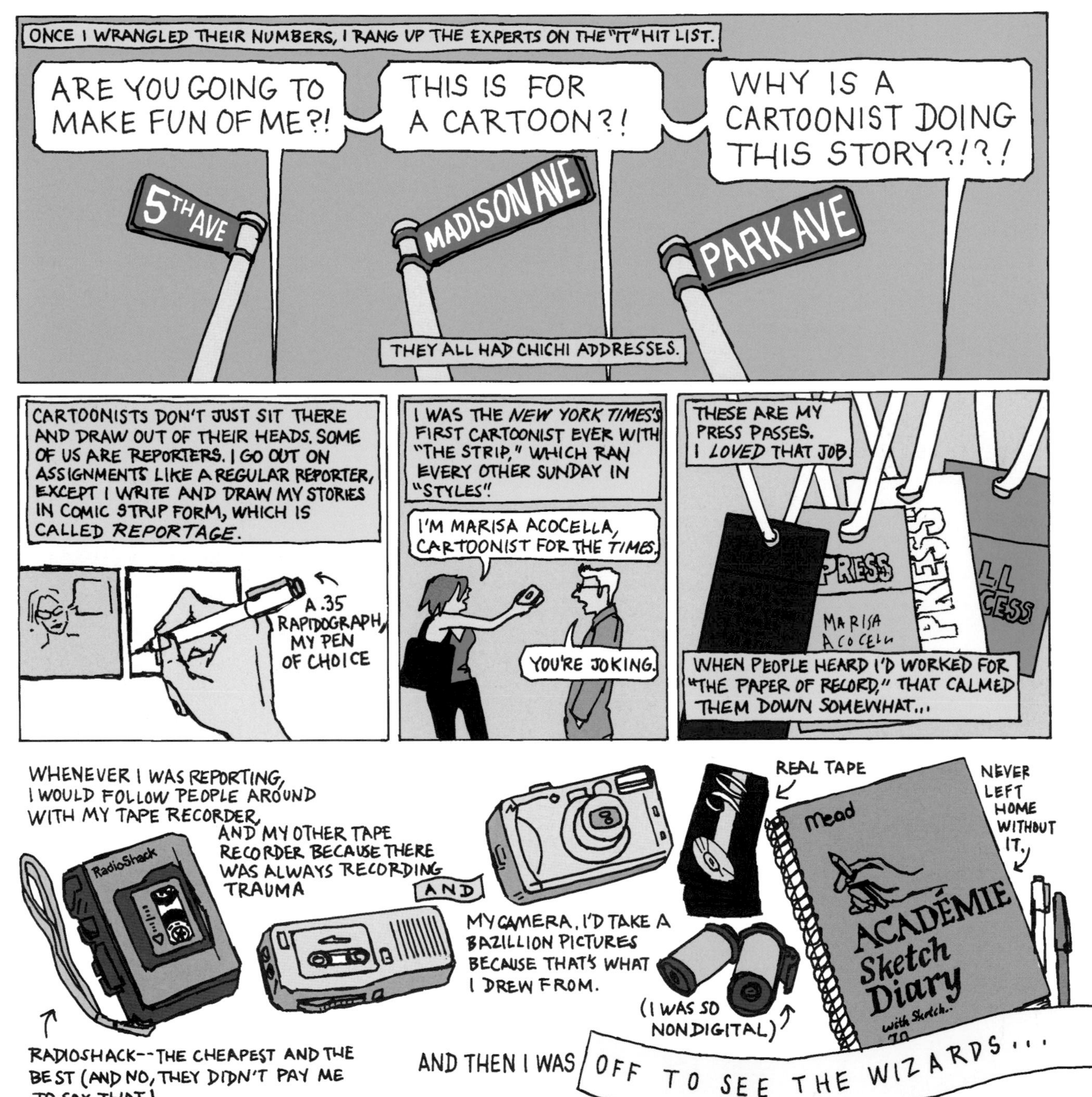
ONCE I WRANGLED THEIR NUMBERS, I RANG UP THE EXPERTS ON THE "IT" HIT LIST.
ARE YOU GOING TO MAKE FUN OF ME?!
THIS IS FOR A CARTOON?!
WHY IS A CARTOONIST DOING THIS STORY?!?!
5TH AVE
MADISON AVE
PARK AVE
THEY ALL HAD CHICHI ADDRESSES.
CARTOONISTS DON'T JUST SIT THERE AND DRAW OUT OF THEIR HEADS. SOME OF US ARE REPORTERS. I GO OUT ON ASSIGNMENTS LIKE A REGULAR REPORTER, EXCEPT I WRITE AND DRAW MY STORIES IN COMIC STRIP FORM, WHICH IS CALLED *REPORTAGE*.
A .35 RAPIDOGRAPH, MY PEN OF CHOICE
I WAS THE *NEW YORK TIMES'S* FIRST CARTOONIST EVER WITH "THE STRIP," WHICH RAN EVERY OTHER SUNDAY IN "STYLES."
I'M MARISA ACOCELLA, CARTOONIST FOR THE *TIMES*.
YOU'RE JOKING.
THESE ARE MY PRESS PASSES. I *LOVED* THAT JOB.
PRESS
MARISA ACOCELLA
PRESS
LL CESS
WHEN PEOPLE HEARD I'D WORKED FOR "THE PAPER OF RECORD," THAT CALMED THEM DOWN SOMEWHAT...
WHENEVER I WAS REPORTING, I WOULD FOLLOW PEOPLE AROUND WITH MY TAPE RECORDER,
AND MY OTHER TAPE RECORDER BECAUSE THERE WAS ALWAYS RECORDING TRAUMA
RadioShack
AND
MY CAMERA. I'D TAKE A BAZILLION PICTURES BECAUSE THAT'S WHAT I DREW FROM.
REAL TAPE
(I WAS SO NONDIGITAL)
NEVER LEFT HOME WITHOUT IT.
Mead
ACADÉMIE
Sketch Diary
RADIOSHACK--THE CHEAPEST AND THE BEST (AND NO, THEY DIDN'T PAY ME TO SAY THAT)
AND THEN I WAS OFF TO SEE THE WIZARDS...

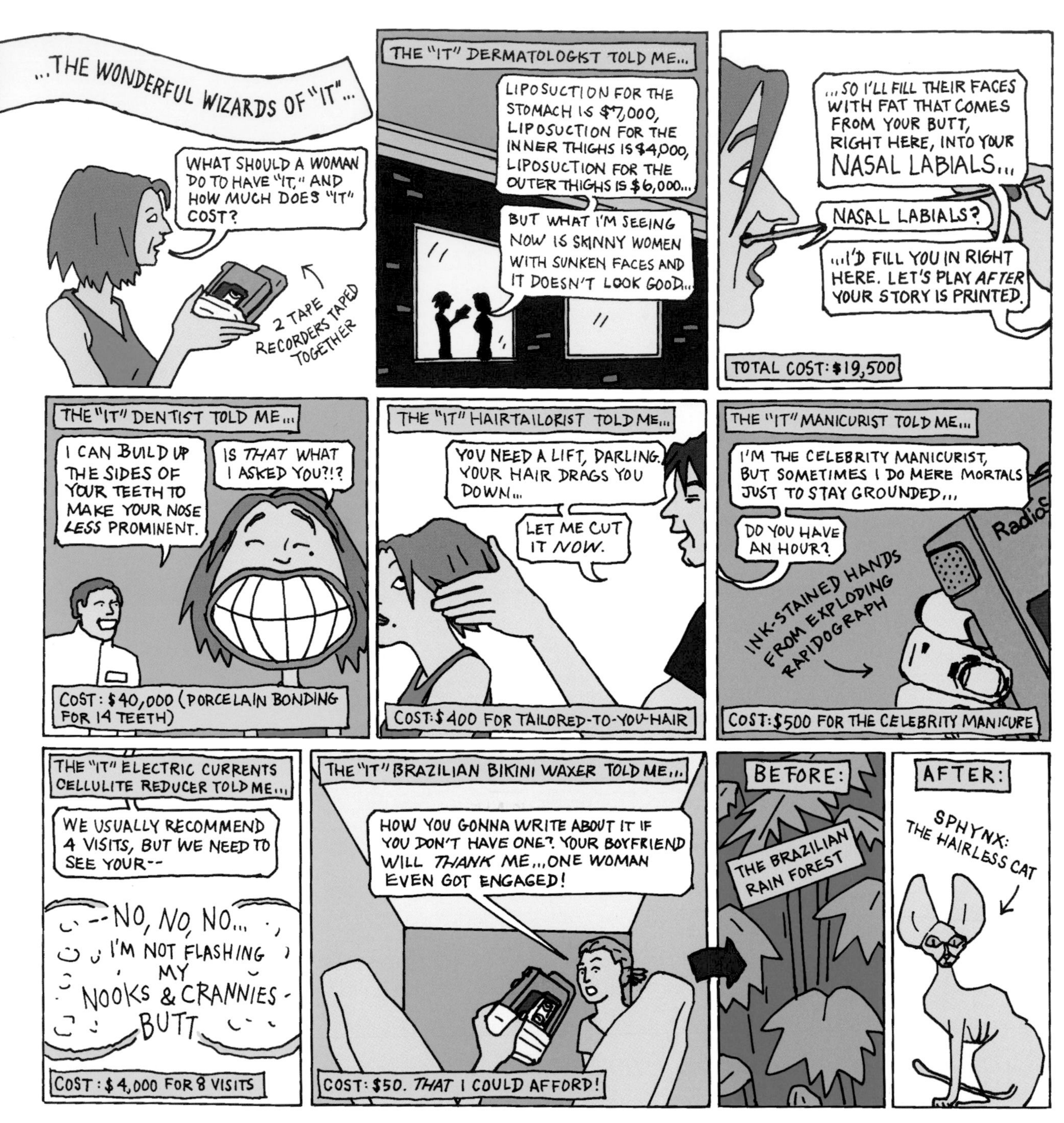
...THE WONDERFUL WIZARDS OF "IT"...
WHAT SHOULD A WOMAN DO TO HAVE "IT," AND HOW MUCH DOES "IT" COST?
2 TAPE RECORDERS TAPED TOGETHER
THE "IT" DERMATOLOGIST TOLD ME...
LIPOSUCTION FOR THE STOMACH IS $7,000, LIPOSUCTION FOR THE INNER THIGHS IS $4,000, LIPOSUCTION FOR THE OUTER THIGHS IS $6,000...
BUT WHAT I'M SEEING NOW IS SKINNY WOMEN WITH SUNKEN FACES AND IT DOESN'T LOOK GOOD...
...SO I'LL FILL THEIR FACES WITH FAT THAT COMES FROM YOUR BUTT, RIGHT HERE, INTO YOUR NASAL LABIALS...
NASAL LABIALS?
...I'D FILL YOU IN RIGHT HERE. LET'S PLAY *AFTER* YOUR STORY IS PRINTED.
TOTAL COST: $19,500
THE "IT" DENTIST TOLD ME...
I CAN BUILD UP THE SIDES OF YOUR TEETH TO MAKE YOUR NOSE *LESS* PROMINENT.
IS *THAT* WHAT I ASKED YOU?!?
COST: $40,000 (PORCELAIN BONDING FOR 14 TEETH)
THE "IT" HAIRTAILORIST TOLD ME...
YOU NEED A LIFT, DARLING. YOUR HAIR DRAGS YOU DOWN...
LET ME CUT IT *NOW*.
COST: $400 FOR TAILORED-TO-YOU-HAIR
THE "IT" MANICURIST TOLD ME...
I'M THE CELEBRITY MANICURIST, BUT SOMETIMES I DO MERE MORTALS JUST TO STAY GROUNDED...
DO YOU HAVE AN HOUR?
INK-STAINED HANDS FROM EXPLODING RAPIDOGRAPH
COST: $500 FOR THE CELEBRITY MANICURE
THE "IT" ELECTRIC CURRENTS CELLULITE REDUCER TOLD ME...
WE USUALLY RECOMMEND 4 VISITS, BUT WE NEED TO SEE YOUR--
--NO, NO, NO... I'M NOT FLASHING MY NOOKS & CRANNIES BUTT
COST: $4,000 FOR 8 VISITS
THE "IT" BRAZILIAN BIKINI WAXER TOLD ME...
HOW YOU GONNA WRITE ABOUT IT IF YOU DON'T HAVE ONE? YOUR BOYFRIEND WILL *THANK* ME... ONE WOMAN EVEN GOT ENGAGED!
COST: $50. *THAT* I COULD AFFORD!
BEFORE:
THE BRAZILIAN RAIN FOREST
AFTER:
SPHYNX: THE HAIRLESS CAT

1 DEFORESTED RAIN FOREST LATER, I RANG MY *THEN* BOYFRIEND, THE ACTOR...
HEY, GUESS WHO GOT A BRAZILIAN BIKINI WAX...
I COULD COME...
BEEP!
...OVER.
5TH AVE
I WASN'T SUPRISED HE DIDN'T PICK UP. HE WAS SO SELF-ABSORBED, HE *NEVER* PICKED UP ON ANYTHING.
THANK GOD FOR CALL WAITING...
I JUST GOT A CANCELLATION, MAREESE, HOW GOES IT?
THE MADISON AVENUE SALON WHERE "IT" HAIRCOLORIST SHARON WORKS.

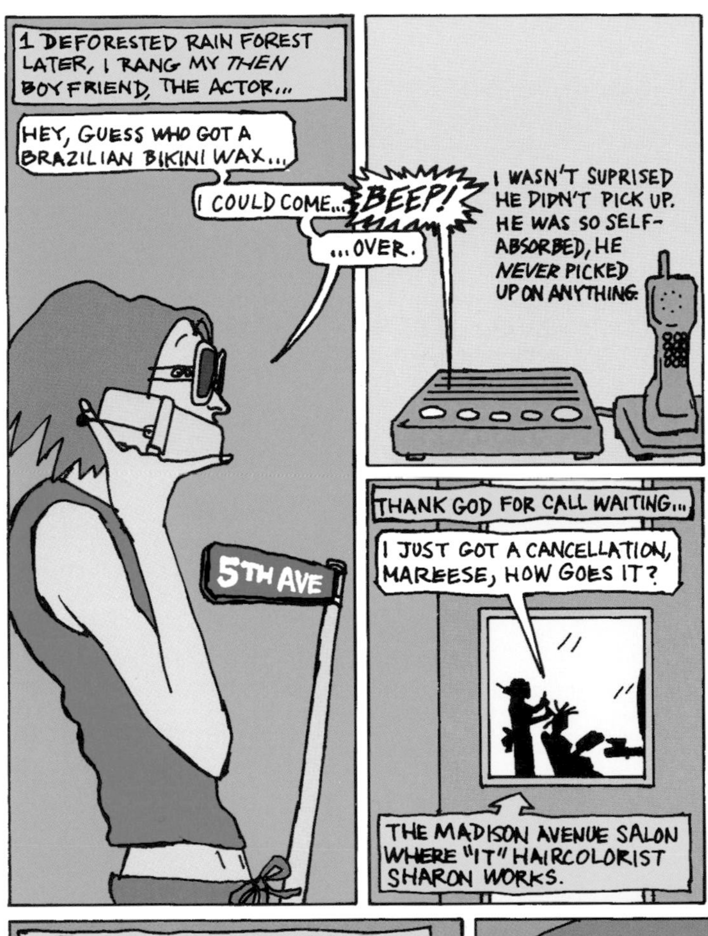

THE PURSUIT OF "IT" IS DRIVING ME NUTS! I HAVEN'T FOUND THE "IT" BAG, THE "IT" WATCH, THE "IT" PHONE--BUT I DO HAVE THE "IT" COLLAGEN, LIPOSUCTION, FAT INJECTIONS, LIP AUGMENTATIONS, EXFOLIATIONS, DERMABRASIONS, BOTOX, ELECTROSHOCK CELLULITE REMOVAL, ELECTROSHOCK FACIALS, STRING FACIALS, LASER FACIALS, FOOT FACIALS, LASER FOOT FACIALS, LASER COLLAGEN SOFT PILLOWS IN THE BALLS OF YOUR FEET, MEDIPEELS, MEDIPEDIS, MEDIMANIS, EYEBROWS TINTED, INDIVIDUAL FALSE EYELASHES APPLIED 1 AT A TIME, EYELASH TINTING, EYELASH PERMING, LASER HAIR REMOVAL, TIT JOB, NOSE JOB, BUT YOU NEED IT BECAUSE IN THIS TOWN YOU'RE EITHER A NOBODY OR A GREAT BODY AND IT ALREADY COSTS $179,546 AND I'M NOT EVEN DONE WITH IT. YOU GET 1 THING DONE THEN ANOTHER THING DONE. THIS IS AN ENDLESS SLIPPERY SLOPE CHASING THE UNATTAINABLE "IT" AND AS SOON AS YOU HAVE "IT"-- IT'S GONE! IT'S CRAZY!

THAT'S HOW GOES IT!

SHARON'S STATION, 11 MINUTES LATER:
DOING THE *BEAUTY* STORY HAS MADE ME FEEL REALLY *UGLY*... THE EXPERTS FOUND FLAWS I DIDN'T EVEN KNOW I HAD!

YOU'RE LOOKING A LITTLE MOUSEY.
COST: $450 FOR HIGHLIGHTS

OH SHARON...
NOT YOU, TOO!
I GUESS IT'S THE NATURE OF THE BEAUTY BEAST?

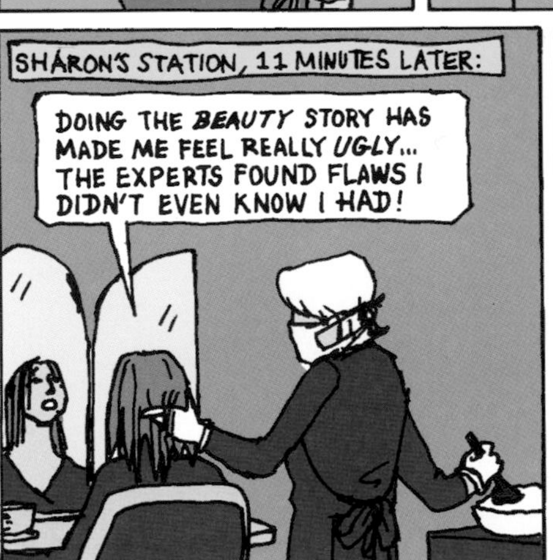

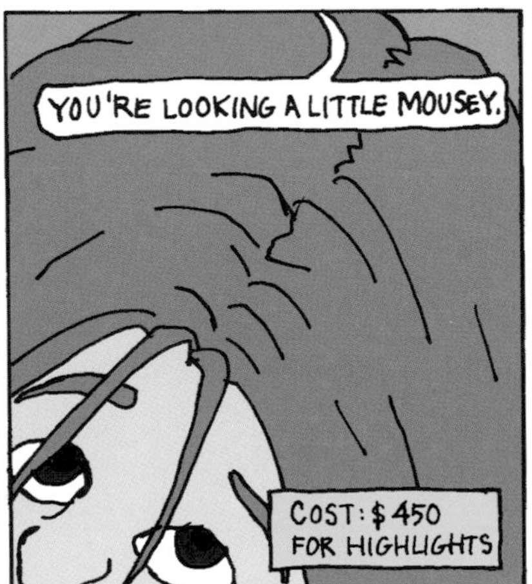

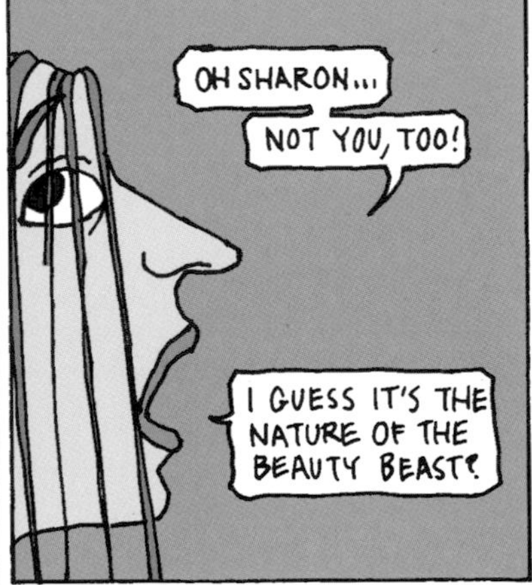

WHY ARE YOU COMPLAINING? IF YOU WRITE ABOUT IT, YOU GET TO HAVE IT, THAT'S HOW THE BUSINESS WORKS... AS LONG AS YOUR PIECE IS PRINTED.
SCRATCH MY BACK, I'LL WAX, NIP, TUCK, PLUCK, BLEACH YOURS?

RING! RING!
GOOD LUCK FINDING ANYTHING IN THIS BAG.
OH, HERE IT IS...

IT'S MY NEXT APPOINTMENT.
Da Silvano
Connected

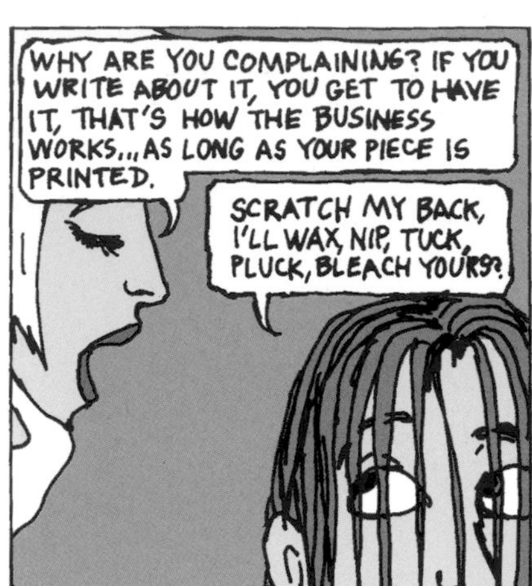

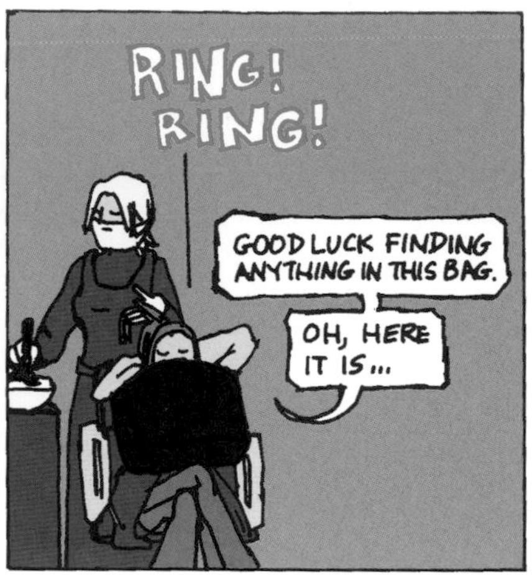

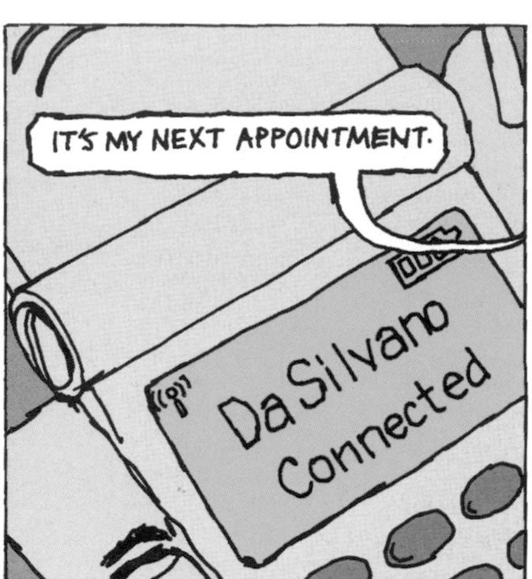

SO OFF I WENT TO INTERVIEW THE "IT" RESTAURATEUR, SILVANO MARCHETTO.
IT JUST SO HAPPENS THAT THE "IT" RESTAURANT HAS BEEN MY "IT" PLACE SINCE I WAS 17.

Da Sil
SILVANO, HOW DO I GET AN "A"* TABLE?
*FYI: YOU WOULD NEVER SAY "IT" TABLE, YOU JUST WOULDN'T.

MARISA, EVERY TABLE'S AN "A" TABLE.
KITCHEN
BAR
ANTIPASTO TABLE
WINES
DA SILVANO FLOOR PLAN

C'MON. THIS IS AN "A" TABLE?
MADONNA WAS 'ERE LAST NIGHT AND SHE SAT IN YOUR SEAT.

MADONNA SAT HERE? WHO WAS SHE WITH? WHAT DID SHE EAT?
GUY RITCHIE AND SHE 'AD THE LAMB CHOP AND SAID IT WAS FANTASTIC.

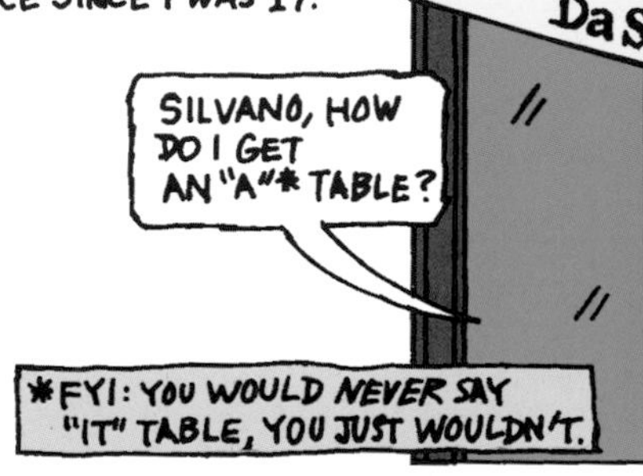

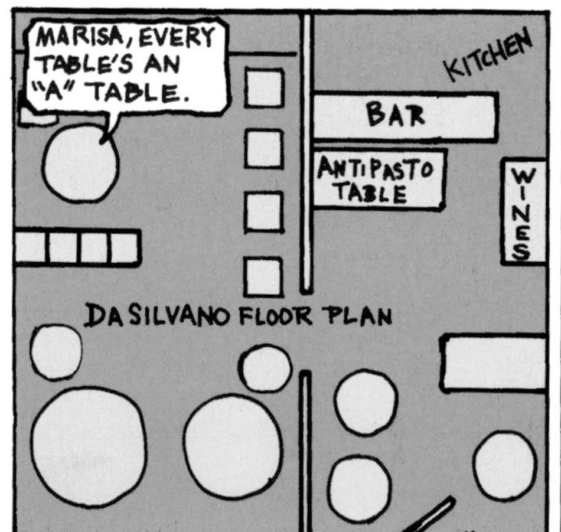

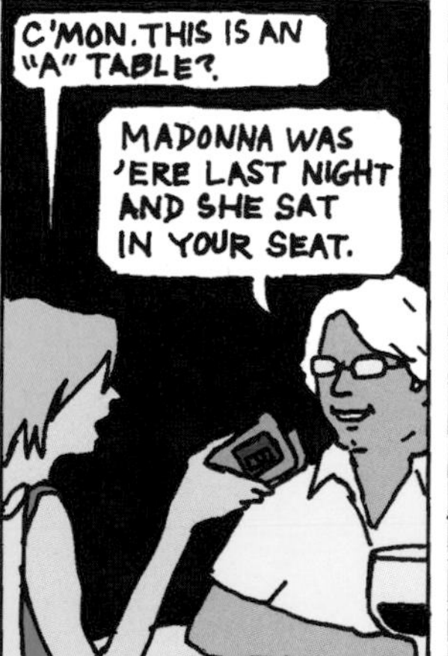

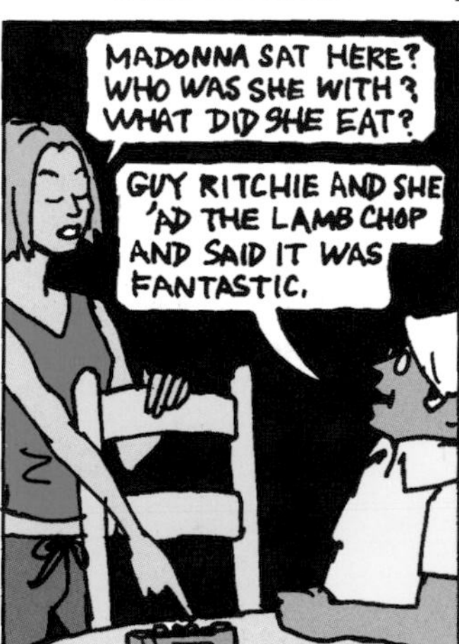

MAYBE SOME OF HER MADONNA-NESS WILL RUB OFF ON ME.

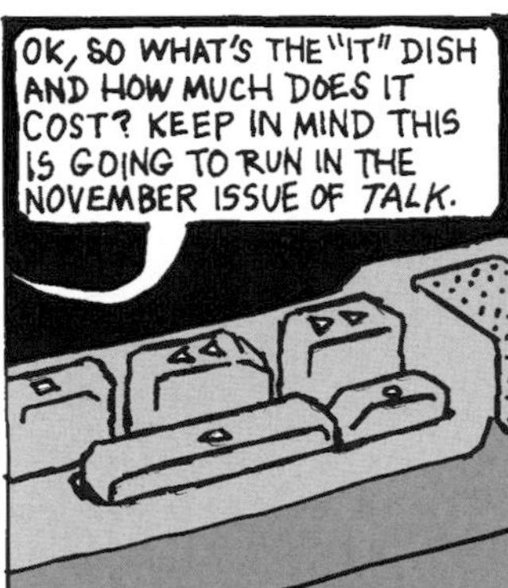
OK, SO WHAT'S THE "IT" DISH AND HOW MUCH DOES IT COST? KEEP IN MIND THIS IS GOING TO RUN IN THE NOVEMBER ISSUE OF *TALK*.

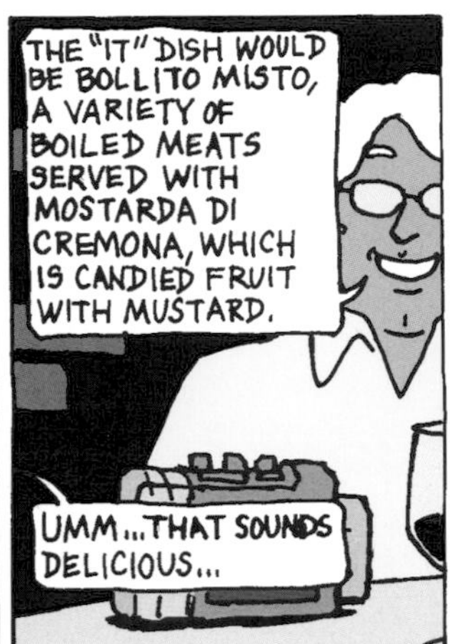
THE "IT" DISH WOULD BE BOLLITO MISTO, A VARIETY OF BOILED MEATS SERVED WITH MOSTARDA DI CREMONA, WHICH IS CANDIED FRUIT WITH MUSTARD.
UMM... THAT SOUNDS DELICIOUS...

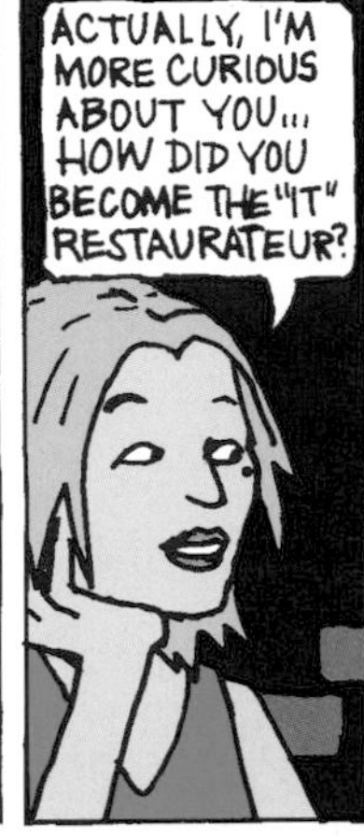
ACTUALLY, I'M MORE CURIOUS ABOUT YOU... HOW DID YOU BECOME THE "IT" RESTAURATEUR?

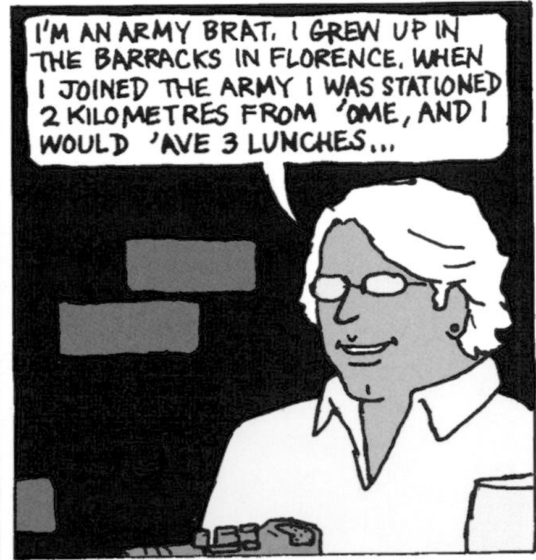
I'M AN ARMY BRAT. I GREW UP IN THE BARRACKS IN FLORENCE. WHEN I JOINED THE ARMY I WAS STATIONED 2 KILOMETRES FROM 'OME, AND I WOULD 'AVE 3 LUNCHES...

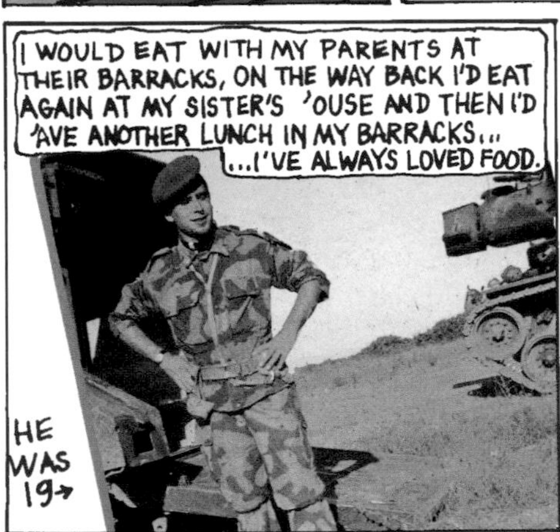
I WOULD EAT WITH MY PARENTS AT THEIR BARRACKS, ON THE WAY BACK I'D EAT AGAIN AT MY SISTER'S 'OUSE AND THEN I'D 'AVE ANOTHER LUNCH IN MY BARRACKS...
...I'VE ALWAYS LOVED FOOD.
HE WAS 19→

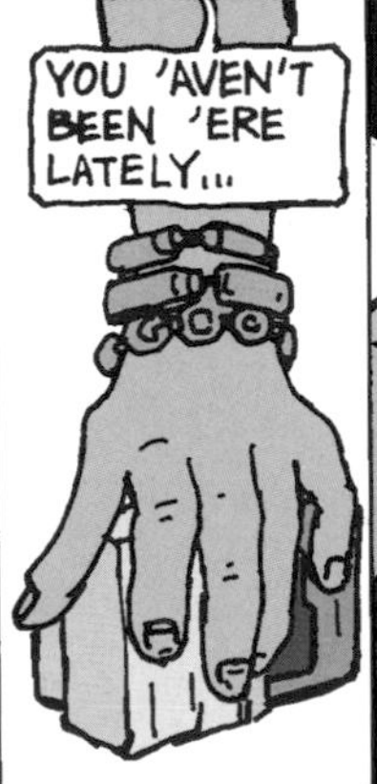
YOU 'AVEN'T BEEN 'ERE LATELY...

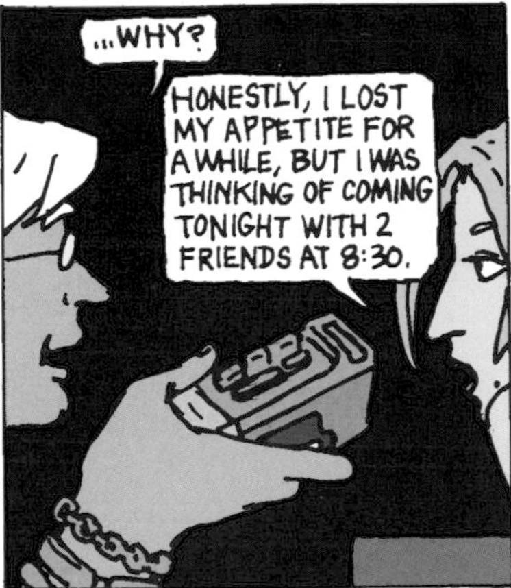
...WHY?
HONESTLY, I LOST MY APPETITE FOR A WHILE, BUT I WAS THINKING OF COMING TONIGHT WITH 2 FRIENDS AT 8:30.

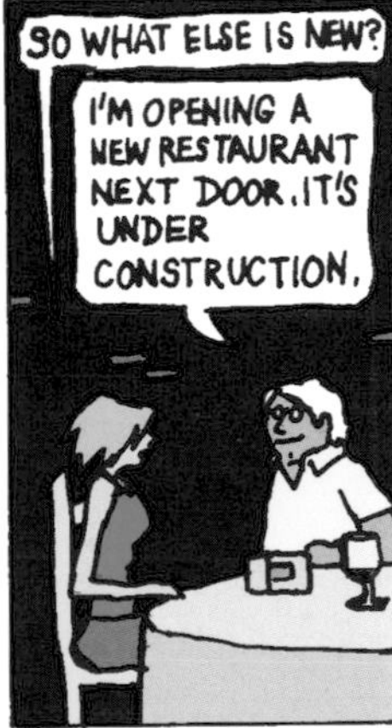
SO WHAT ELSE IS NEW?
I'M OPENING A NEW RESTAURANT NEXT DOOR. IT'S UNDER CONSTRUCTION.

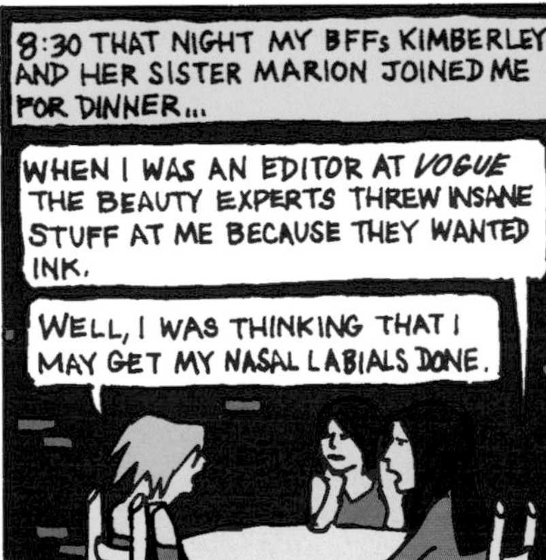
8:30 THAT NIGHT MY BFFs KIMBERLEY AND HER SISTER MARION JOINED ME FOR DINNER...
WHEN I WAS AN EDITOR AT *VOGUE* THE BEAUTY EXPERTS THREW INSANE STUFF AT ME BECAUSE THEY WANTED INK.
WELL, I WAS THINKING THAT I MAY GET MY NASAL LABIALS DONE.

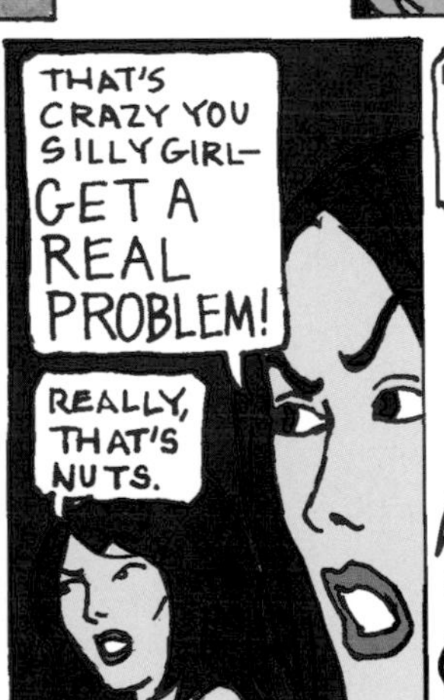
THAT'S CRAZY YOU SILLY GIRL– GET A REAL PROBLEM!
REALLY, THAT'S NUTS.

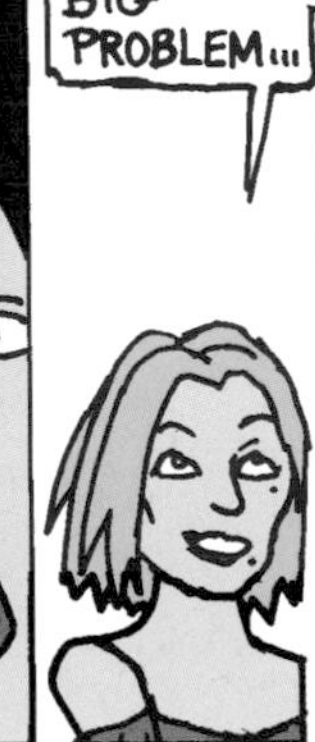
MY NOSE IS A REAL BIG PROBLEM...

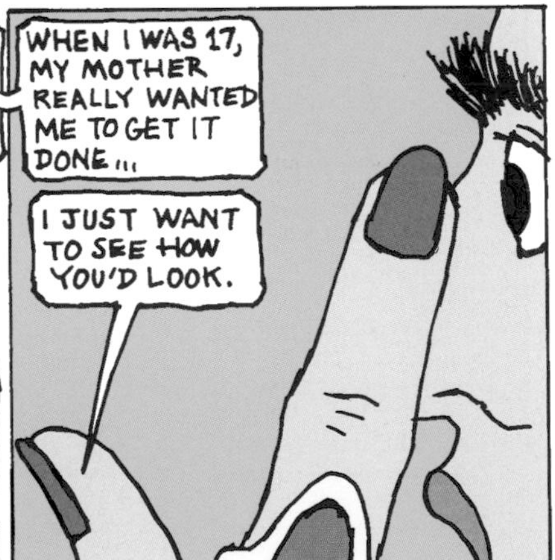
WHEN I WAS 17, MY MOTHER REALLY WANTED ME TO GET IT DONE...
I JUST WANT TO SEE HOW YOU'D LOOK.

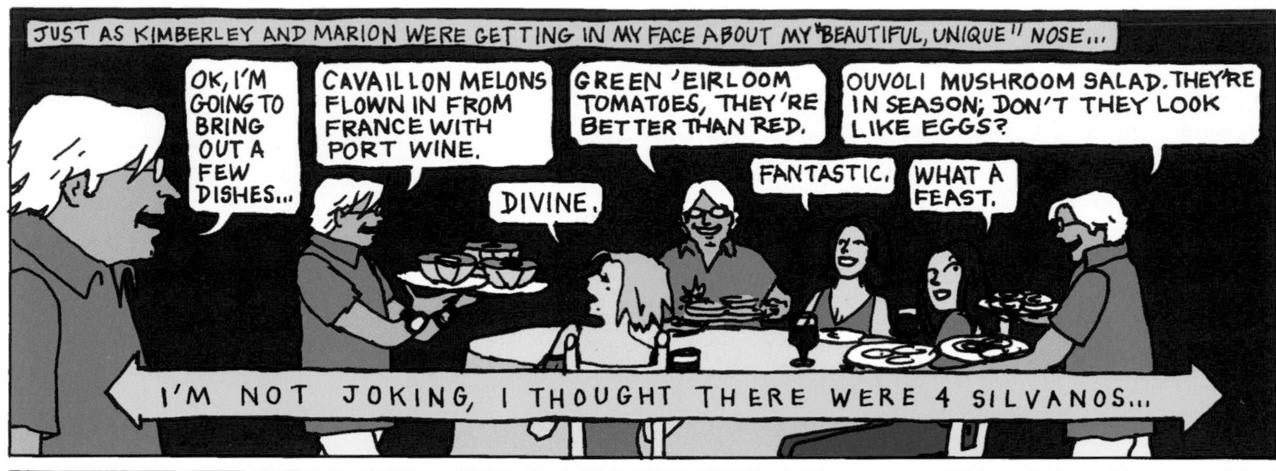
JUST AS KIMBERLEY AND MARION WERE GETTING IN MY FACE ABOUT MY "BEAUTIFUL, UNIQUE" NOSE...
OK, I'M GOING TO BRING OUT A FEW DISHES...
CAVAILLON MELONS FLOWN IN FROM FRANCE WITH PORT WINE.
DIVINE.
GREEN 'EIRLOOM TOMATOES, THEY'RE BETTER THAN RED.
FANTASTIC.
OUVOLI MUSHROOM SALAD. THEY'RE IN SEASON; DON'T THEY LOOK LIKE EGGS?
WHAT A FEAST.
I'M NOT JOKING, I THOUGHT THERE WERE 4 SILVANOS...

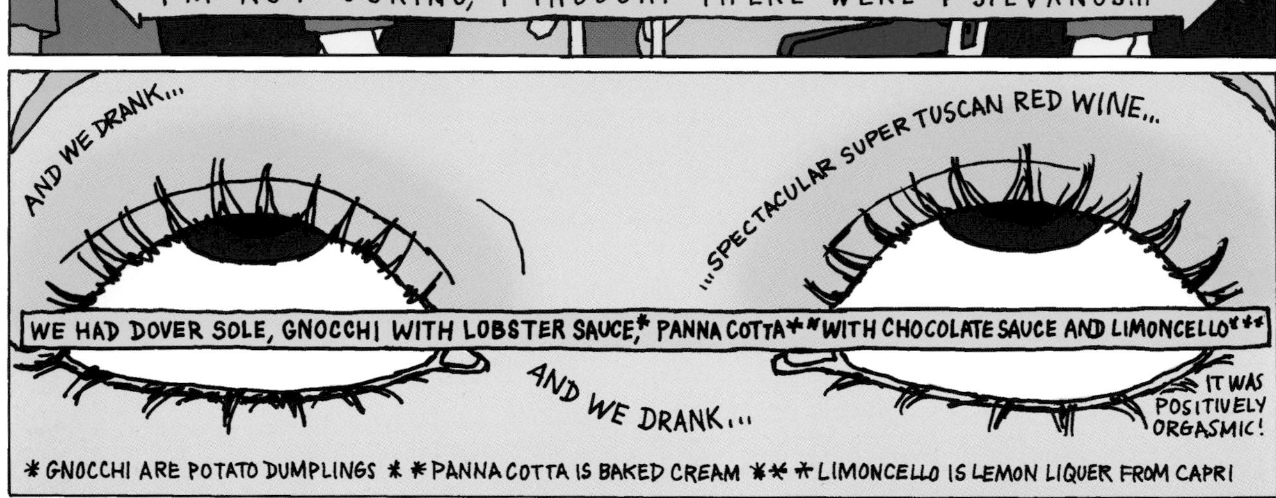
AND WE DRANK...
...SPECTACULAR SUPER TUSCAN RED WINE...
WE HAD DOVER SOLE, GNOCCHI WITH LOBSTER SAUCE,* PANNA COTTA** WITH CHOCOLATE SAUCE AND LIMONCELLO***
AND WE DRANK...
IT WAS POSITIVELY ORGASMIC!
* GNOCCHI ARE POTATO DUMPLINGS ** PANNA COTTA IS BAKED CREAM *** LIMONCELLO IS LEMON LIQUER FROM CAPRI

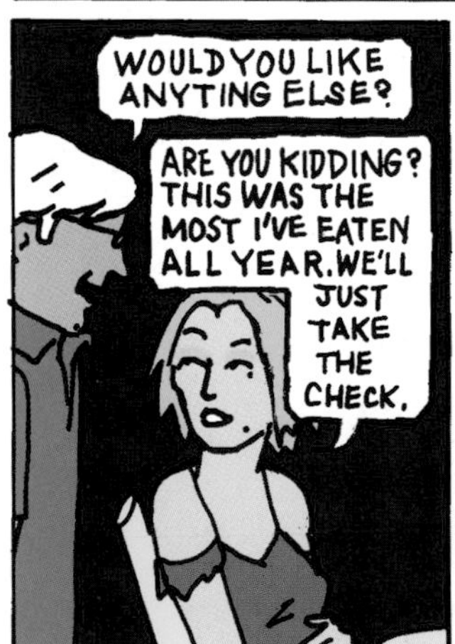
WOULD YOU LIKE ANYTING ELSE?
ARE YOU KIDDING? THIS WAS THE MOST I'VE EATEN ALL YEAR. WE'LL JUST TAKE THE CHECK.

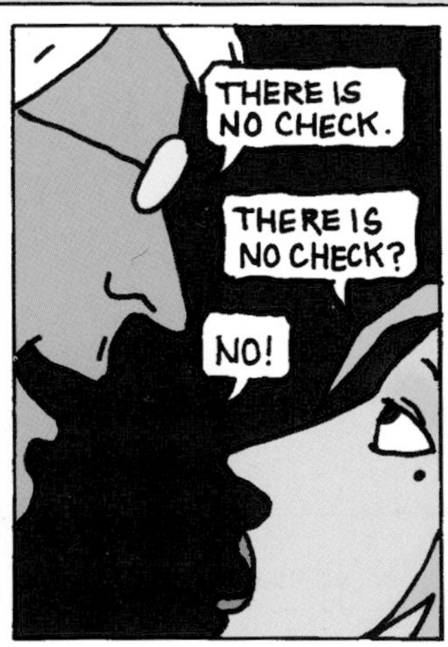
THERE IS NO CHECK.
THERE IS NO CHECK?
NO!

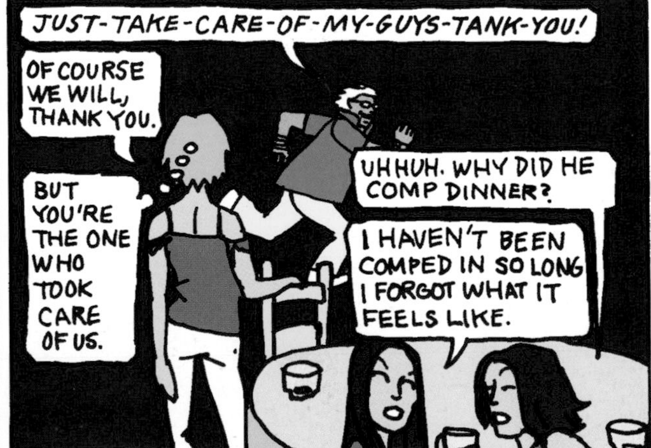
JUST-TAKE-CARE-OF-MY-GUYS-TANK-YOU!
OF COURSE WE WILL, THANK YOU.
BUT YOU'RE THE ONE WHO TOOK CARE OF US.
UHHUH. WHY DID HE COMP DINNER?
I HAVEN'T BEEN COMPED IN SO LONG I FORGOT WHAT IT FEELS LIKE.

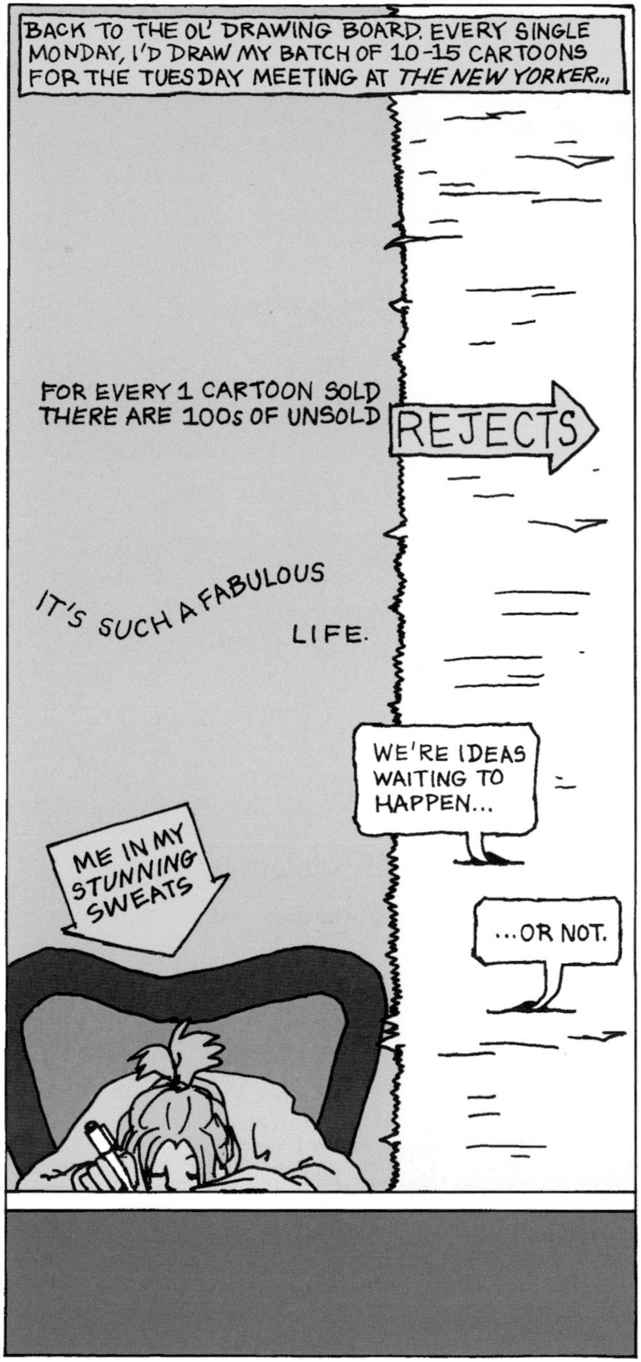

BACK TO THE OL' DRAWING BOARD. EVERY SINGLE MONDAY, I'D DRAW MY BATCH OF 10-15 CARTOONS FOR THE TUESDAY MEETING AT *THE NEW YORKER*...

FOR EVERY 1 CARTOON SOLD THERE ARE 100s OF UNSOLD

REJECTS

IT'S SUCH A FABULOUS LIFE.

WE'RE IDEAS WAITING TO HAPPEN...

ME IN MY STUNNING SWEATS

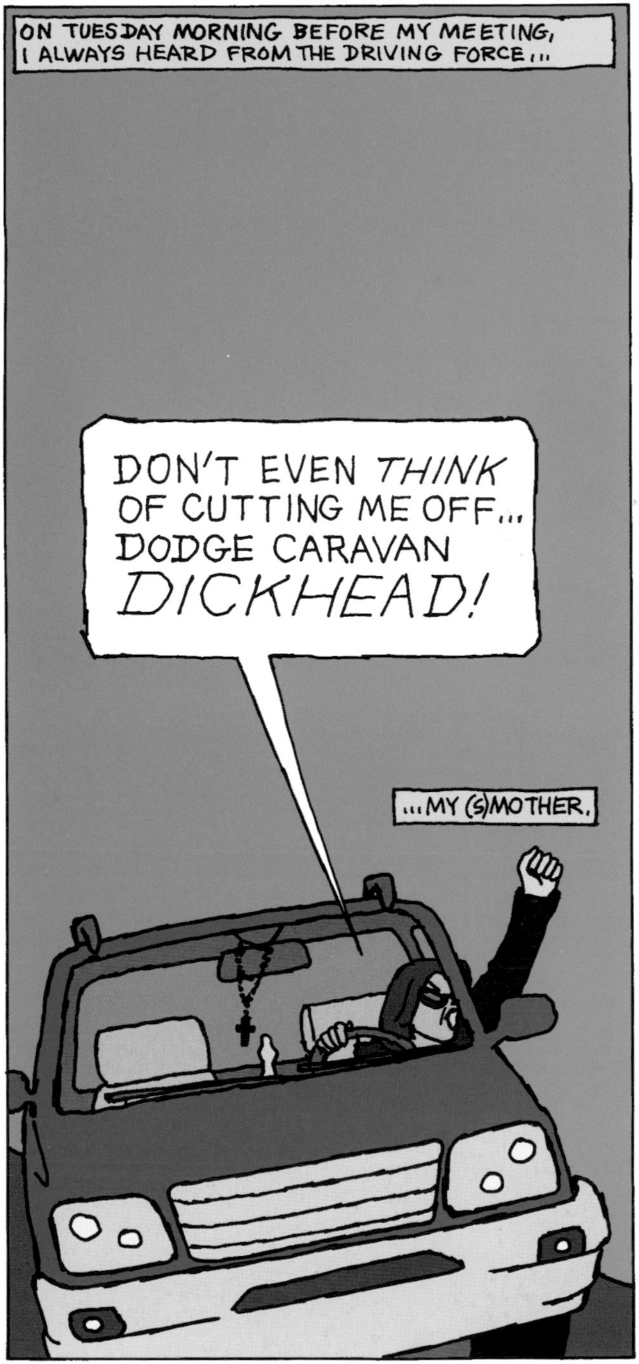

...OR NOT.

ON TUESDAY MORNING BEFORE MY MEETING, I ALWAYS HEARD FROM THE DRIVING FORCE...

DON'T EVEN *THINK* OF CUTTING ME OFF... DODGE CARAVAN *DICKHEAD!*

...MY (S)MOTHER.

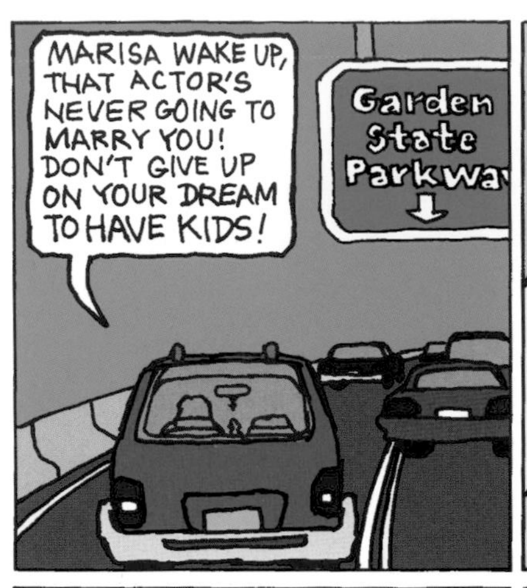
MARISA WAKE UP, THAT ACTOR'S NEVER GOING TO MARRY YOU! DON'T GIVE UP ON YOUR DREAM TO HAVE KIDS!
Garden State Parkwa
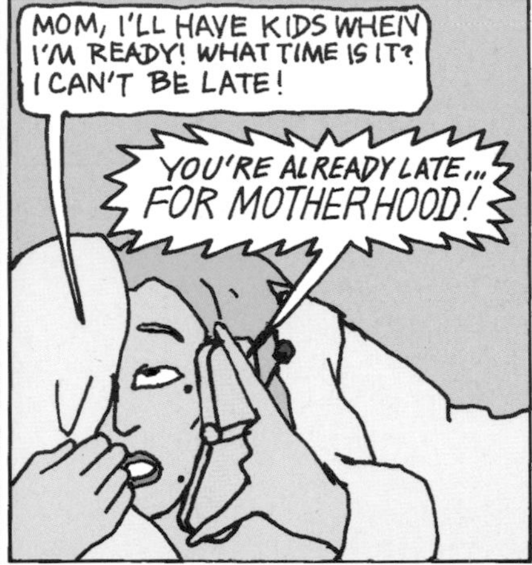
MOM, I'LL HAVE KIDS WHEN I'M READY! WHAT TIME IS IT? I CAN'T BE LATE!
YOU'RE ALREADY LATE... FOR MOTHERHOOD!
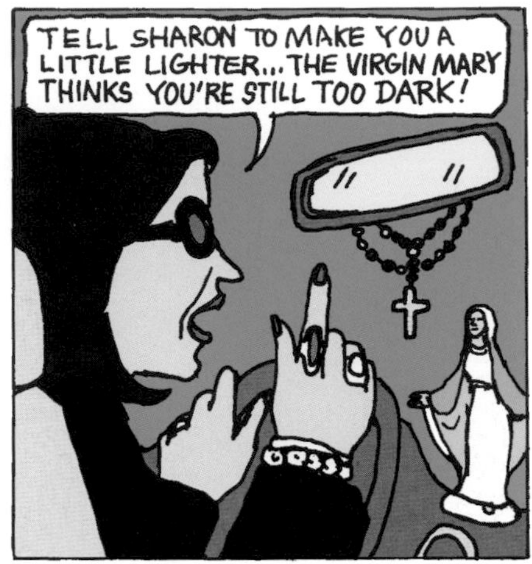
TELL SHARON TO MAKE YOU A LITTLE LIGHTER... THE VIRGIN MARY THINKS YOU'RE STILL TOO DARK!
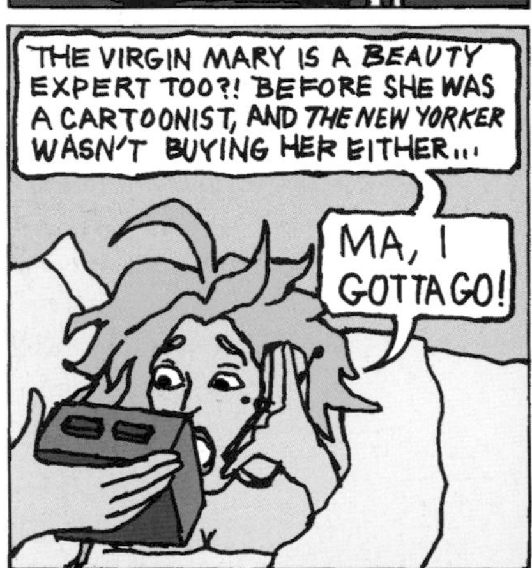
THE VIRGIN MARY IS A *BEAUTY EXPERT* TOO?! BEFORE SHE WAS A CARTOONIST, AND *THE NEW YORKER* WASN'T BUYING HER EITHER...
MA, I GOTTA GO!
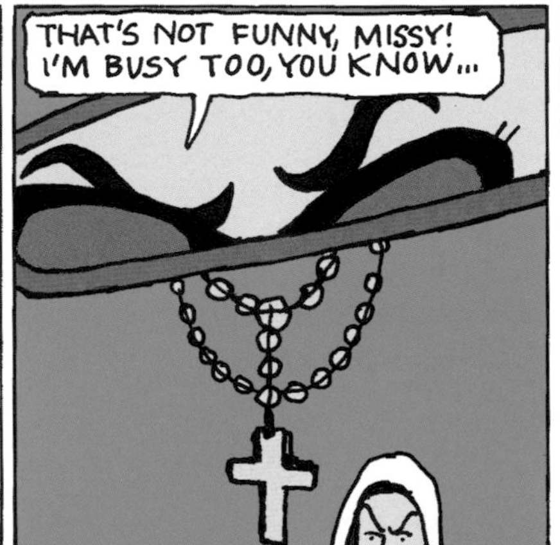
THAT'S NOT FUNNY, MISSY! I'M BUSY TOO, YOU KNOW...
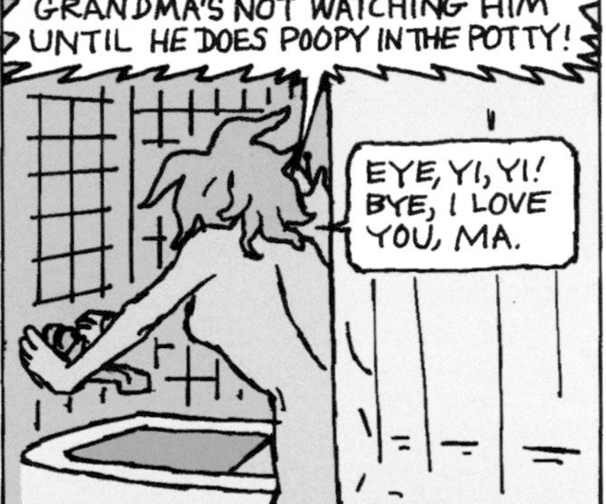
YOUR SISTER'S TRYING TO CON ME INTO BABYSITTING JOHNNY, BUT GRANDMA'S NOT WATCHING HIM UNTIL HE DOES POOPY IN THE POTTY!
EYE, YI, YI! BYE, I LOVE YOU, MA.
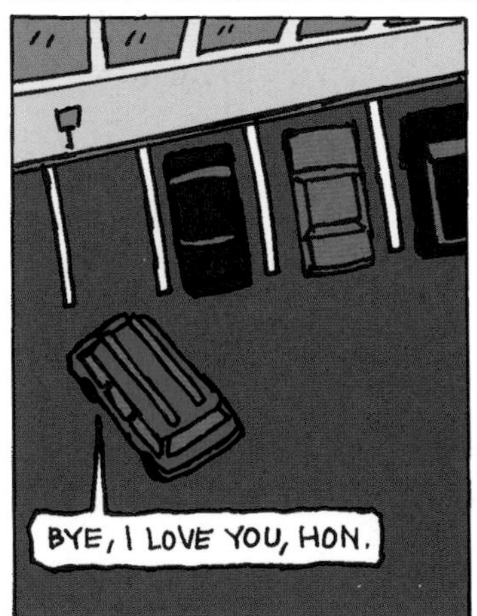
BYE, I LOVE YOU, HON.
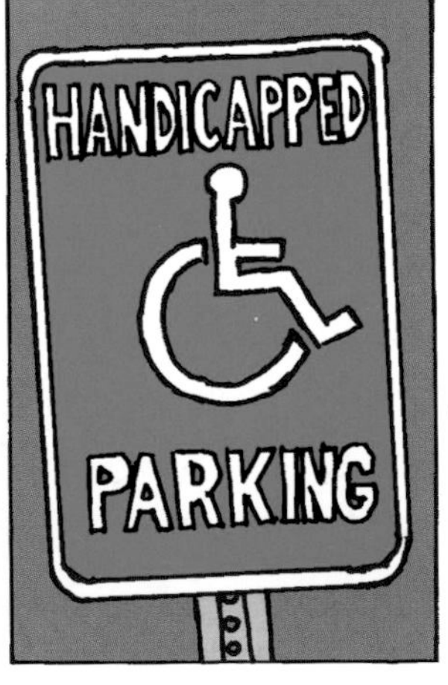
HANDICAPPED
PARKING
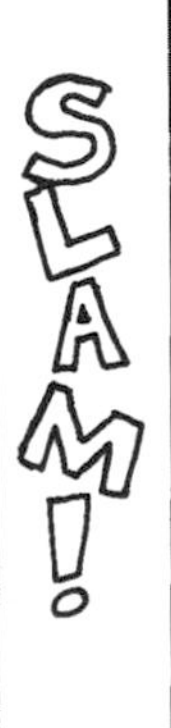
SLAM!
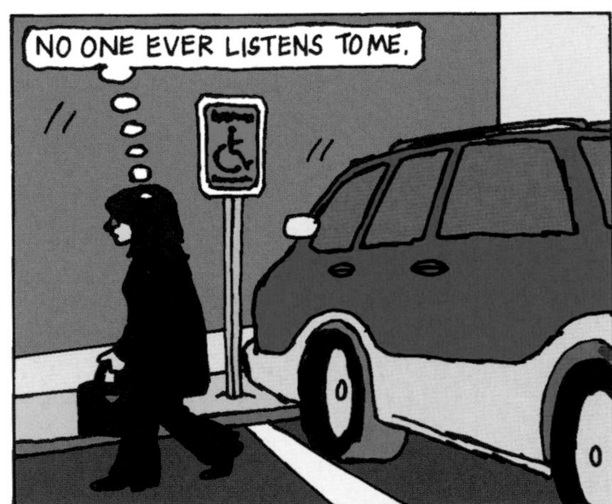
NO ONE EVER LISTENS TO ME.

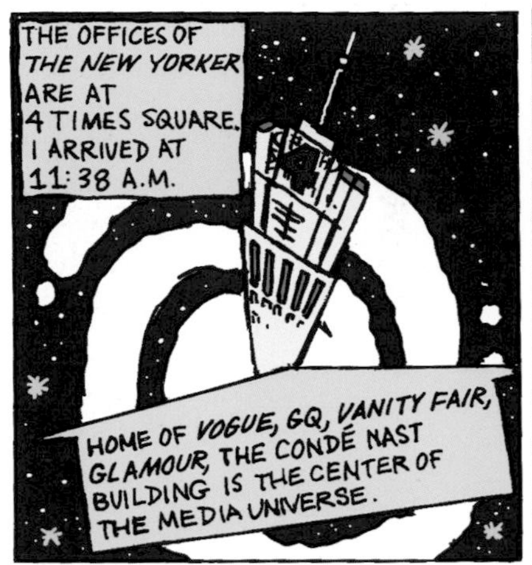
THE OFFICES OF *THE NEW YORKER* ARE AT 4 TIMES SQUARE. I ARRIVED AT 11:38 A.M.
HOME OF *VOGUE, GQ, VANITY FAIR, GLAMOUR*, THE CONDÉ NAST BUILDING IS THE CENTER OF THE MEDIA UNIVERSE.

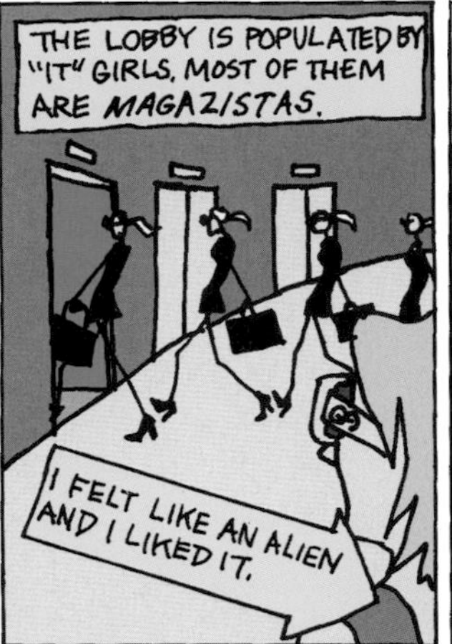
THE LOBBY IS POPULATED BY "IT" GIRLS, MOST OF THEM ARE *MAGAZISTAS*.
I FELT LIKE AN ALIEN AND I LIKED IT.

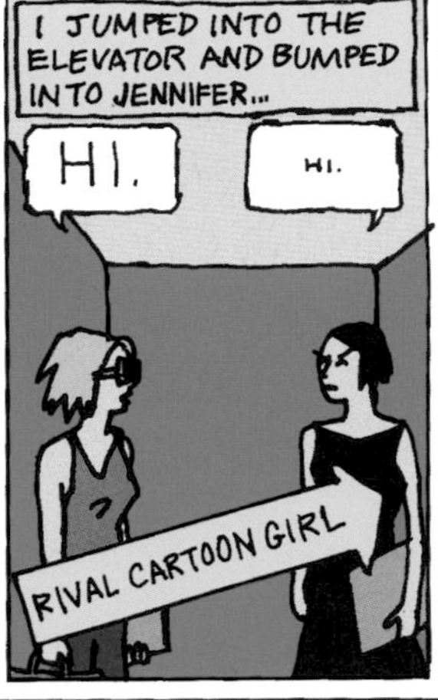
I JUMPED INTO THE ELEVATOR AND BUMPED INTO JENNIFER...
HI.
HI.
RIVAL CARTOON GIRL

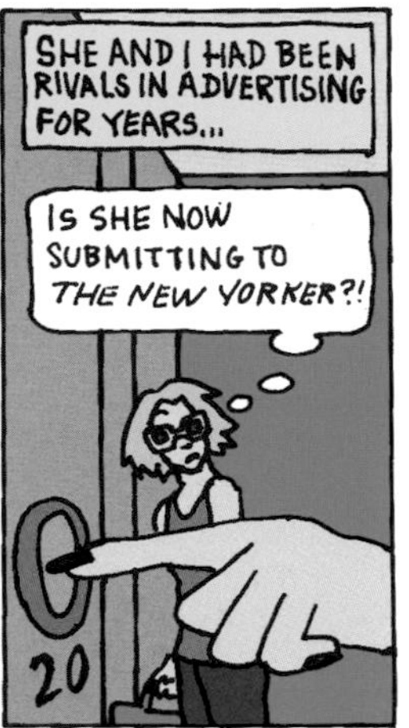
SHE AND I HAD BEEN RIVALS IN ADVERTISING FOR YEARS...
IS SHE NOW SUBMITTING TO *THE NEW YORKER*?!
20

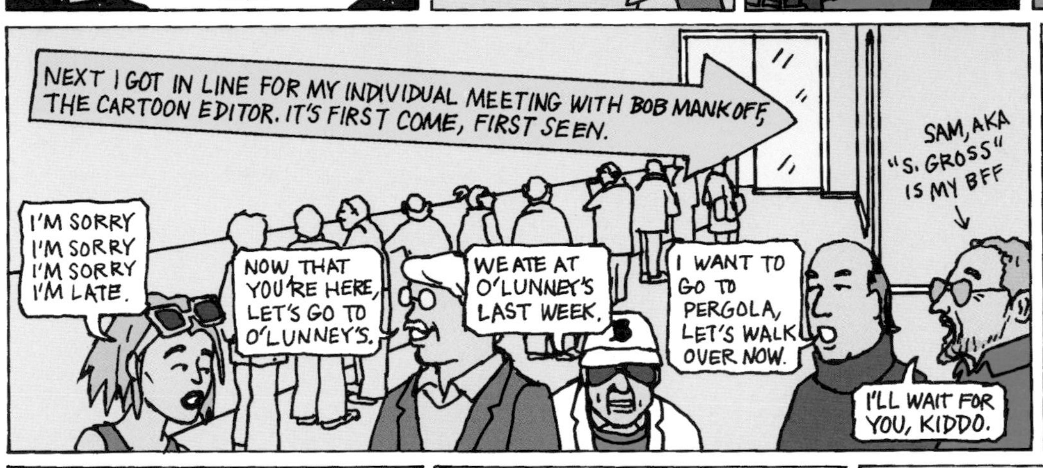
NEXT I GOT IN LINE FOR MY INDIVIDUAL MEETING WITH BOB MANKOFF, THE CARTOON EDITOR. IT'S FIRST COME, FIRST SEEN.
I'M SORRY I'M SORRY I'M SORRY I'M LATE.
NOW THAT YOU'RE HERE, LET'S GO TO O'LUNNEY'S.
WE ATE AT O'LUNNEY'S LAST WEEK.
I WANT TO GO TO PERGOLA, LET'S WALK OVER NOW.
SAM, AKA "S. GROSS" IS MY BFF
I'LL WAIT FOR YOU, KIDDO.

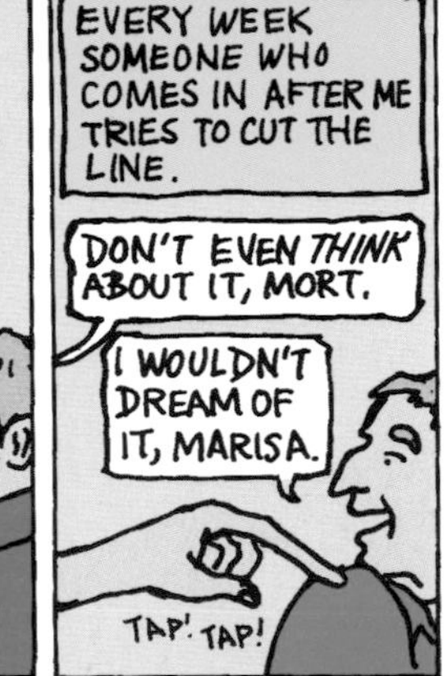
EVERY WEEK SOMEONE WHO COMES IN AFTER ME TRIES TO CUT THE LINE.
DON'T EVEN *THINK* ABOUT IT, MORT.
I WOULDN'T DREAM OF IT, MARISA.
TAP! TAP!

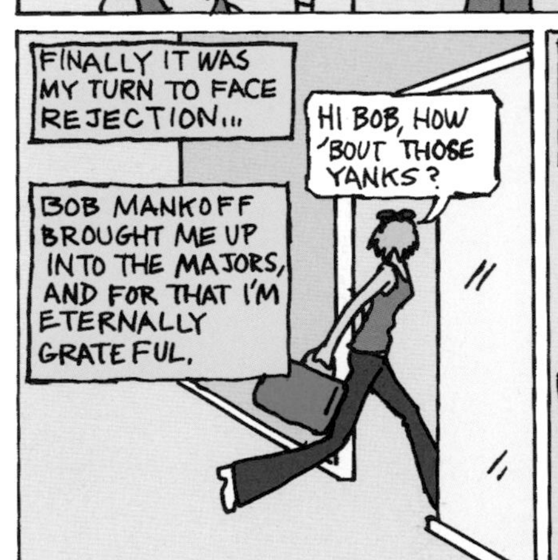
FINALLY IT WAS MY TURN TO FACE REJECTION...
HI BOB, HOW 'BOUT THOSE YANKS?
BOB MANKOFF BROUGHT ME UP INTO THE MAJORS, AND FOR THAT I'M ETERNALLY GRATEFUL.

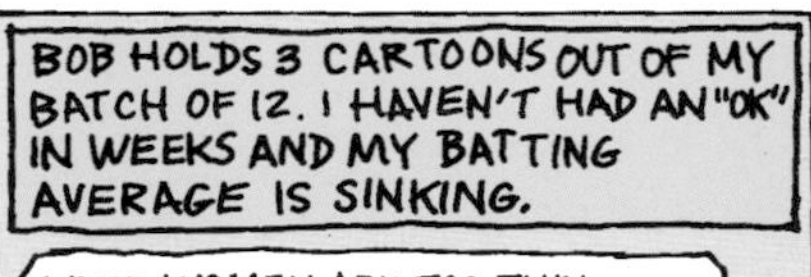
BOB HOLDS 3 CARTOONS OUT OF MY BATCH OF 12. I HAVEN'T HAD AN "OK" IN WEEKS AND MY BATTING AVERAGE IS SINKING.
YOUR WOMEN ARE TOO THIN, TOO PRETTY, THEY'RE NOT REAL AND I CAN'T RELATE TO THEM.

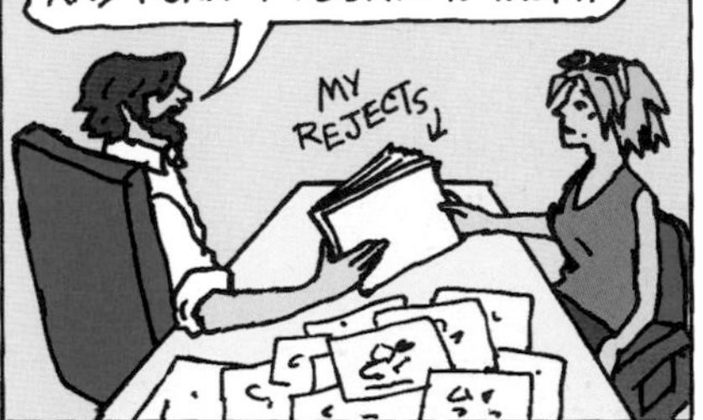
MY REJECTS

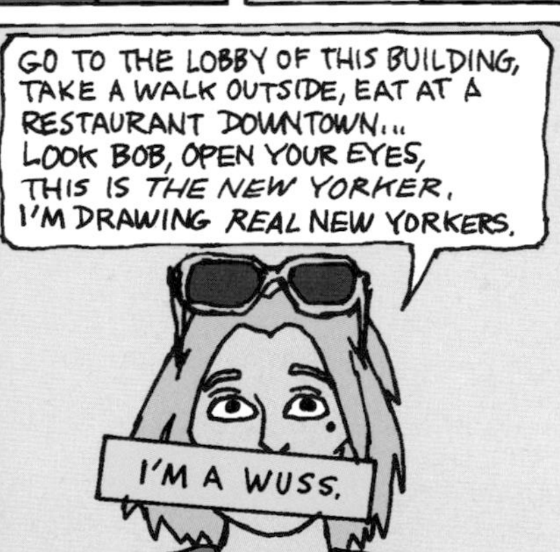
GO TO THE LOBBY OF THIS BUILDING, TAKE A WALK OUTSIDE, EAT AT A RESTAURANT DOWNTOWN... LOOK BOB, OPEN YOUR EYES, THIS IS *THE NEW YORKER*, I'M DRAWING *REAL* NEW YORKERS.
I'M A WUSS.
I REALLY DIDN'T SAY THAT.

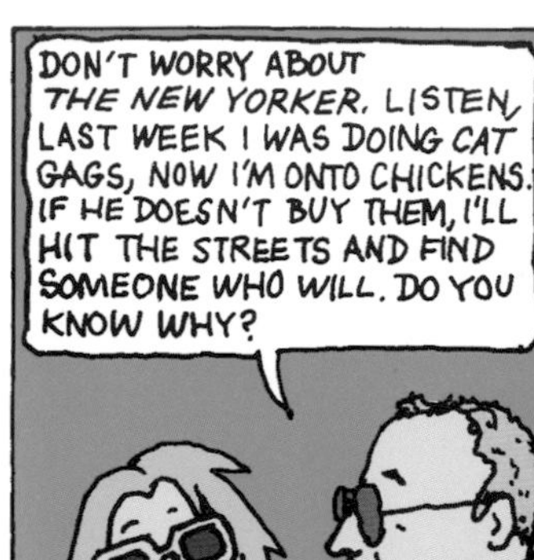
DON'T WORRY ABOUT *THE NEW YORKER.* LISTEN, LAST WEEK I WAS DOING CAT GAGS, NOW I'M ONTO CHICKENS. IF HE DOESN'T BUY THEM, I'LL HIT THE STREETS AND FIND SOMEONE WHO WILL. DO YOU KNOW WHY?

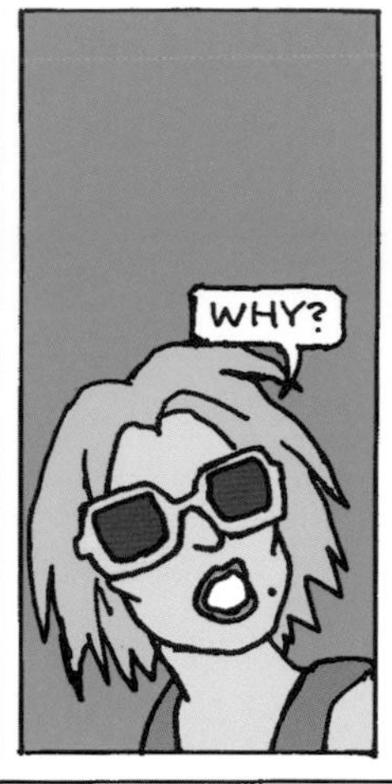
WHY?

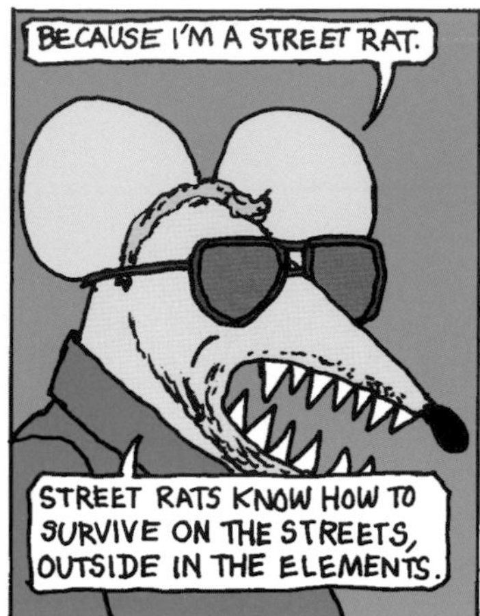
BECAUSE I'M A STREET RAT.
STREET RATS KNOW HOW TO SURVIVE ON THE STREETS, OUTSIDE IN THE ELEMENTS.

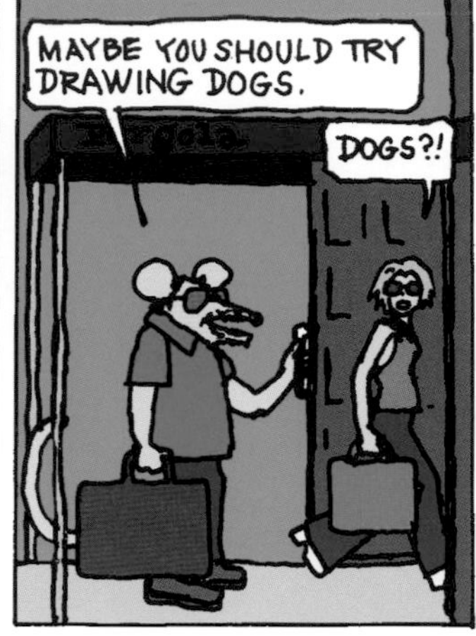
MAYBE YOU SHOULD TRY DRAWING DOGS.
DOGS?!

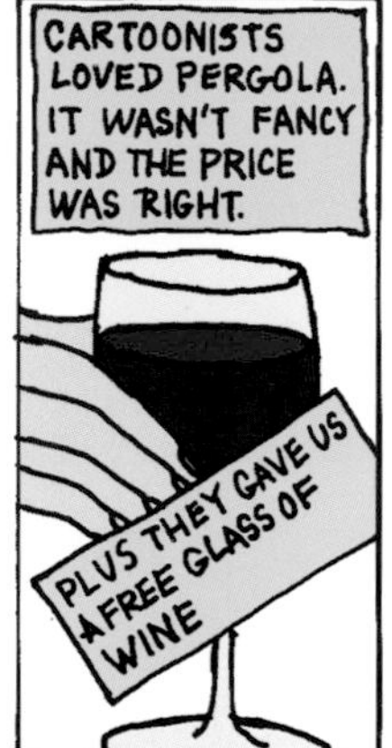
CARTOONISTS LOVED PERGOLA. IT WASN'T FANCY AND THE PRICE WAS RIGHT.
PLUS THEY GAVE US A FREE GLASS OF WINE

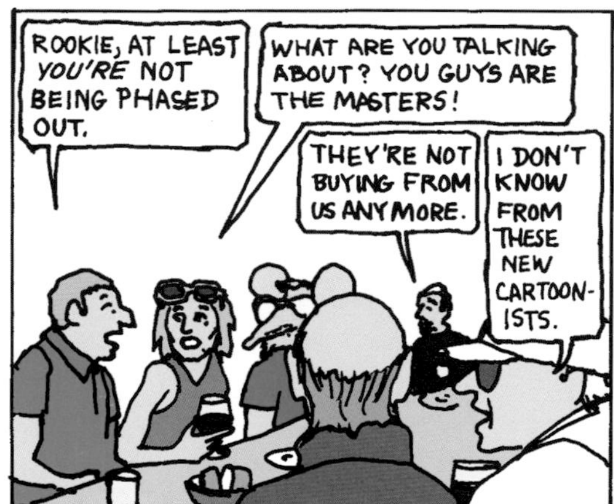
ROOKIE, AT LEAST *YOU'RE* NOT BEING PHASED OUT.
WHAT ARE YOU TALKING ABOUT? YOU GUYS ARE THE MASTERS!
THEY'RE NOT BUYING FROM US ANYMORE.
I DON'T KNOW FROM THESE NEW CARTOON-ISTS.

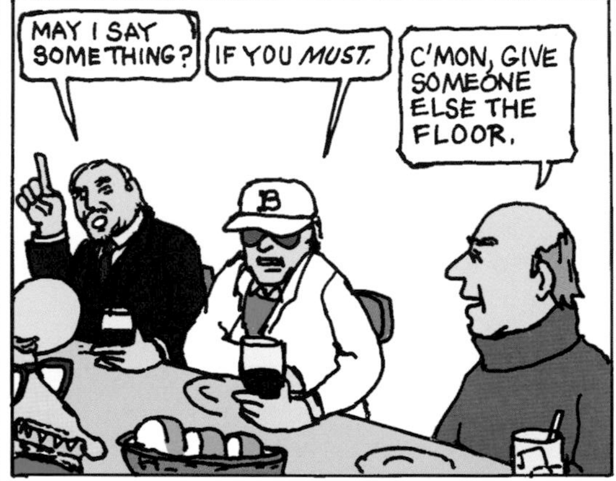
MAY I SAY SOMETHING?
IF YOU *MUST.*
C'MON, GIVE SOMEONE ELSE THE FLOOR.

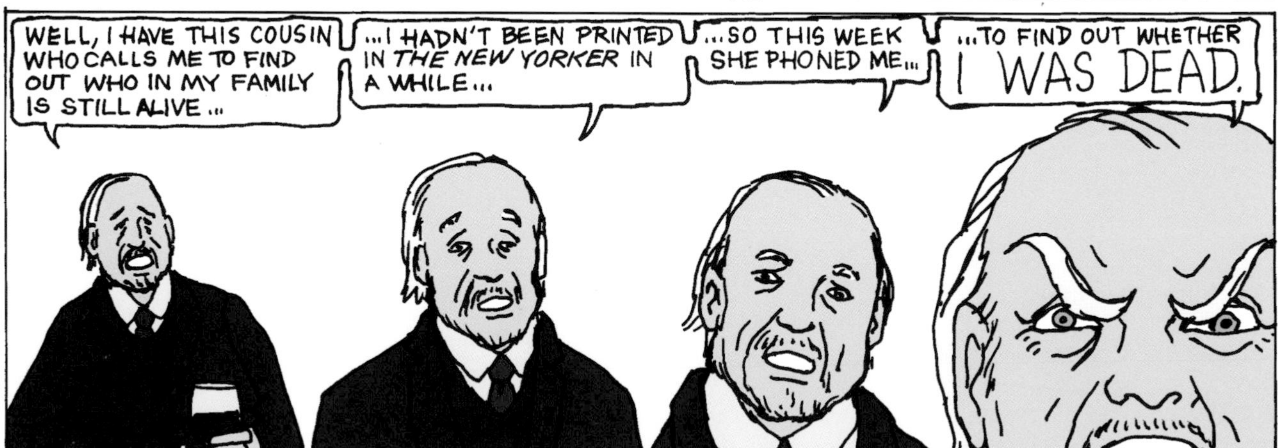
WELL, I HAVE THIS COUSIN WHO CALLS ME TO FIND OUT WHO IN MY FAMILY IS STILL ALIVE...
...I HADN'T BEEN PRINTED IN *THE NEW YORKER* IN A WHILE...
...SO THIS WEEK SHE PHONED ME...
...TO FIND OUT WHETHER I WAS DEAD.

THEN, ANOTHER MONDAY NIGHT A FEW WEEKS LATER.
SEPTEMBER 11, 3:06 A.M.
I WAS ON DEADLINE FOR *THE NEW YORKER*, WATCHING MY PARENTS' YORKIE WHILE THEY WERE AWAY.

GRRRRR...
PRECIOUS HAD A VERY SUBTLE WAY OF TELLING ME SHE WAS IRKED I WAS STILL UP
OK GIRLIE GIRL, I GOT THE MESSAGE.
C'MON PRECIOUS, TIME FOR BED.

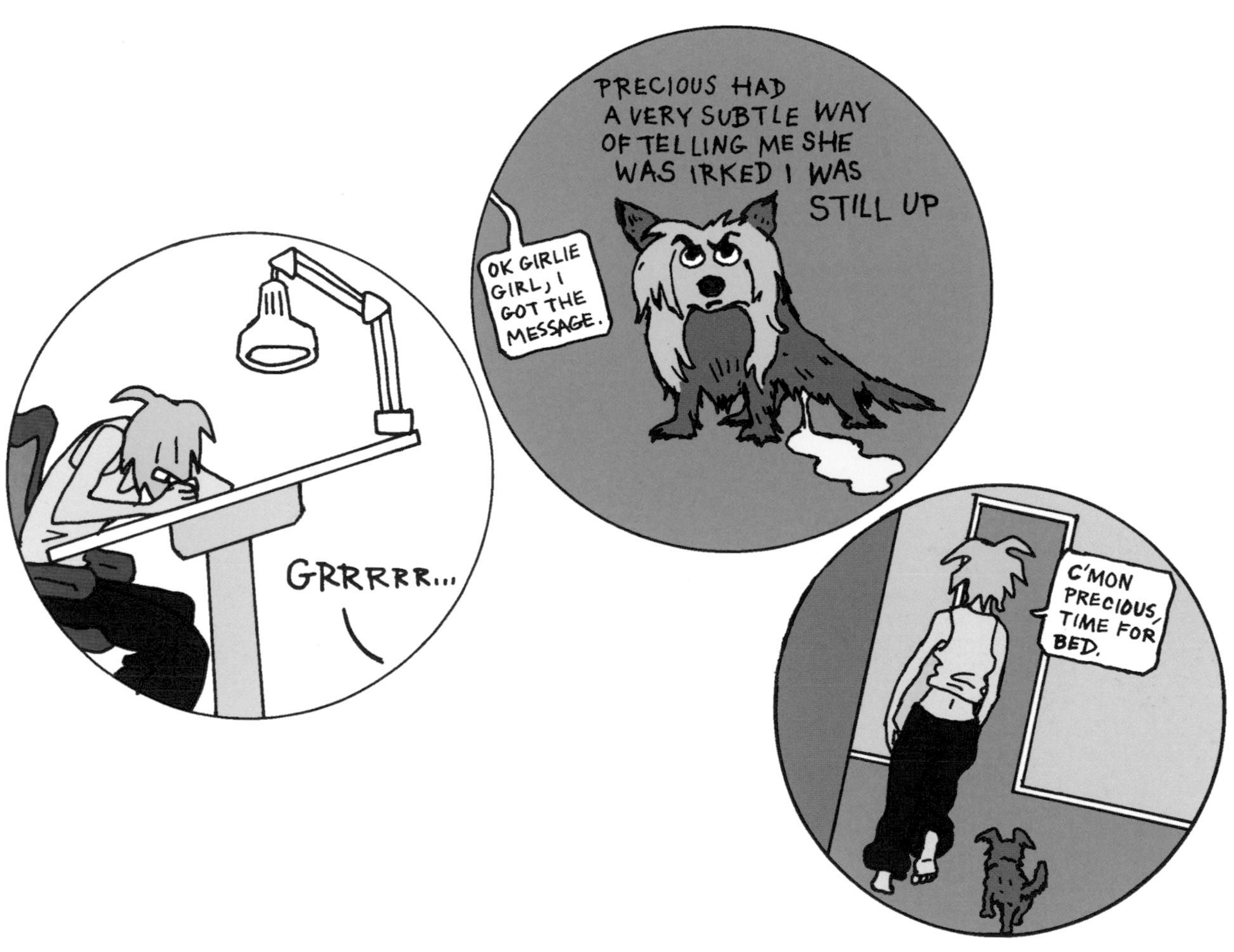

8:47 A.M. I WAS WOKEN OUT OF A DEEP SLEEP.
MAN, THAT WAS ONE LOUD PLANE...
THE JET SOUNDED LIKE IT FLEW RIGHT OVER MY APARTMENT.

12 MINUTES LATER...
IT'S KIMBERLEY— NEW YORK IS UNDER ATTACK! COME TO CONNECTICUT RIGHT NOW!

I CAN'T, I HAVE PRECIOUS AND I HAVE TO GO TO THE NEW YORKER.
THERE IS NO NEW YORKER!

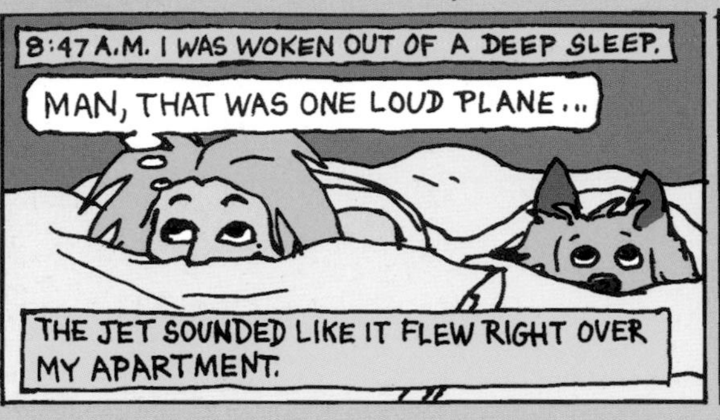

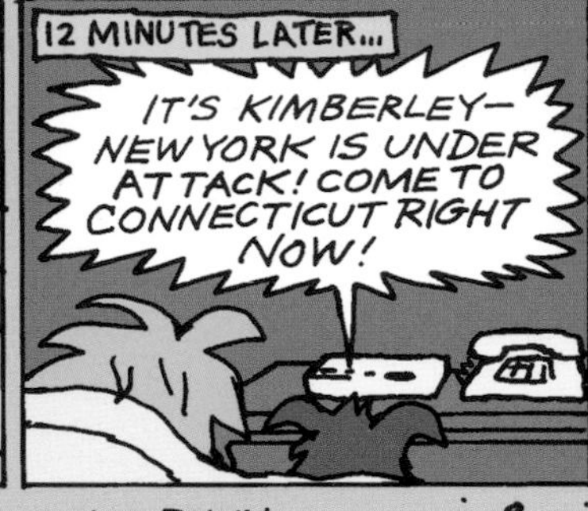

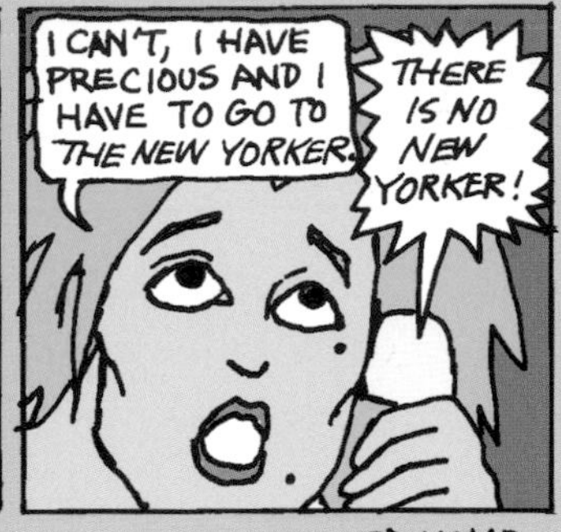

KIMBERLEY WAS RIGHT. *THE NEW YORKER* WAS SHUT DOWN. IMMEDIATELY AFTER THE FIRST PLANE HIT, I SAW PEOPLE COVERED WITH DUST RUNNING UP THE STREETS FROM DOWNTOWN.

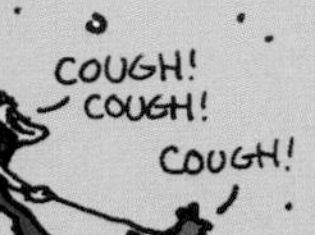

I RUSHED HOME, WORRIED ABOUT PRECIOUS'S LITTLE LUNGS.

1:32 P.M. MY *TALK* EDITOR DREW CALLED ME ON MY LAND LINE. CELL PHONES DIDN'T WORK BECAUSE THE ANTENNA WAS ON TOP OF TOWER 2.
MARISA, WE'RE RIPPING APART THE MAGAZINE AND WE'RE SENDING EVERYONE TO GROUND ZERO... CAN YOU COVER IT FROM YOUR END?!?!

...AND BY THE WAY, YOUR STORY "WHAT 'IT' COSTS" IS DEAD. IT'S TOO SUPERFICIAL RIGHT NOW.
EVERYTHING IS SUPERFICIAL RIGHT NOW.

OK PRECIOUS, I'LL SEE YOU IN A BIT.
SOB! SOB!
SOB! SOB!

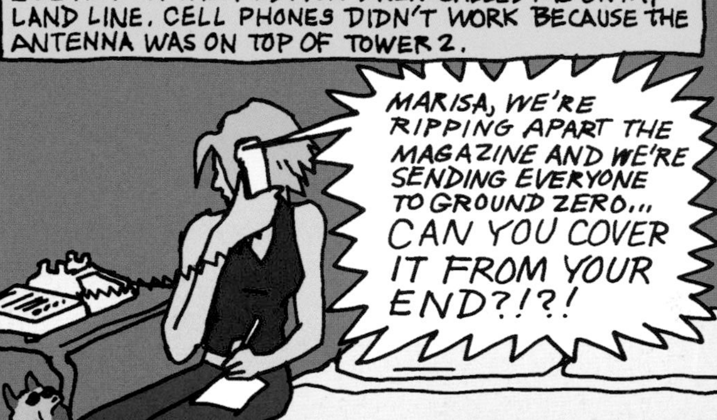

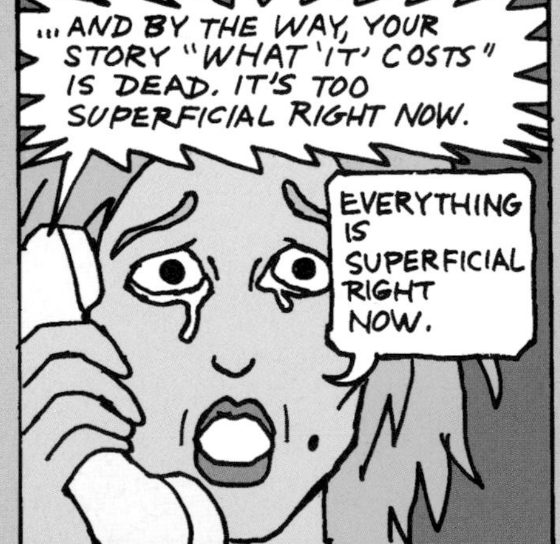

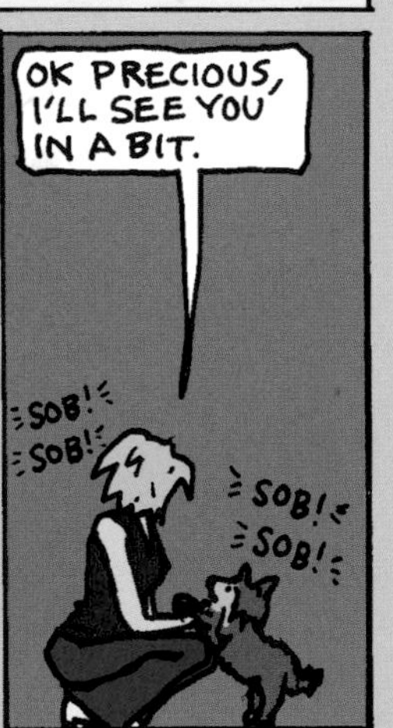

THEN I GRABBED MY TAPE RECORDER, CAMERA, FILM, BLANK TAPES, PENS AND SKETCH PAD AND TREKKED DOWNTOWN TO GROUND ZERO...

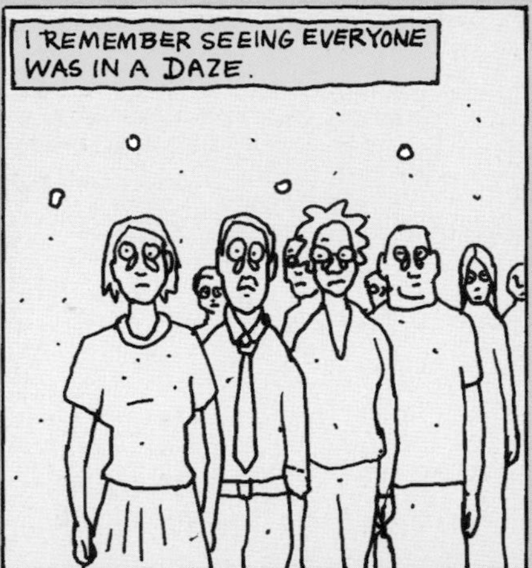
I REMEMBER SEEING EVERYONE WAS IN A DAZE.

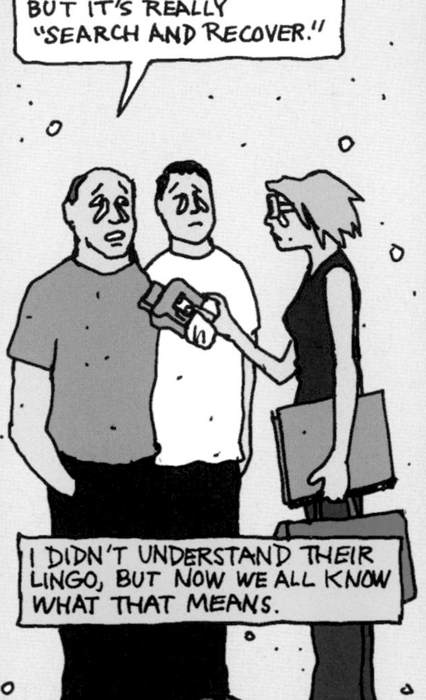
THE NATIONAL GUARD KNEW EARLY ON...
THEY SENT US DOWN TO "SEARCH AND RESCUE," BUT IT'S REALLY "SEARCH AND RECOVER."
I DIDN'T UNDERSTAND THEIR LINGO, BUT NOW WE ALL KNOW WHAT THAT MEANS.

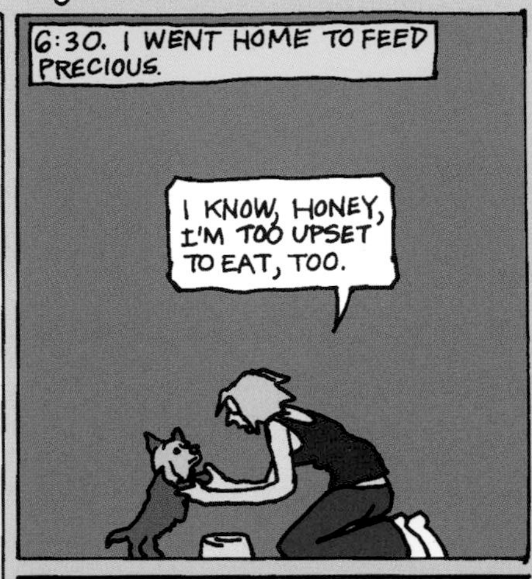
6:30. I WENT HOME TO FEED PRECIOUS.
I KNOW, HONEY, I'M TOO UPSET TO EAT, TOO.

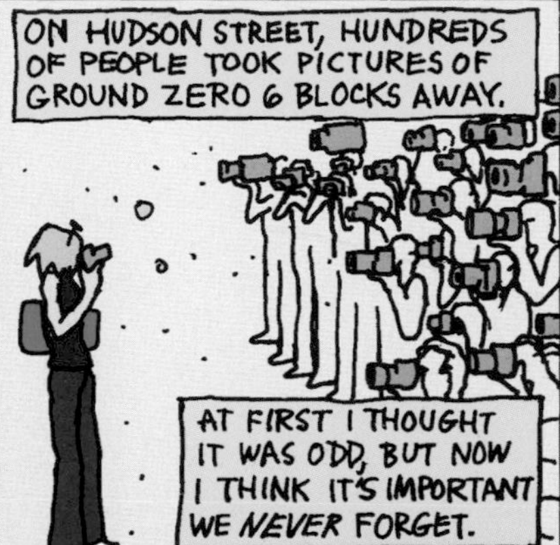
ON HUDSON STREET, HUNDREDS OF PEOPLE TOOK PICTURES OF GROUND ZERO 6 BLOCKS AWAY.
AT FIRST I THOUGHT IT WAS ODD, BUT NOW I THINK IT'S IMPORTANT WE NEVER FORGET.

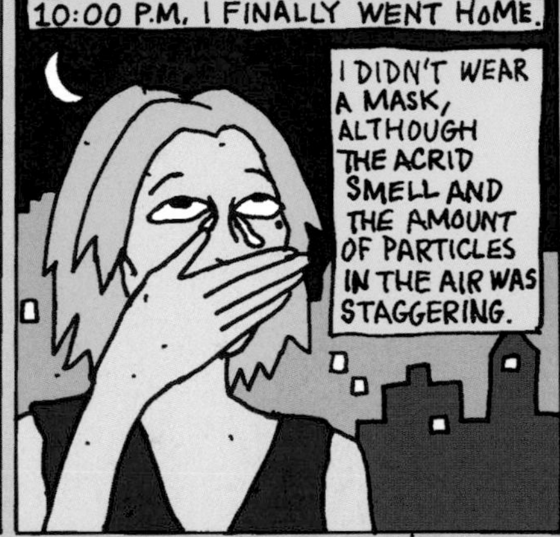
10:00 P.M. I FINALLY WENT HOME.
I DIDN'T WEAR A MASK, ALTHOUGH THE ACRID SMELL AND THE AMOUNT OF PARTICLES IN THE AIR WAS STAGGERING.

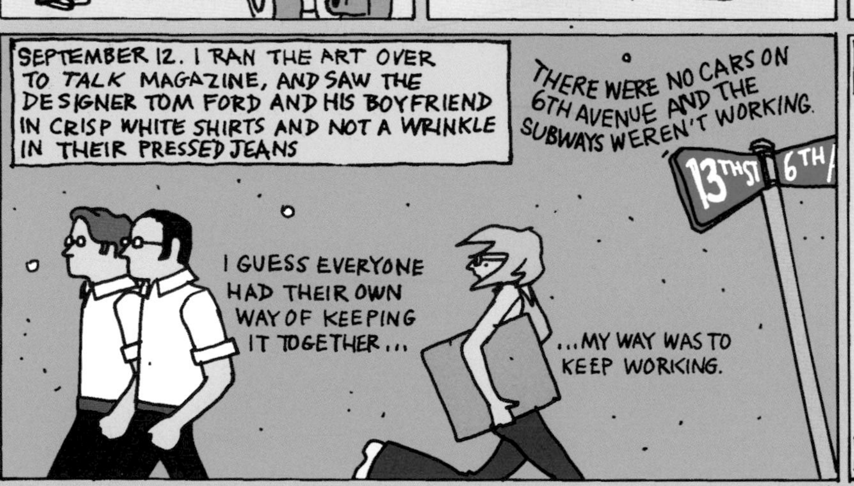
SEPTEMBER 12. I RAN THE ART OVER TO TALK MAGAZINE, AND SAW THE DESIGNER TOM FORD AND HIS BOYFRIEND IN CRISP WHITE SHIRTS AND NOT A WRINKLE IN THEIR PRESSED JEANS
THERE WERE NO CARS ON 6TH AVENUE AND THE SUBWAYS WEREN'T WORKING.
13TH ST
6TH
I GUESS EVERYONE HAD THEIR OWN WAY OF KEEPING IT TOGETHER...
...MY WAY WAS TO KEEP WORKING.

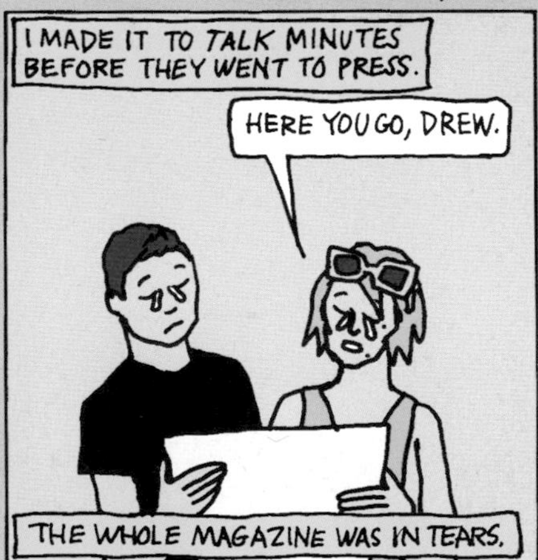
I MADE IT TO TALK MINUTES BEFORE THEY WENT TO PRESS.
HERE YOU GO, DREW.
THE WHOLE MAGAZINE WAS IN TEARS.

HERE'S WHAT RAN IN *TALK* MAGAZINE.
(IT'S STILL ONE OF
THE THINGS I'M MOST PROUD OF.)

TALKING PICTURES
BY MARISA ACOCELLA
9/11/01
ALL DIALOGUE 100% AUTHENTIC
8:48 AM THE FIRST PLANE HITS TOWER 1
9:03 THE SECOND PLANE HITS TOWER 2
9:59 TOWER 2 COLLAPSES
10:28 TOWER 1 COLLAPSES
2:05 ON THAT FATEFUL DAY NO ONE WILL FORGET, I LEAVE MY APARTMENT AND WALK TOWARDS GROUND ZERO. A VISUAL JOURNEY OF LIFE DURING
F-16s FLEW OVERHEAD. PEOPLE DUCKED
SEVENTH AVE SOUTH
ST. VINCENT'S
W 12
W 11
1
I SAW BOTH TOWERS FALL. MY TWO BEST FRIENDS WERE THERE AND I'VE HEARD *NOTHING*.
2:07 DON COPA, MY NEIGHBOR, ON HIS 3rd BEER
2
I WAS IN THE BASEMENT OF TOWER TWO WHEN IT HAPPENED
HE DOESN'T WANT TO TALK ABOUT IT.
2:11 BEDFORD ST.
3
FREE BREAD FROM MURRAY'S
2:20 A GIFT FOUND ON BLEECKER STREET
4
MY BUILDING WAS EVACUATED. I LIVE ON WALL STREET. SO I WALKED TO EMMA KATES AND THE BOMB SQUAD KNOCKED ON *HER* DOOR AND HER BUILDING WAS EVACUATED.
EMMA KATE
2:37 KING STREET. 22 BLOCKS FROM THE TOWERS, 2 BLOCKS FROM ME
6
A FIRE FIGHTER COVERED IN SOOT.
FDNY
5
I JUST WALKED FROM

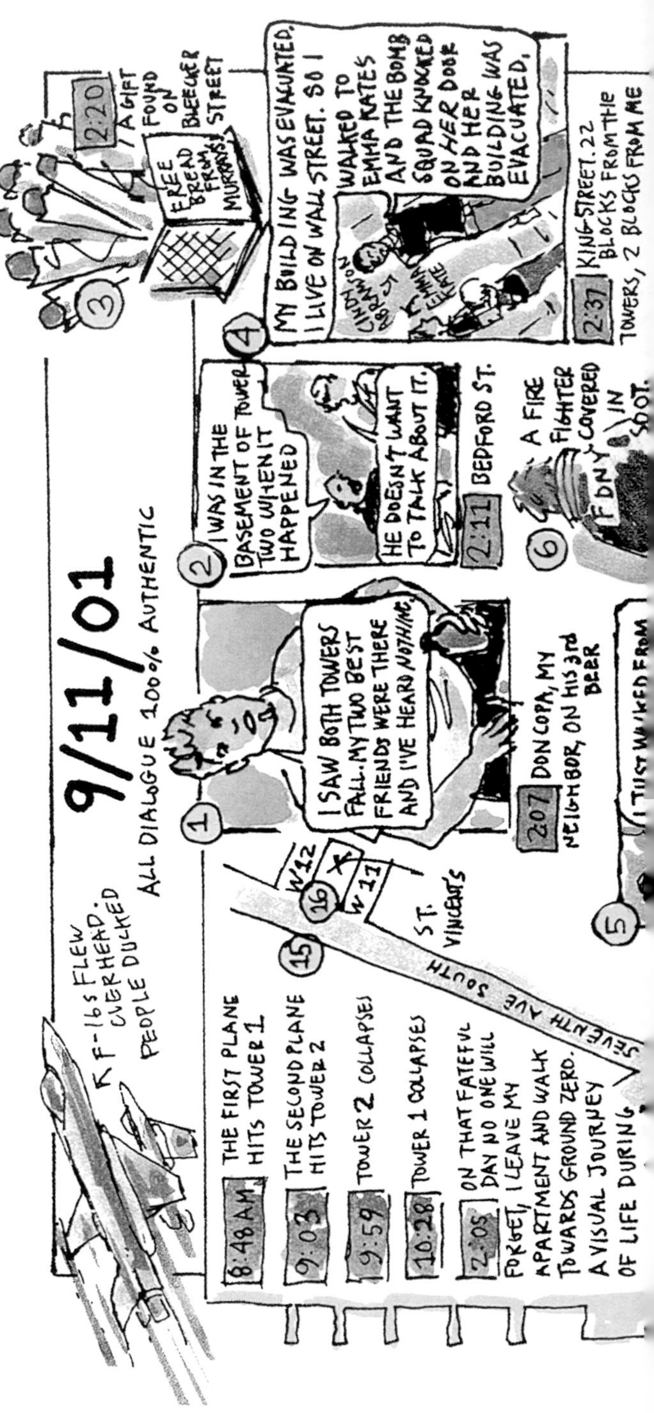

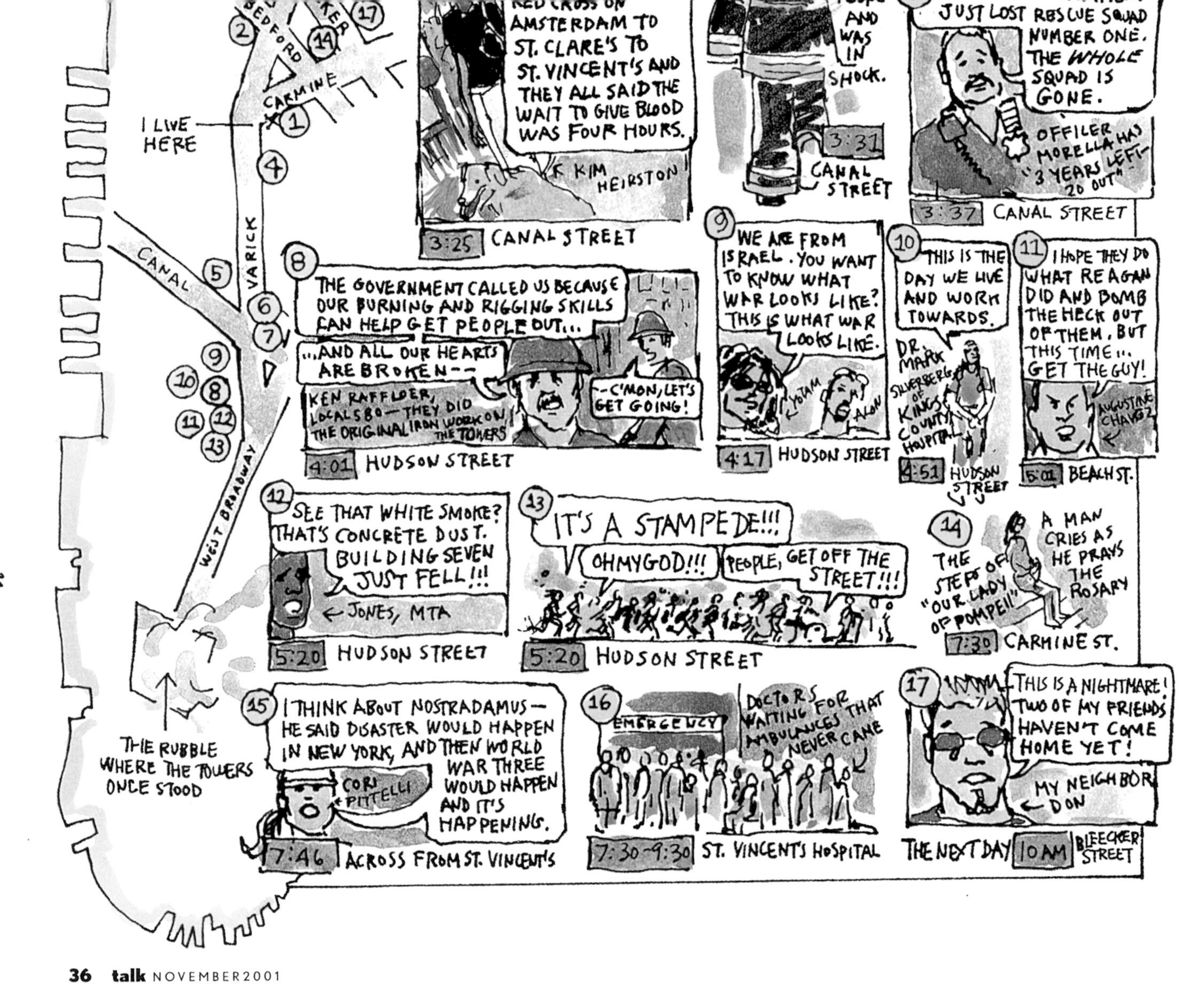

I LIVE HERE
BEDFORD
CARMINE
VARICK
CANAL
WEST BROADWAY
THE RUBBLE WHERE THE TOWERS ONCE STOOD
AMSTERDAM TO ST. CLARE'S TO ST. VINCENT'S AND THEY ALL SAID THE WAIT TO GIVE BLOOD WAS FOUR HOURS.
KIM HEIRSTON
3:25 CANAL STREET
AND WAS IN SHOCK.
3:31 CANAL STREET
JUST LOST RESCUE SQUAD NUMBER ONE. THE WHOLE SQUAD IS GONE.
OFFILER MORELLA HAS "3 YEARS LEFT - 20 OUT"
3:37 CANAL STREET
8
THE GOVERNMENT CALLED US BECAUSE OUR BURNING AND RIGGING SKILLS CAN HELP GET PEOPLE OUT...
...AND ALL OUR HEARTS ARE BROKEN--
--C'MON, LET'S GET GOING!
KEN RAFFLOER, LOCAL 580 — THEY DID THE ORIGINAL IRON WORK ON THE TOWERS
4:01 HUDSON STREET
9
WE ARE FROM ISRAEL. YOU WANT TO KNOW WHAT WAR LOOKS LIKE? THIS IS WHAT WAR LOOKS LIKE.
YOTAM
ALON
4:17 HUDSON STREET
10
THIS IS THE DAY WE LIVE AND WORK TOWARDS.
DR. MARK SILVERBERG OF KINGS COUNTY HOSPITAL
4:51 HUDSON STREET
11
I HOPE THEY DO WHAT REAGAN DID AND BOMB THE HECK OUT OF THEM, BUT THIS TIME... GET THE GUY!
AUGUSTINE CHAVEZ
5:01 BEACH ST.
12
SEE THAT WHITE SMOKE? THAT'S CONCRETE DUST. BUILDING SEVEN JUST FELL!!!
JONES, MTA
5:20 HUDSON STREET
13
IT'S A STAMPEDE!!!
OHMYGOD!!!
PEOPLE, GET OFF THE STREET!!!
5:20 HUDSON STREET
14
THE STEPS OF "OUR LADY OF POMPEII"
A MAN CRIES AS HE PRAYS THE ROSARY
7:30 CARMINE ST.
15
I THINK ABOUT NOSTRADAMUS — HE SAID DISASTER WOULD HAPPEN IN NEW YORK, AND THEN WORLD WAR THREE WOULD HAPPEN AND IT'S HAPPENING.
CORI PITTELLI
7:46 ACROSS FROM ST. VINCENT'S
16
EMERGENCY
DOCTORS WAITING FOR AMBULANCES THAT NEVER CAME
7:30-9:30 ST. VINCENT'S HOSPITAL
17
THIS IS A NIGHTMARE! TWO OF MY FRIENDS HAVEN'T COME HOME YET!
MY NEIGHBOR DON
THE NEXT DAY 10 AM BLEECKER STREET

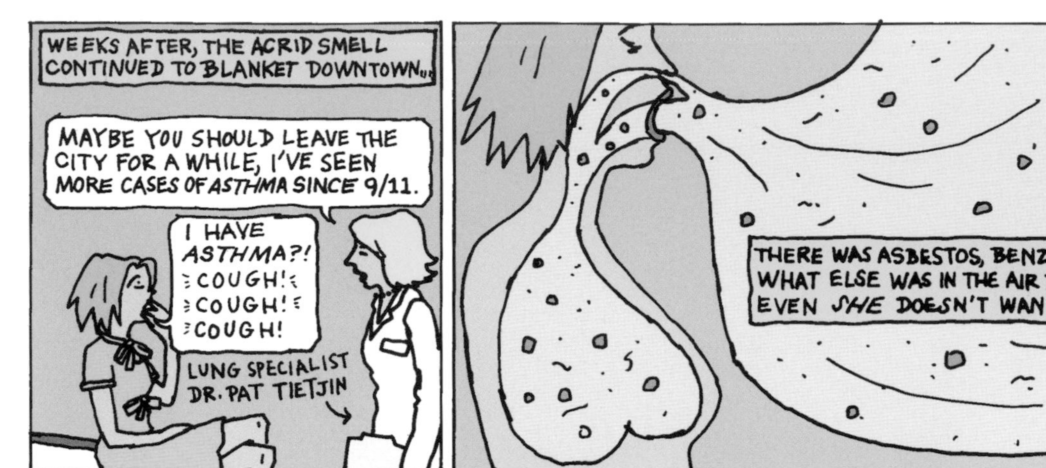

SO WHEN I FIRST GOT THE DIAGNOSIS... FAST FORWARD

FF

WE'RE JUMPING AHEAD TO 2004...

I ASKED THE NUMBER 1 QUESTION:
IS *THAT* WHY I GOT CANCER?!
9/11 COULD BE A FACTOR, BUT MARISA...

...DO YOU REALLY WANT TO DRIVE YOURSELF CRAZY PLAYING *THAT* GAME?!

YOU THINK THIS IS A *GAME*?!

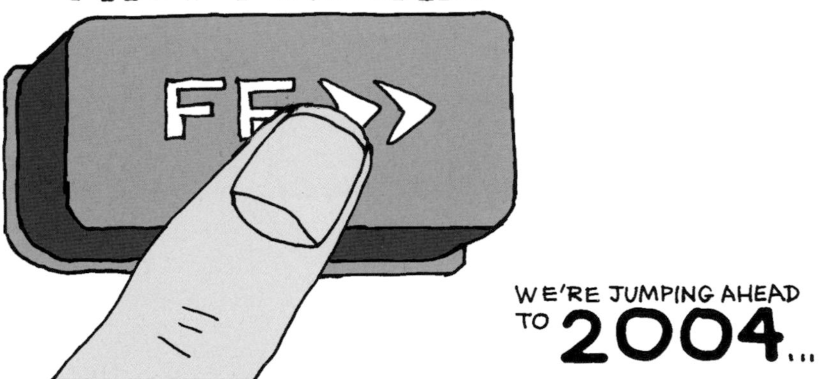

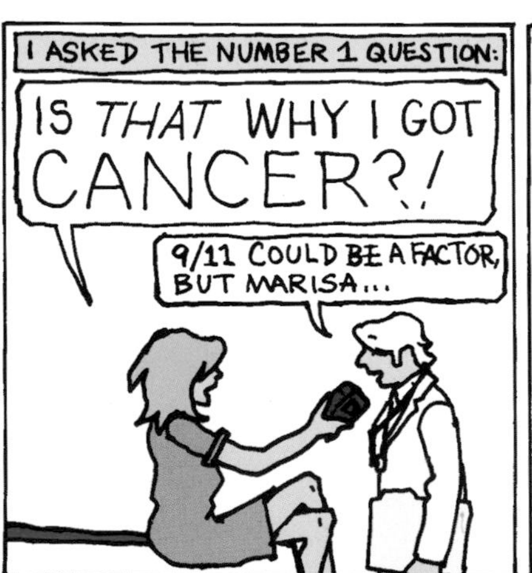

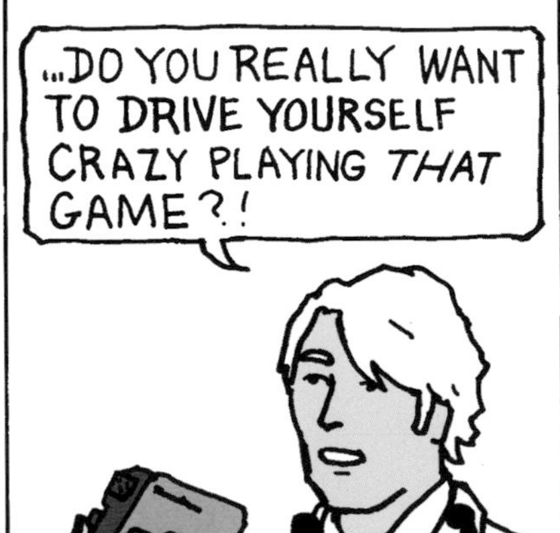

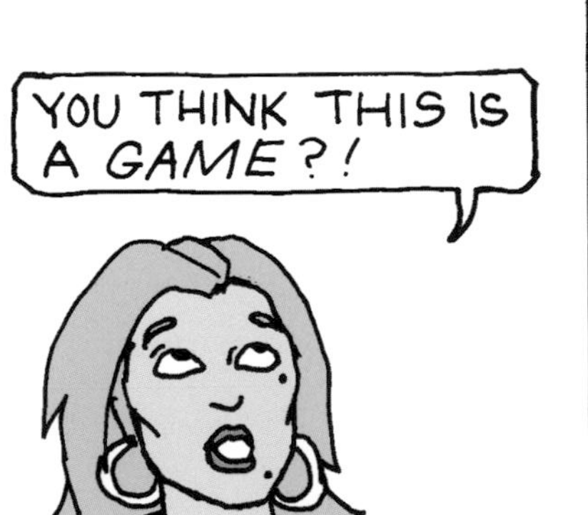

LATER:

Google

Web Images Groups News Froogle Local more»

breast cancer - causes

Google Search I'm Feeling Lucky

Advanced Search
Preferences
Language Tools

CLICK!

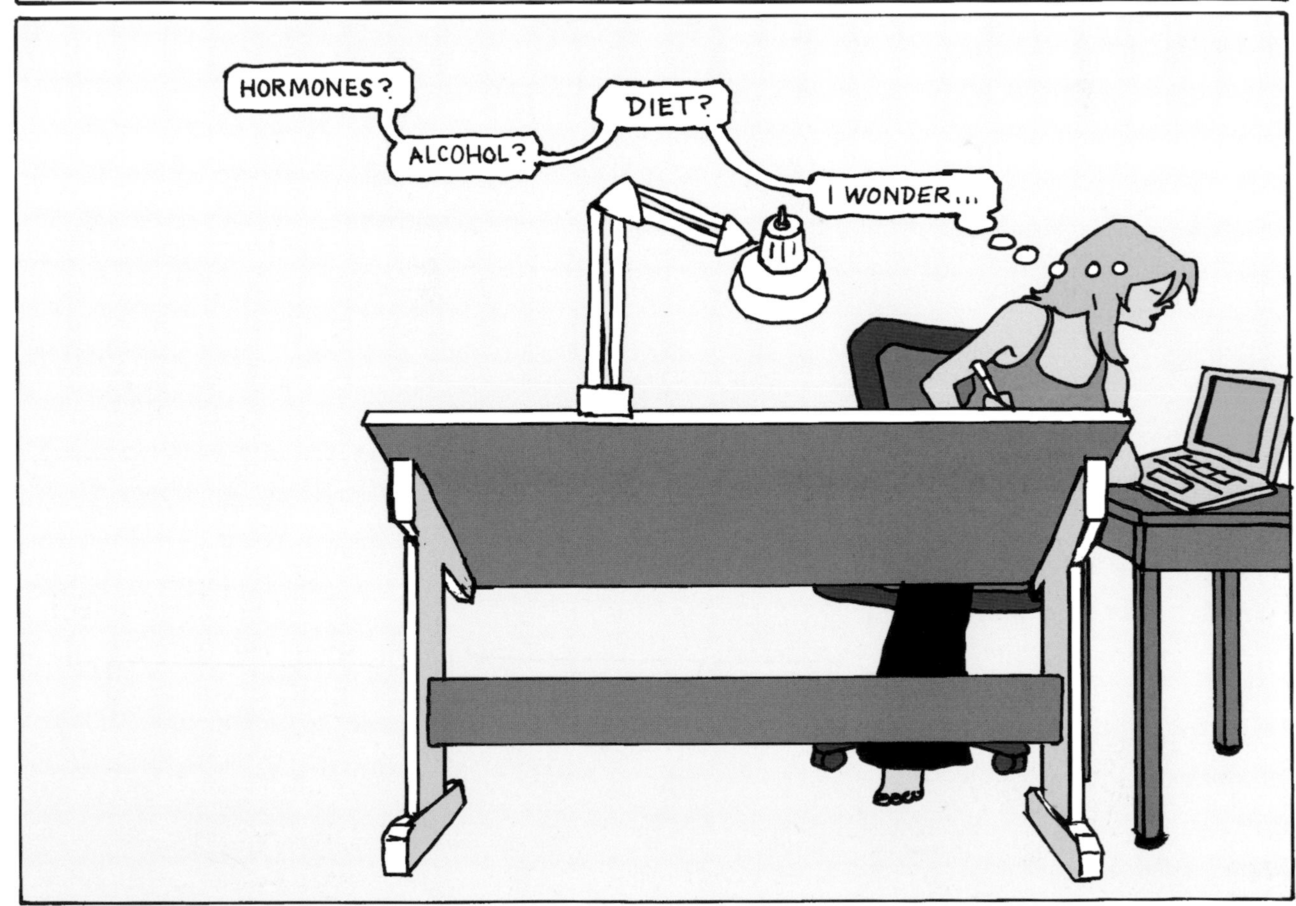

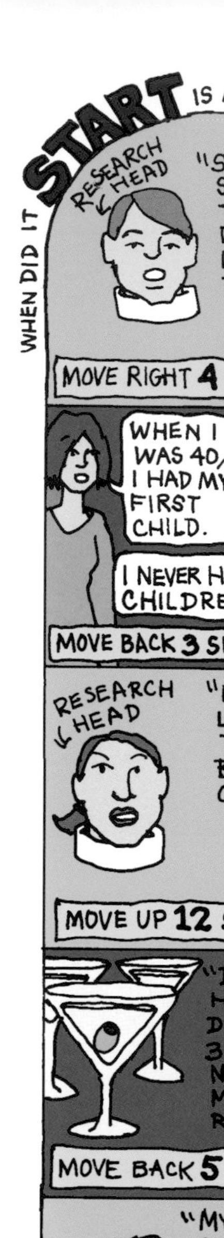
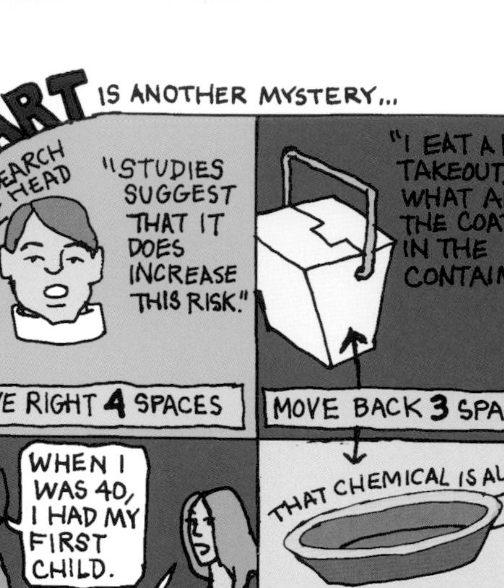
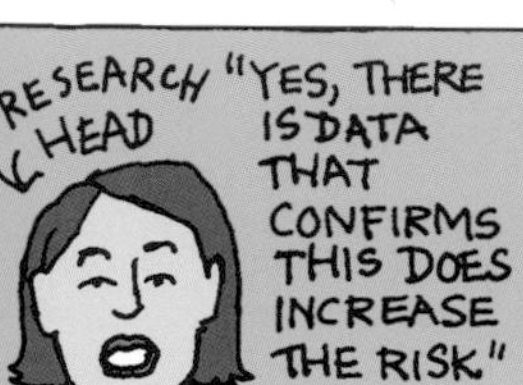
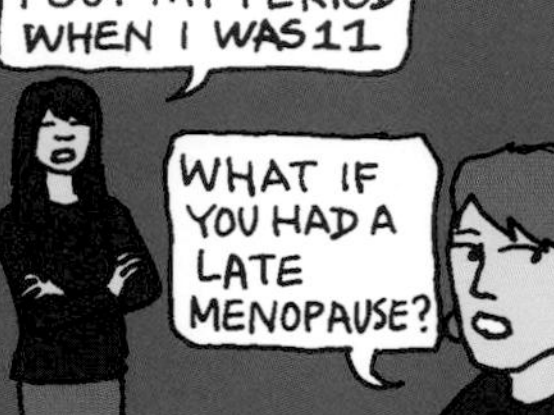
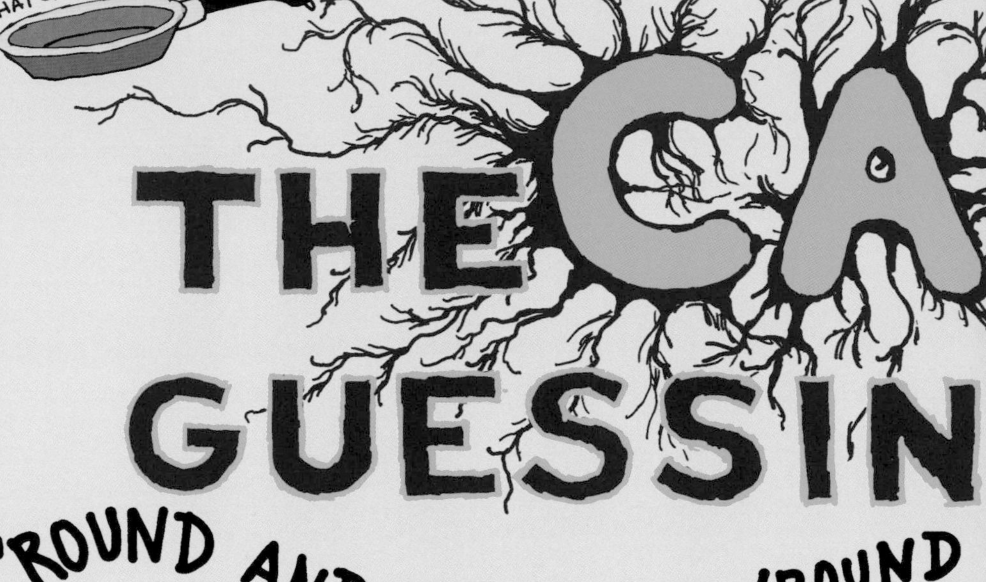
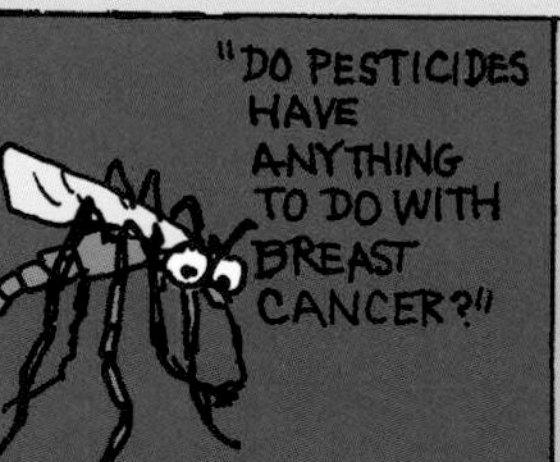
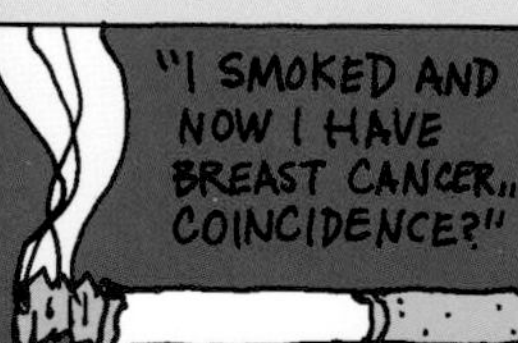
WHEN DID IT START IS ANOTHER MYSTERY...
RESEARCH HEAD
"STUDIES SUGGEST THAT IT DOES INCREASE THIS RISK."
MOVE RIGHT 4 SPACES
"I EAT A LOT OF TAKEOUT, WHAT ABOUT THE COATING IN THE CONTAINERS?"
MOVE BACK 3 SPACES
RESEARCH HEAD
"YES, THERE IS DATA THAT CONFIRMS THIS DOES INCREASE THE RISK."
MOVE UP 4 SPACES
I GOT MY PERIOD WHEN I WAS 11
WHAT IF YOU HAD A LATE MENOPAUSE?
MOVE BACK 1 SPACE
RESEARCH HEAD
MOVE BACK
WHEN I WAS 40, I HAD MY FIRST CHILD.
I NEVER HAD CHILDREN.
MOVE BACK 3 SPACES
THAT CHEMICAL IS ALSO ON TEFLON PANS
THE CA
GUESSIN
'ROUND AND 'ROUND AND 'ROUND
RESEARCH HEAD
"IT IS LIKELY TO CAUSE BREAST CANCER."
MOVE UP 12 SPACES
"DOES HAVING A DRINK OR 3 EVERY NIGHT PUT ME AT RISK?"
MOVE BACK 5 SPACES
"MY MOTHER HAD BREAST CANCER, DO I HAVE THE GENE?"
MOVE BACK 6 SPACES
"DO PESTICIDES HAVE ANYTHING TO DO WITH BREAST CANCER?"
MOVE BACK 5 SPACES
"WOMEN WHO STOPPED USING THE PILL MORE THAN 10 YEARS AGO DO NOT SEEM TO HAVE AN INCREASED RISK, BUT IF YOU TOOK THE HIGHER DOSES IN THE LATE 70s, YOU COULD STILL BE AT RISK."
RESEARCH HEAD
MOVE UP 9 SPACES
"I SMOKED AND NOW I HAVE BREAST CANCER... COINCIDENCE?"
MOVE BACK 7 SPACES
CORPORATE HEAD
MOVE UP

"THERE IS NO CLEAR LINK FOUND."
4 SPACES

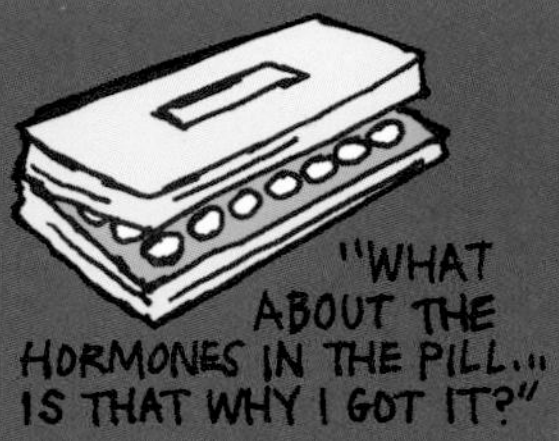
"WHAT ABOUT THE HORMONES IN THE PILL... IS THAT WHY I GOT IT?"
MOVE BACK 11 SPACES

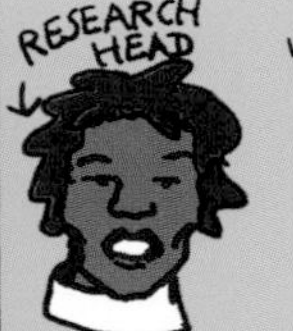
RESEARCH HEAD
"SOME WOMEN WHO HAVE RISK FACTORS NEVET GET BREAST CANCER."
MOVE BACK 4 SPACES

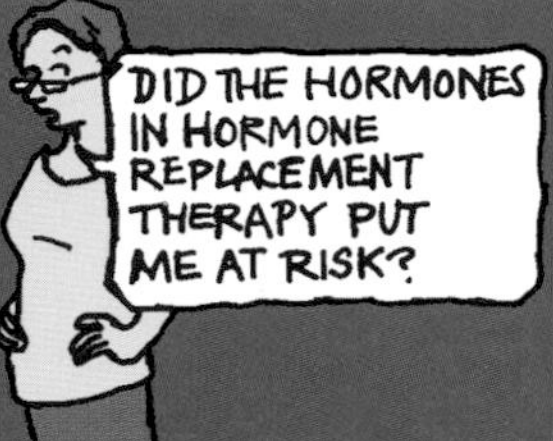
DID THE HORMONES IN HORMONE REPLACEMENT THERAPY PUT ME AT RISK?
MOVE BACK 7 SPACES

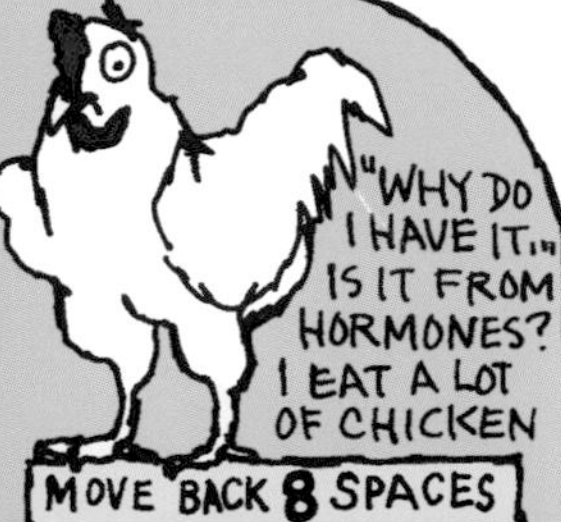
"WHY DO I HAVE IT... IS IT FROM HORMONES? I EAT A LOT OF CHICKEN
MOVE BACK 8 SPACES

RESEARCH HEAD
"OUR RESULTS FOUND THAT ORAL CONTRACEPTIVES DID NOT SIGNIFICANTLY INCREASE THE RISK OF BREAST CANCER."
MOVE DOWN 9 SPACES
NCER
G GAME
WHAT ABOUT THE UNDERWIRE IN UNDERWIRE BRAS?
YOU GO...HOW YOU GET IT NOBODY KNOWS!
"THE EVIDENCE SUGGESTS IT DOES NOT CAUSE CANCER."
CORPORATE HEAD
MOVE BACK 12 SPACES

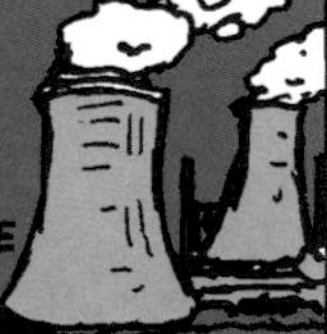
"WE LIVE NEAR A NUCLEAR REACTOR, IS THAT THE REASON?"
MOVE UP 1 SPACE

"PARABENS HAVE A VERY, VERY GOOD SAFETY PROFILE."
4 SPACES
"DO ANTIBIOTICS HAVE ANYTHING TO DO WITH BREAST CANCER? I WAS ALWAYS ON THEM AS A KID."
MOVE BACK 11 SPACES
"WHAT'S THE STORY ON ANTIPERSPIRANTS? THE PARABENS IN IT MIMIC ESTROGEN, AND ESTROGEN PROMOTES BREAST CANCER CELLS."
MOVE BACK 2 SPACES
"IS BEING OVERWEIGHT, ESPECIALLY IF THE WEIGHT IS IN YOUR STOMACH, A BREAST CANCER FACTOR?"
MOVE BACK 13 SPACES

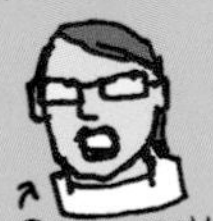
"OUR STUDY INDICATES MORE RESEARCH IS NEEDED... TRACES OF PARABENS HAVE BEEN FOUND IN TUMOR SAMPLES."
RESEARCH HEAD
MOVE BACK 4 SPACES

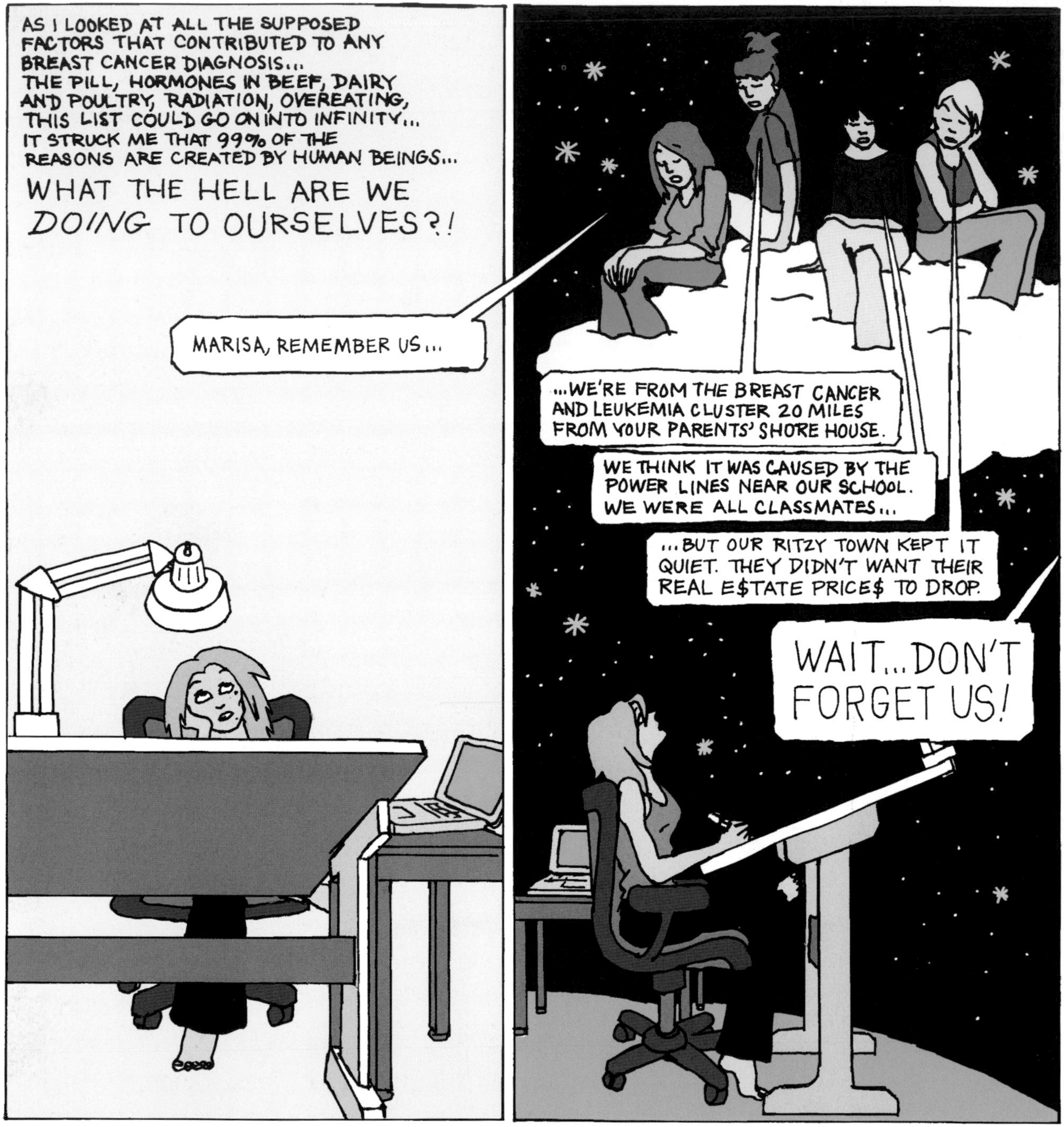

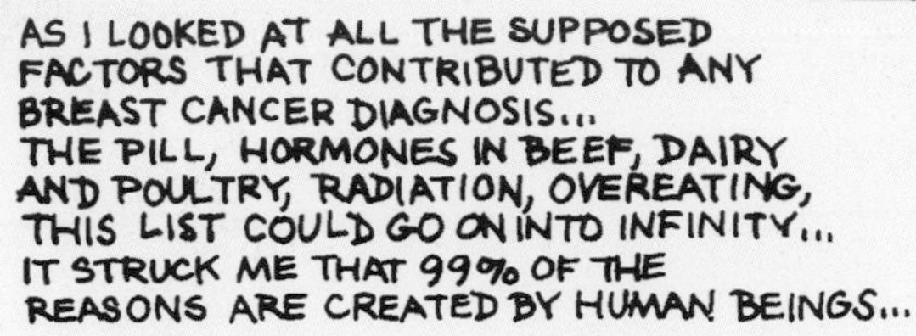

MARISA, REMEMBER US...

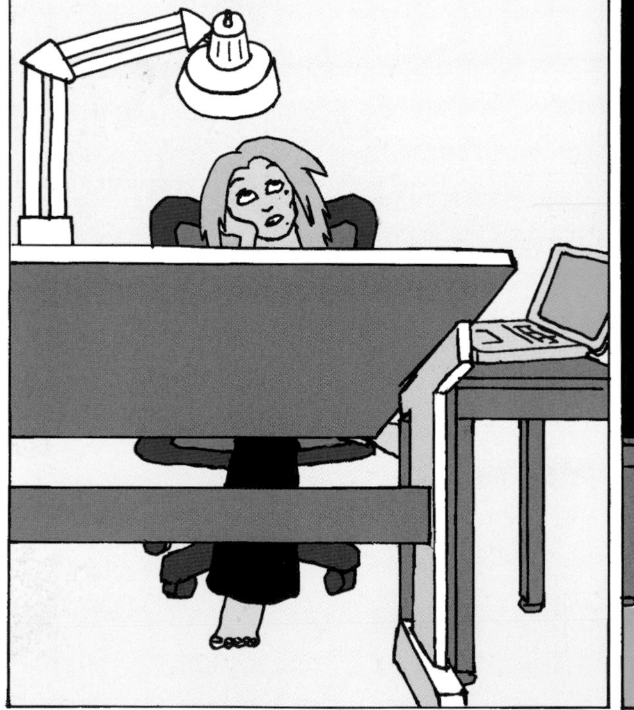

...WE'RE FROM THE BREAST CANCER AND LEUKEMIA CLUSTER 20 MILES FROM YOUR PARENTS' SHORE HOUSE.

WE THINK IT WAS CAUSED BY THE POWER LINES NEAR OUR SCHOOL. WE WERE ALL CLASSMATES...

...BUT OUR RITZY TOWN KEPT IT QUIET. THEY DIDN'T WANT THEIR REAL E$TATE PRICE$ TO DROP.

WAIT...DON'T FORGET US!

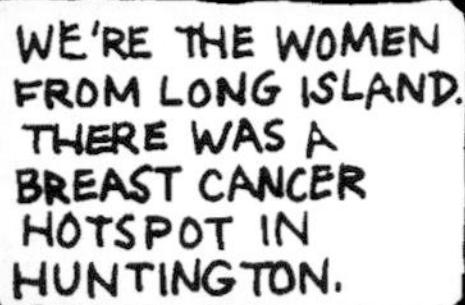
WE'RE THE WOMEN FROM LONG ISLAND. THERE WAS A BREAST CANCER HOTSPOT IN HUNTINGTON.
WE'RE FROM BOSTON. THERE'S A BREAST CANCER CLUSTER THERE, TOO.
I CAME FROM A CLUSTER CALLED "THE LOVE CANAL."
A MOUNTAIN OF TOXIC GARBAGE STUNK UP OUR AIR AND POLLUTED OUR WATER. WHEN I DIED OF LEUKEMIA, I WAS ALMOST 10 YEARS OLD.
THEY SAY IT WAS A COINCIDENCE, I SAY IT WAS A CANCER CLUSTER.
I WAS 10.
I WAS 15.
THERE WAS A LEUKEMIA CLUSTER IN NEVADA WHERE I LIVED, TOO. JET FUEL WAS DUMPED INTO OUR DRINKING WATER FROM THE NEARBY NAVAL BASE...
THAT CHEMICAL WAS BENZENE, AND IT'S SMELLING UP THE AIR.
NOW I WONDER ABOUT GROUND ZERO...
I LIVED NEAR A MILITARY BASE IN ARIZONA. A LEUKEMIA CLUSTER WAS FOUND THERE AS WELL.
11
IN CALIFORNIA, WHERE I COME FROM, THEY FOUND BRAIN CANCER CLUSTERS.
THEY SAY IT WAS CAUSED BY *PESTICIDES*.
RADIOACTIVE DUST STRAYED FROM A NEARBY NUCLEAR PLANT WHERE I LIVED IN PENNSYLVANIA. THAT CAUSED A CANCER CLUSTER.
15 OF US COME FROM SOUTH JERSEY. THEY FOUND WASTE PRODUCTS IN OUR WATER. THERE WAS A SETTLEMENT WITH THE CHEMICAL COMPANY...
...BUT OUR FAMILIES DECLINED IT, AND NOW THERE'S A CLASS ACTION SUIT.
THERE WAS A CANCER CLUSTER IN MY NEIGHBORHOOD IN NEW JERSEY TOO... BUT IT WAS *NEVER* PROVEN...
...AREN'T WE *ENOUGH* EVIDENCE???

A MOMENT OF SILENCE.

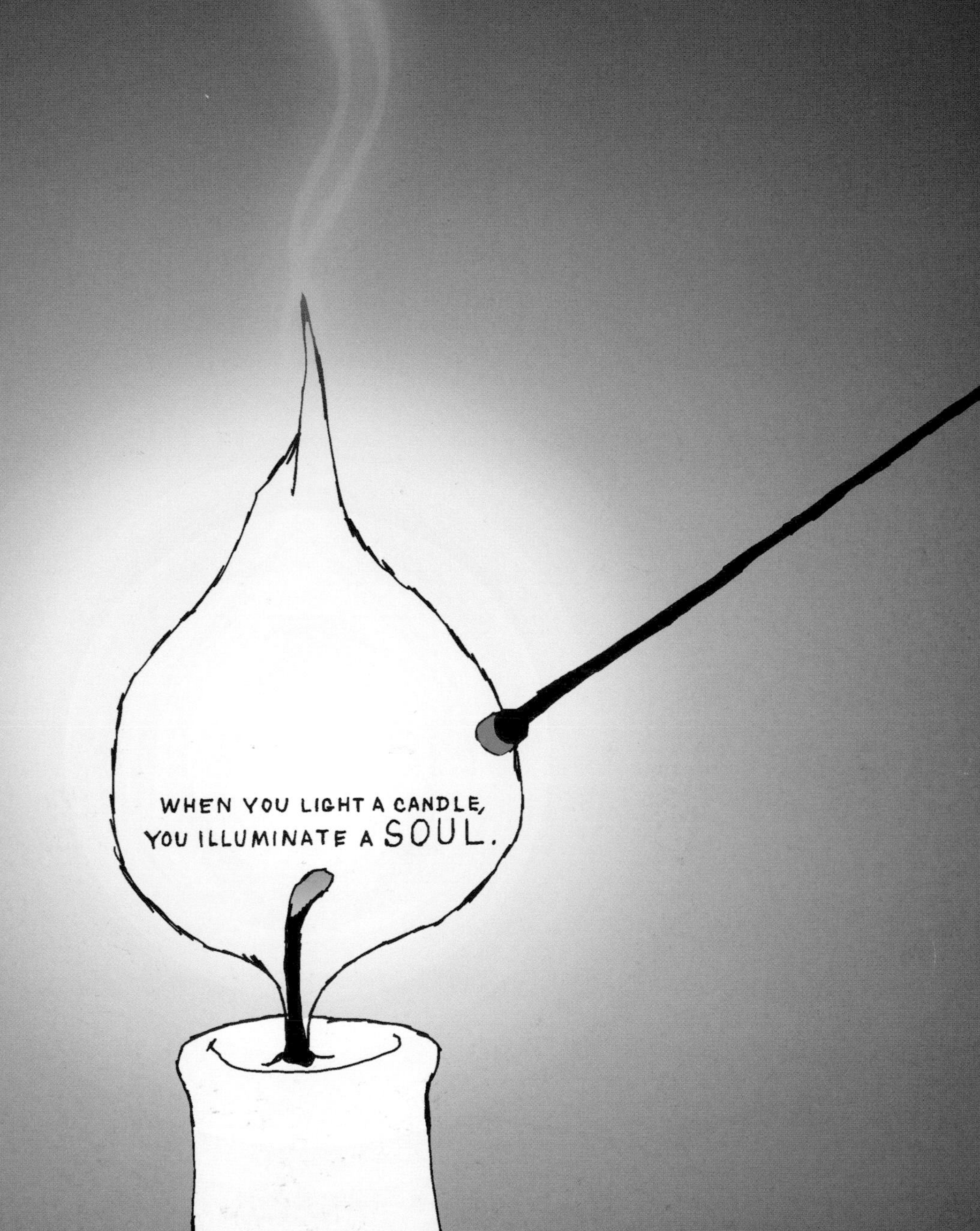
WHEN YOU LIGHT A CANDLE,
YOU ILLUMINATE A SOUL.

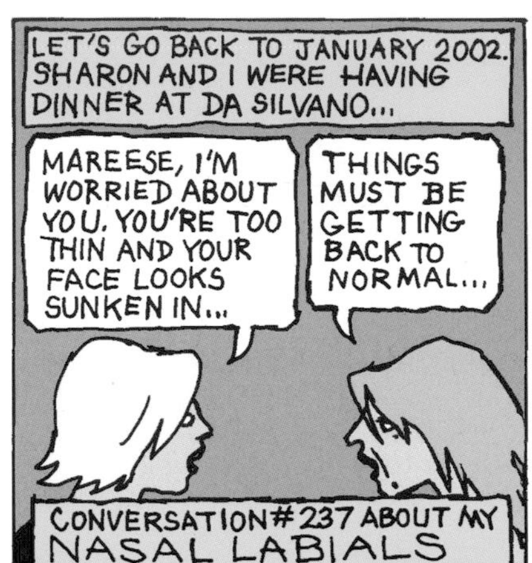
LET'S GO BACK TO JANUARY 2002. SHARON AND I WERE HAVING DINNER AT DA SILVANO...
MAREESE, I'M WORRIED ABOUT YOU. YOU'RE TOO THIN AND YOUR FACE LOOKS SUNKEN IN...
THINGS MUST BE GETTING BACK TO NORMAL...
CONVERSATION #237 ABOUT MY NASAL LABIALS

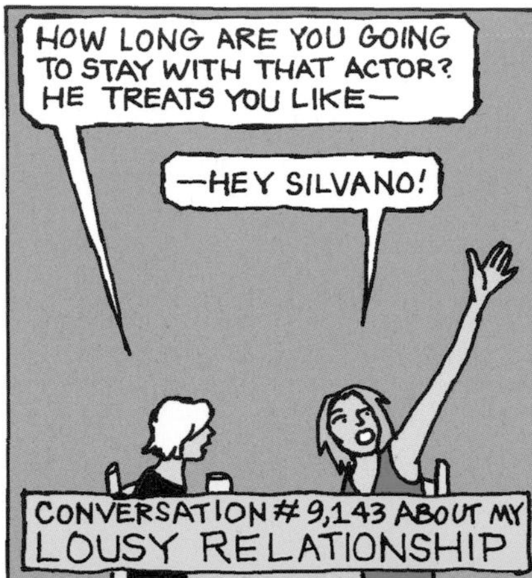
HOW LONG ARE YOU GOING TO STAY WITH THAT ACTOR? HE TREATS YOU LIKE—
—HEY SILVANO!
CONVERSATION #9,143 ABOUT MY LOUSY RELATIONSHIP

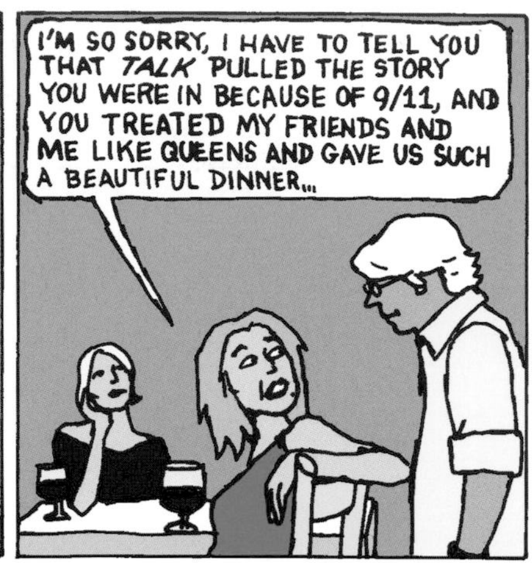
I'M SO SORRY, I HAVE TO TELL YOU THAT TALK PULLED THE STORY YOU WERE IN BECAUSE OF 9/11, AND YOU TREATED MY FRIENDS AND ME LIKE QUEENS AND GAVE US SUCH A BEAUTIFUL DINNER...

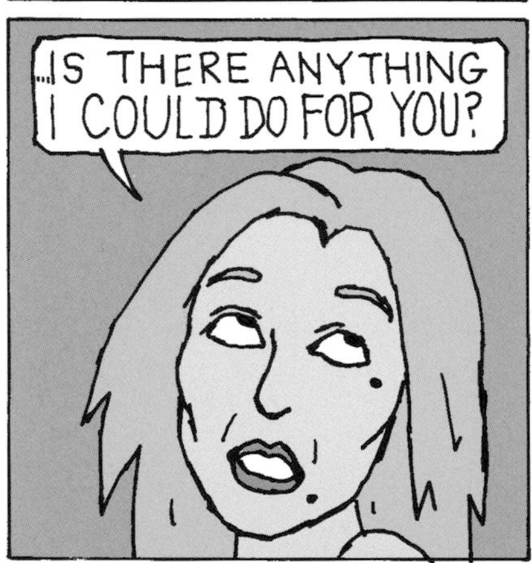
...IS THERE ANYTHING I COULD DO FOR YOU?

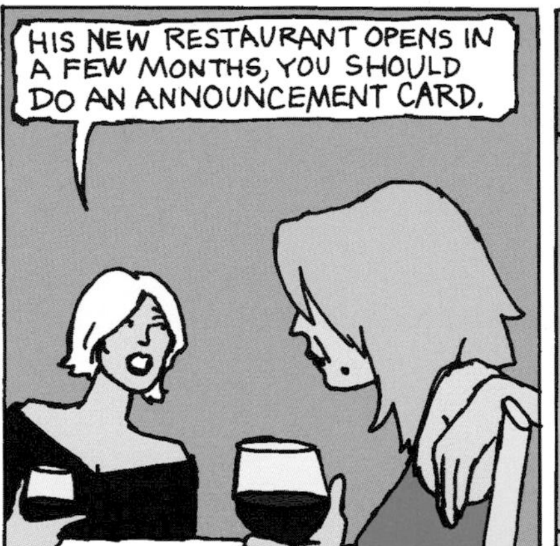
HIS NEW RESTAURANT OPENS IN A FEW MONTHS, YOU SHOULD DO AN ANNOUNCEMENT CARD.

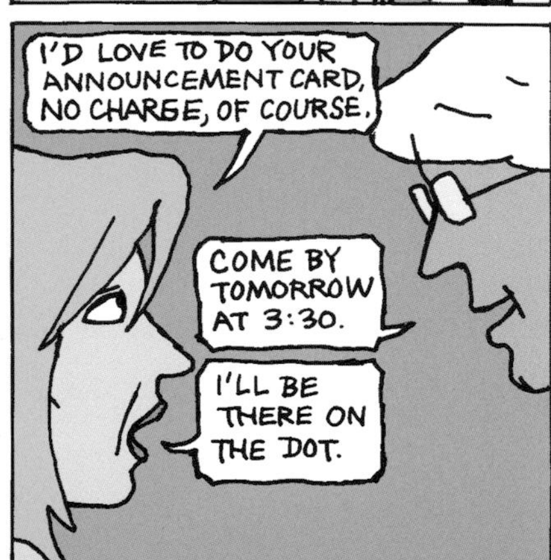
I'D LOVE TO DO YOUR ANNOUNCEMENT CARD, NO CHARGE, OF COURSE.
COME BY TOMORROW AT 3:30.
I'LL BE THERE ON THE DOT.

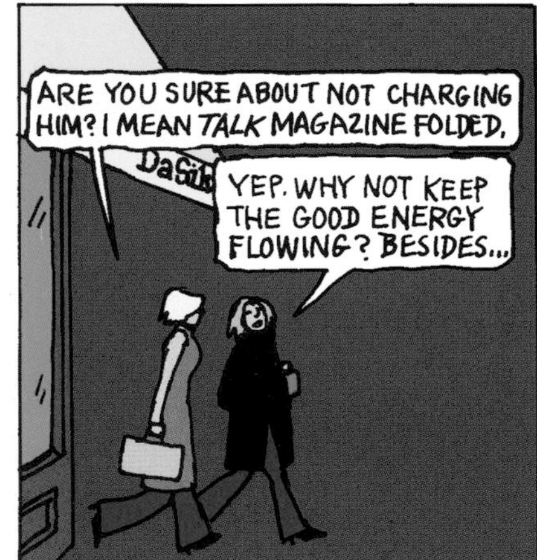
ARE YOU SURE ABOUT NOT CHARGING HIM? I MEAN TALK MAGAZINE FOLDED.
YEP. WHY NOT KEEP THE GOOD ENERGY FLOWING? BESIDES...

YOU PUT GOOD THINGS OUT THERE...
YOU'LL GET IT BACK SOMEDAY...
THIS UNIVERSAL LAW ALSO WORKS CONVERSELY...

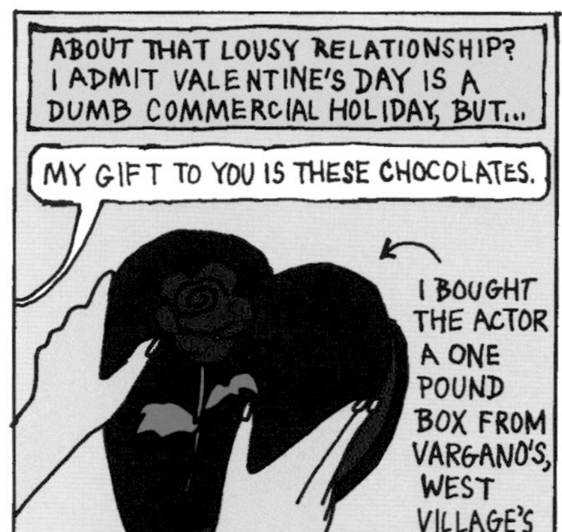
ABOUT THAT LOUSY RELATIONSHIP? I ADMIT VALENTINE'S DAY IS A DUMB COMMERCIAL HOLIDAY, BUT...
MY GIFT TO YOU IS THESE CHOCOLATES.
I BOUGHT THE ACTOR A ONE POUND BOX FROM VARGANO'S, WEST VILLAGE'S FINEST

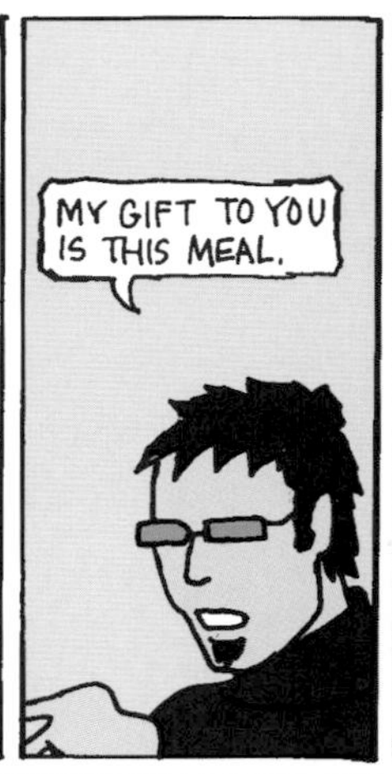
MY GIFT TO YOU IS THIS MEAL.

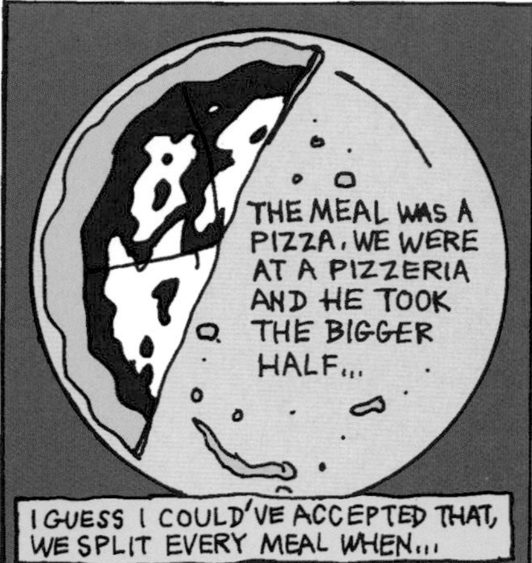
THE MEAL WAS A PIZZA. WE WERE AT A PIZZERIA AND HE TOOK THE BIGGER HALF...
I GUESS I COULD'VE ACCEPTED THAT, WE SPLIT EVERY MEAL WHEN...

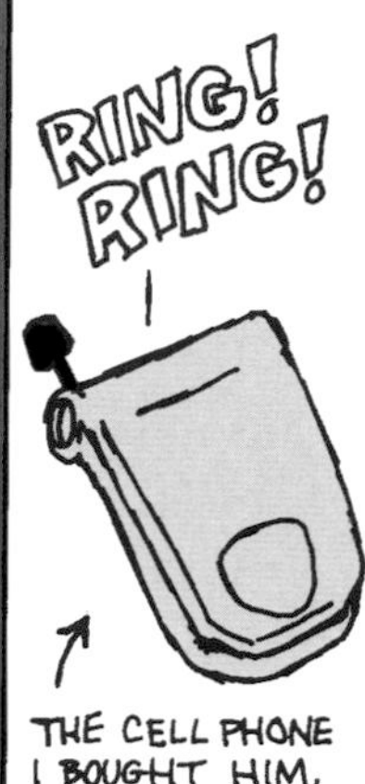
RING! RING!
THE CELL PHONE I BOUGHT HIM.

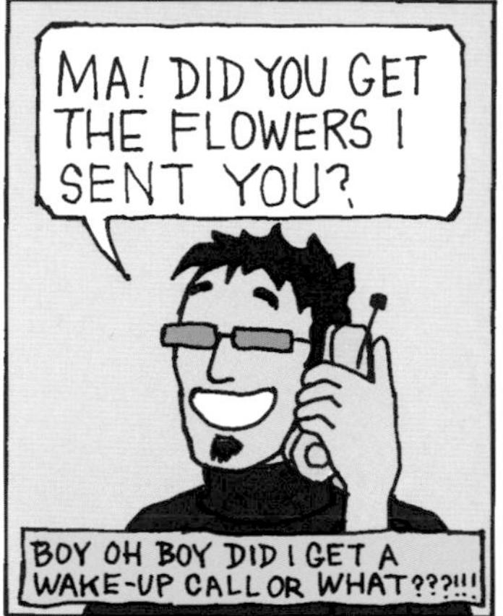
MA! DID YOU GET THE FLOWERS I SENT YOU?
BOY OH BOY DID I GET A WAKE-UP CALL OR WHAT???!!!

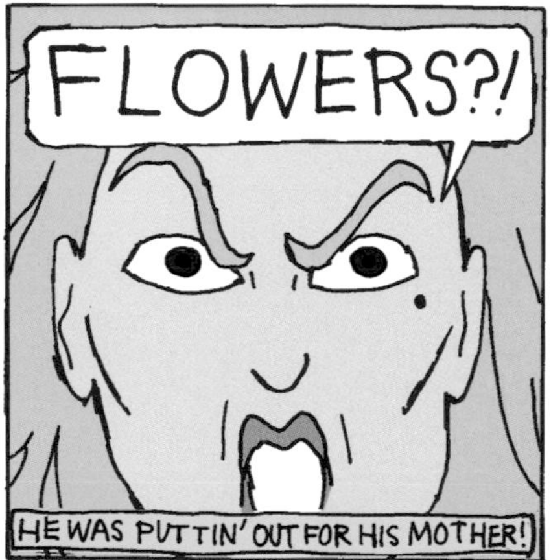
FLOWERS?!
HE WAS PUTTIN' OUT FOR HIS MOTHER!

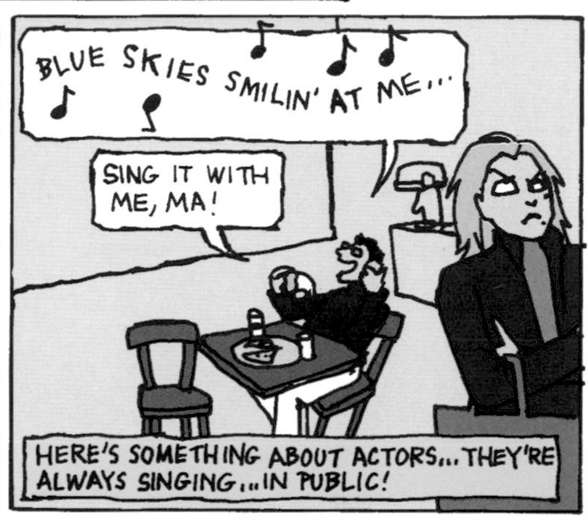
BLUE SKIES SMILIN' AT ME...
SING IT WITH ME, MA!
HERE'S SOMETHING ABOUT ACTORS... THEY'RE ALWAYS SINGING... IN PUBLIC!

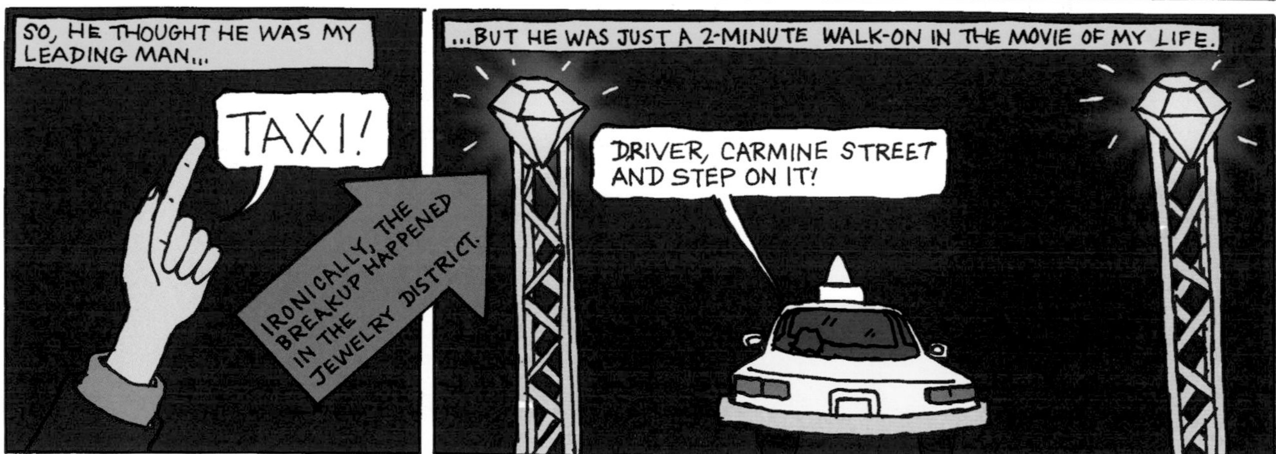
SO, HE THOUGHT HE WAS MY LEADING MAN...
TAXI!
IRONICALLY, THE BREAKUP HAPPENED IN THE JEWELRY DISTRICT.
...BUT HE WAS JUST A 2-MINUTE WALK-ON IN THE MOVIE OF MY LIFE.
DRIVER, CARMINE STREET AND STEP ON IT!

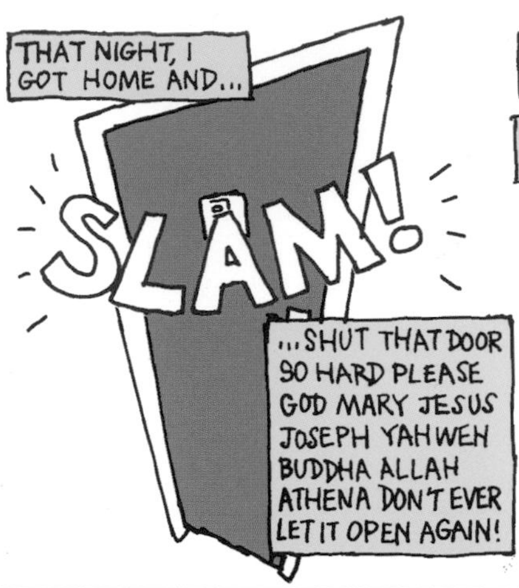
THAT NIGHT, I GOT HOME AND...
SLAM!
...SHUT THAT DOOR SO HARD PLEASE GOD MARY JESUS JOSEPH YAHWEH BUDDHA ALLAH ATHENA DON'T EVER LET IT OPEN AGAIN!

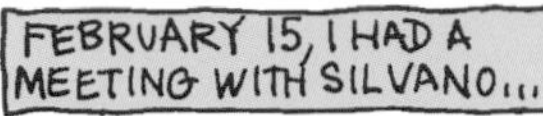
FEBRUARY 15, I HAD A MEETING WITH SILVANO...
I'D DRAWN UP 4 IDEAS, HOPEFULLY HE'D LIKE 1...

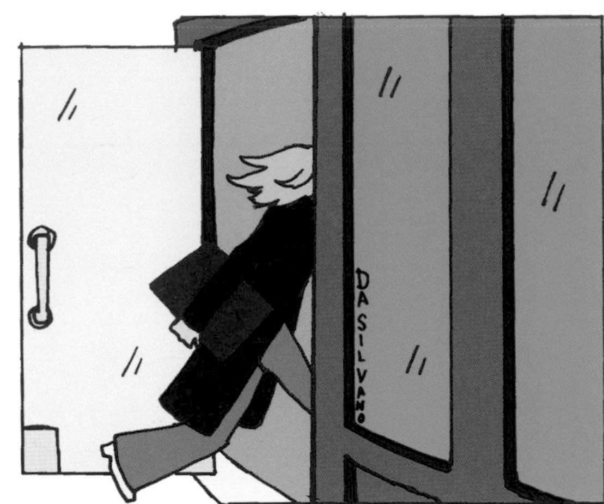
DA SILVANO

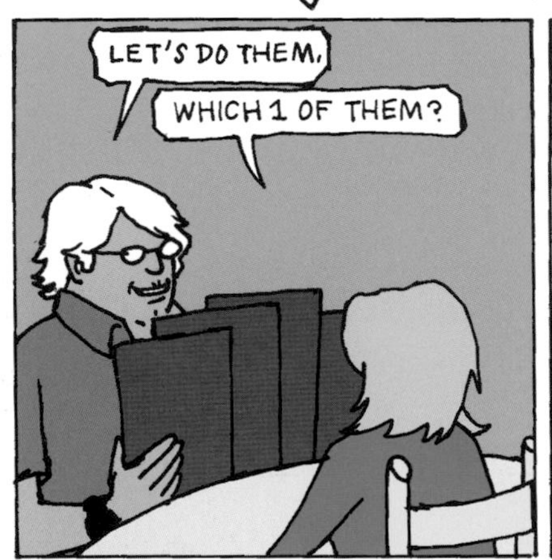
LET'S DO THEM.
WHICH 1 OF THEM?

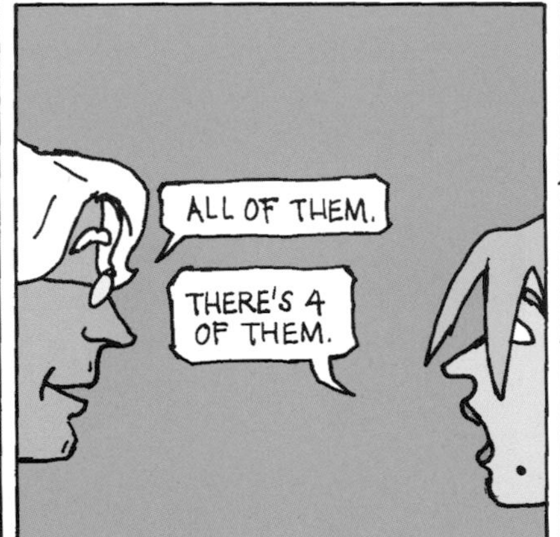
ALL OF THEM.
THERE'S 4 OF THEM.

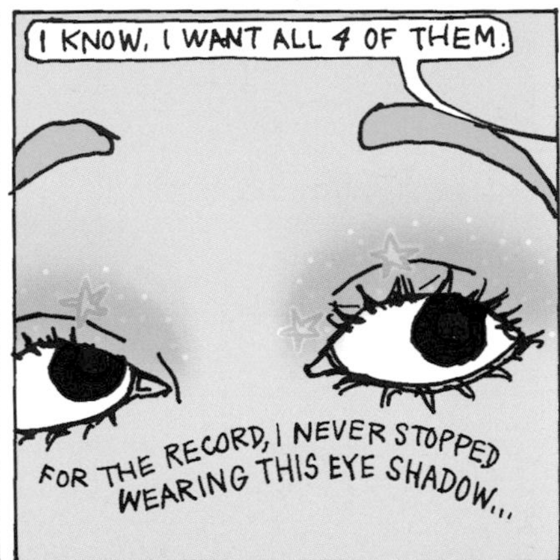
I KNOW. I WANT ALL 4 OF THEM.
FOR THE RECORD, I NEVER STOPPED WEARING THIS EYE SHADOW...

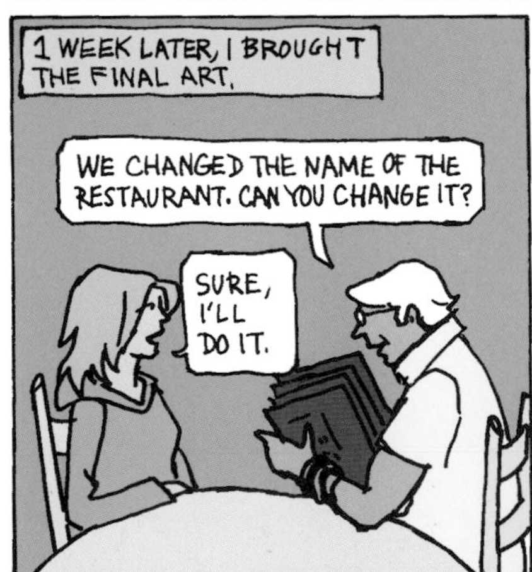
1 WEEK LATER, I BROUGHT THE FINAL ART.
WE CHANGED THE NAME OF THE RESTAURANT. CAN YOU CHANGE IT?
SURE, I'LL DO IT.

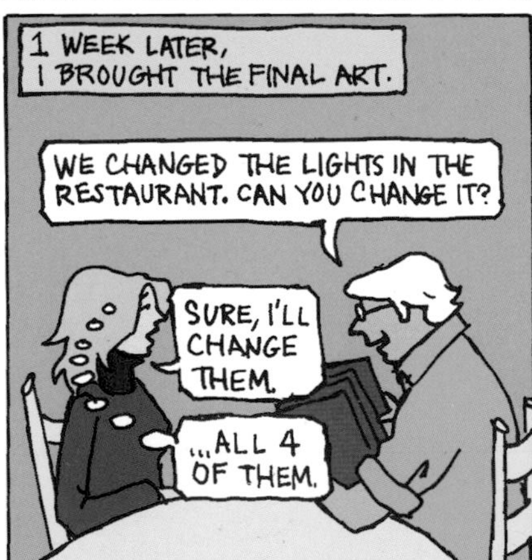
1 WEEK LATER, I BROUGHT THE FINAL ART.
WE CHANGED THE LIGHTS IN THE RESTAURANT. CAN YOU CHANGE IT?
SURE, I'LL CHANGE THEM.
...ALL 4 OF THEM.

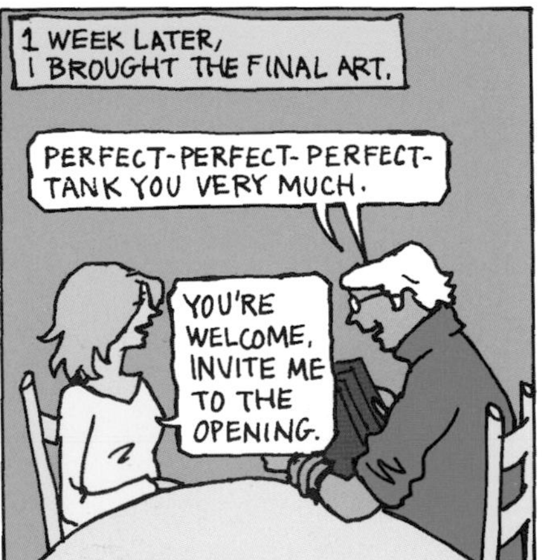
1 WEEK LATER, I BROUGHT THE FINAL ART.
PERFECT-PERFECT-PERFECT-TANK YOU VERY MUCH.
YOU'RE WELCOME. INVITE ME TO THE OPENING.

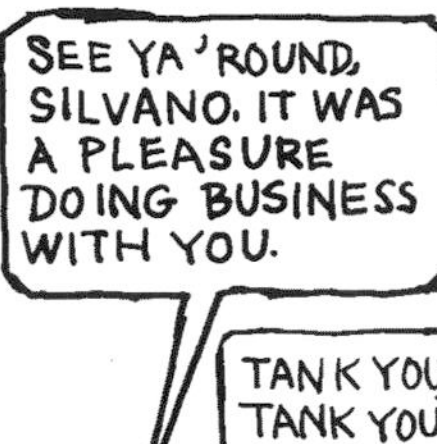
SEE YA 'ROUND, SILVANO. IT WAS A PLEASURE DOING BUSINESS WITH YOU.
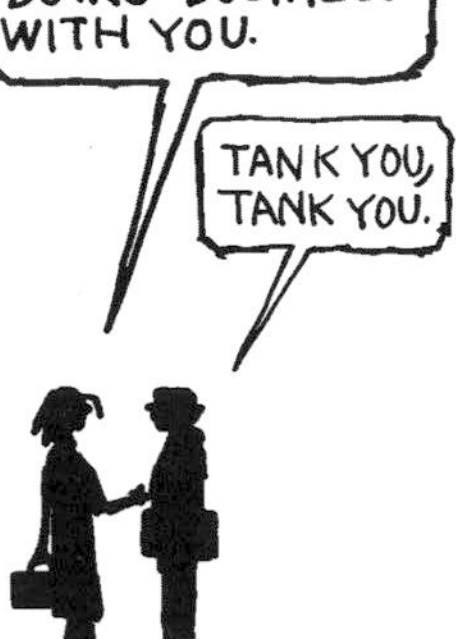
TANK YOU, TANK YOU.
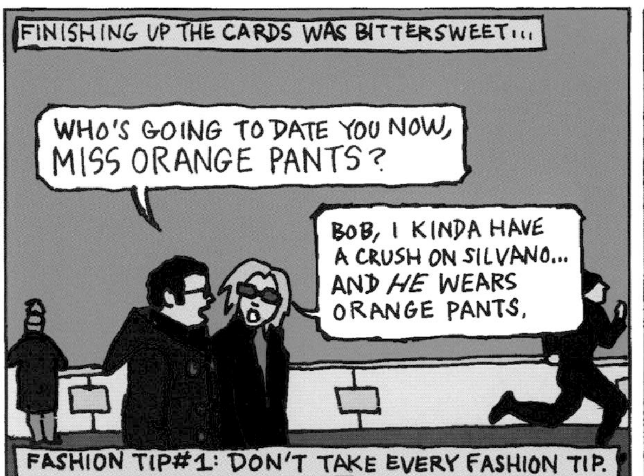
FINISHING UP THE CARDS WAS BITTERSWEET...
WHO'S GOING TO DATE YOU NOW, MISS ORANGE PANTS?
BOB, I KINDA HAVE A CRUSH ON SILVANO... AND HE WEARS ORANGE PANTS.
FASHION TIP#1: DON'T TAKE EVERY FASHION TIP.
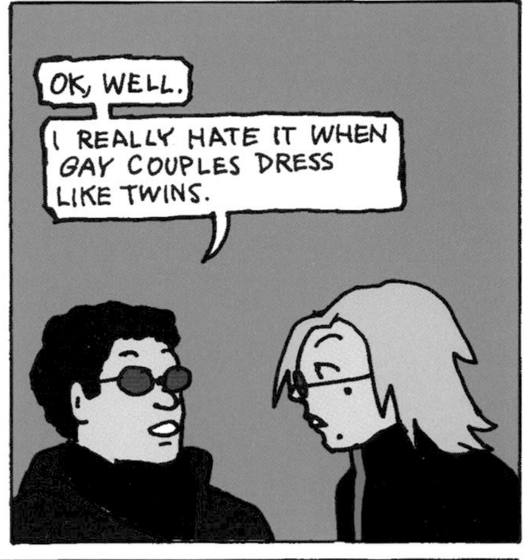
OK, WELL.
I REALLY HATE IT WHEN GAY COUPLES DRESS LIKE TWINS.
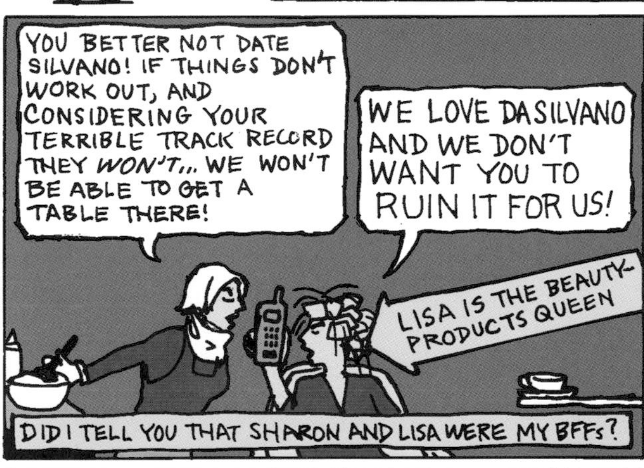
YOU BETTER NOT DATE SILVANO! IF THINGS DON'T WORK OUT, AND CONSIDERING YOUR TERRIBLE TRACK RECORD THEY WON'T... WE WON'T BE ABLE TO GET A TABLE THERE!
WE LOVE DA SILVANO AND WE DON'T WANT YOU TO RUIN IT FOR US!
LISA IS THE BEAUTY-PRODUCTS QUEEN
DID I TELL YOU THAT SHARON AND LISA WERE MY BFFs?
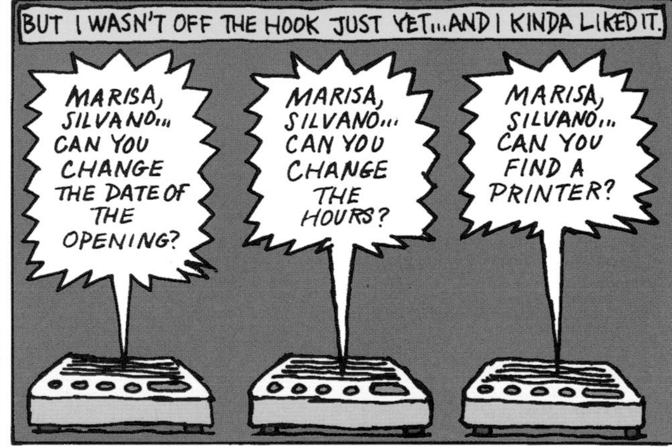
BUT I WASN'T OFF THE HOOK JUST YET... AND I KINDA LIKED IT.
MARISA, SILVANO... CAN YOU CHANGE THE DATE OF THE OPENING?
MARISA, SILVANO... CAN YOU CHANGE THE HOURS?
MARISA, SILVANO... CAN YOU FIND A PRINTER?
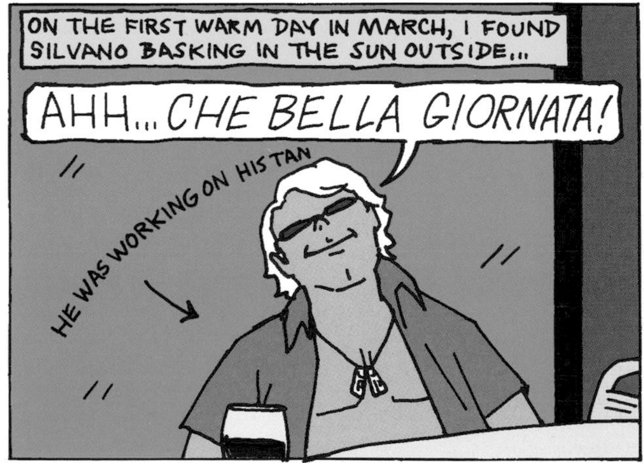
ON THE FIRST WARM DAY IN MARCH, I FOUND SILVANO BASKING IN THE SUN OUTSIDE...
AHH... CHE BELLA GIORNATA!
HE WAS WORKING ON HIS TAN
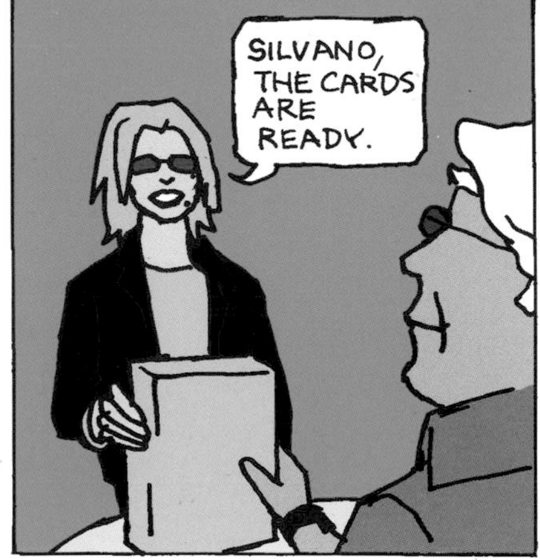
SILVANO, THE CARDS ARE READY.
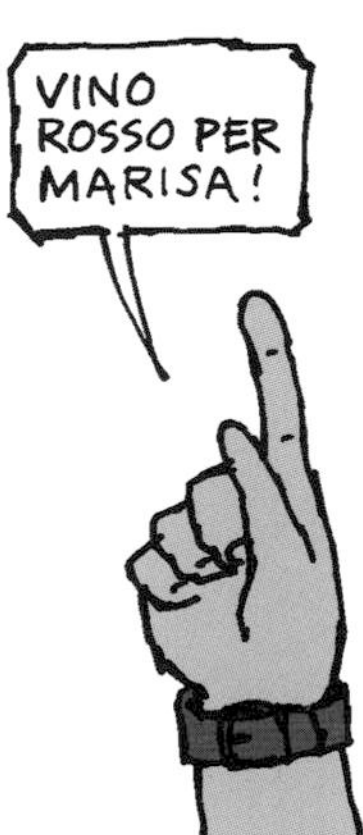
VINO ROSSO PER MARISA!

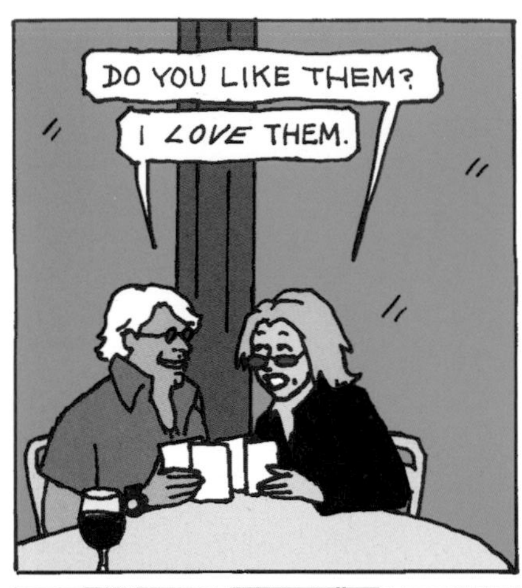
DO YOU LIKE THEM?
I LOVE THEM.

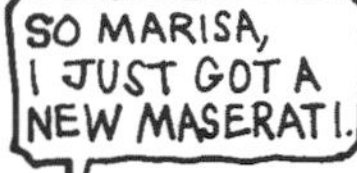
SO MARISA, I JUST GOT A NEW MASERATI.

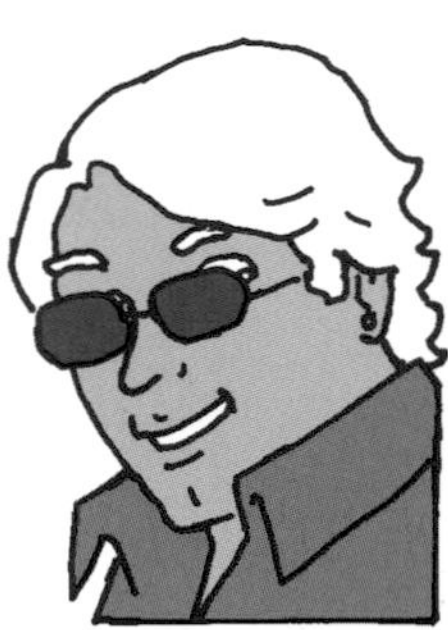

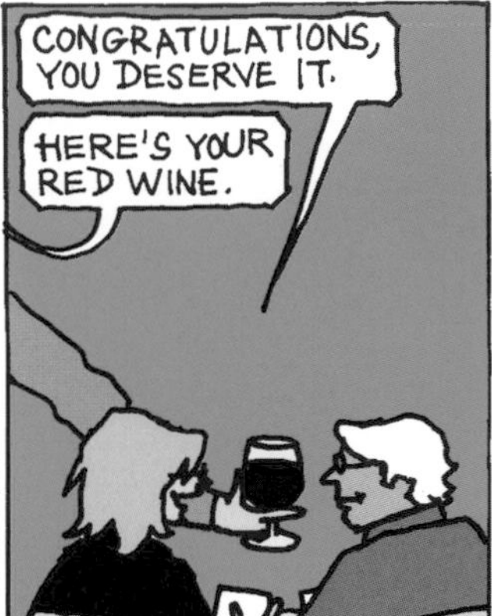
CONGRATULATIONS, YOU DESERVE IT.
HERE'S YOUR RED WINE.

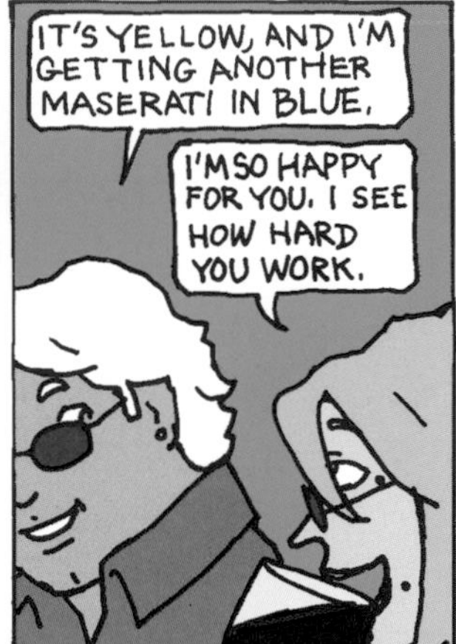
IT'S YELLOW, AND I'M GETTING ANOTHER MASERATI IN BLUE.
I'M SO HAPPY FOR YOU. I SEE HOW HARD YOU WORK.

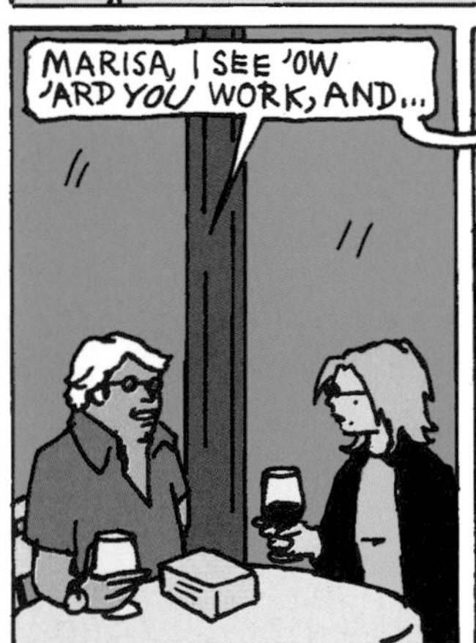
MARISA, I SEE 'OW 'ARD YOU WORK, AND...

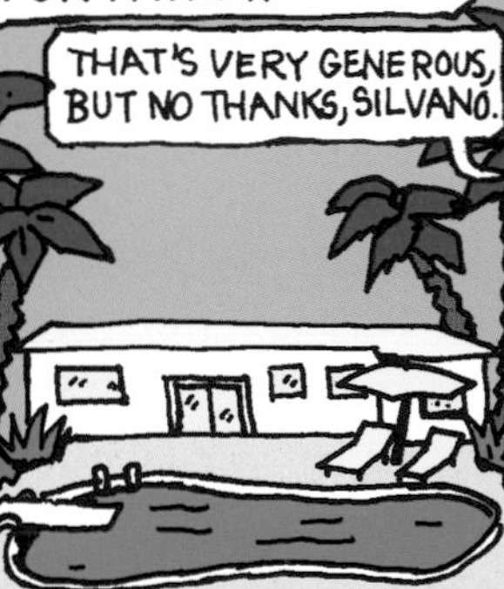
...I'D LIKE TO OFFER YOU MY 'OUSE IN FLORIDA FOR A WEEK.
THAT'S VERY GENEROUS, BUT NO THANKS, SILVANO.

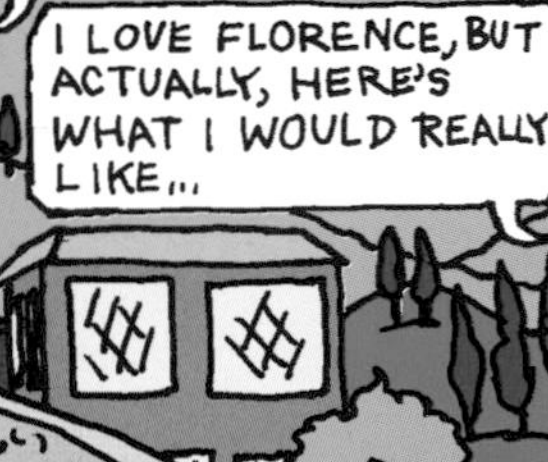
THEN LET ME OFFER YOU MY 'OUSE IN TUSCANY FOR A WEEK...
I LOVE FLORENCE, BUT ACTUALLY, HERE'S WHAT I WOULD REALLY LIKE...

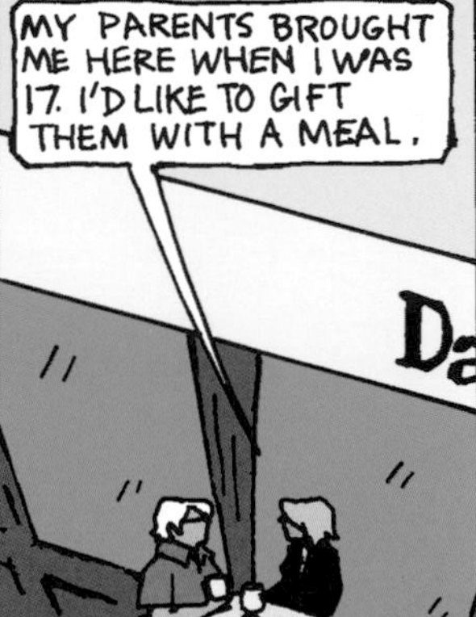
MY PARENTS BROUGHT ME HERE WHEN I WAS 17. I'D LIKE TO GIFT THEM WITH A MEAL.

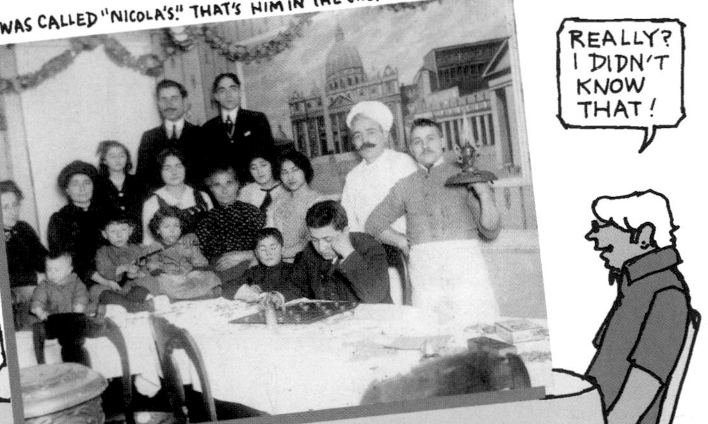
I DON'T KNOW IF I EVER TOLD YOU THIS...
MY GREAT-GRANDFATHER AND HIS BROTHER WERE CHEFS...
...AND HE STARTED ONE OF THE FIRST ITALIAN RESTAURANTS HERE IN 1901.
IT WAS CALLED "NICOLA'S." THAT'S HIM IN THE CHEF'S HAT
REALLY? I DIDN'T KNOW THAT!

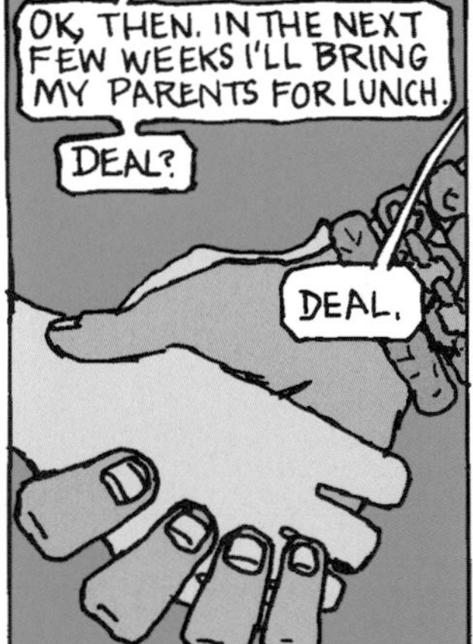
OK, THEN. IN THE NEXT FEW WEEKS I'LL BRING MY PARENTS FOR LUNCH.
DEAL?
DEAL.

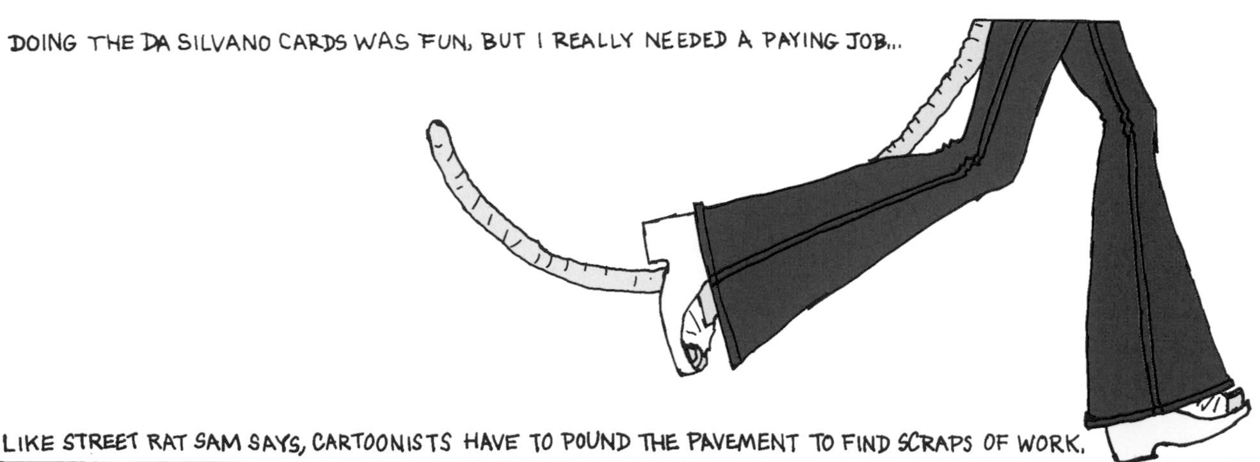
DOING THE DA SILVANO CARDS WAS FUN, BUT I REALLY NEEDED A PAYING JOB...
LIKE STREET RAT SAM SAYS, CARTOONISTS HAVE TO POUND THE PAVEMENT TO FIND SCRAPS OF WORK.

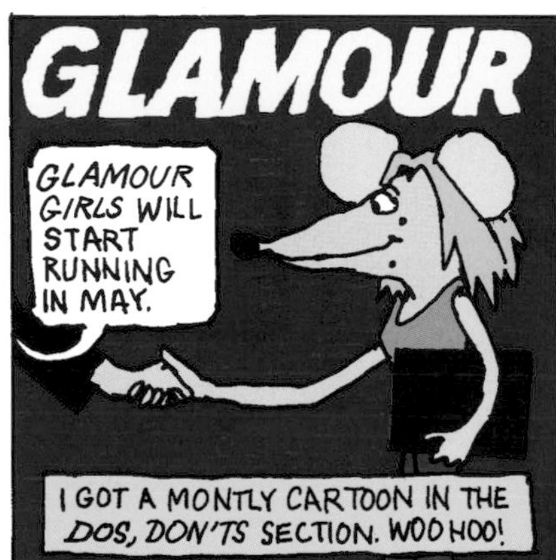
GLAMOUR
GLAMOUR GIRLS WILL START RUNNING IN MAY.
I GOT A MONTLY CARTOON IN THE DOS, DON'TS SECTION. WOO HOO!

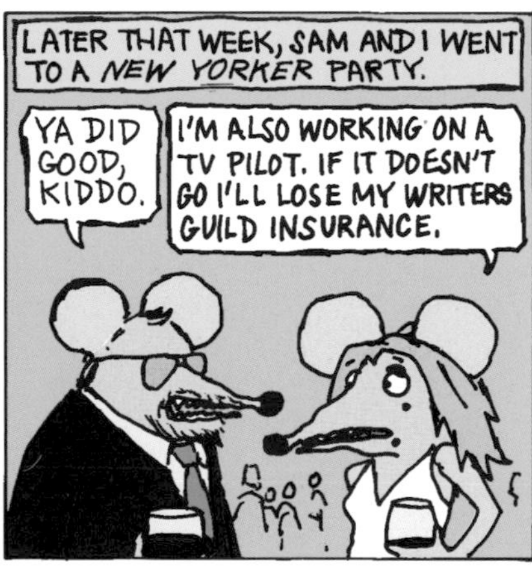
LATER THAT WEEK, SAM AND I WENT TO A NEW YORKER PARTY.
YA DID GOOD, KIDDO.
I'M ALSO WORKING ON A TV PILOT. IF IT DOESN'T GO I'LL LOSE MY WRITERS GUILD INSURANCE.

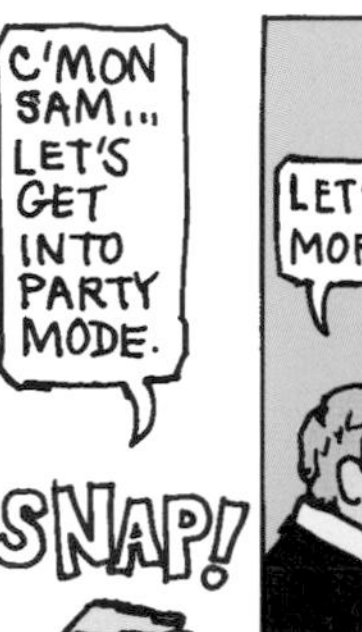
C'MON SAM... LET'S GET INTO PARTY MODE.
SNAP!

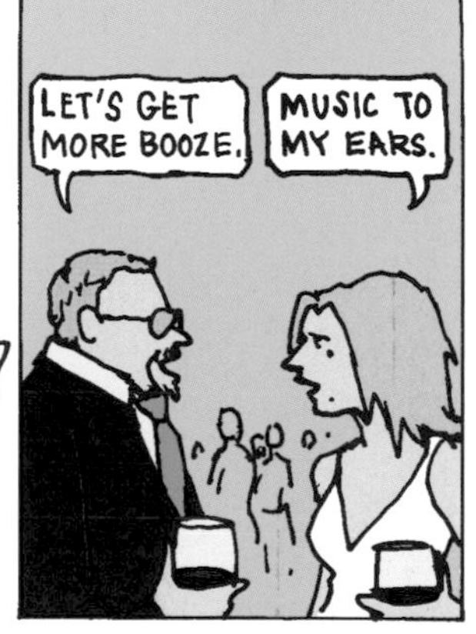
LET'S GET MORE BOOZE.
MUSIC TO MY EARS.

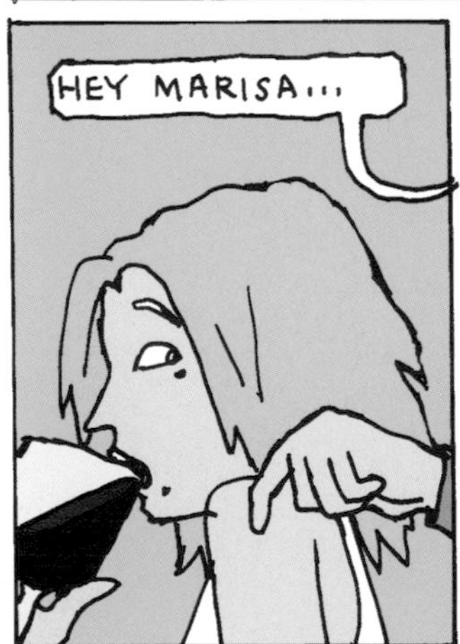
HEY MARISA...

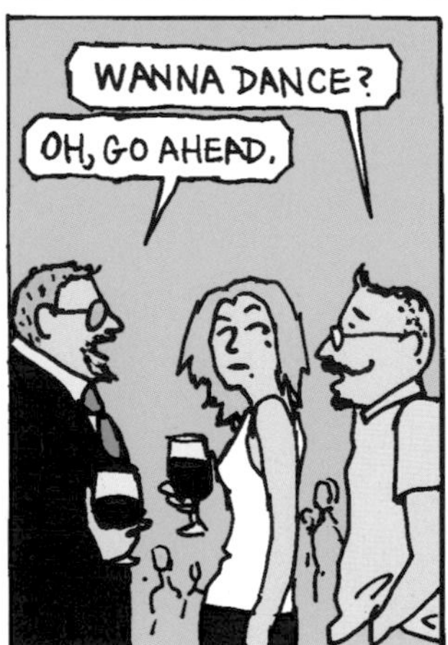
WANNA DANCE?
OH, GO AHEAD.

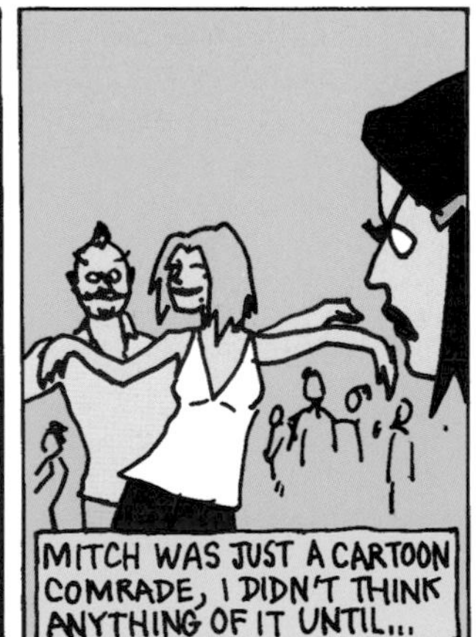
MITCH WAS JUST A CARTOON COMRADE, I DIDN'T THINK ANYTHING OF IT UNTIL...

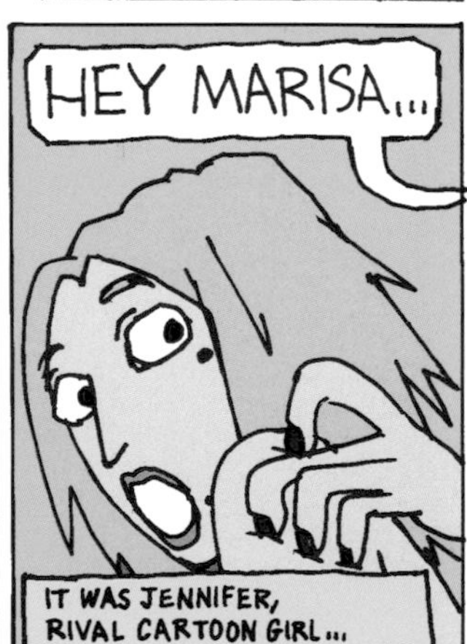
HEY MARISA...
IT WAS JENNIFER, RIVAL CARTOON GIRL...

YOU'RE A STUPID ****ING ****!!!*
*SORRY. I DON'T WANT THOSE UGLY WORDS OF RIVAL CARTOON GIRL IN MY BOOK.

I HATE YOU BECAUSE YOU ALWAYS HAVE A BOYFRIEND!

WHAT THE HELL DID I START?

...AND BECAUSE YOU CAN WEAR LEATHER PANTS!
WHAT GRADE ARE YOU IN?!?
C'MON, LET'S GO.
WHAT GRADE WAS I IN?

COME ON, I'M SEPARATING YOU TWO...
WHAT THE HELL IS YOUR PROBLEM?
BUT I WILL SAY THAT I'VE NEVER BEEN CALLED ANYTHING LIKE THAT. EVER.

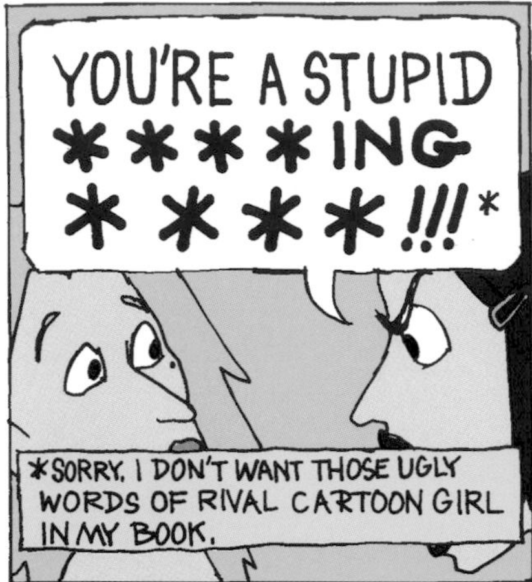

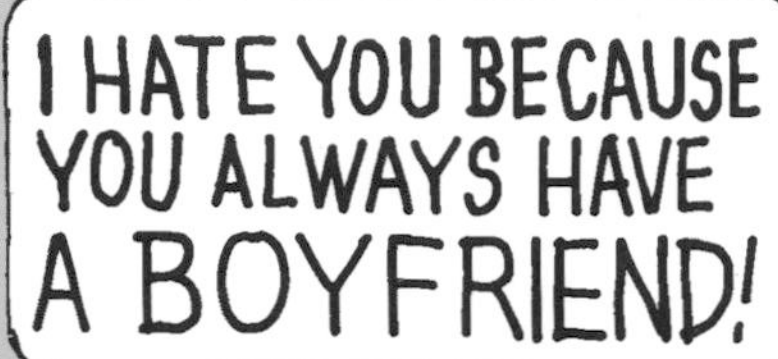

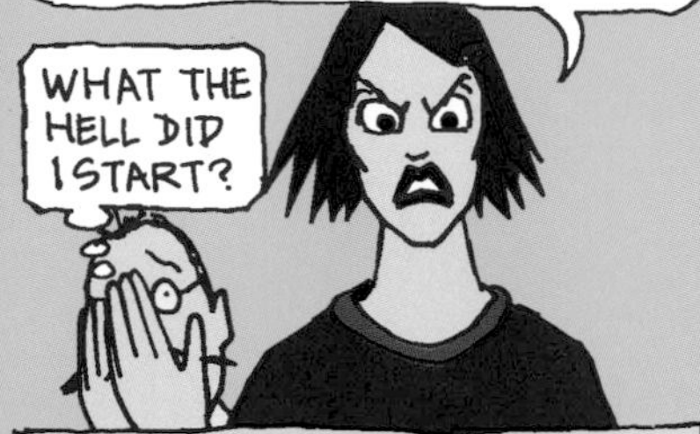

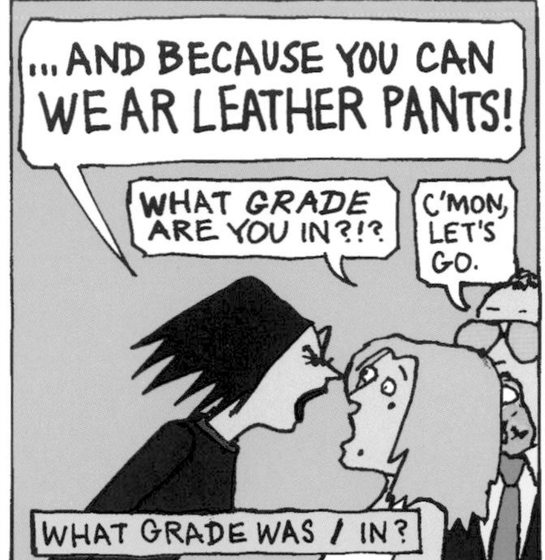

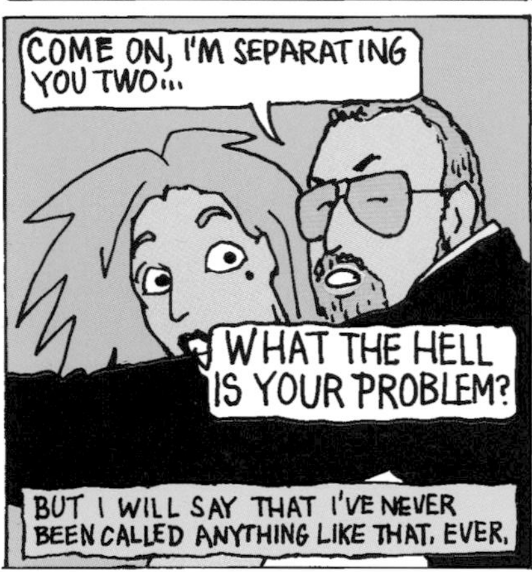

BACK THEN, ON A SCALE OF 1 TO 10 OF THE TERRIBLE THINGS THAT HAPPEN IN LIFE, THIS WAS AN 11. I HATED THAT WE WERE SO UNPROFESSIONAL AT A *NEW YORKER* PARTY, THE MAGAZINE WE BOTH KILLED OURSELVES TO GET INTO. I HATED HAVING A NEMESIS, AND I HATED HOW WOMEN HATE EACH OTHER IN BUSINESS.

THERE ARE OVER 50 MALE CARTOONISTS, AND I DON'T SEE YOU GUYS GETTING INTO CAT FIGHTS.
DIFFEE, I'M GONNA SCRATCH YOUR EYES OUT.
SHUT UP, ERIC.

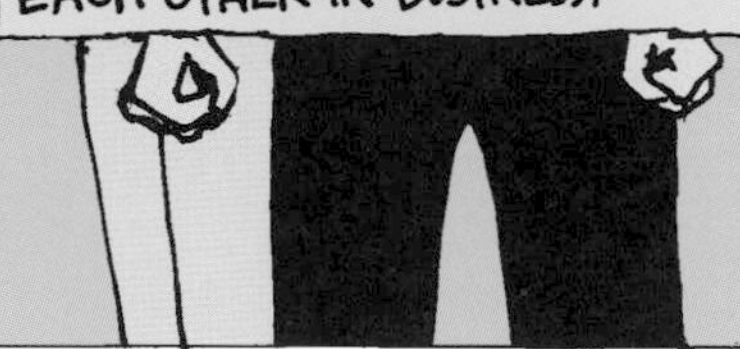

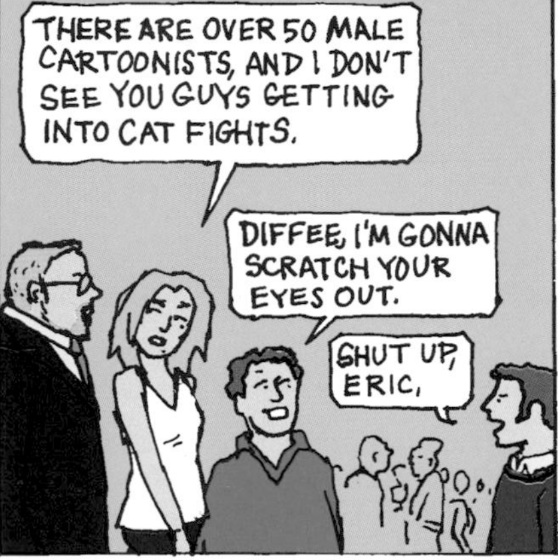

SPEAKING OF CREATING A SCENE, SILVANO PUT UP HIS NEW SHINGLE, AND MY FRIENDS AND I HAD AN 8 O'CLOCK RESERVATION...

IT WAS AN AUTOMATIC HOT SPOT. THERE WAS A WAIT...

WHEN I GOT THERE, SILVANO TOOK ME AROUND...
MARISA, THIS IS MY DAUGHTER LEYLA, AND MY LAWYER, STEVE GARDNER. I WANTED THEM TO MEET YOU.
HELLO.
HELLO.
HELLO.

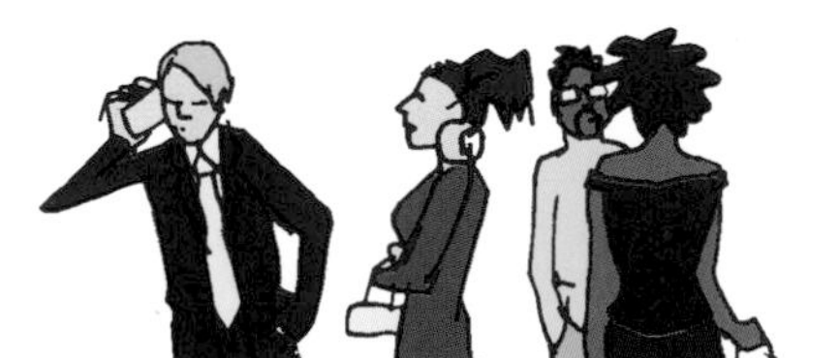

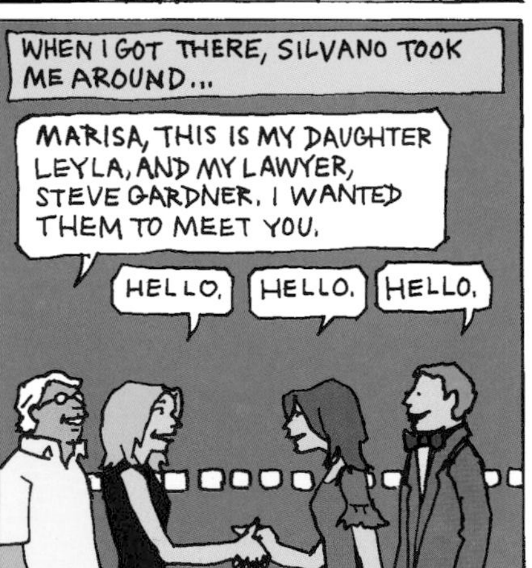

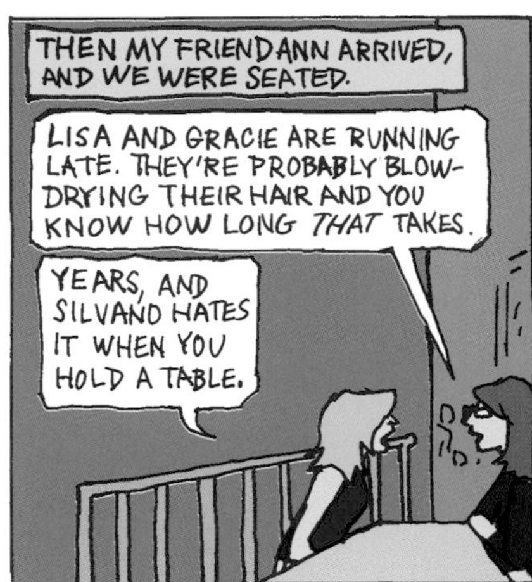
THEN MY FRIEND ANN ARRIVED, AND WE WERE SEATED.
LISA AND GRACIE ARE RUNNING LATE. THEY'RE PROBABLY BLOW-DRYING THEIR HAIR AND YOU KNOW HOW LONG *THAT* TAKES.
YEARS, AND SILVANO HATES IT WHEN YOU HOLD A TABLE.

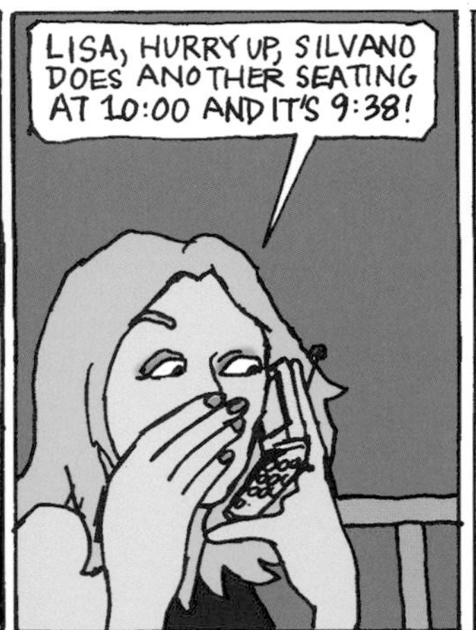
LISA, HURRY UP, SILVANO DOES ANOTHER SEATING AT 10:00 AND IT'S 9:38!

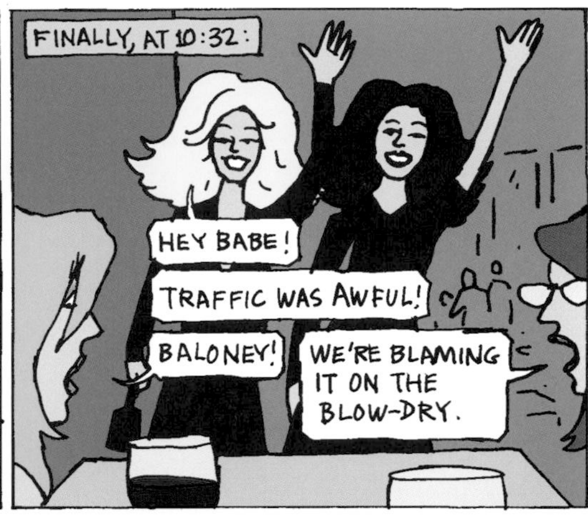
FINALLY, AT 10:32:
HEY BABE!
TRAFFIC WAS AWFUL!
BALONEY!
WE'RE BLAMING IT ON THE BLOW-DRY.

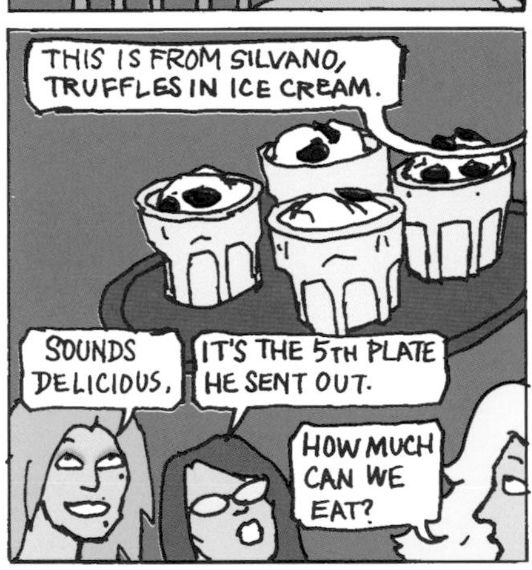
THIS IS FROM SILVANO, TRUFFLES IN ICE CREAM.
SOUNDS DELICIOUS.
IT'S THE 5TH PLATE HE SENT OUT.
HOW MUCH CAN WE EAT?

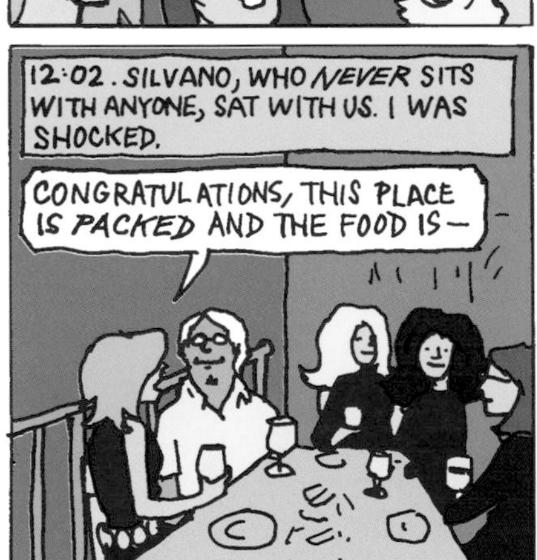
12:02. SILVANO, WHO *NEVER* SITS WITH ANYONE, SAT WITH US. I WAS SHOCKED.
CONGRATULATIONS, THIS PLACE IS *PACKED* AND THE FOOD IS—

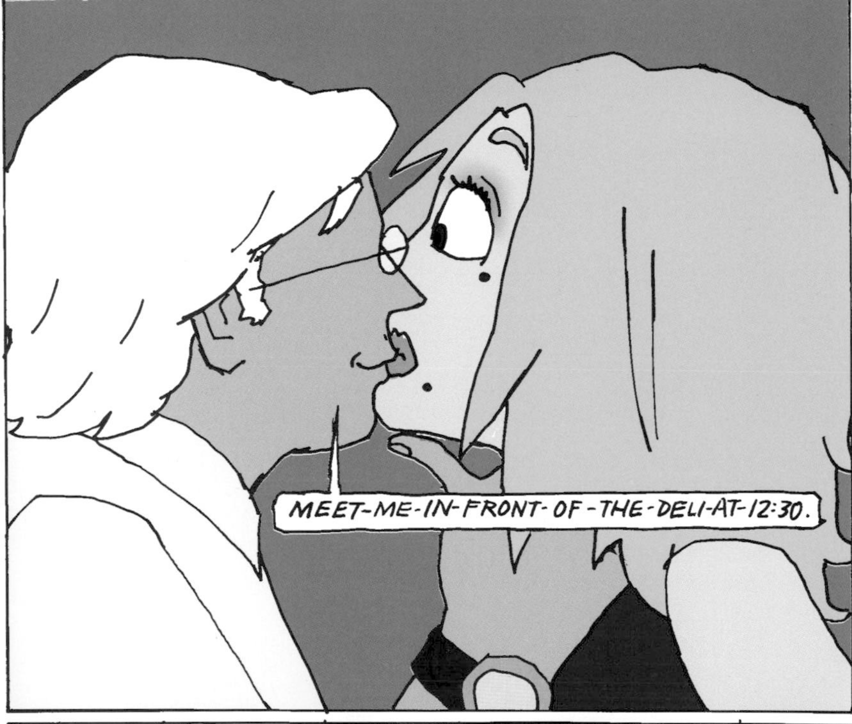
MEET-ME-IN-FRONT-OF-THE-DELI-AT-12:30.

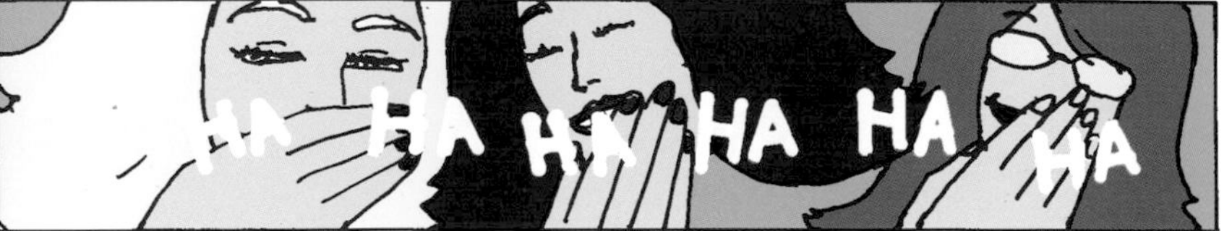
HA HA HA HA HA HA HA

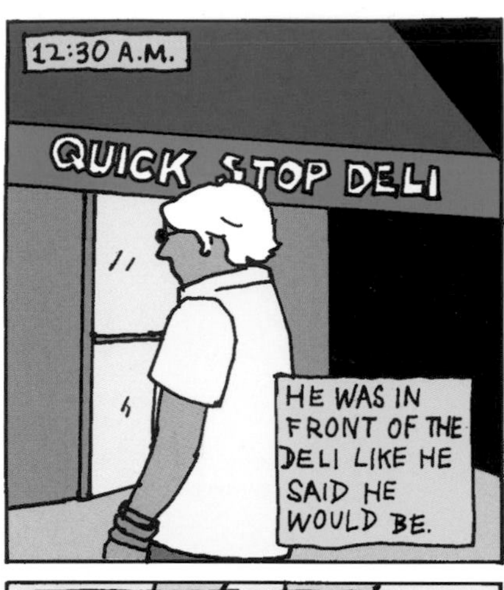
12:30 A.M.
QUICK STOP DELI
HE WAS IN FRONT OF THE DELI LIKE HE SAID HE WOULD BE.

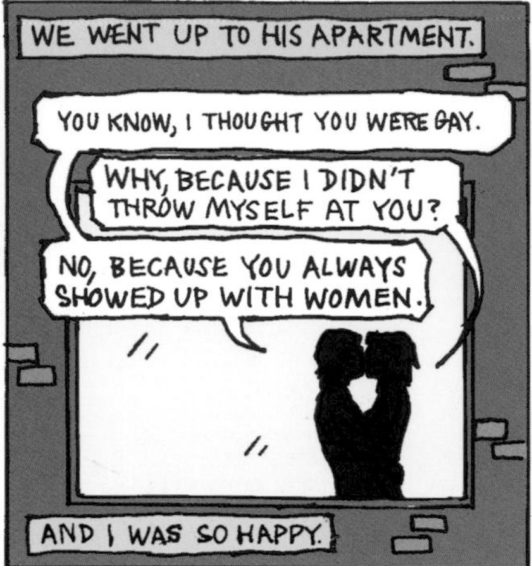
WE WENT UP TO HIS APARTMENT.
YOU KNOW, I THOUGHT YOU WERE GAY.
WHY, BECAUSE I DIDN'T THROW MYSELF AT YOU?
NO, BECAUSE YOU ALWAYS SHOWED UP WITH WOMEN.
AND I WAS SO HAPPY.

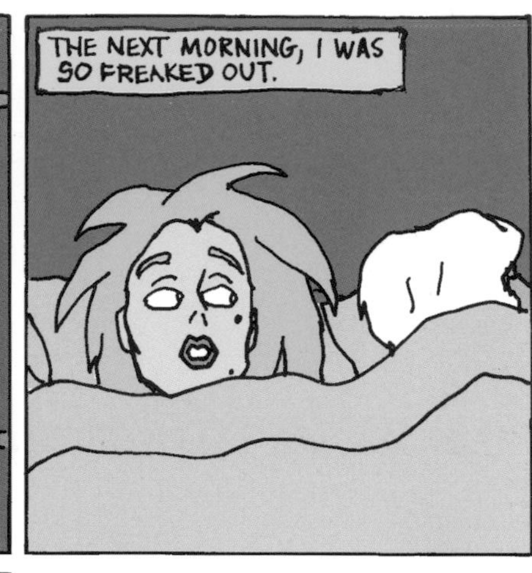
THE NEXT MORNING, I WAS SO FREAKED OUT.

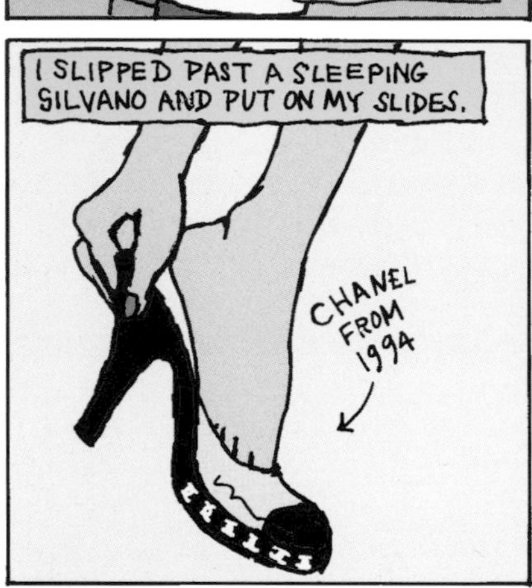
I SLIPPED PAST A SLEEPING SILVANO AND PUT ON MY SLIDES.
CHANEL FROM 1994

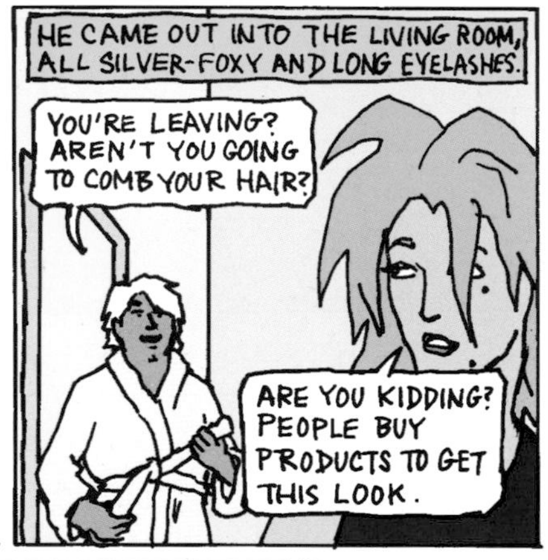
HE CAME OUT INTO THE LIVING ROOM, ALL SILVER-FOXY AND LONG EYELASHES.
YOU'RE LEAVING? AREN'T YOU GOING TO COMB YOUR HAIR?
ARE YOU KIDDING? PEOPLE BUY PRODUCTS TO GET THIS LOOK.

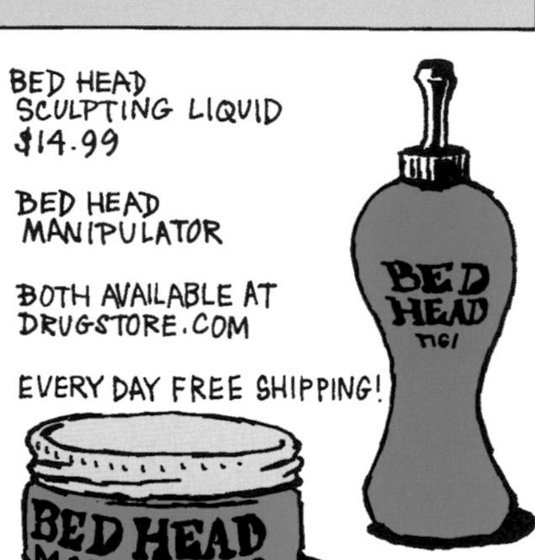
BED HEAD SCULPTING LIQUID
$14.99
BED HEAD MANIPULATOR
BOTH AVAILABLE AT DRUGSTORE.COM
EVERY DAY FREE SHIPPING!
BED HEAD
TIGI
BED HEAD MANIPULATOR

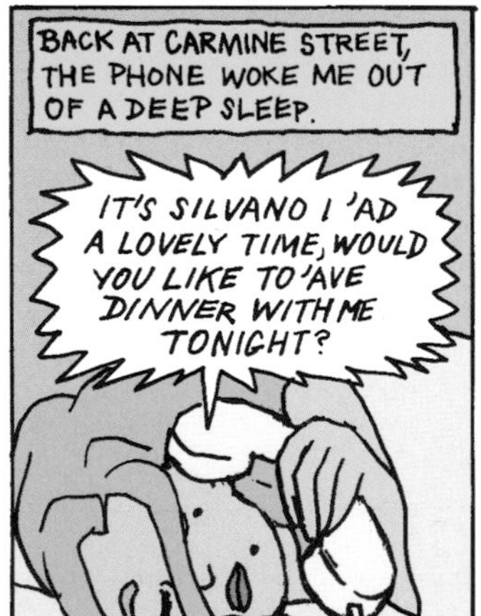
BACK AT CARMINE STREET, THE PHONE WOKE ME OUT OF A DEEP SLEEP.
IT'S SILVANO I 'AD A LOVELY TIME, WOULD YOU LIKE TO 'AVE DINNER WITH ME TONIGHT?

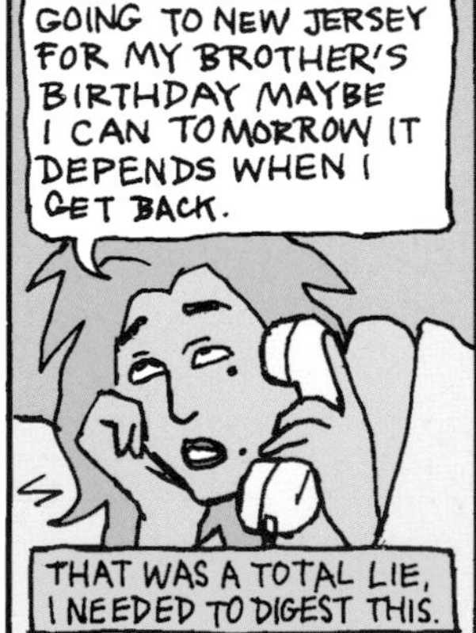
I CAN'T TONIGHT I'M GOING TO NEW JERSEY FOR MY BROTHER'S BIRTHDAY MAYBE I CAN TOMORROW IT DEPENDS WHEN I GET BACK.
THAT WAS A TOTAL LIE, I NEEDED TO DIGEST THIS.

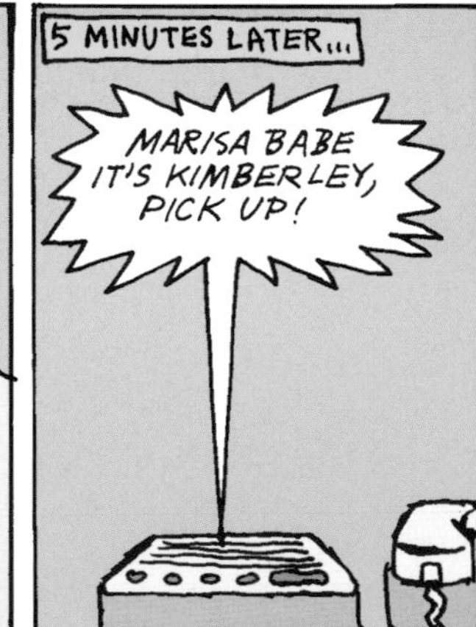
5 MINUTES LATER...
MARISA BABE IT'S KIMBERLEY, PICK UP!

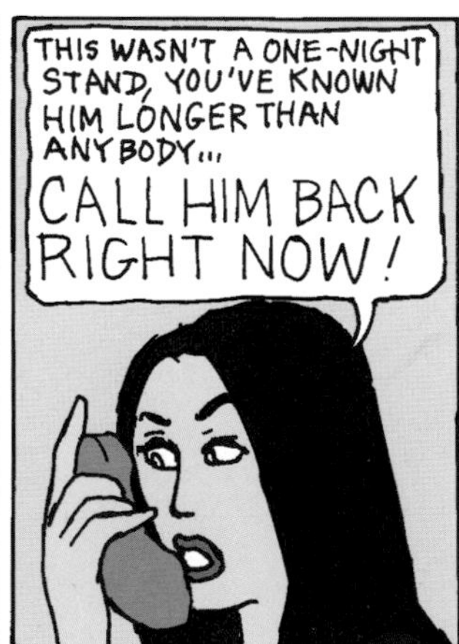
THIS WASN'T A ONE-NIGHT STAND, YOU'VE KNOWN HIM LONGER THAN ANYBODY...
CALL HIM BACK RIGHT NOW!

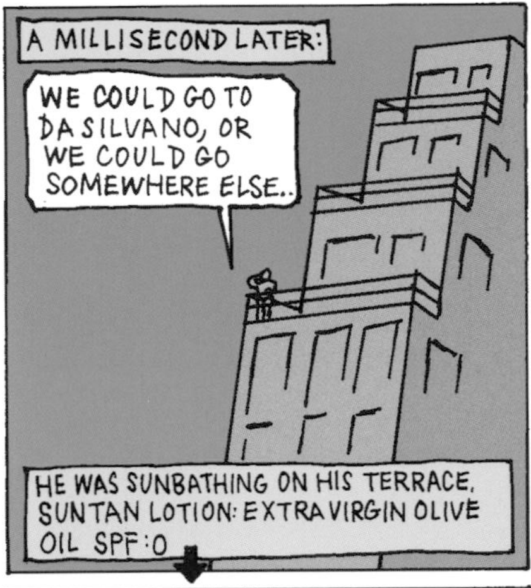
A MILLISECOND LATER:
WE COULD GO TO DA SILVANO, OR WE COULD GO SOMEWHERE ELSE..
HE WAS SUNBATHING ON HIS TERRACE. SUNTAN LOTION: EXTRA VIRGIN OLIVE OIL SPF:0

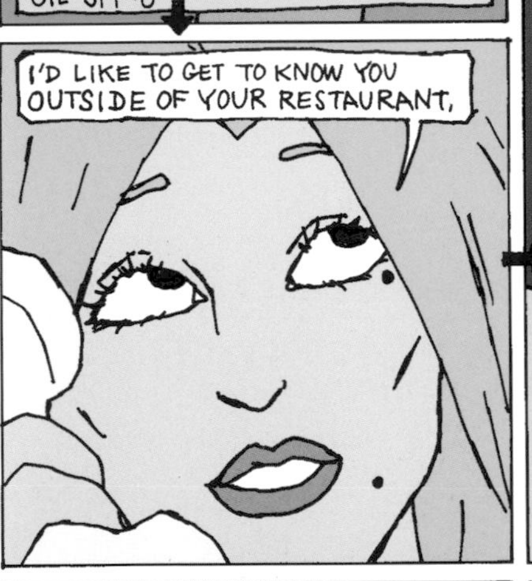
I'D LIKE TO GET TO KNOW YOU OUTSIDE OF YOUR RESTAURANT,

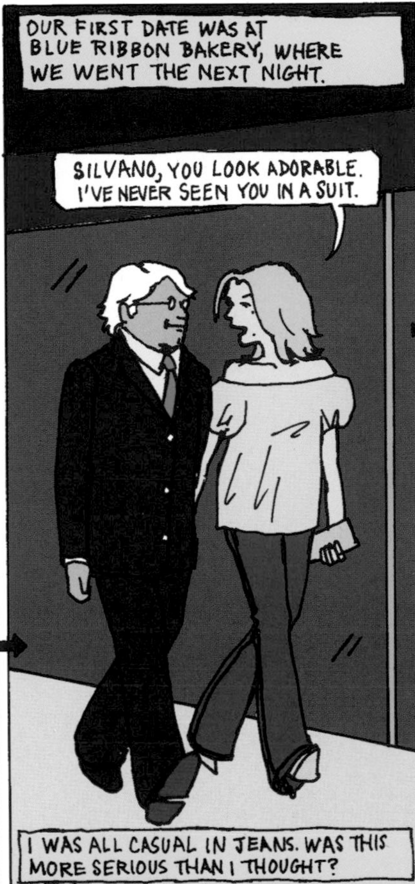
OUR FIRST DATE WAS AT BLUE RIBBON BAKERY, WHERE WE WENT THE NEXT NIGHT.
SILVANO, YOU LOOK ADORABLE. I'VE NEVER SEEN YOU IN A SUIT.
I WAS ALL CASUAL IN JEANS. WAS THIS MORE SERIOUS THAN I THOUGHT?

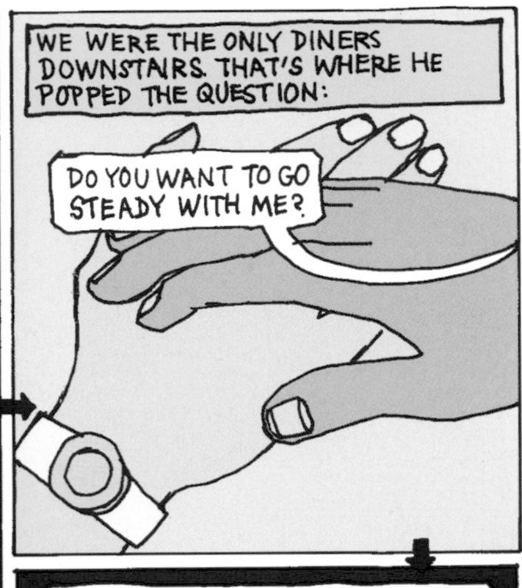
WE WERE THE ONLY DINERS DOWNSTAIRS. THAT'S WHERE HE POPPED THE QUESTION:
DO YOU WANT TO GO STEADY WITH ME?

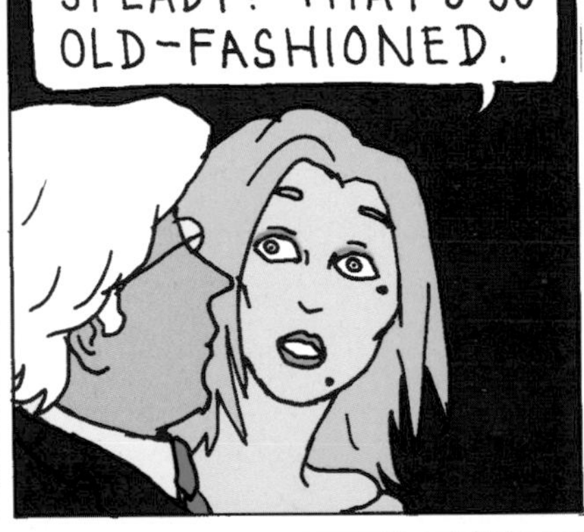
STEADY? THAT'S SO OLD-FASHIONED.

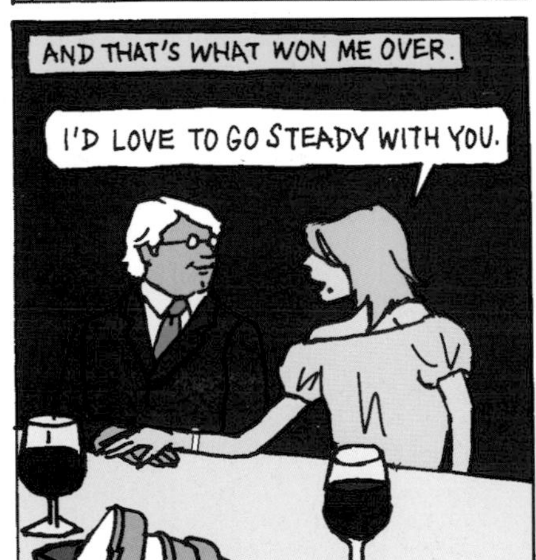
AND THAT'S WHAT WON ME OVER.
I'D LOVE TO GO STEADY WITH YOU.

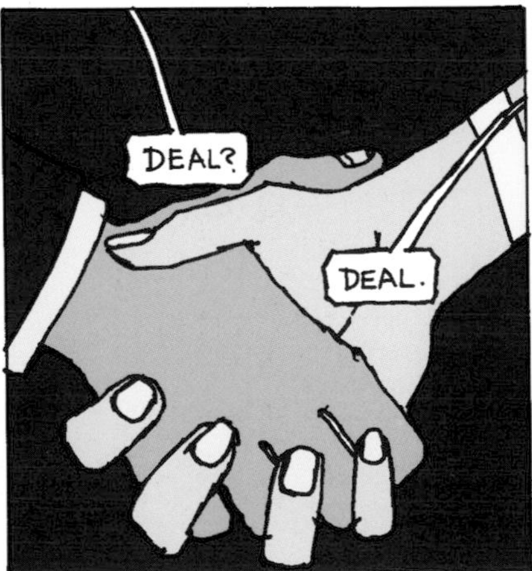
DEAL?
DEAL.

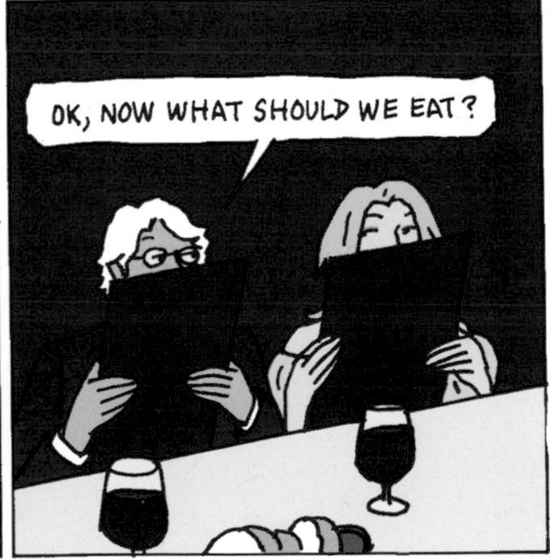
OK, NOW WHAT SHOULD WE EAT?

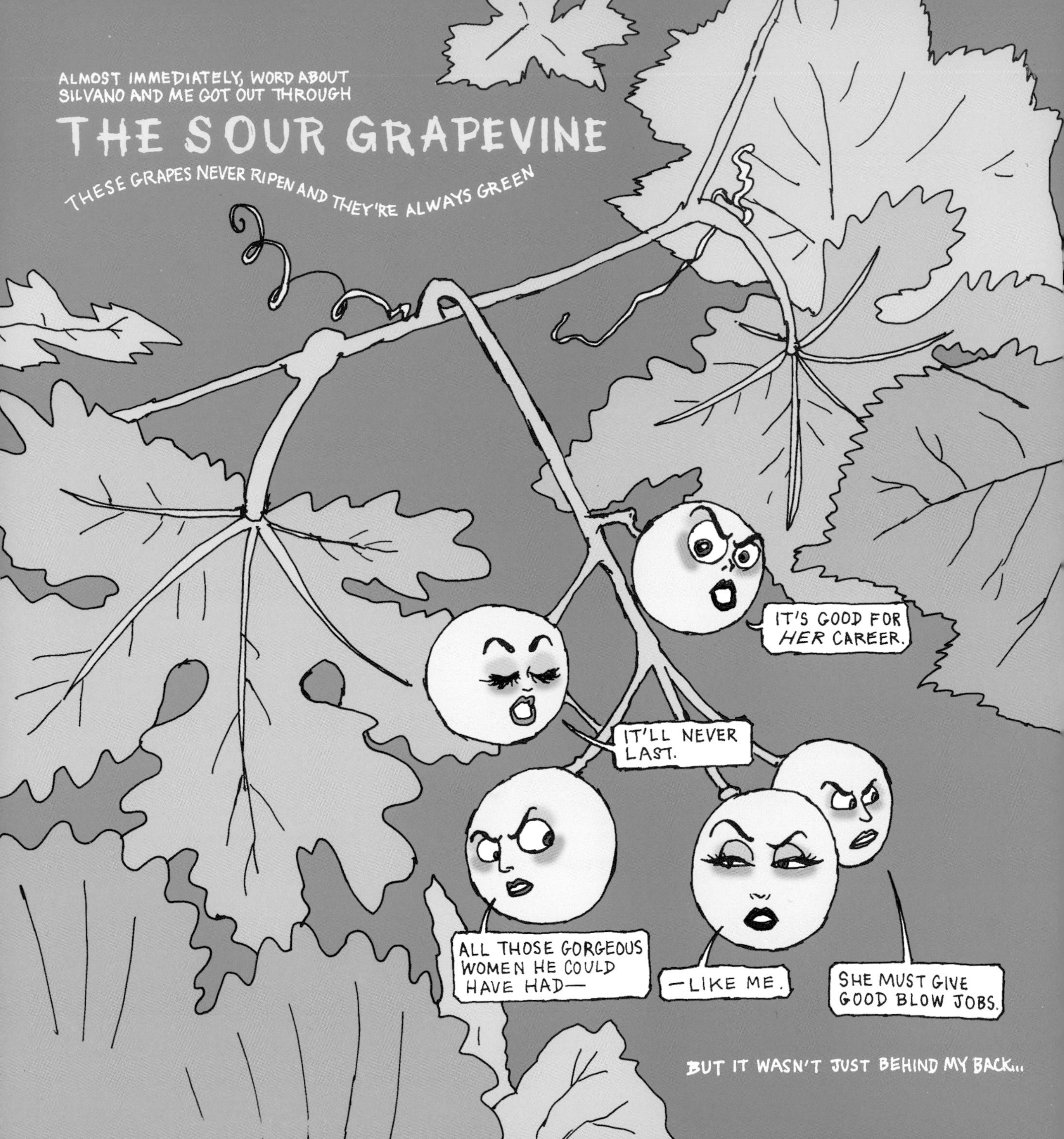
ALMOST IMMEDIATELY, WORD ABOUT SILVANO AND ME GOT OUT THROUGH
THE SOUR GRAPEVINE
THESE GRAPES NEVER RIPEN AND THEY'RE ALWAYS GREEN
IT'S GOOD FOR *HER* CAREER.
IT'LL NEVER LAST.
ALL THOSE GORGEOUS WOMEN HE COULD HAVE HAD—
—LIKE ME.
SHE MUST GIVE GOOD BLOW JOBS.
BUT IT WASN'T JUST BEHIND MY BACK...

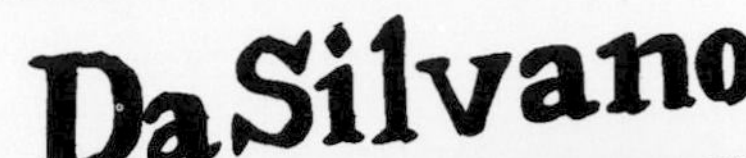

IF NEW YORK CITY IS HIGH SCHOOL, THIS IS ITS CAFETERIA*...

THE POPULAR GIRLS—THE "IT" GIRLS; THE DRAMA DEPARTMENT—"A" LIST ACTORS; THE MUSIC DEPARTMENT—ROCK STARS; THE JOCKS—HALL OF FAME ATHLETES; THE NEWS PAPER—THE MEDIA ELITE, GOSSIP MEISTERS AND BLOGGER MONGERS WHO WATCH AND OVERHEAR EVERYONE'S EVERY MOVE AND REPORT IT; THE A.V. SQUAD—FILM, TV AND RECORD EXECUTIVES; THE HOMECOMING KING? SILVANO. AND ME? AS "THE GIRL FRIEND" I WAS THE NEW KID IN TOWN. YOU KNOW WHAT THAT MEANS. THAT WAS MY BIGGEST CHALLENGE. HERE'S WHAT HAPPENED WHEN I WENT TO SCHOOL...

* WITH FABULOUS FOOD, OF COURSE.

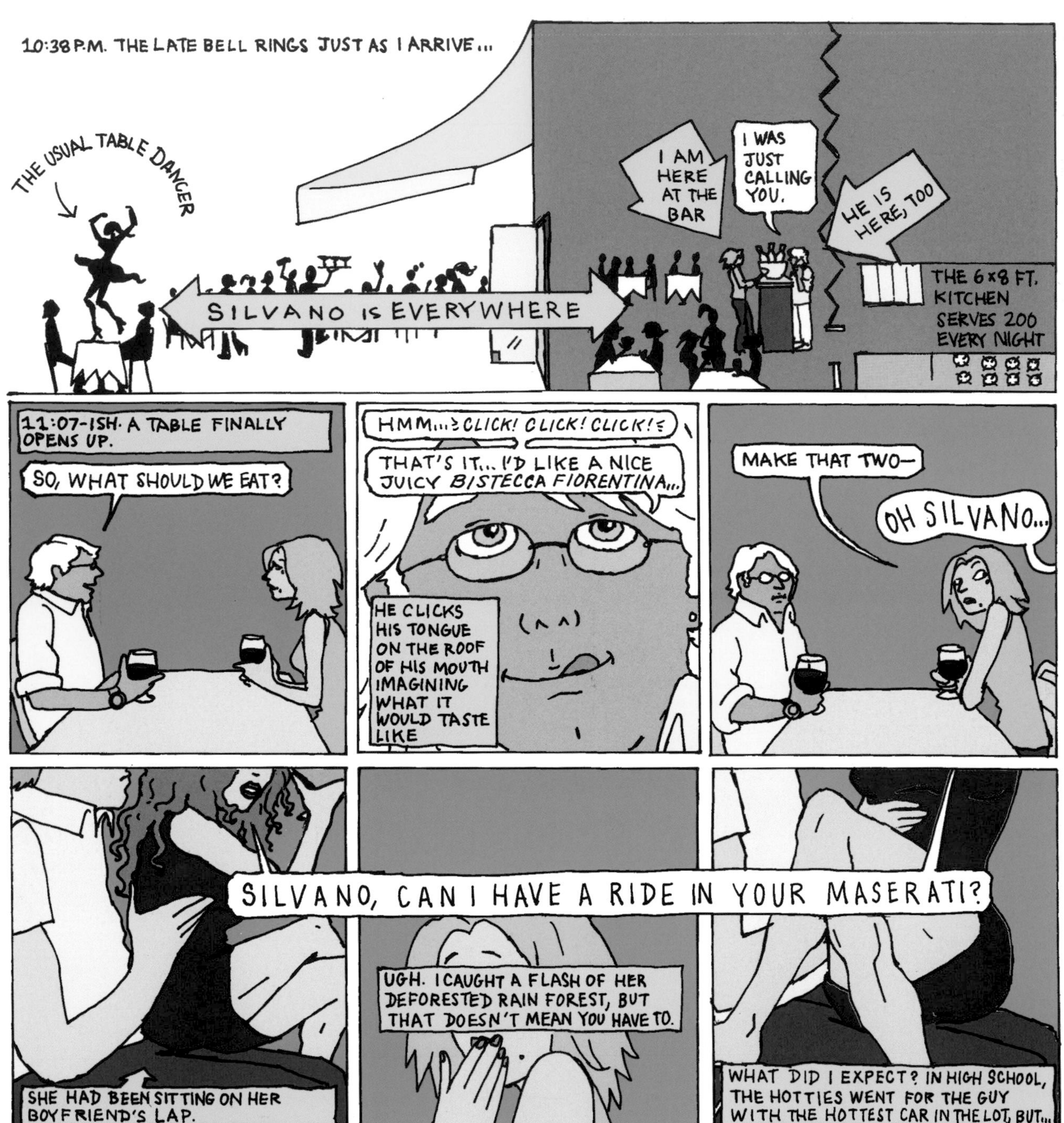
10:38 P.M. THE LATE BELL RINGS JUST AS I ARRIVE...
THE USUAL TABLE DANCER
SILVANO IS EVERYWHERE
I AM HERE AT THE BAR
I WAS JUST CALLING YOU.
HE IS HERE, TOO
THE 6×8 FT. KITCHEN SERVES 200 EVERY NIGHT
11:07-ISH. A TABLE FINALLY OPENS UP.
SO, WHAT SHOULD WE EAT?
HMM... CLICK! CLICK! CLICK!
THAT'S IT... I'D LIKE A NICE JUICY BISTECCA FIORENTINA...
HE CLICKS HIS TONGUE ON THE ROOF OF HIS MOUTH IMAGINING WHAT IT WOULD TASTE LIKE
MAKE THAT TWO—
OH SILVANO...
SILVANO, CAN I HAVE A RIDE IN YOUR MASERATI?
SHE HAD BEEN SITTING ON HER BOYFRIEND'S LAP.
UGH. I CAUGHT A FLASH OF HER DEFORESTED RAIN FOREST, BUT THAT DOESN'T MEAN YOU HAVE TO.
WHAT DID I EXPECT? IN HIGH SCHOOL, THE HOTTIES WENT FOR THE GUY WITH THE HOTTEST CAR IN THE LOT, BUT...

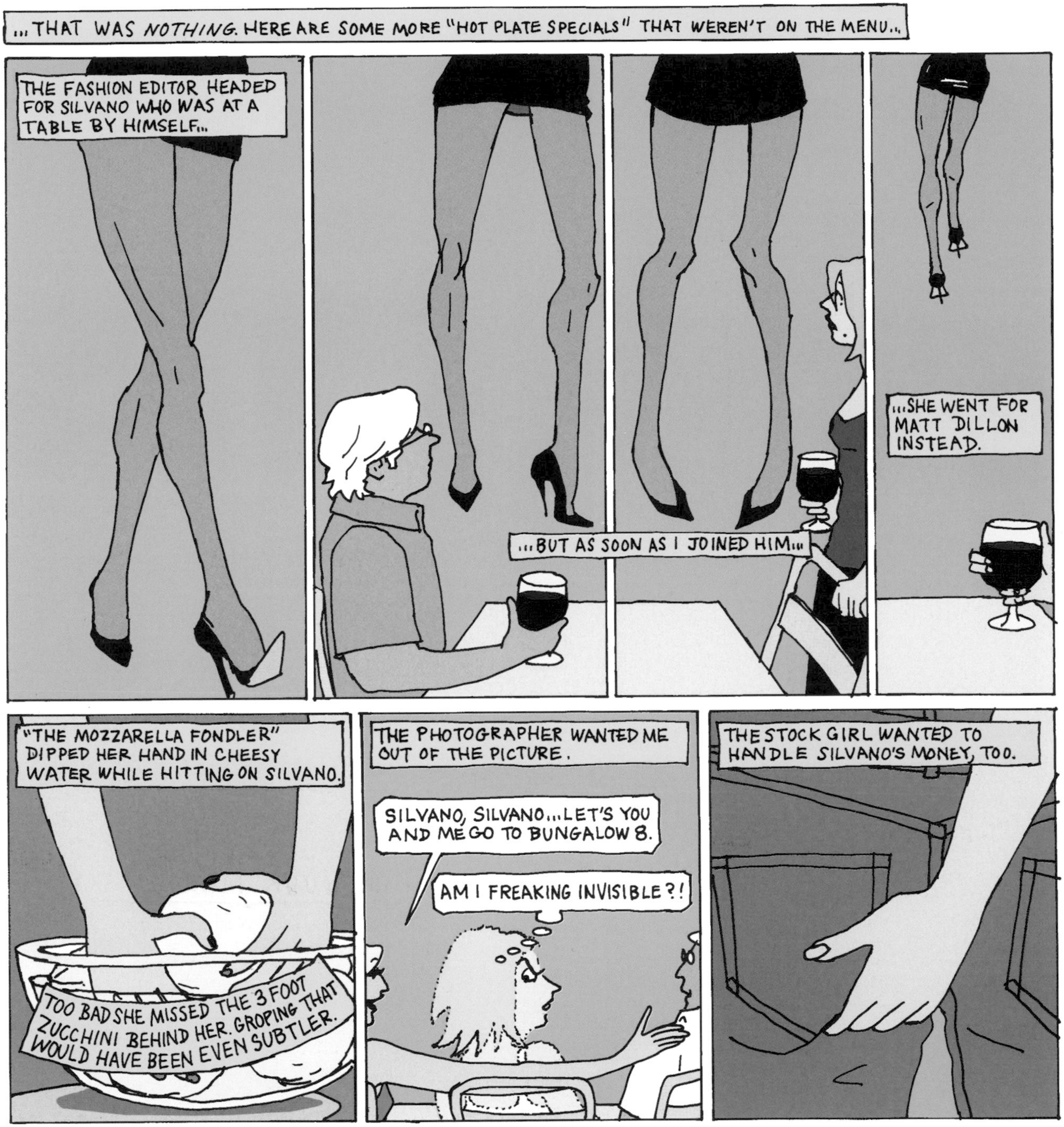

...THAT WAS *NOTHING*. HERE ARE SOME MORE "HOT PLATE SPECIALS" THAT WEREN'T ON THE MENU...

THE FASHION EDITOR HEADED FOR SILVANO WHO WAS AT A TABLE BY HIMSELF...

...BUT AS SOON AS I JOINED HIM...

...SHE WENT FOR MATT DILLON INSTEAD.

"THE MOZZARELLA FONDLER" DIPPED HER HAND IN CHEESY WATER WHILE HITTING ON SILVANO.
TOO BAD SHE MISSED THE 3 FOOT ZUCCHINI BEHIND HER. GROPING THAT WOULD HAVE BEEN EVEN SUBTLER.

THE PHOTOGRAPHER WANTED ME OUT OF THE PICTURE.
SILVANO, SILVANO...LET'S YOU AND ME GO TO BUNGALOW 8.
AM I FREAKING INVISIBLE?!

THE STOCK GIRL WANTED TO HANDLE SILVANO'S MONEY, TOO.

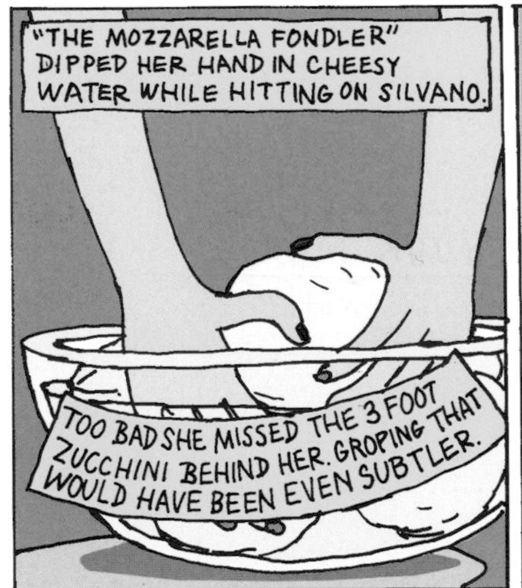

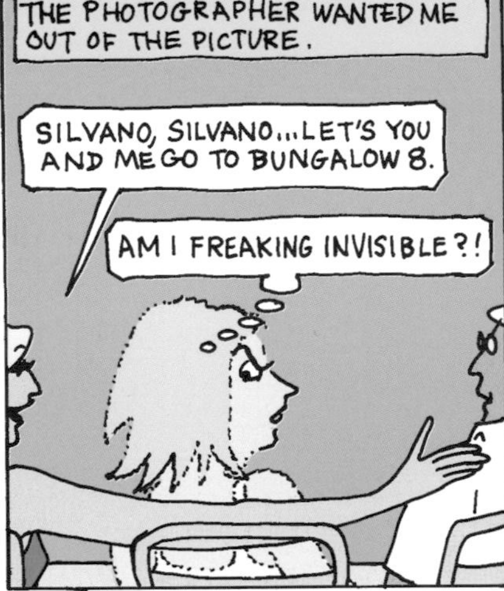

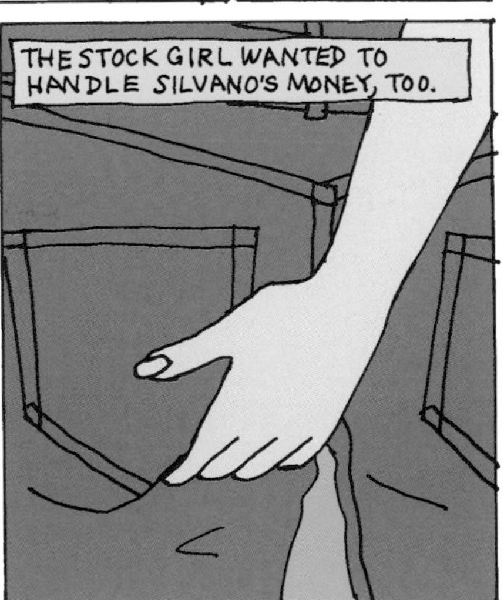

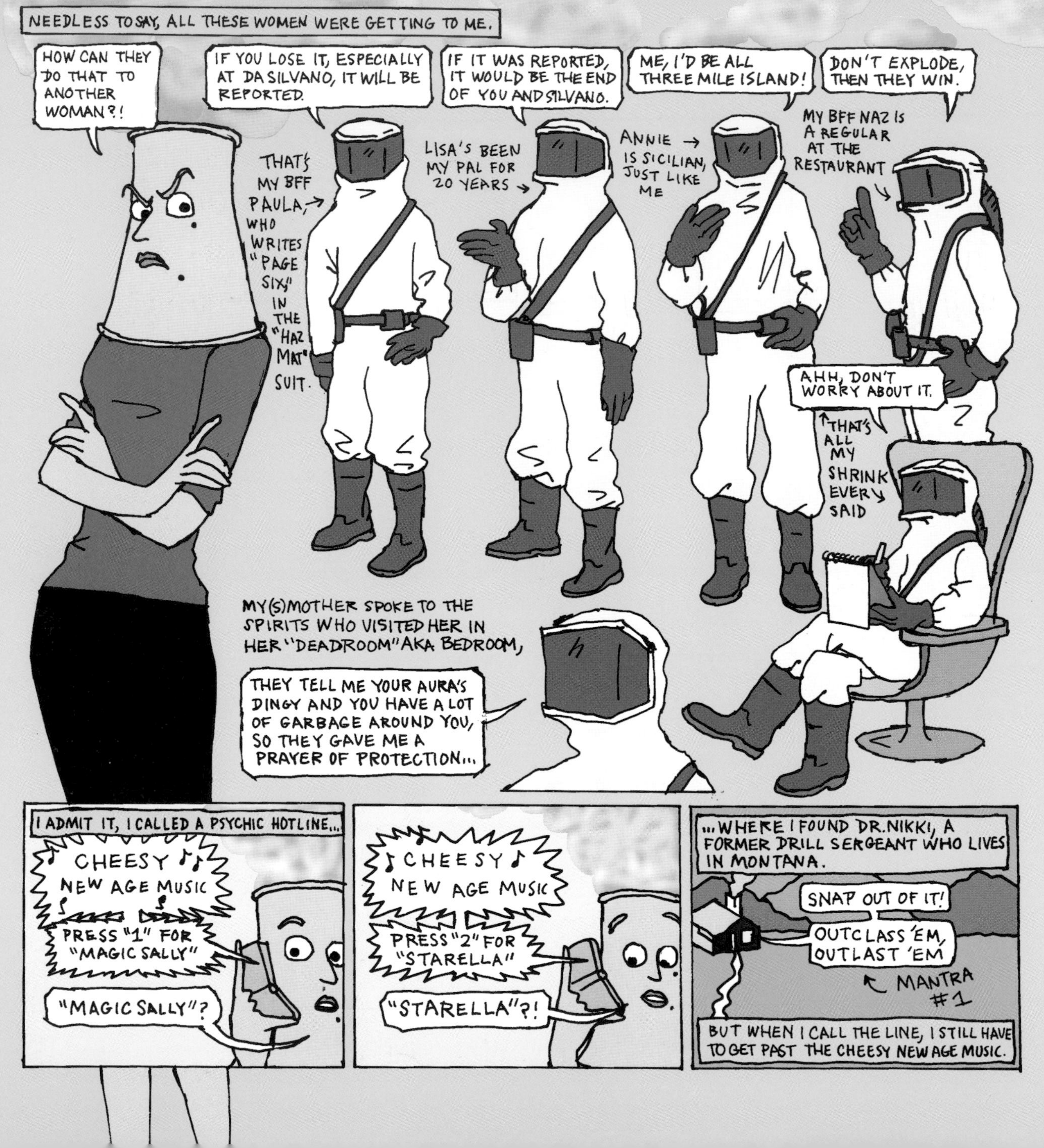

NEEDLESS TO SAY, ALL THESE WOMEN WERE GETTING TO ME.

HOW CAN THEY DO THAT TO ANOTHER WOMAN?!

IF YOU LOSE IT, ESPECIALLY AT DA SILVANO, IT WILL BE REPORTED.

IF IT WAS REPORTED, IT WOULD BE THE END OF YOU AND SILVANO.

ME, I'D BE ALL THREE MILE ISLAND!

DON'T EXPLODE, THEN THEY WIN.

THAT'S MY BFF PAULA, WHO WRITES "PAGE SIX" IN THE "HAZ MAT" SUIT.

LISA'S BEEN MY PAL FOR 20 YEARS

ANNIE IS SICILIAN, JUST LIKE ME

MY BFF NAZ IS A REGULAR AT THE RESTAURANT

AHH, DON'T WORRY ABOUT IT.

THAT'S ALL MY SHRINK EVERY SAID

MY(S)MOTHER SPOKE TO THE SPIRITS WHO VISITED HER IN HER "DEADROOM" AKA BEDROOM,

THEY TELL ME YOUR AURA'S DINGY AND YOU HAVE A LOT OF GARBAGE AROUND YOU, SO THEY GAVE ME A PRAYER OF PROTECTION...

I ADMIT IT, I CALLED A PSYCHIC HOTLINE...
CHEESY NEW AGE MUSIC
PRESS "1" FOR "MAGIC SALLY"
"MAGIC SALLY"?

CHEESY NEW AGE MUSIC
PRESS "2" FOR "STARELLA"
"STARELLA"?!

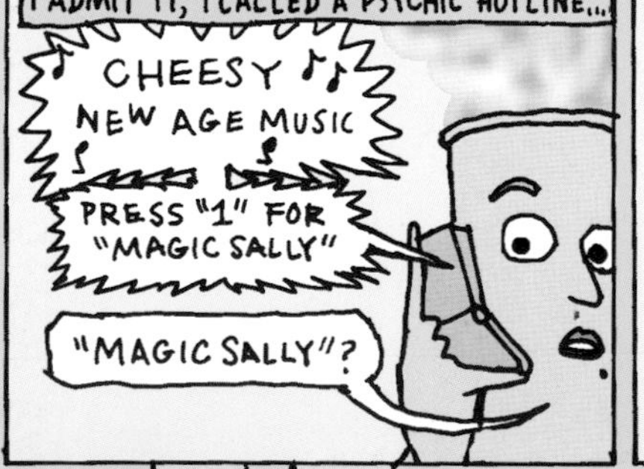

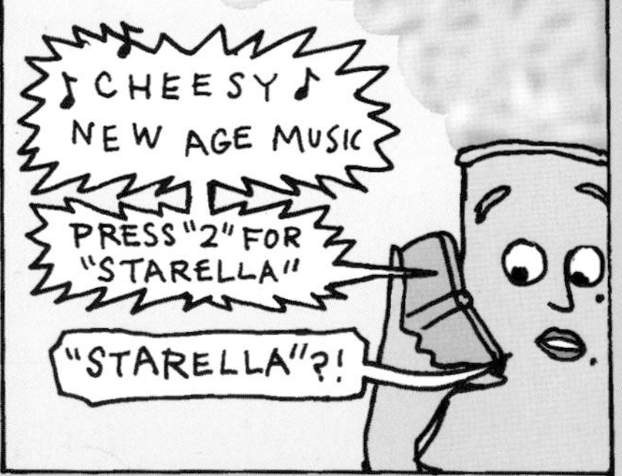

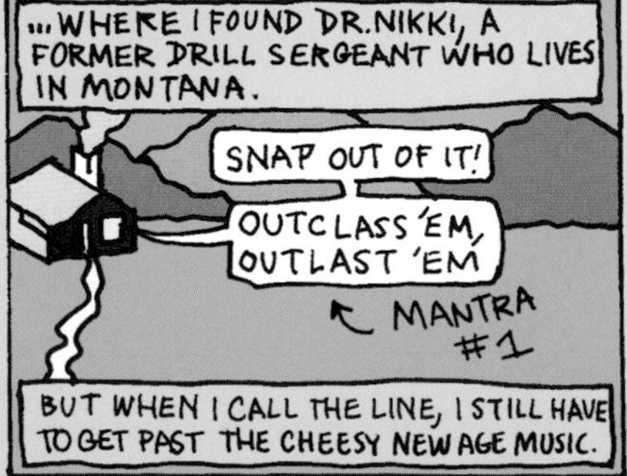

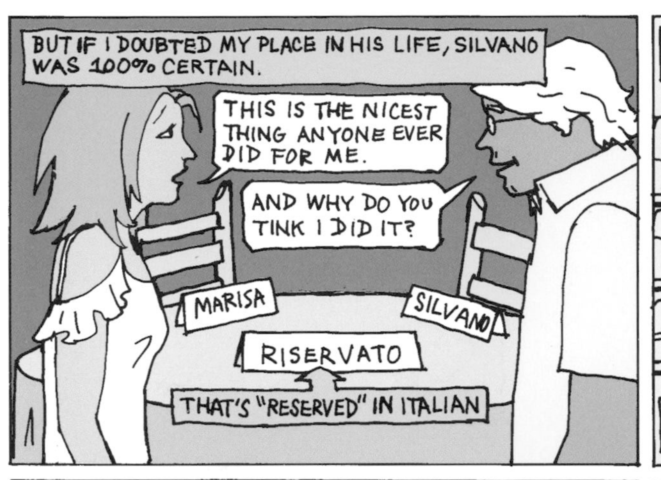
BUT IF I DOUBTED MY PLACE IN HIS LIFE, SILVANO WAS 100% CERTAIN.
THIS IS THE NICEST THING ANYONE EVER DID FOR ME.
AND WHY DO YOU TINK I DID IT?
MARISA
SILVANO
RISERVATO
THAT'S "RESERVED" IN ITALIAN

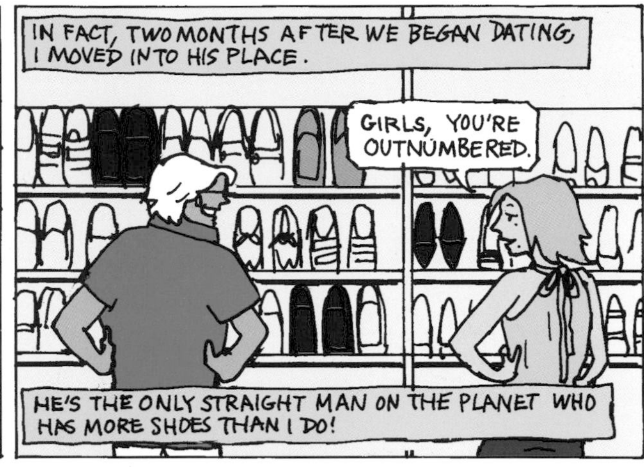
IN FACT, TWO MONTHS AFTER WE BEGAN DATING, I MOVED INTO HIS PLACE.
GIRLS, YOU'RE OUTNUMBERED.
HE'S THE ONLY STRAIGHT MAN ON THE PLANET WHO HAS MORE SHOES THAN I DO!

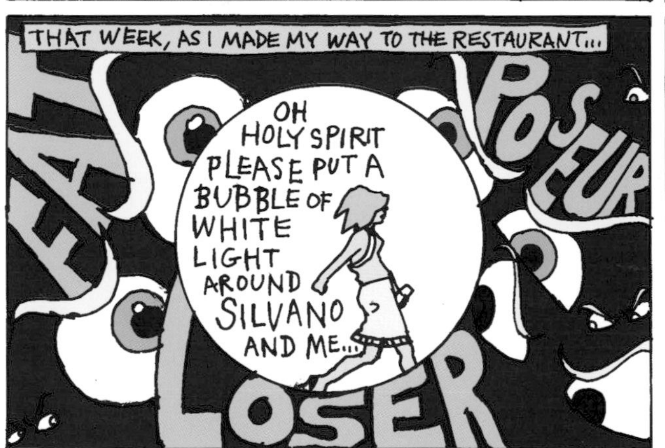
THAT WEEK, AS I MADE MY WAY TO THE RESTAURANT...
OH HOLY SPIRIT PLEASE PUT A BUBBLE OF WHITE LIGHT AROUND SILVANO AND ME...
FAT
POSEUR
LOSER

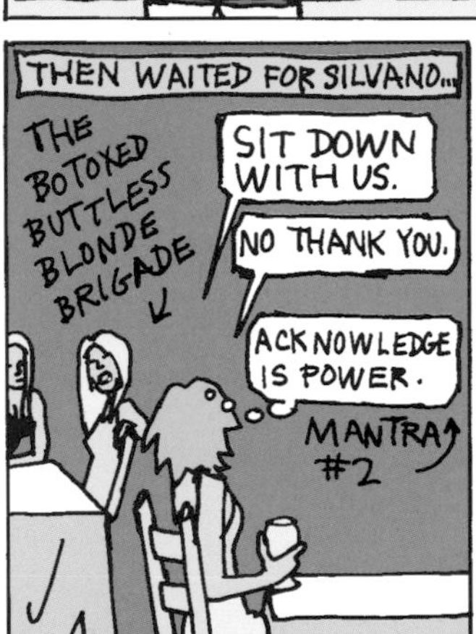
THEN WAITED FOR SILVANO...
THE BOTOXED BUTTLESS BLONDE BRIGADE
SIT DOWN WITH US.
NO THANK YOU.
ACKNOWLEDGE IS POWER.
MANTRA #2

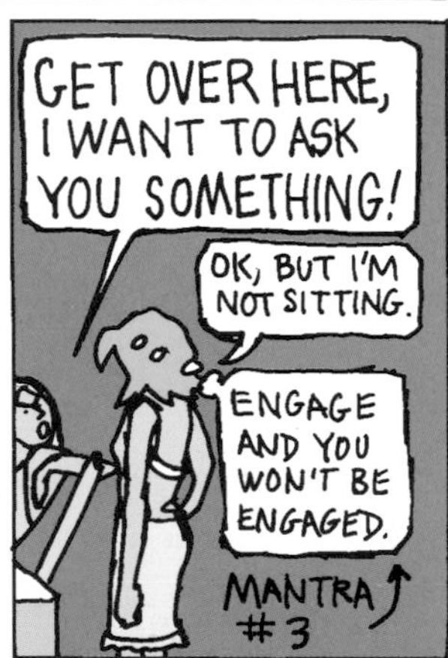
GET OVER HERE, I WANT TO ASK YOU SOMETHING!
OK, BUT I'M NOT SITTING.
ENGAGE AND YOU WON'T BE ENGAGED.
MANTRA #3

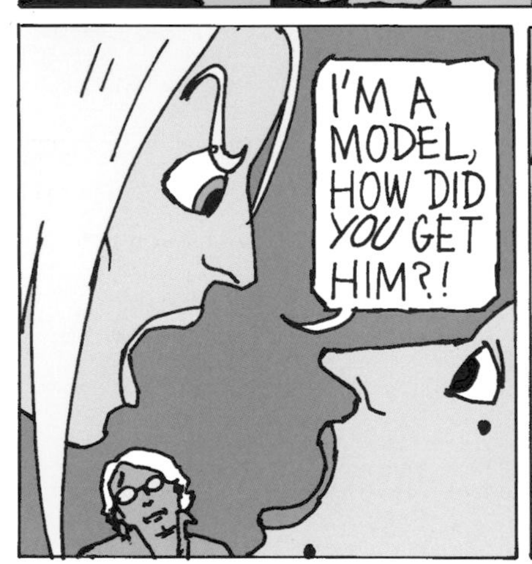
I'M A MODEL, HOW DID YOU GET HIM?!

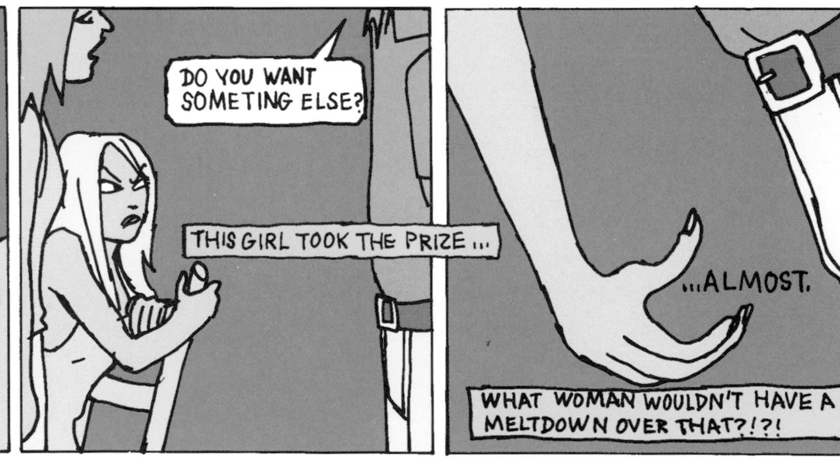
DO YOU WANT SOMETING ELSE?
THIS GIRL TOOK THE PRIZE...
...ALMOST.
WHAT WOMAN WOULDN'T HAVE A MELTDOWN OVER THAT?!?!

HOW CAN YOU DO THAT
TO ANOTHER WOMAN?!

ALL MY FRIENDS ARE *MODELS* AND WE'VE BEEN HITTING ON SILVANO FOR *15 YEARS!* HOW DID *YOU* GET HIM?

HOW DID I GET HIM?
RRRIP!

BY BEING A *GOOD* PERSON.
THWOP!

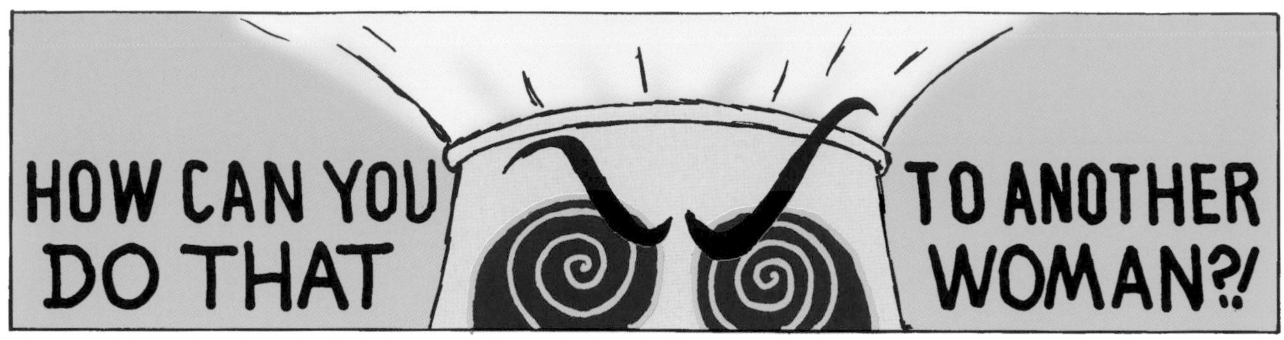

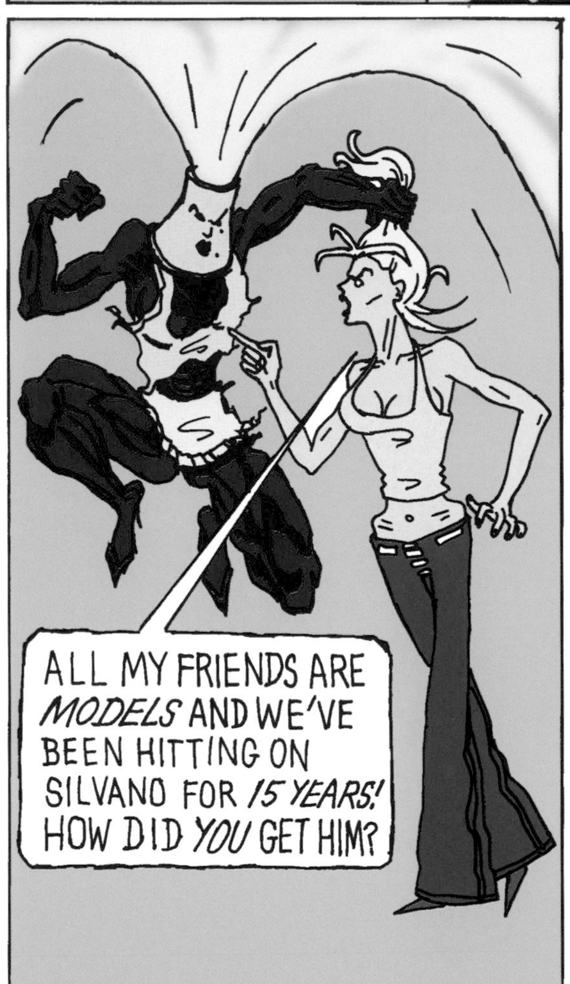

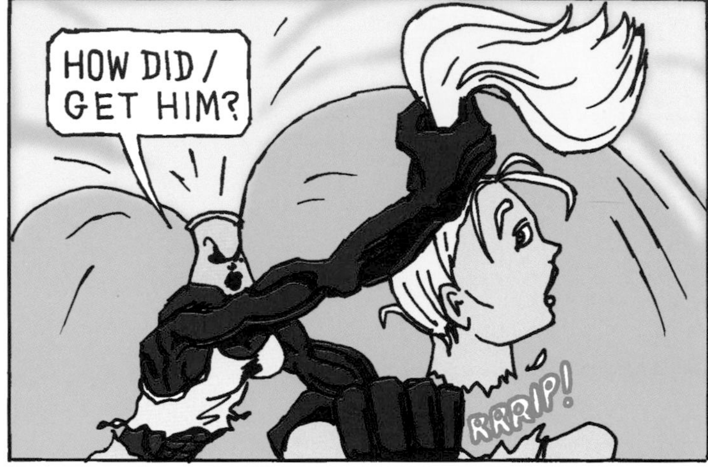

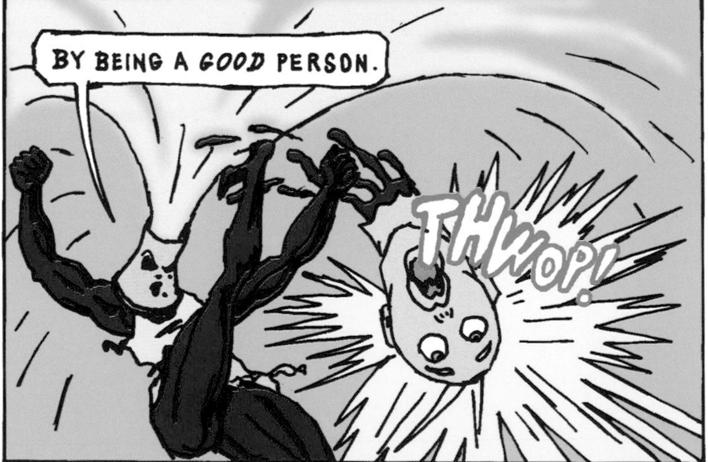

OF COURSE I REALLY DIDN'T DO THIS, BUT I DID *THINK* ABOUT IT.

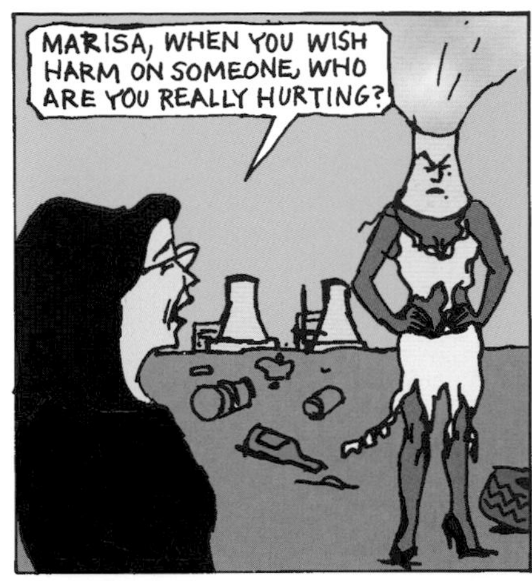
MARISA, WHEN YOU WISH HARM ON SOMEONE, WHO ARE YOU REALLY HURTING?
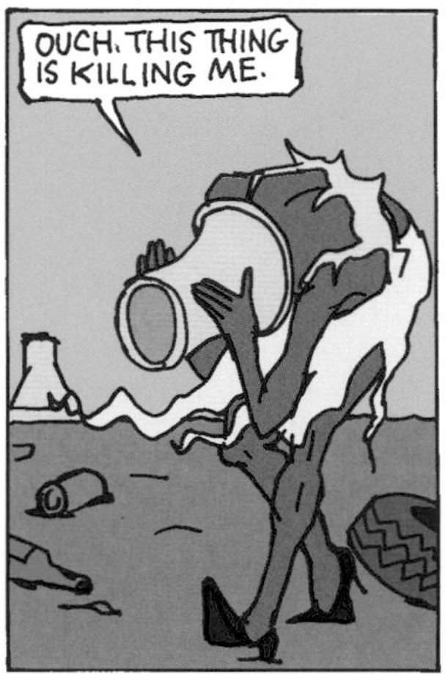
OUCH. THIS THING IS KILLING ME.
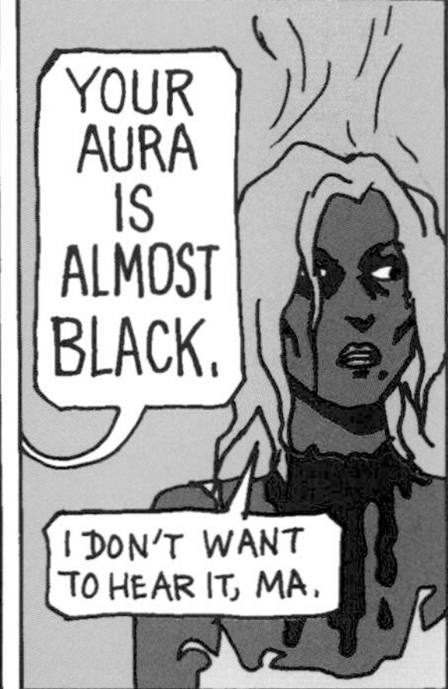
YOUR AURA IS ALMOST BLACK.
I DON'T WANT TO HEAR IT, MA.
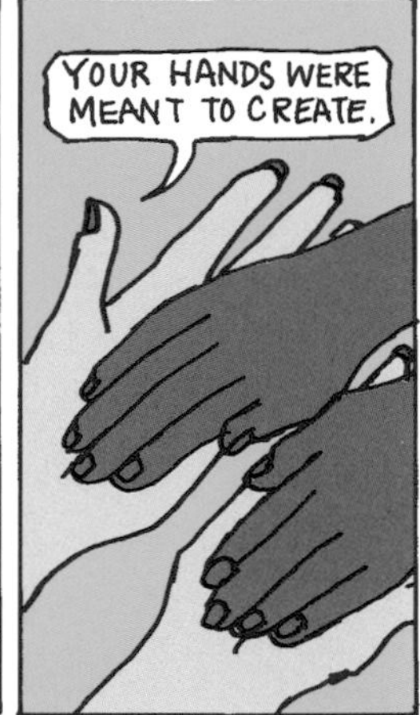
YOUR HANDS WERE MEANT TO CREATE.
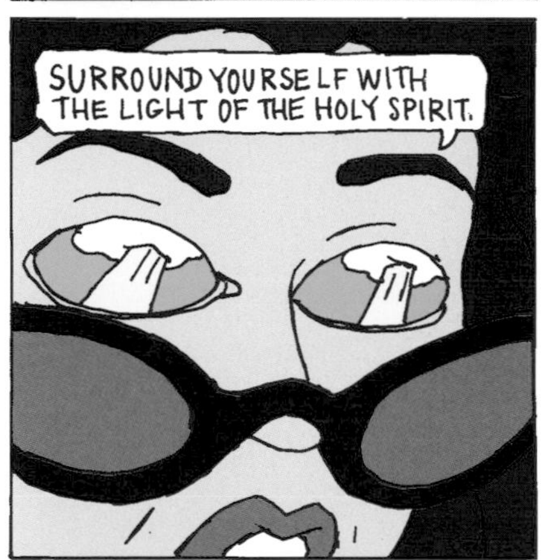
SURROUND YOURSELF WITH THE LIGHT OF THE HOLY SPIRIT.
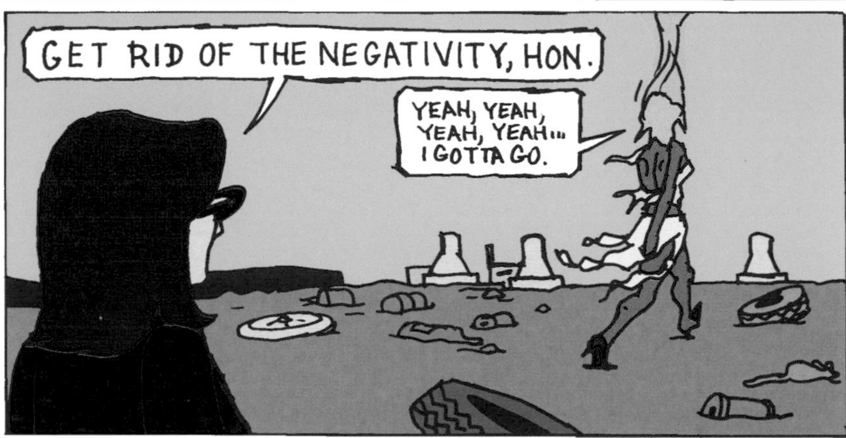
GET RID OF THE NEGATIVITY, HON.
YEAH, YEAH, YEAH, YEAH... I GOTTA GO.
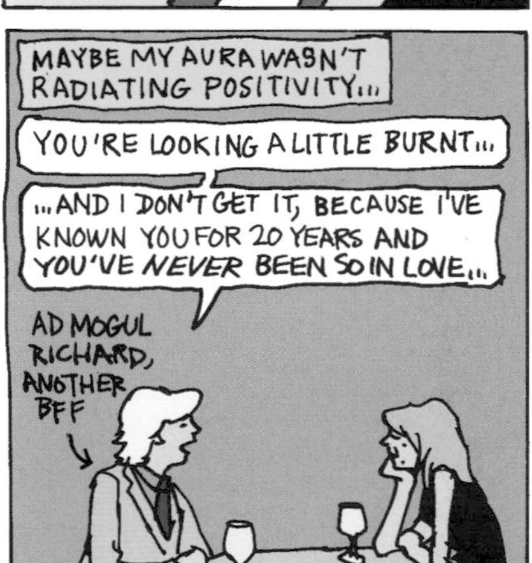
MAYBE MY AURA WASN'T RADIATING POSITIVITY...
YOU'RE LOOKING A LITTLE BURNT...
...AND I DON'T GET IT, BECAUSE I'VE KNOWN YOU FOR 20 YEARS AND YOU'VE NEVER BEEN SO IN LOVE...
AD MOGUL RICHARD, ANOTHER BFF
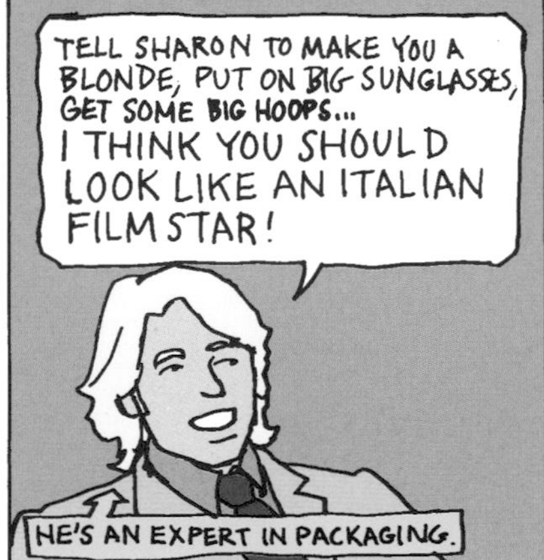
TELL SHARON TO MAKE YOU A BLONDE, PUT ON BIG SUNGLASSES, GET SOME BIG HOOPS... I THINK YOU SHOULD LOOK LIKE AN ITALIAN FILM STAR!
HE'S AN EXPERT IN PACKAGING.
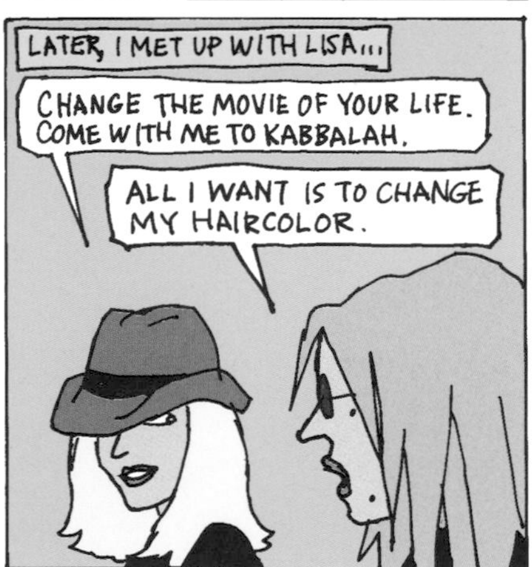
LATER, I MET UP WITH LISA...
CHANGE THE MOVIE OF YOUR LIFE. COME WITH ME TO KABBALAH.
ALL I WANT IS TO CHANGE MY HAIRCOLOR.

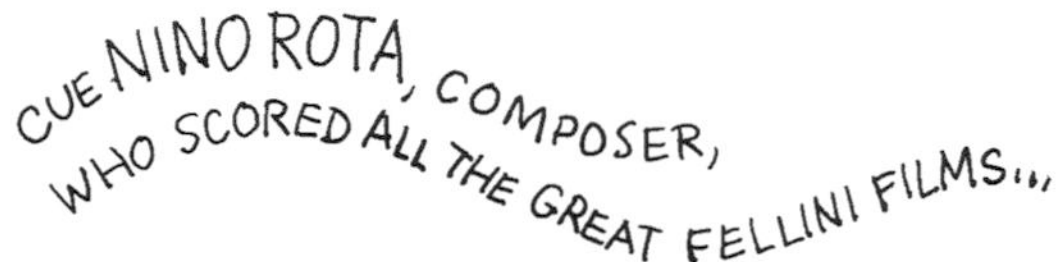
BUT MY MOVIE SEEMED TO HAVE A LIFE OF ITS OWN, AND I WAS REALLY LUCKY...
CUE NINO ROTA, COMPOSER, WHO SCORED ALL THE GREAT FELLINI FILMS...

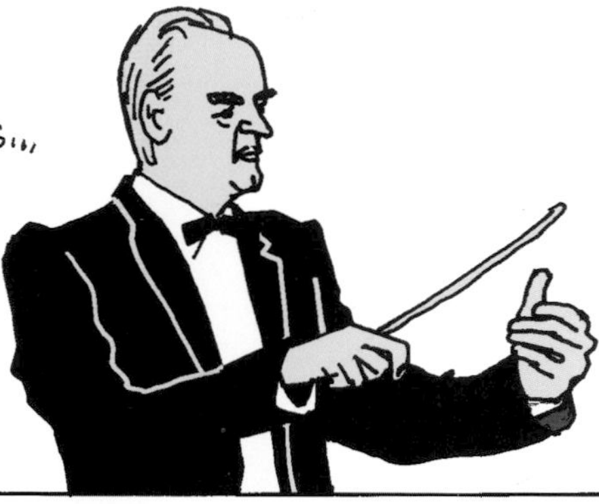
LIGHTS DOWN, CAMERA ON, LET'S ROLL PICTURE...

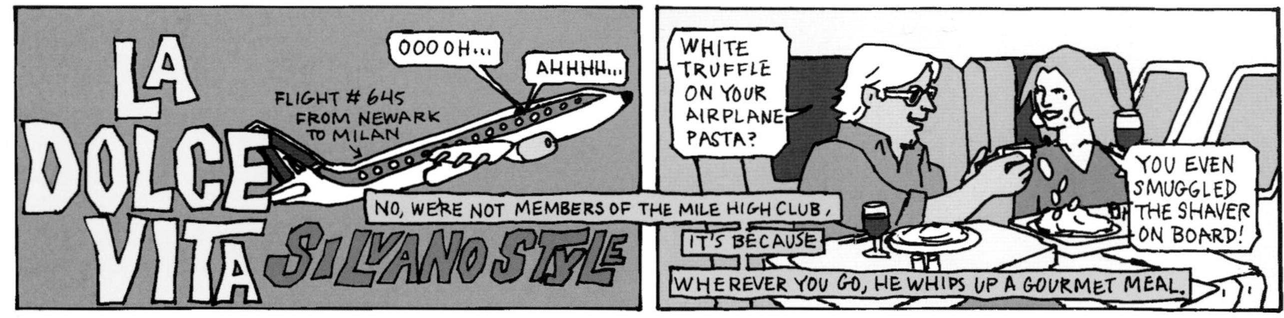
LA DOLCE VITA
SILVANO STYLE
FLIGHT # 645 FROM NEWARK TO MILAN
OOOOH...
AHHHH...
NO, WE'RE NOT MEMBERS OF THE MILE HIGH CLUB,
IT'S BECAUSE
WHITE TRUFFLE ON YOUR AIRPLANE PASTA?
YOU EVEN SMUGGLED THE SHAVER ON BOARD!
WHEREVER YOU GO, HE WHIPS UP A GOURMET MEAL.

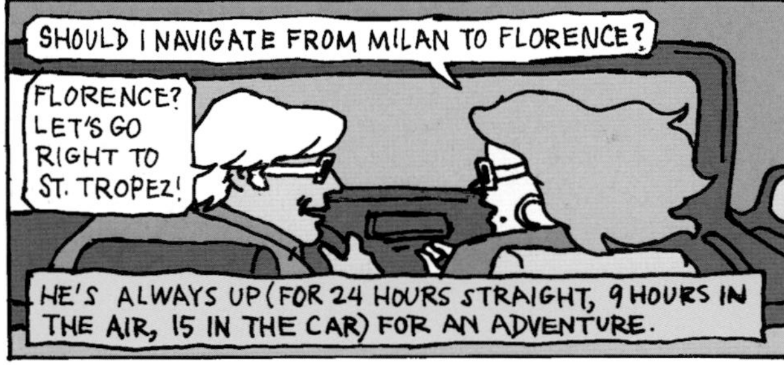
SHOULD I NAVIGATE FROM MILAN TO FLORENCE?
FLORENCE? LET'S GO RIGHT TO ST. TROPEZ!
HE'S ALWAYS UP (FOR 24 HOURS STRAIGHT, 9 HOURS IN THE AIR, 15 IN THE CAR) FOR AN ADVENTURE.

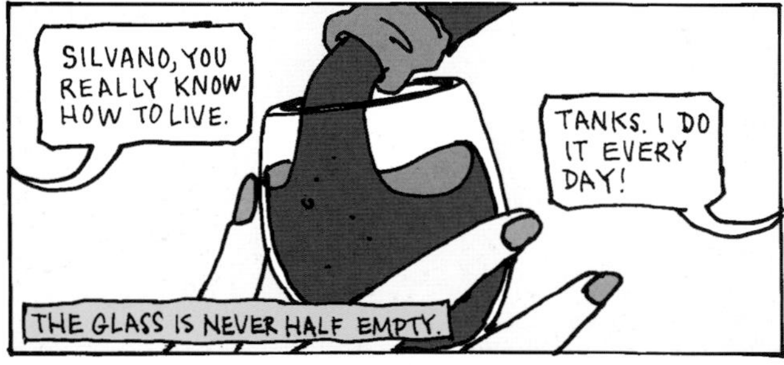
SILVANO, YOU REALLY KNOW HOW TO LIVE.
TANKS. I DO IT EVERY DAY!
THE GLASS IS NEVER HALF EMPTY.

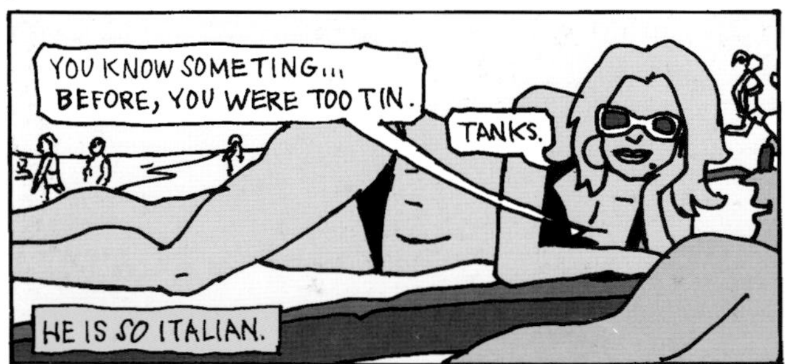
YOU KNOW SOMETING... BEFORE, YOU WERE TOO TIN.
TANKS.
HE IS SO ITALIAN.

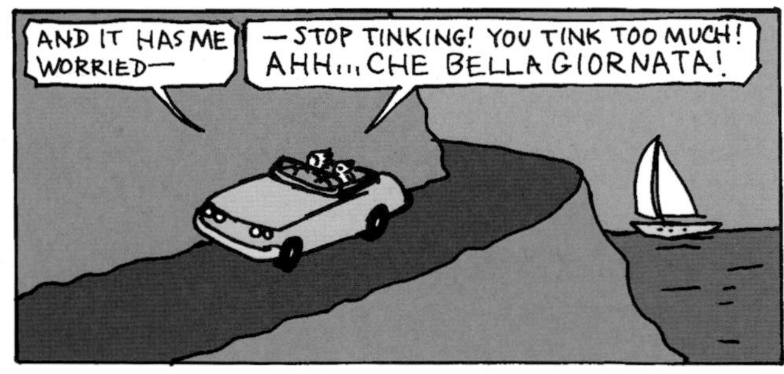
AND IT HAS ME WORRIED—
—STOP TINKING! YOU TINK TOO MUCH! AHH... CHE BELLA GIORNATA!

ITALIAN MOVIE STAR
PAPARAZZI
POP!
POP!
POP!
POPPING OFF
WHY DO YOU LOVE ME?
BECAUSE YOU ARE YOU.
ALLORA... WHAT SHOULD WE EAT?
DID I SAY HE IS SO ITALIAN?

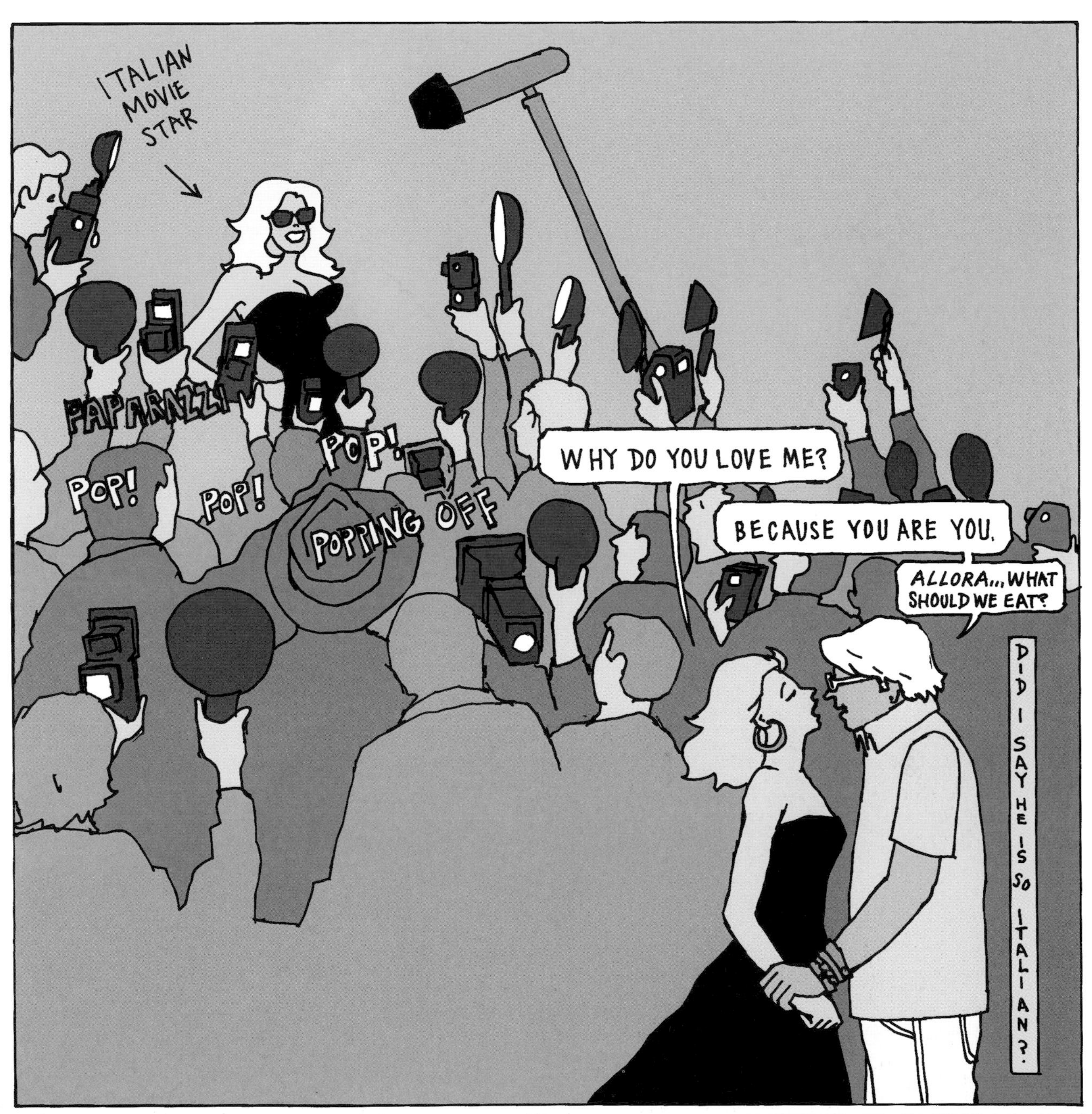

I HAVE TO ADMIT, I DID LOVE BEING SILVANO'S LEADING LADY...

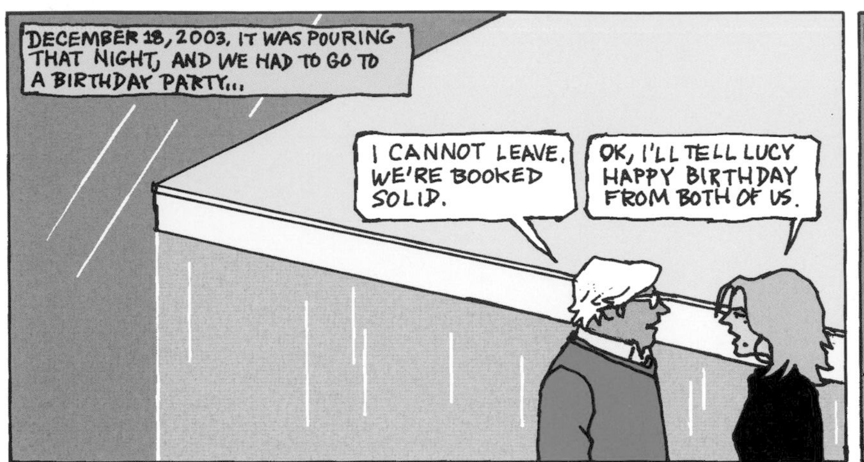
DECEMBER 18, 2003, IT WAS POURING THAT NIGHT, AND WE HAD TO GO TO A BIRTHDAY PARTY...
I CANNOT LEAVE. WE'RE BOOKED SOLID.
OK, I'LL TELL LUCY HAPPY BIRTHDAY FROM BOTH OF US.

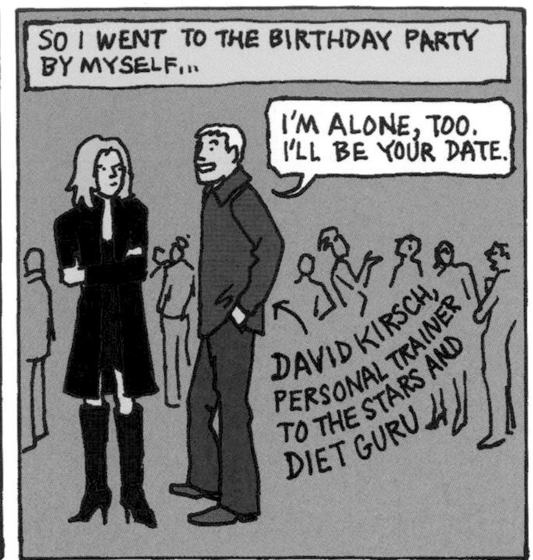
SO I WENT TO THE BIRTHDAY PARTY BY MYSELF...
I'M ALONE, TOO. I'LL BE YOUR DATE.
DAVID KIRSCH, PERSONAL TRAINER TO THE STARS AND DIET GURU

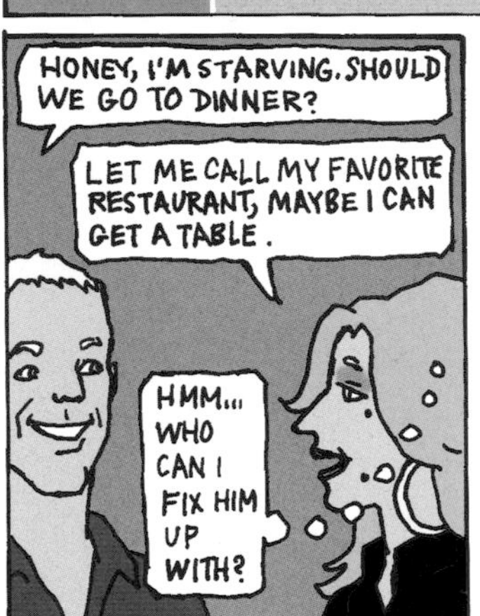
HONEY, I'M STARVING. SHOULD WE GO TO DINNER?
LET ME CALL MY FAVORITE RESTAURANT, MAYBE I CAN GET A TABLE.
HMM... WHO CAN I FIX HIM UP WITH?

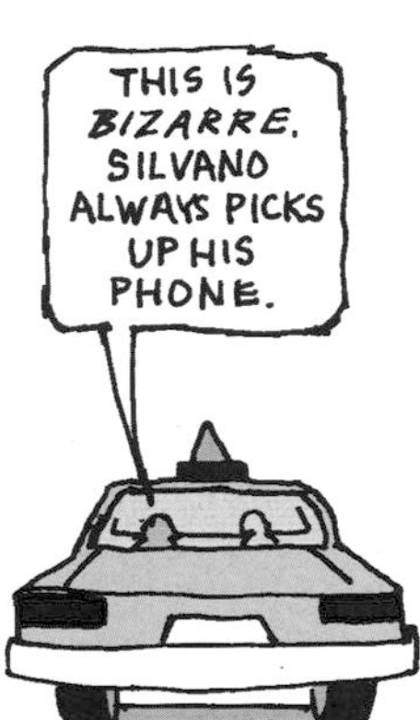
THIS IS *BIZARRE*. SILVANO ALWAYS PICKS UP HIS PHONE.

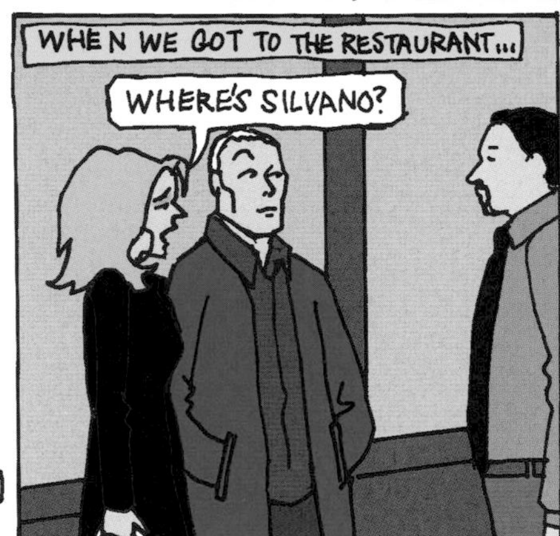
WHEN WE GOT TO THE RESTAURANT...
WHERE'S SILVANO?

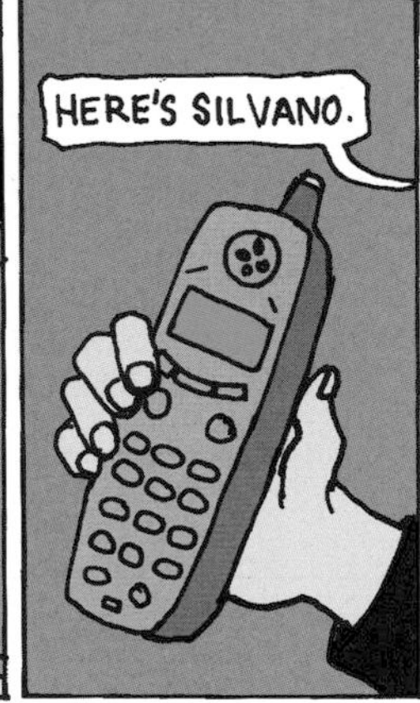
HERE'S SILVANO.

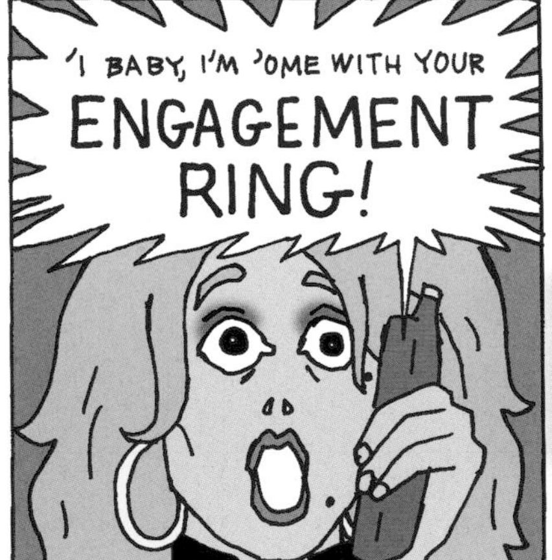
'I BABY, I'M 'OME WITH YOUR ENGAGEMENT RING!

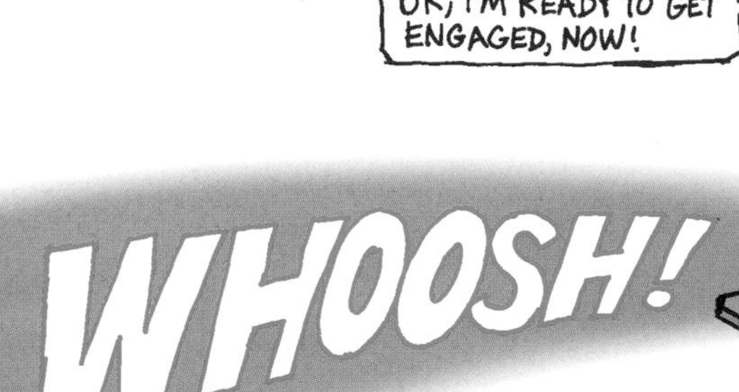
WHOOSH!

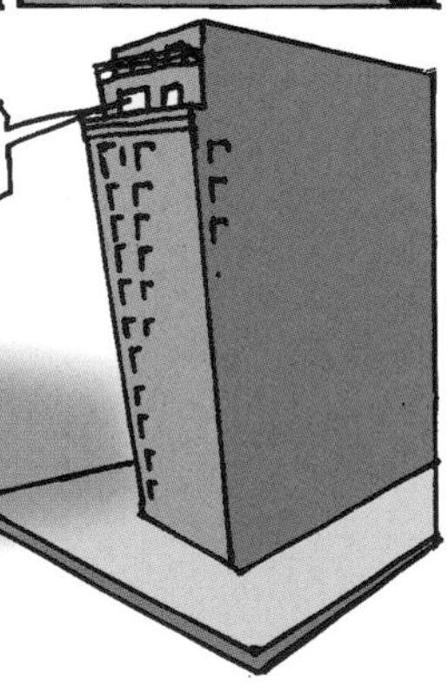
OK, I'M READY TO GET ENGAGED, NOW!

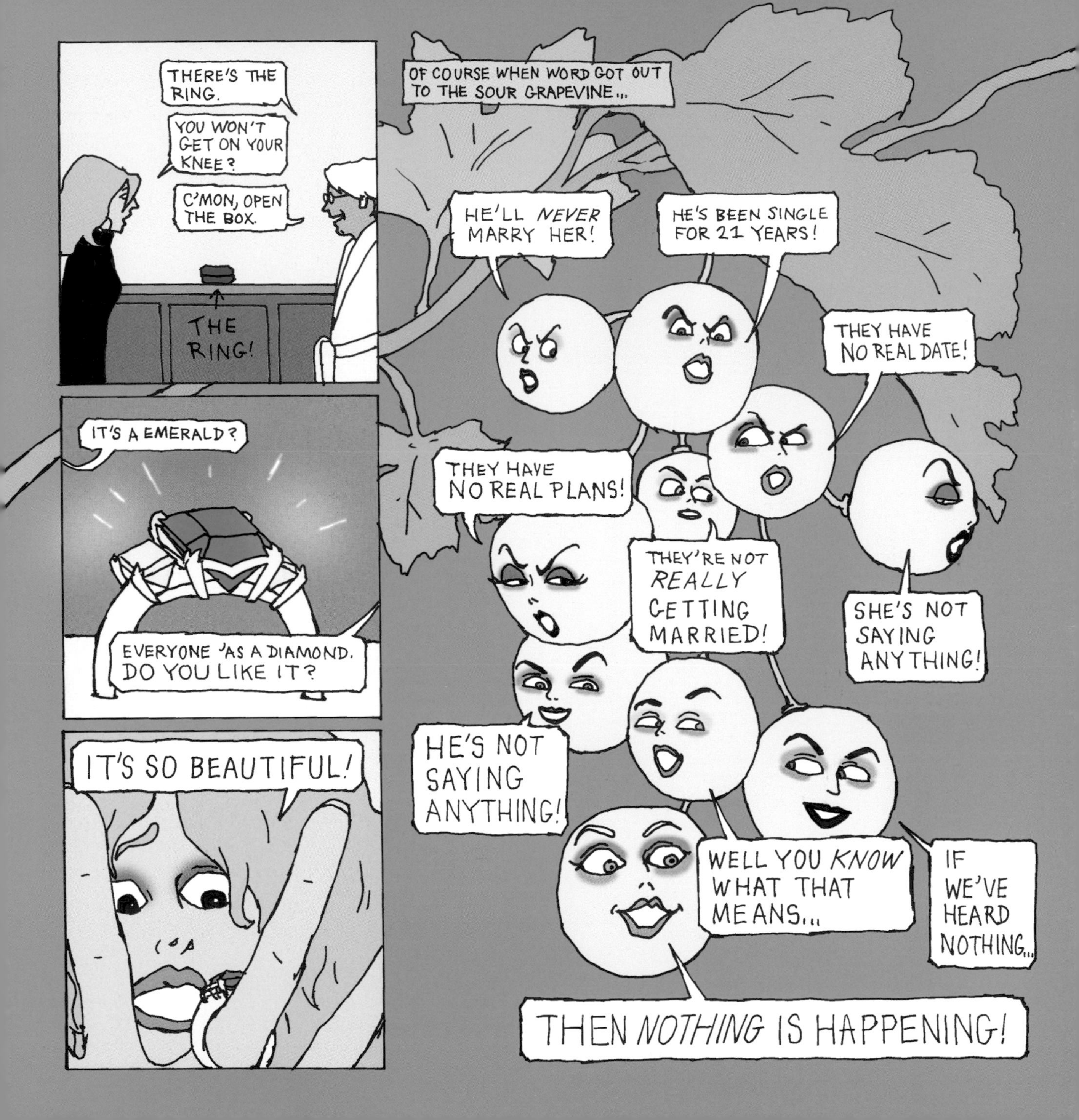

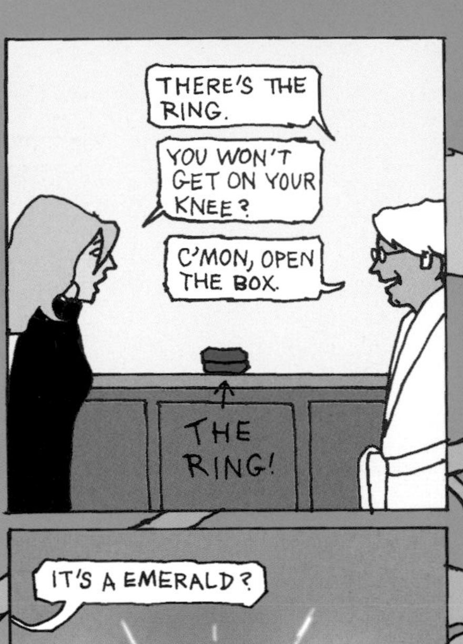
THERE'S THE RING.
YOU WON'T GET ON YOUR KNEE?
C'MON, OPEN THE BOX.
THE RING!

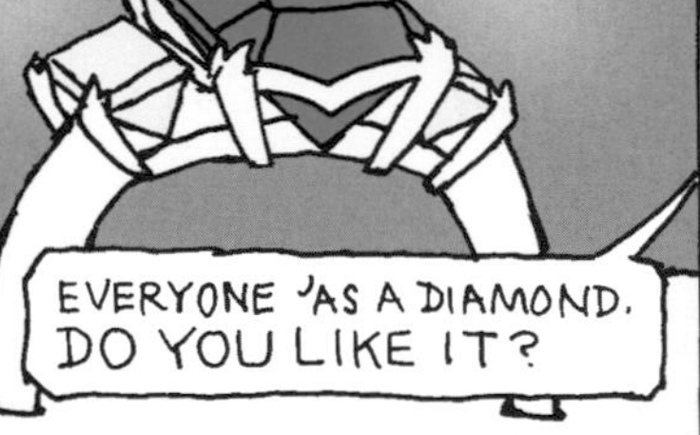
IT'S A EMERALD?
EVERYONE 'AS A DIAMOND. DO YOU LIKE IT?

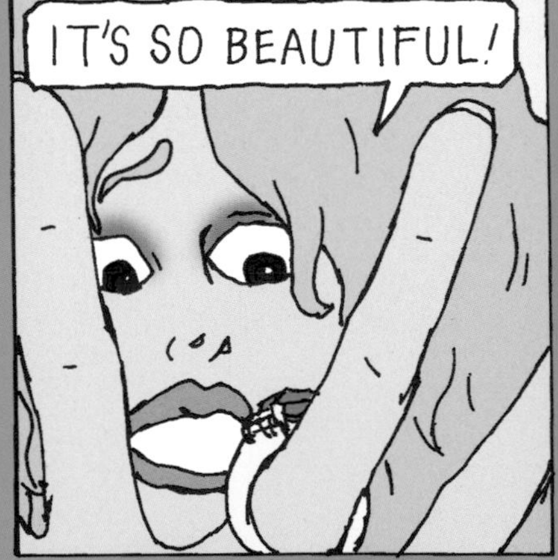
IT'S SO BEAUTIFUL!

OF COURSE WHEN WORD GOT OUT TO THE SOUR GRAPEVINE...
HE'LL *NEVER* MARRY HER!
HE'S BEEN SINGLE FOR 21 YEARS!
THEY HAVE NO REAL DATE!
THEY HAVE NO REAL PLANS!
THEY'RE NOT *REALLY* GETTING MARRIED!
SHE'S NOT SAYING ANYTHING!
HE'S NOT SAYING ANYTHING!
WELL YOU *KNOW* WHAT THAT MEANS...
IF WE'VE HEARD NOTHING...
THEN *NOTHING* IS HAPPENING!

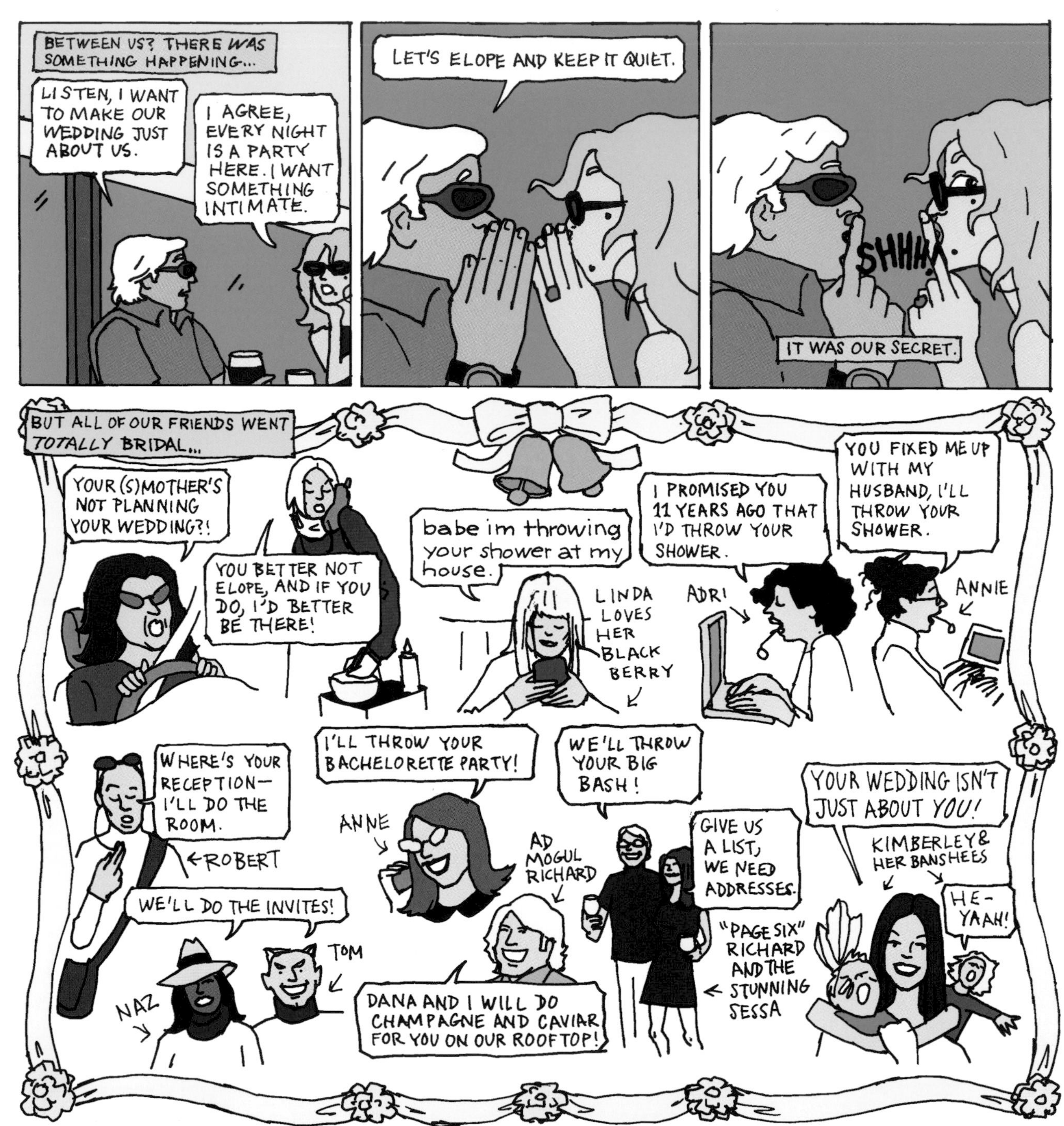
BETWEEN US? THERE WAS SOMETHING HAPPENING...
LISTEN, I WANT TO MAKE OUR WEDDING JUST ABOUT US.
I AGREE, EVERY NIGHT IS A PARTY HERE. I WANT SOMETHING INTIMATE.
LET'S ELOPE AND KEEP IT QUIET.
SHHH!
IT WAS OUR SECRET.
BUT ALL OF OUR FRIENDS WENT TOTALLY BRIDAL...
YOUR (S)MOTHER'S NOT PLANNING YOUR WEDDING?!
YOU BETTER NOT ELOPE, AND IF YOU DO, I'D BETTER BE THERE!
babe im throwing your shower at my house.
LINDA LOVES HER BLACK BERRY
I PROMISED YOU 11 YEARS AGO THAT I'D THROW YOUR SHOWER.
ADRI
YOU FIXED ME UP WITH MY HUSBAND, I'LL THROW YOUR SHOWER.
ANNIE
WHERE'S YOUR RECEPTION— I'LL DO THE ROOM.
ROBERT
WE'LL DO THE INVITES!
TOM
NAZ
I'LL THROW YOUR BACHELORETTE PARTY!
ANNE
AD MOGUL RICHARD
DANA AND I WILL DO CHAMPAGNE AND CAVIAR FOR YOU ON OUR ROOFTOP!
WE'LL THROW YOUR BIG BASH!
GIVE US A LIST, WE NEED ADDRESSES.
"PAGE SIX" RICHARD AND THE STUNNING SESSA
YOUR WEDDING ISN'T JUST ABOUT YOU!
KIMBERLEY & HER BANSHEES
HE-YAAH!

JUST WHEN WE PICKED OUR WEDDING DATE...
JUNE 11?
JUNE 11!
SHHH!
IT WAS OUR SECRET.

JUST WHEN I SOLD A FEW CARTOONS TO *THE NEW YORKER*.

JUST WHEN I PICKED OUT MY SHOES AND BAG...
THEY'RE GOING WITH A WHITE DRESS THAT I HAVEN'T FOUND YET.
BOTH BY GIUSEPPE ZANOTTI

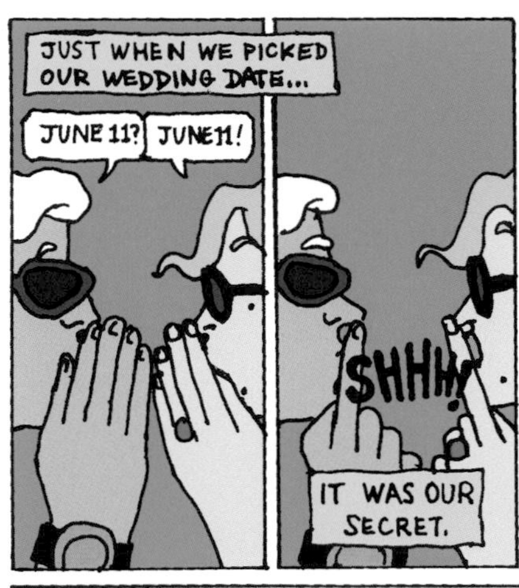

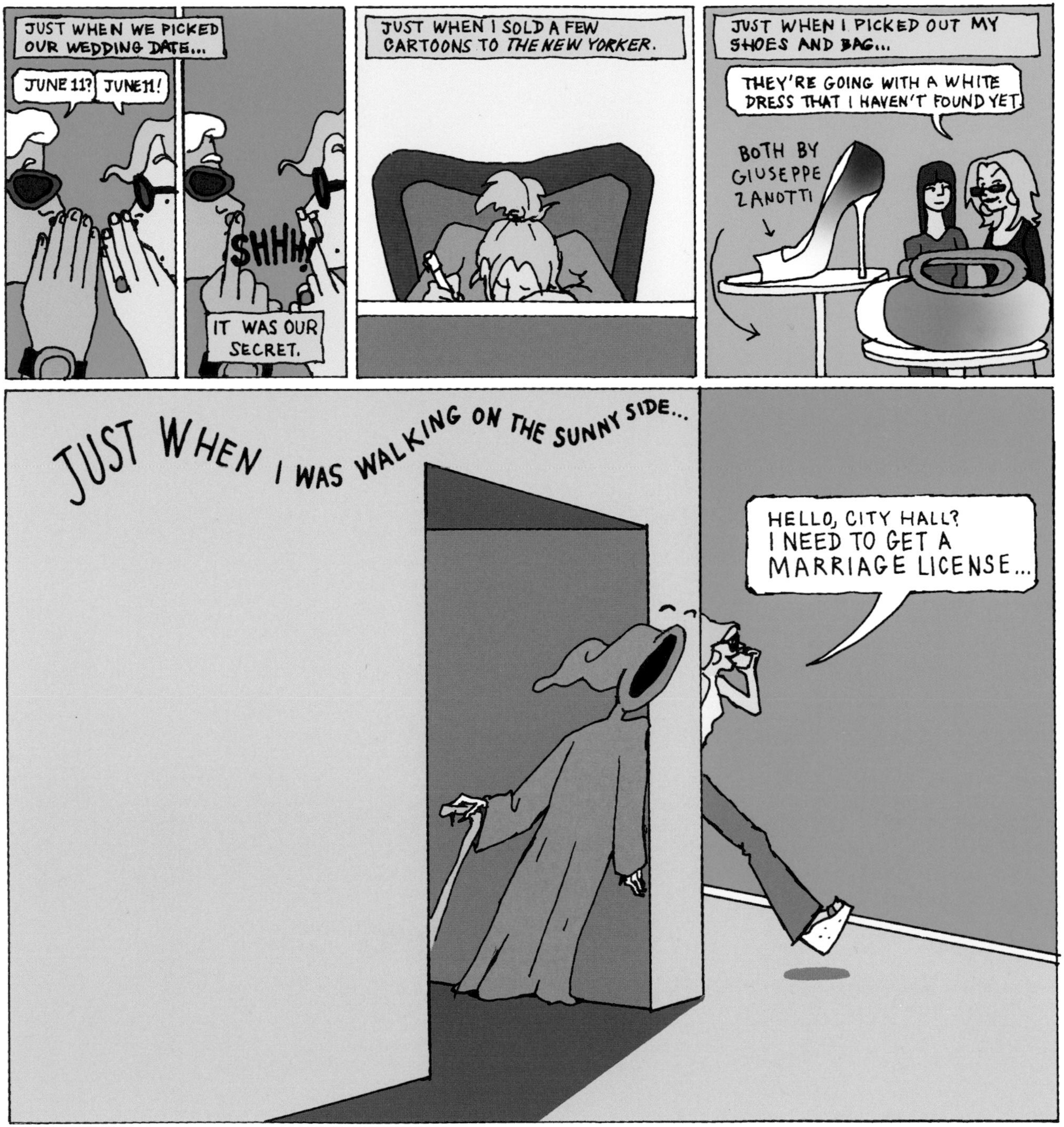

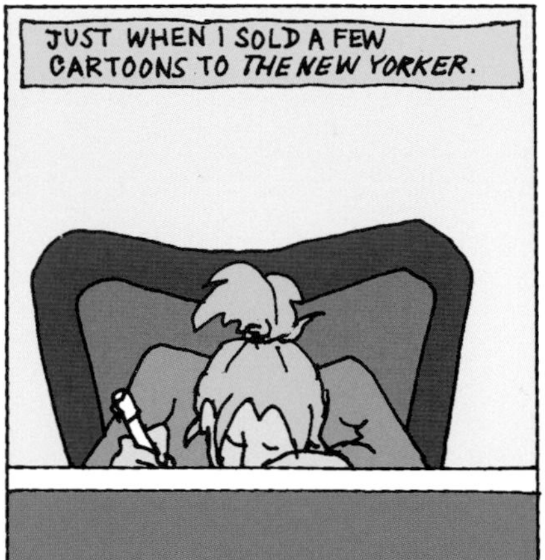

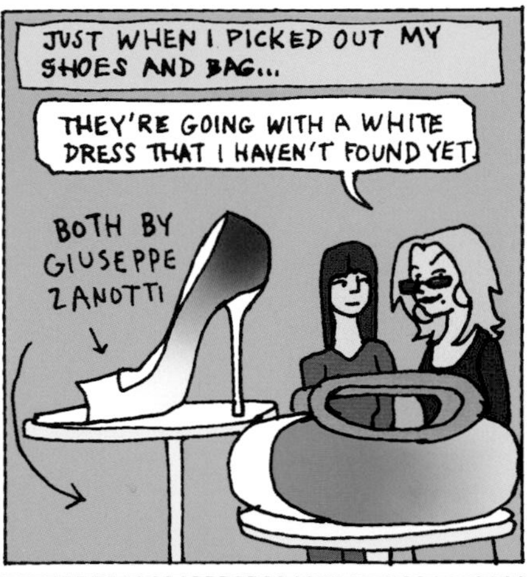

JUST WHEN I WAS WALKING ON THE SUNNY SIDE...

HELLO, CITY HALL? I NEED TO GET A MARRIAGE LICENSE...

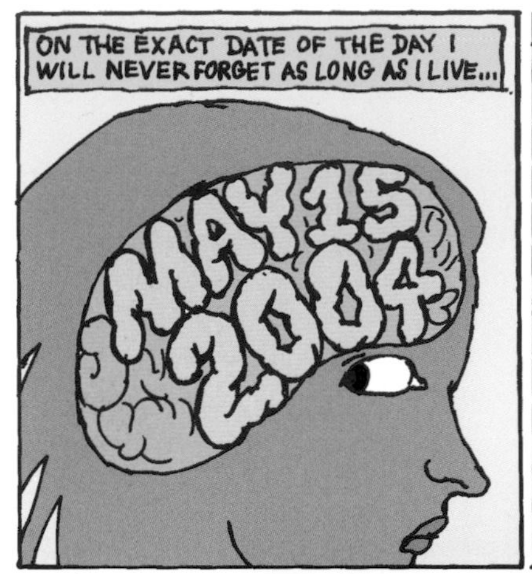

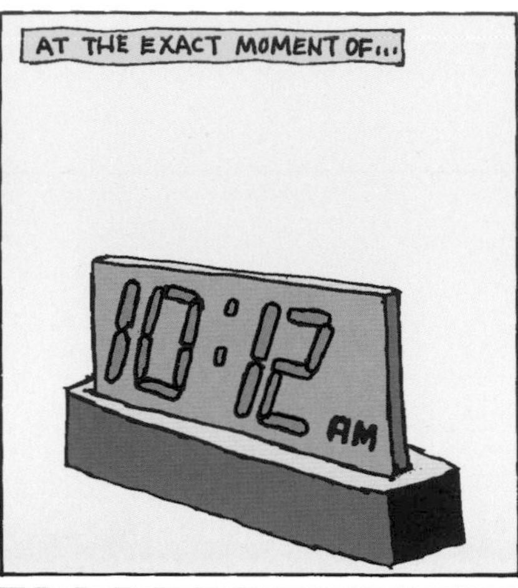

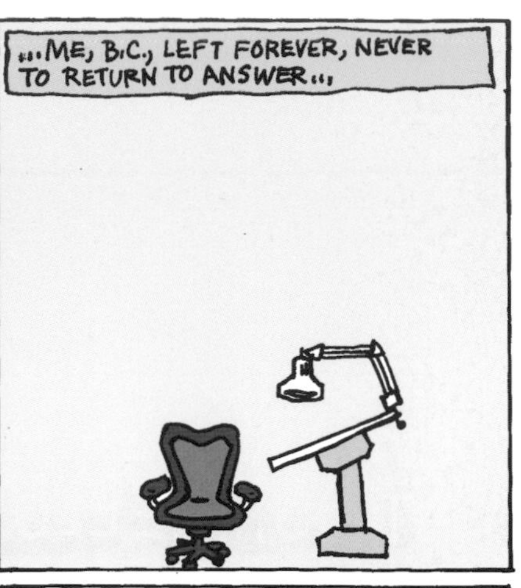

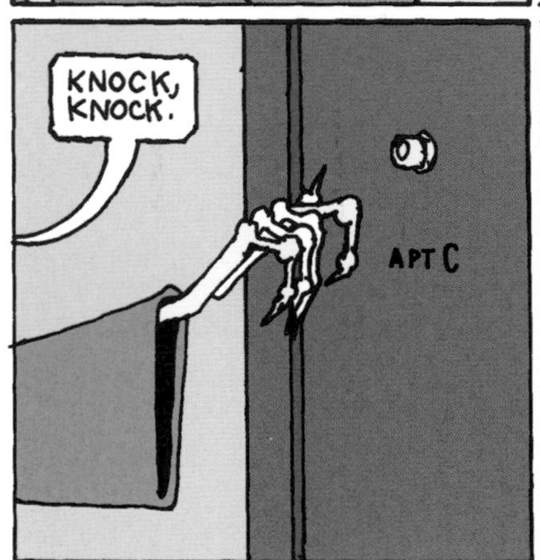

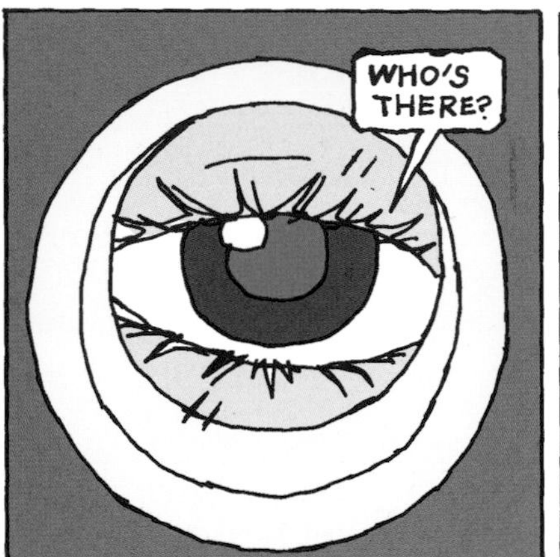

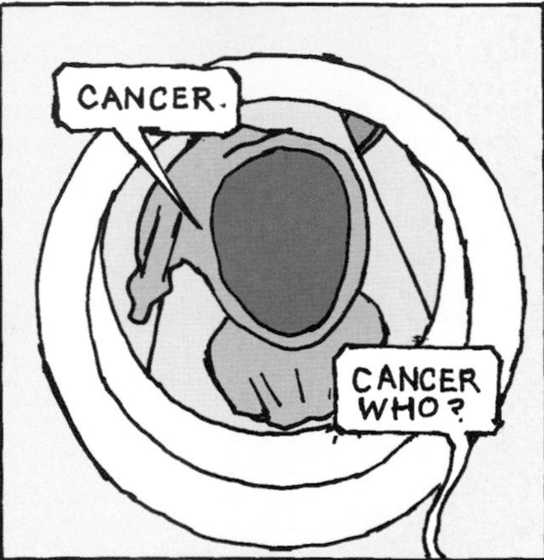

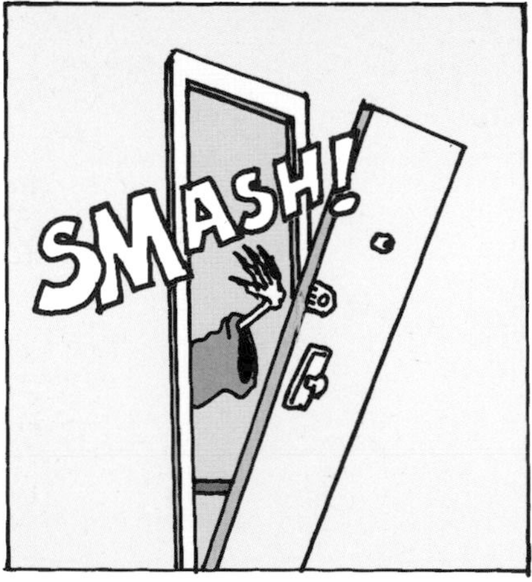

CANCER YOUR WEDDING! CANCER YOUR CAREER! CANCER YOUR LIFE!

WAS IT SOMETHING I SAID?
WAS IT SOMETHING I ATE, DRANK, SMOKED, INHALED, PUT ON, PUT INSIDE MY BODY?
WHY? WHY? WHY? WHY IS THIS HAPPENING NOW, JUST WHEN I'M ABOUT TO GO TO CITY HALL IN 3 WEEKS TO GET MARRIED FOR THE FIRST TIME AT 43...
AT 43...HELLO UP THERE...
THIS IS *KIND* OF A BIG MOMENT FOR ME...

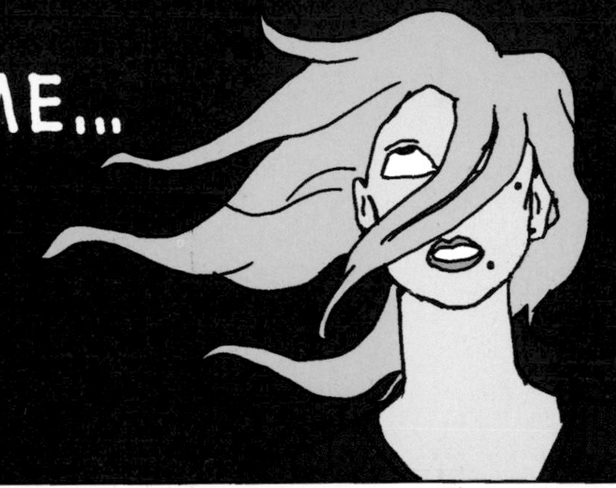

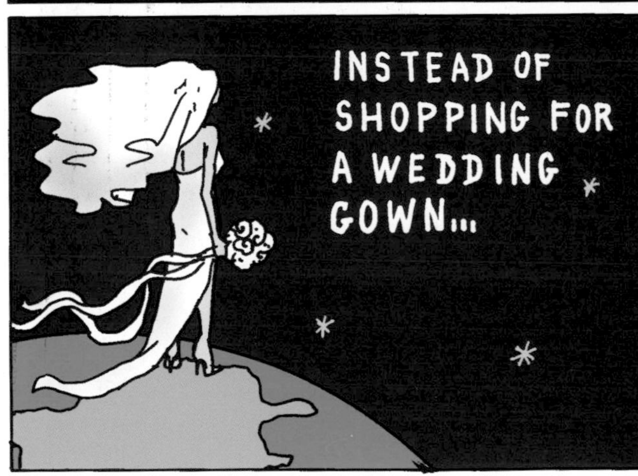

INSTEAD OF SHOPPING FOR A WEDDING GOWN...

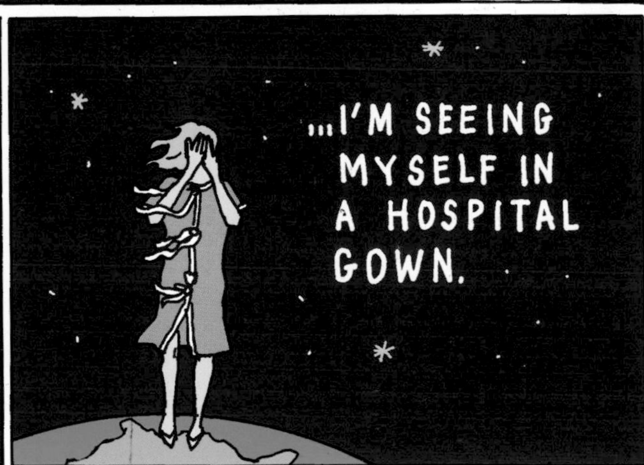

...I'M SEEING MYSELF IN A HOSPITAL GOWN.

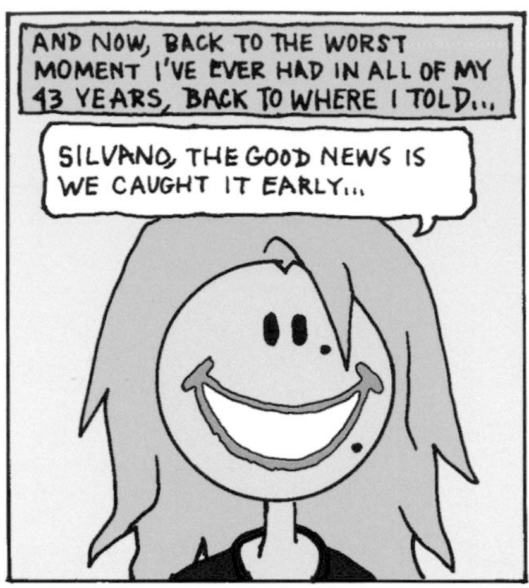
AND NOW, BACK TO THE WORST MOMENT I'VE EVER HAD IN ALL OF MY 43 YEARS, BACK TO WHERE I TOLD...
SILVANO, THE GOOD NEWS IS WE CAUGHT IT EARLY...

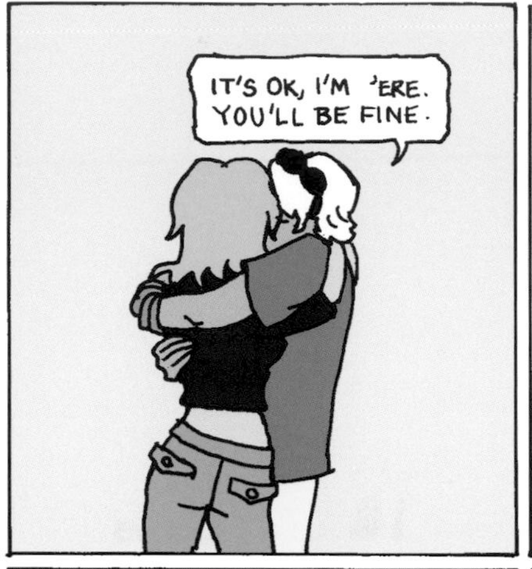
IT'S OK, I'M 'ERE. YOU'LL BE FINE.

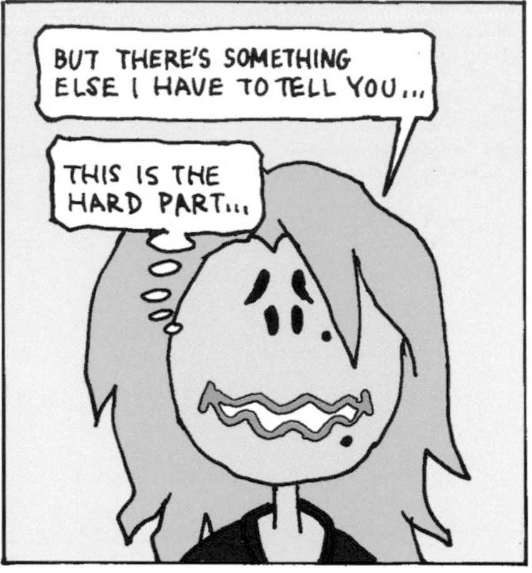
BUT THERE'S SOMETHING ELSE I HAVE TO TELL YOU...
THIS IS THE HARD PART...

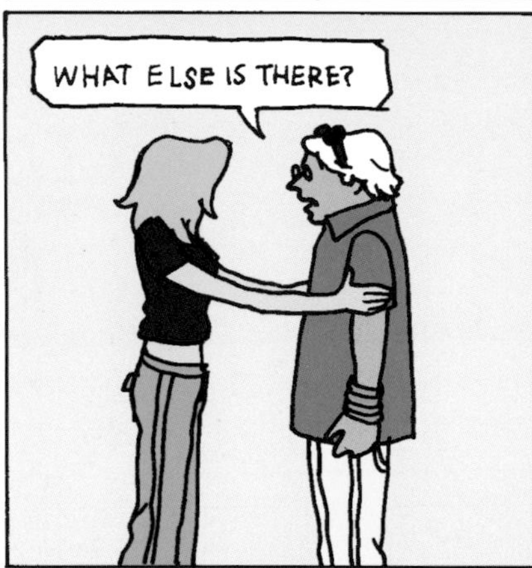
WHAT ELSE IS THERE?

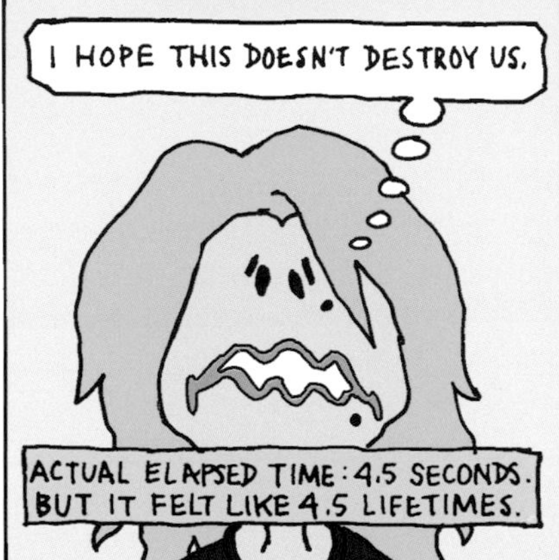
I HOPE THIS DOESN'T DESTROY US.
ACTUAL ELAPSED TIME: 4.5 SECONDS. BUT IT FELT LIKE 4.5 LIFETIMES.

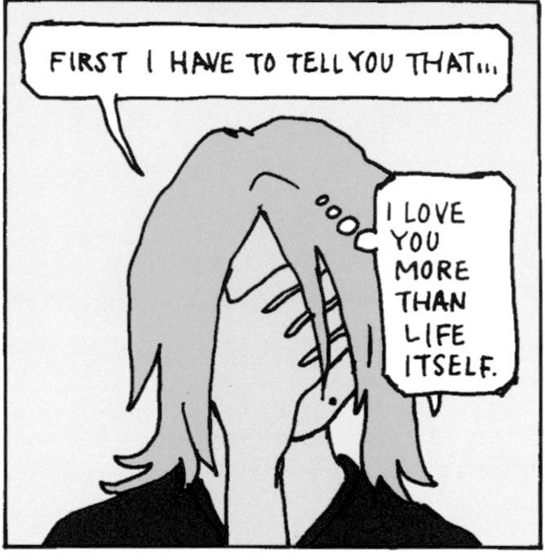
FIRST I HAVE TO TELL YOU THAT...
I LOVE YOU MORE THAN LIFE ITSELF.

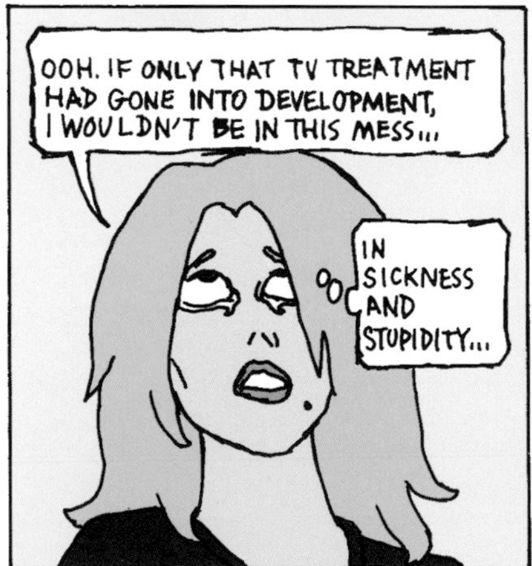
OOH. IF ONLY THAT TV TREATMENT HAD GONE INTO DEVELOPMENT, I WOULDN'T BE IN THIS MESS...
IN SICKNESS AND STUPIDITY...

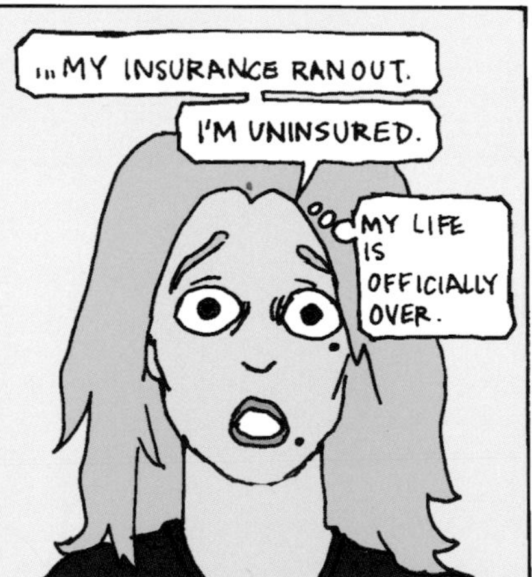
...MY INSURANCE RAN OUT.
I'M UNINSURED.
MY LIFE IS OFFICIALLY OVER.

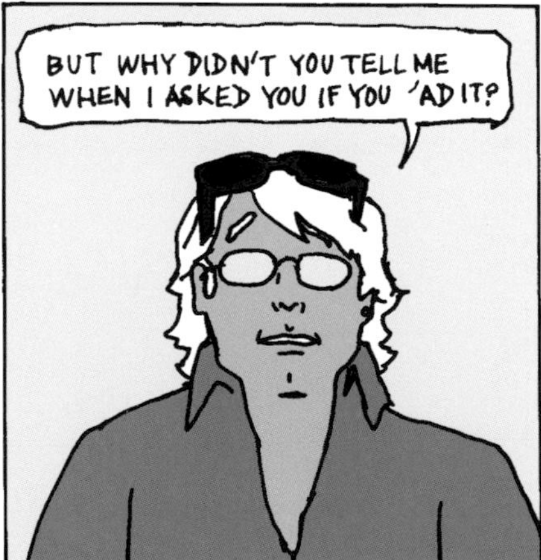
BUT WHY DIDN'T YOU TELL ME WHEN I ASKED YOU IF YOU 'AD IT?

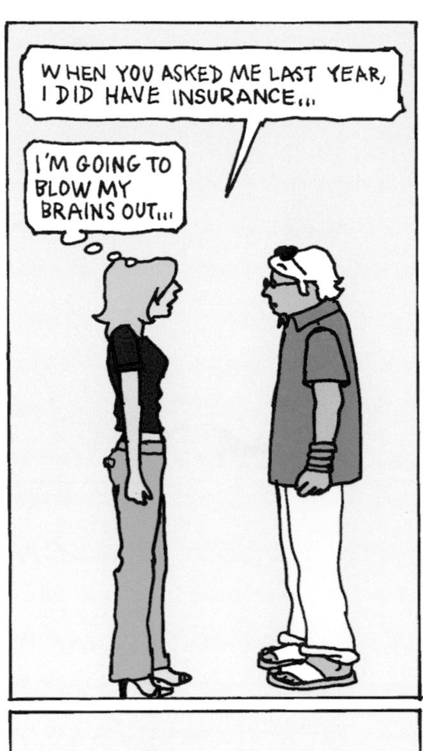
WHEN YOU ASKED ME LAST YEAR, I DID HAVE INSURANCE...
I'M GOING TO BLOW MY BRAINS OUT...

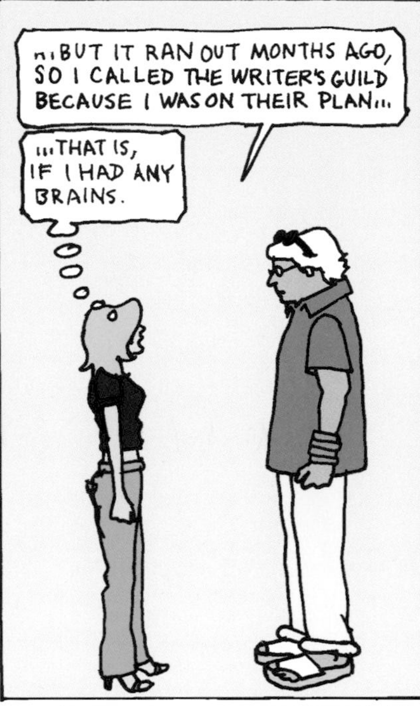
...BUT IT RAN OUT MONTHS AGO, SO I CALLED THE WRITER'S GUILD BECAUSE I WAS ON THEIR PLAN...
...THAT IS, IF I HAD ANY BRAINS.

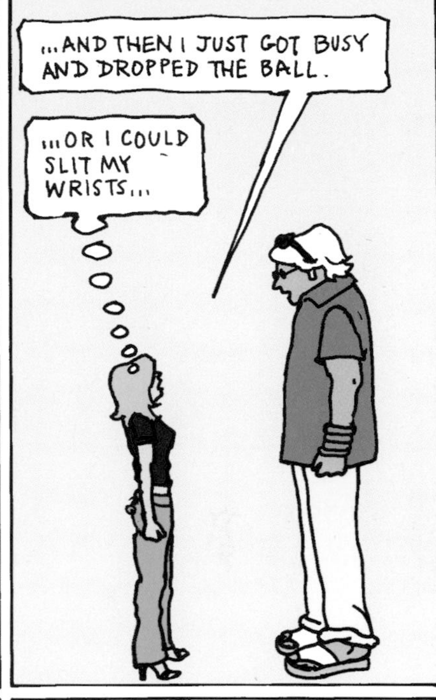
...AND THEN I JUST GOT BUSY AND DROPPED THE BALL.
...OR I COULD SLIT MY WRISTS...

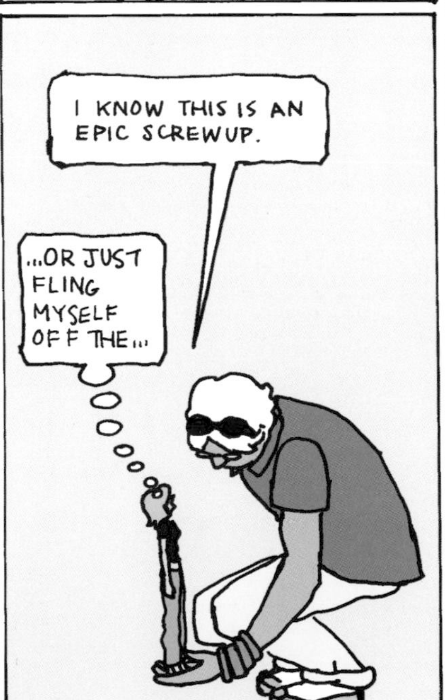
I KNOW THIS IS AN EPIC SCREWUP.
...OR JUST FLING MYSELF OFF THE...

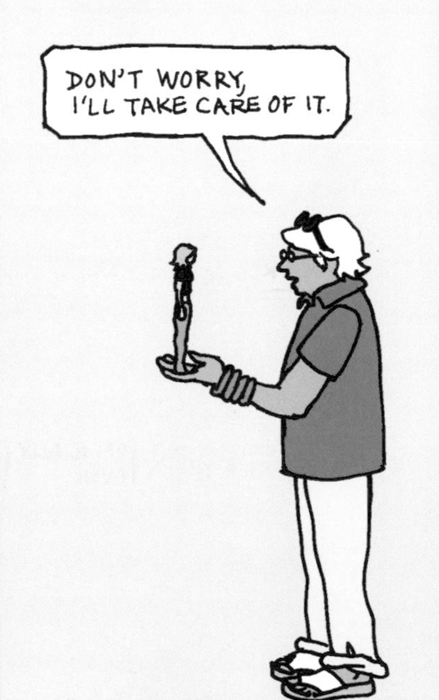
DON'T WORRY, I'LL TAKE CARE OF IT.

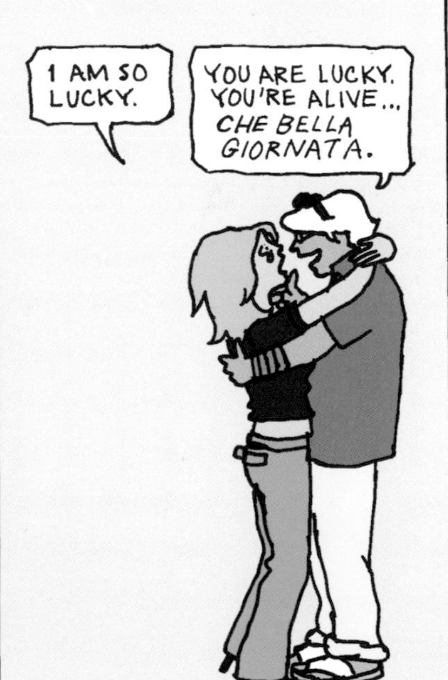
I AM SO LUCKY.
YOU ARE LUCKY. YOU'RE ALIVE... CHE BELLA GIORNATA.

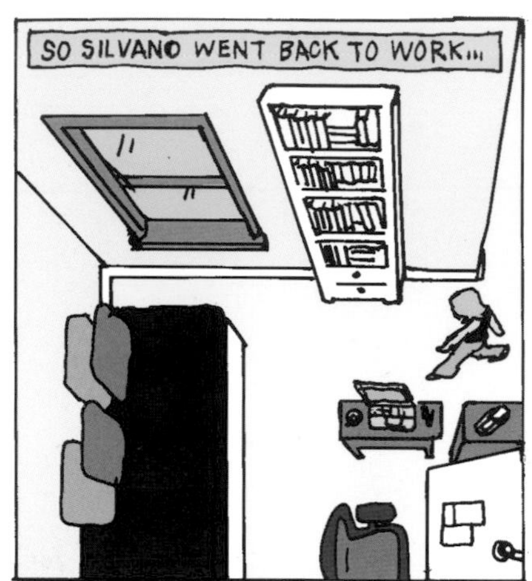

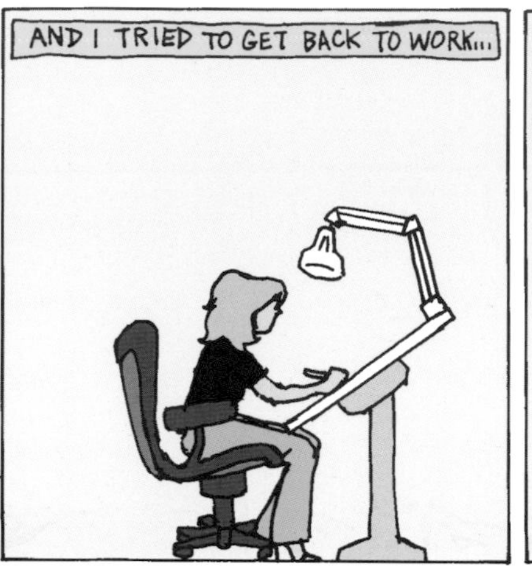

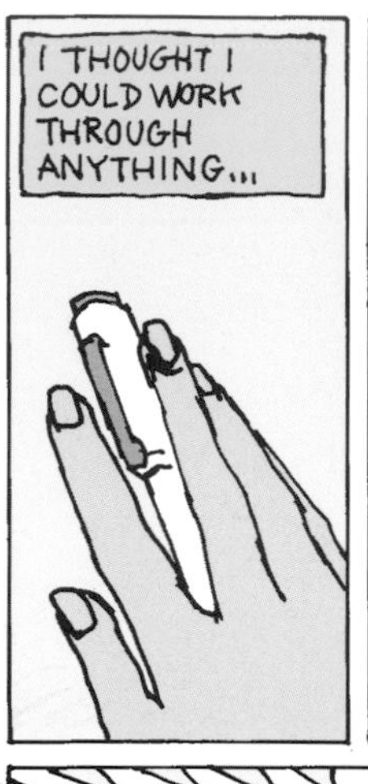

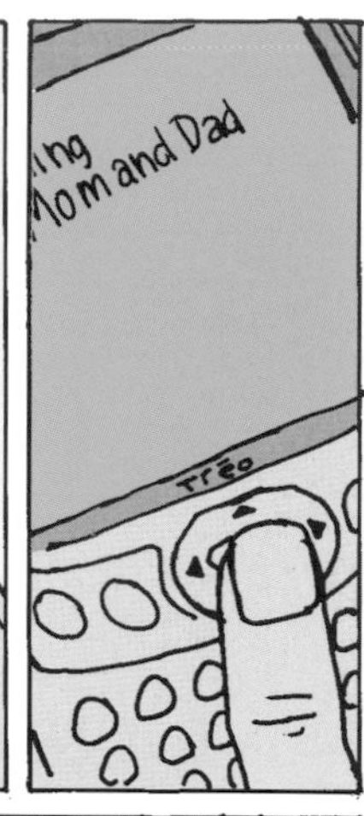

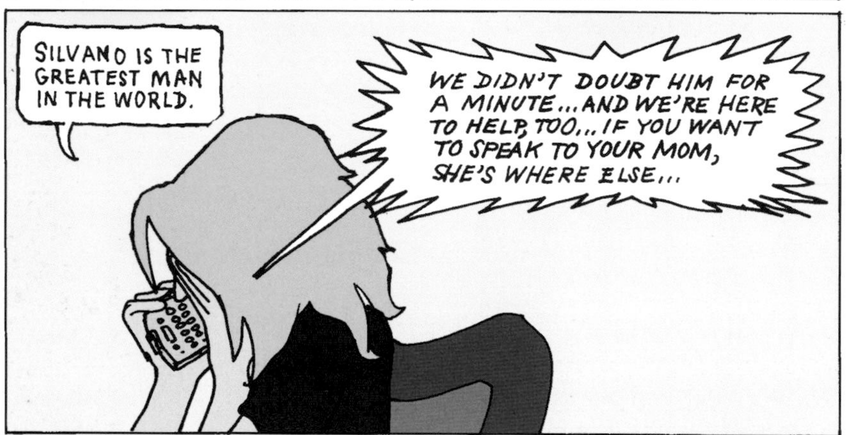

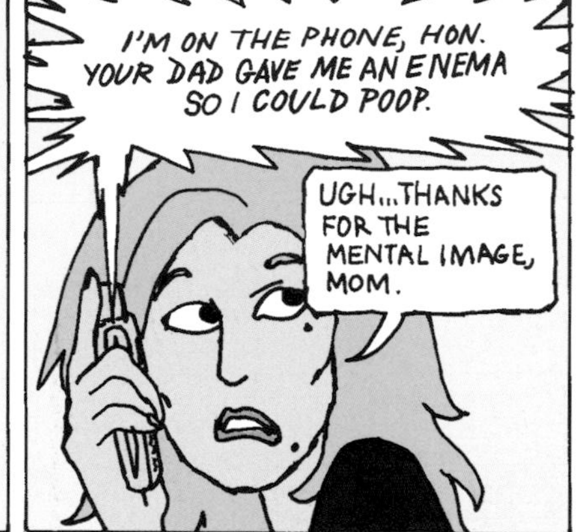

THEN I PHONED MY GAL PALS AND GAVE THEM THE SENSATIONAL SCOOP.

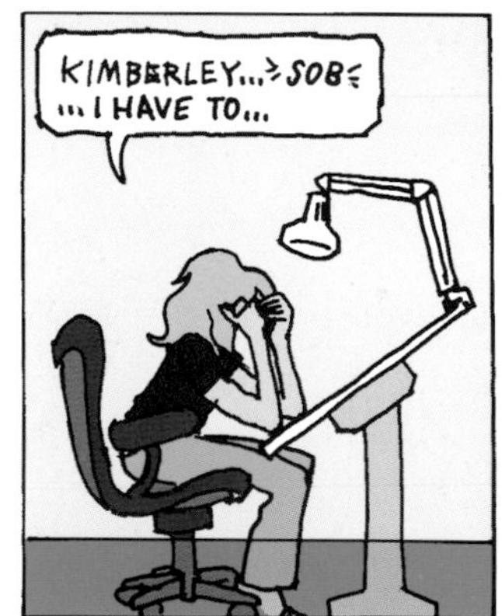

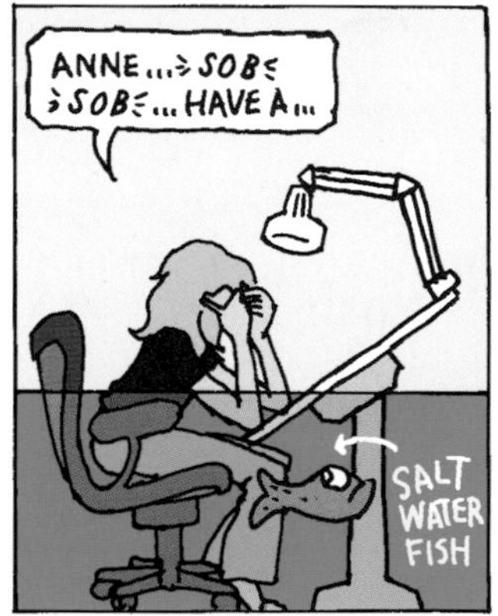

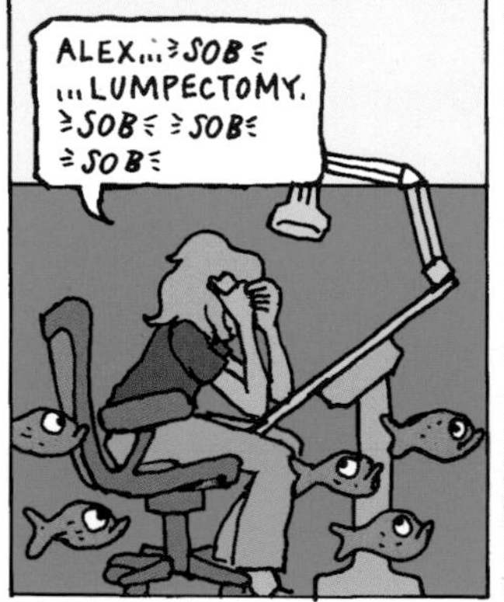

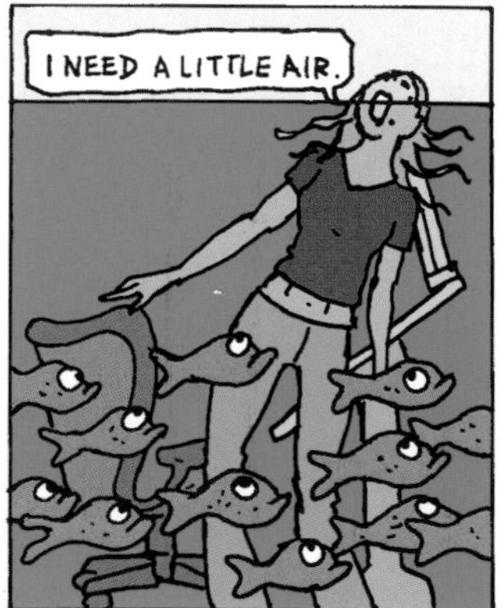

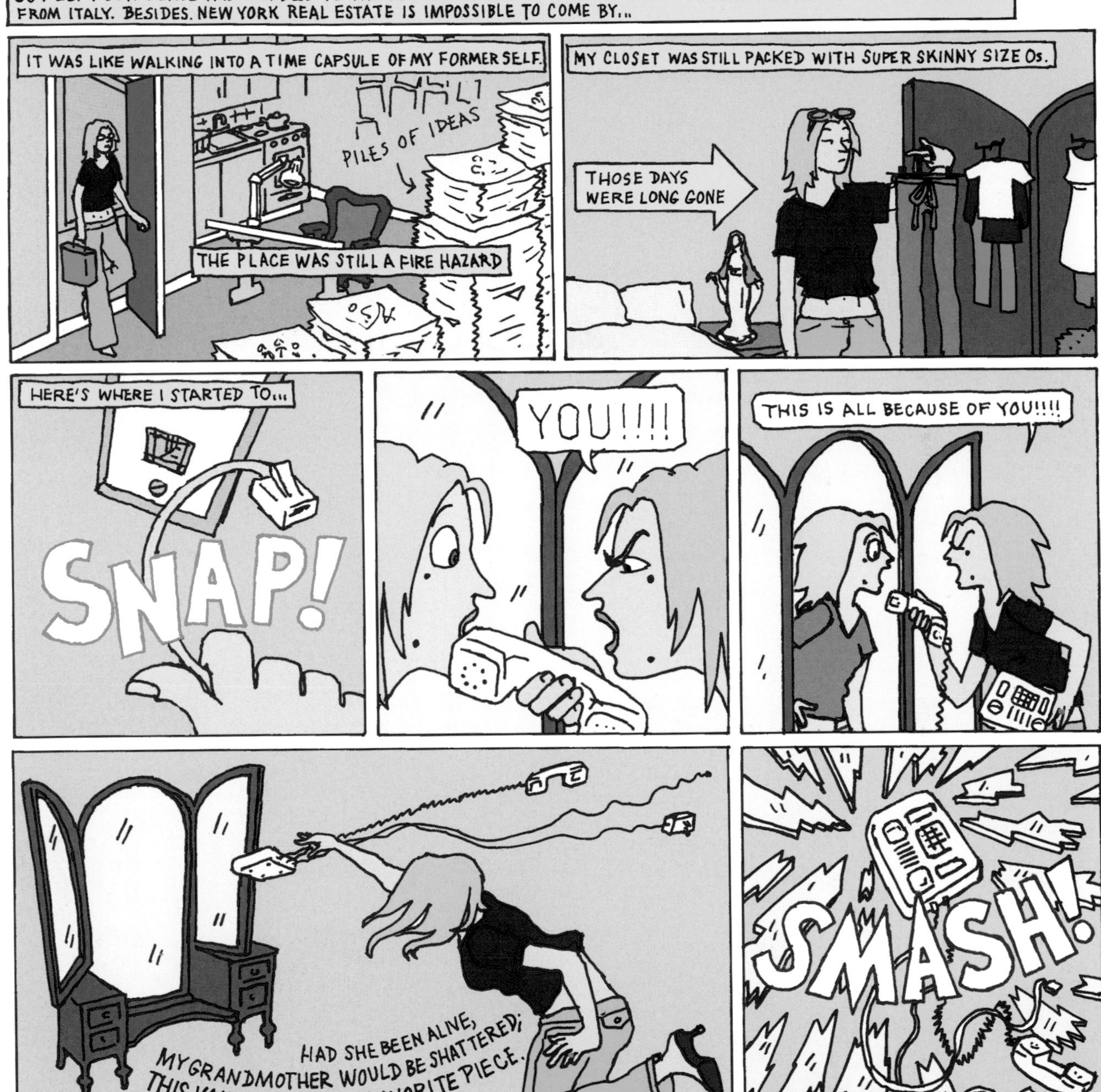
SO I LEFT OUR PLACE AND HEADED TO THE OLD BACHELORETTE PAD. WE KEPT IT FOR STORAGE, AND VISITING RELATIVES FROM ITALY. BESIDES. NEW YORK REAL ESTATE IS IMPOSSIBLE TO COME BY...
IT WAS LIKE WALKING INTO A TIME CAPSULE OF MY FORMER SELF.
PILES OF IDEAS
THE PLACE WAS STILL A FIRE HAZARD
MY CLOSET WAS STILL PACKED WITH SUPER SKINNY SIZE 0s.
THOSE DAYS WERE LONG GONE
HERE'S WHERE I STARTED TO...
SNAP!
YOU!!!!
THIS IS ALL BECAUSE OF YOU!!!!
HAD SHE BEEN ALIVE, MY GRANDMOTHER WOULD BE SHATTERED; THIS VANITY WAS HER FAVORITE PIECE.
SMASH!

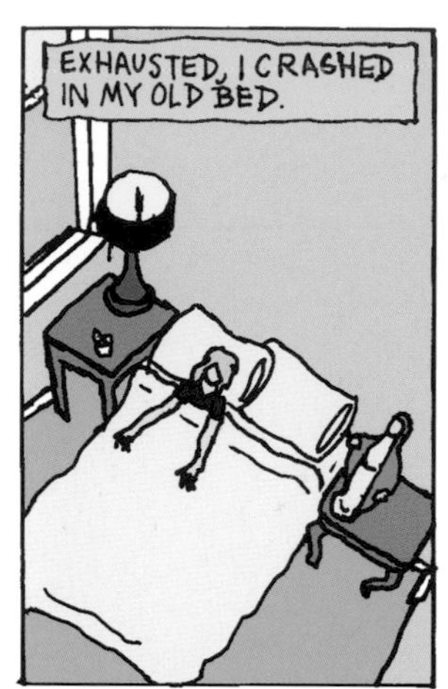
EXHAUSTED, I CRASHED IN MY OLD BED.

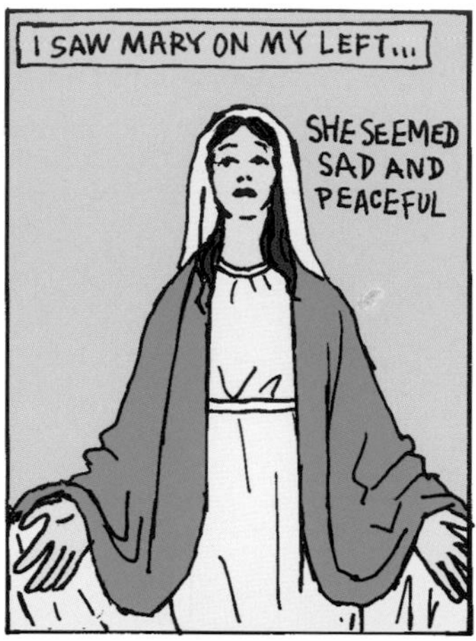
I SAW MARY ON MY LEFT...
SHE SEEMED SAD AND PEACEFUL

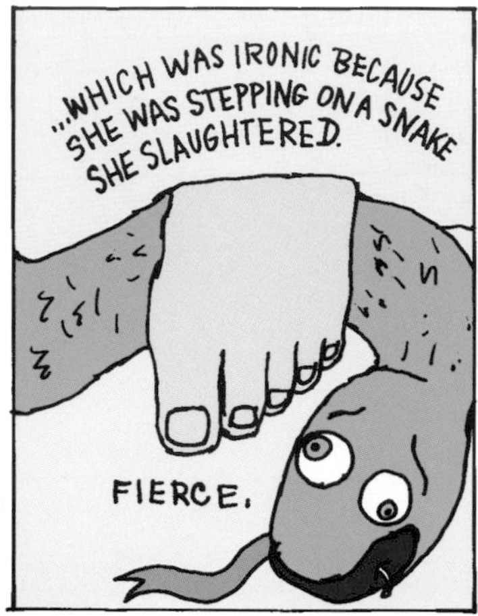
...WHICH WAS IRONIC BECAUSE SHE WAS STEPPING ON A SNAKE SHE SLAUGHTERED.
FIERCE.

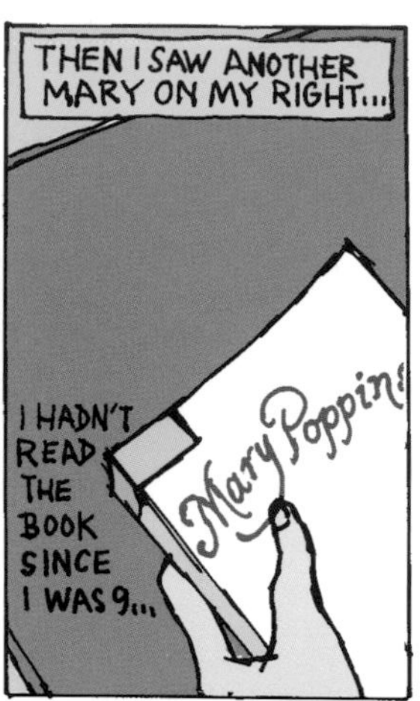
THEN I SAW ANOTHER MARY ON MY RIGHT...
I HADN'T READ THE BOOK SINCE I WAS 9...
Mary Poppins

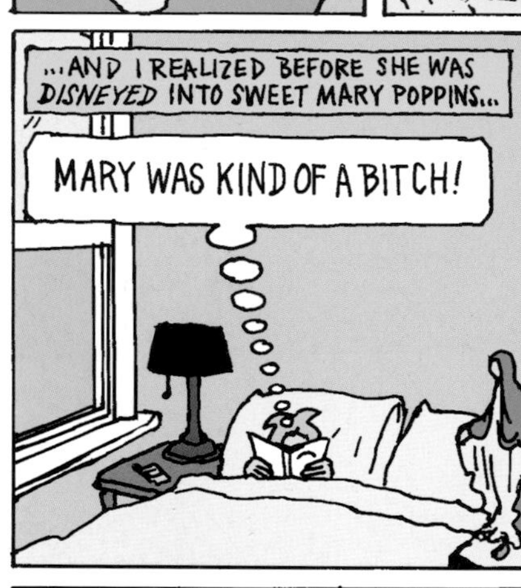
...AND I REALIZED BEFORE SHE WAS DISNEYED INTO SWEET MARY POPPINS...
MARY WAS KIND OF A BITCH!

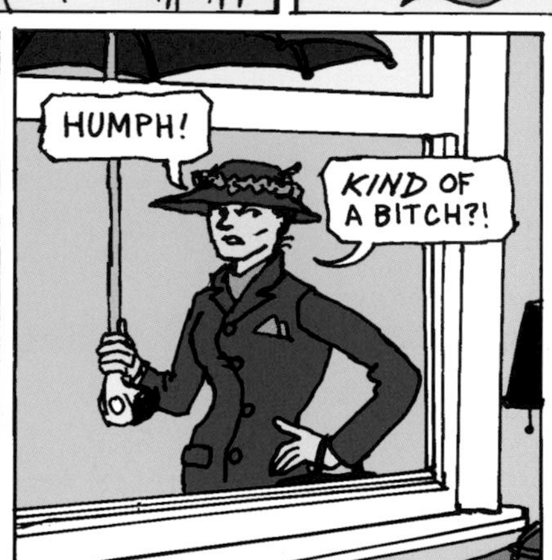
HUMPH!
KIND OF A BITCH?!

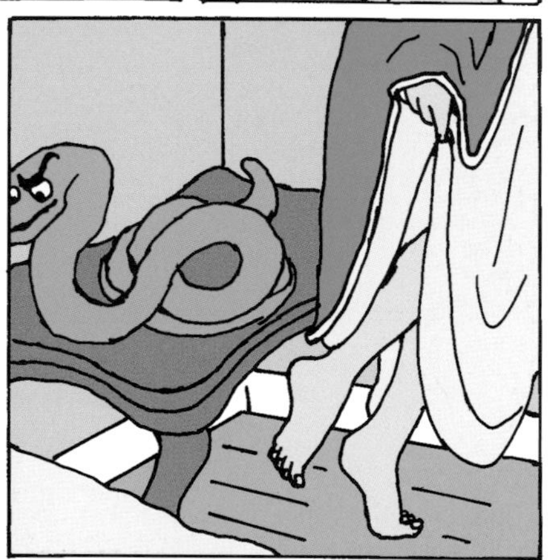

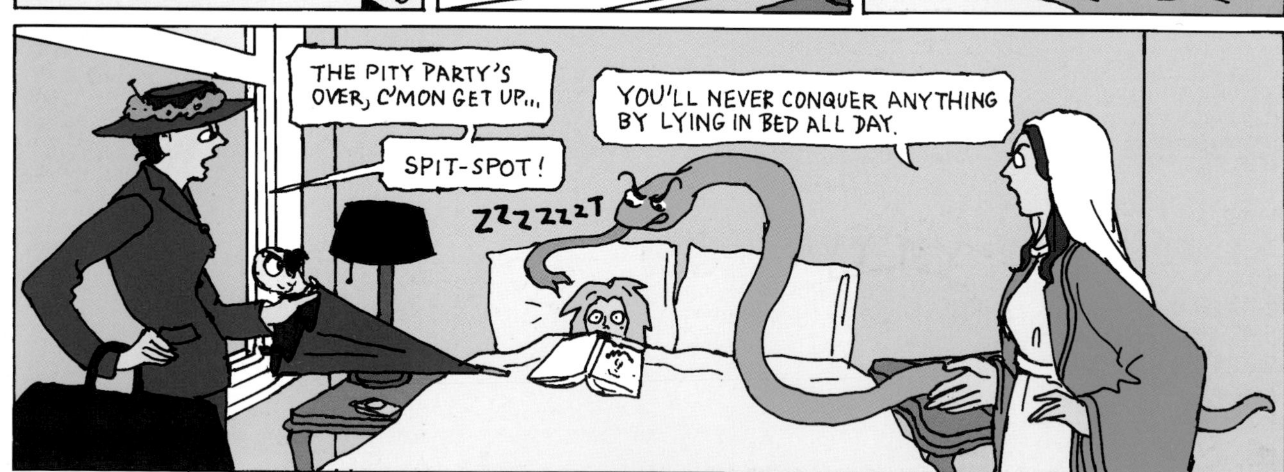
THE PITY PARTY'S OVER, C'MON GET UP...
SPIT-SPOT!
ZZZZZZZT
YOU'LL NEVER CONQUER ANYTHING BY LYING IN BED ALL DAY.

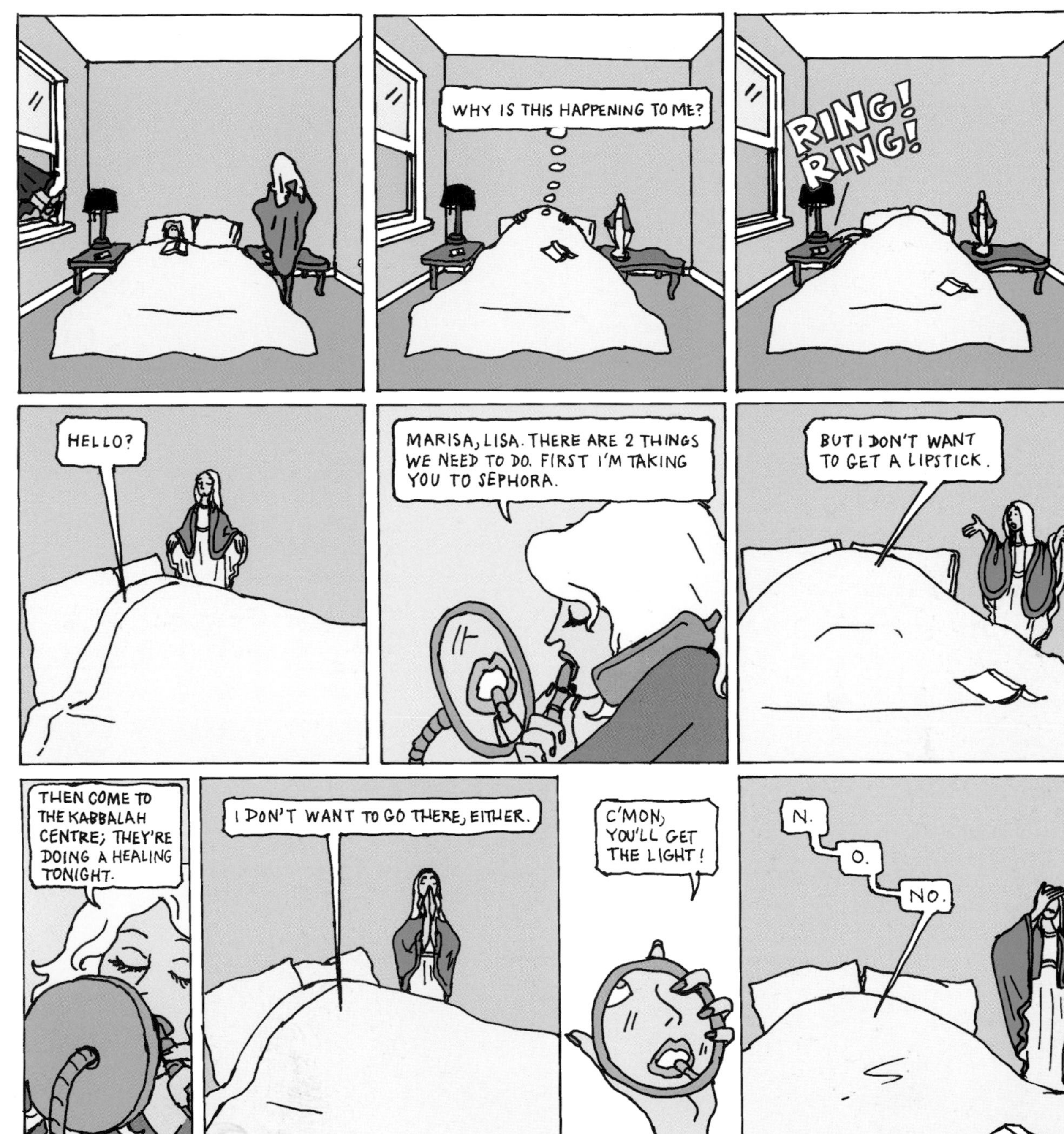
WHY IS THIS HAPPENING TO ME?
RING! RING!
HELLO?
MARISA, LISA. THERE ARE 2 THINGS WE NEED TO DO. FIRST I'M TAKING YOU TO SEPHORA.
BUT I DON'T WANT TO GET A LIPSTICK.
THEN COME TO THE KABBALAH CENTRE; THEY'RE DOING A HEALING TONIGHT.
I DON'T WANT TO GO THERE, EITHER.
C'MON, YOU'LL GET THE LIGHT!
N.
O.
NO.

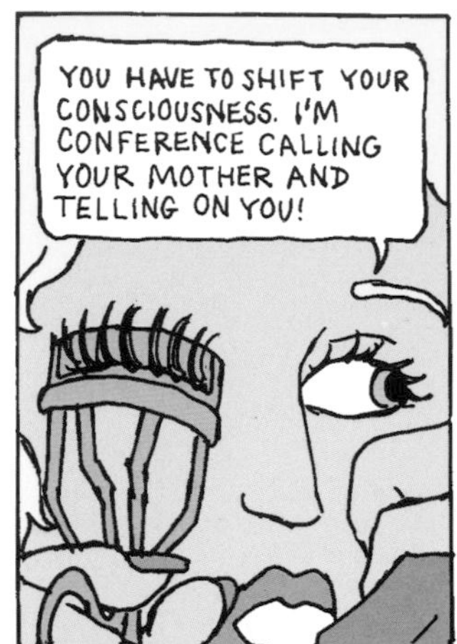
YOU HAVE TO SHIFT YOUR CONSCIOUSNESS. I'M CONFERENCE CALLING YOUR MOTHER AND TELLING ON YOU!

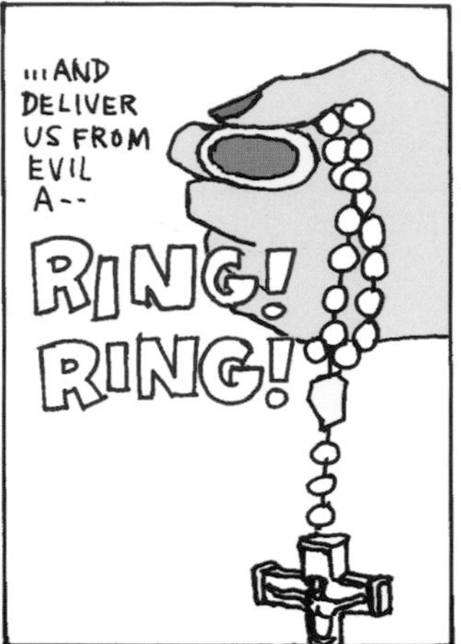
...AND DELIVER US FROM EVIL A--
RING! RING!

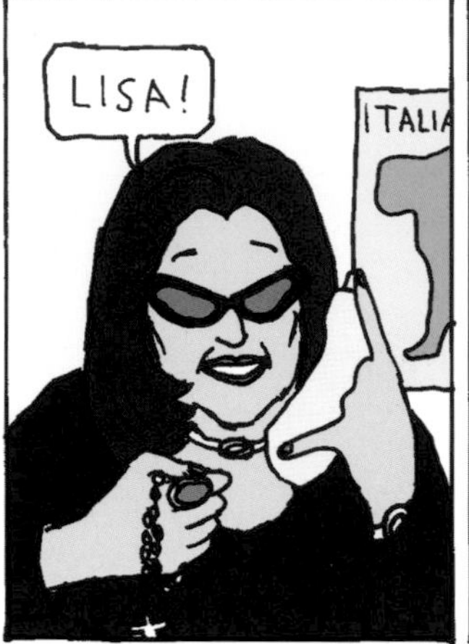
LISA!
ITALIA

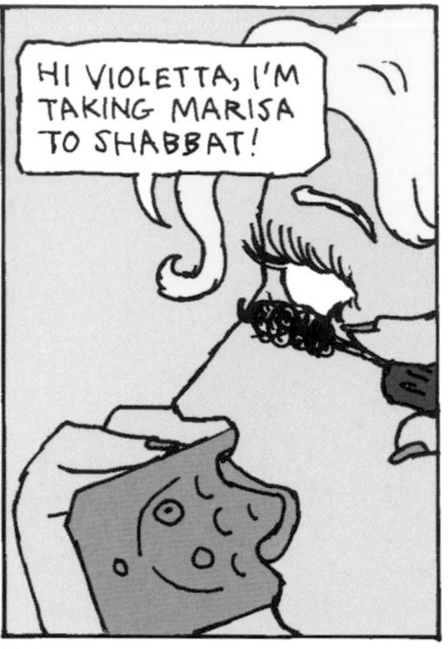
HI VIOLETTA, I'M TAKING MARISA TO SHABBAT!

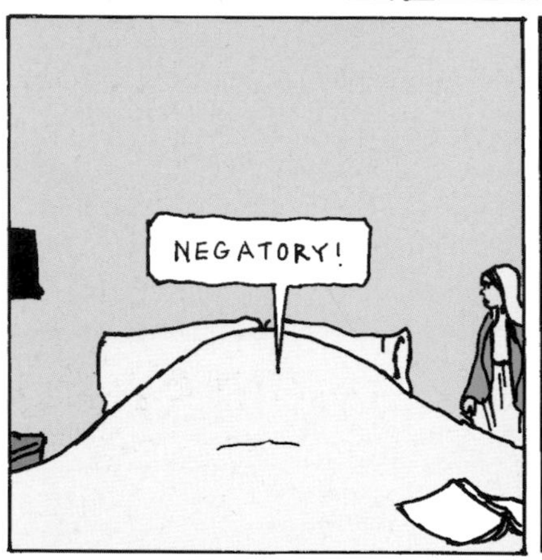
NEGATORY!

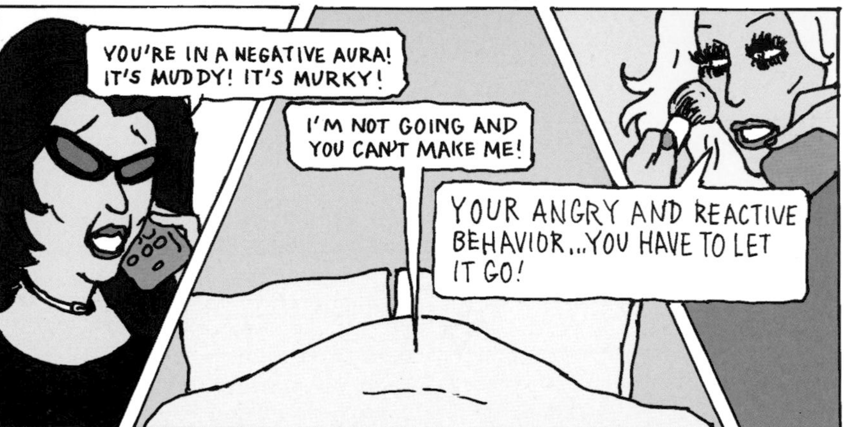
YOU'RE IN A NEGATIVE AURA! IT'S MUDDY! IT'S MURKY!
I'M NOT GOING AND YOU CAN'T MAKE ME!
YOUR ANGRY AND REACTIVE BEHAVIOR...YOU HAVE TO LET IT GO!

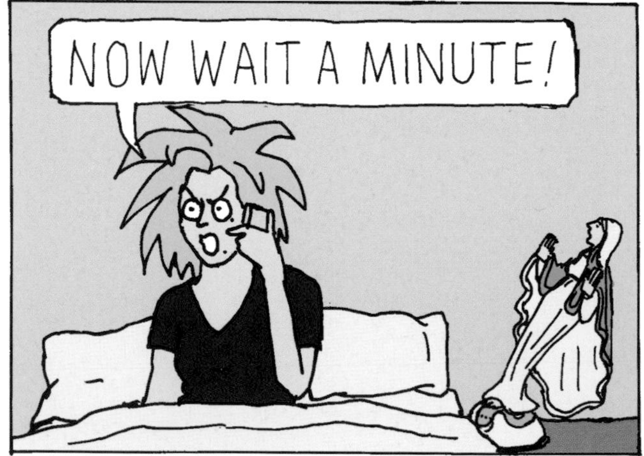
NOW WAIT A MINUTE!

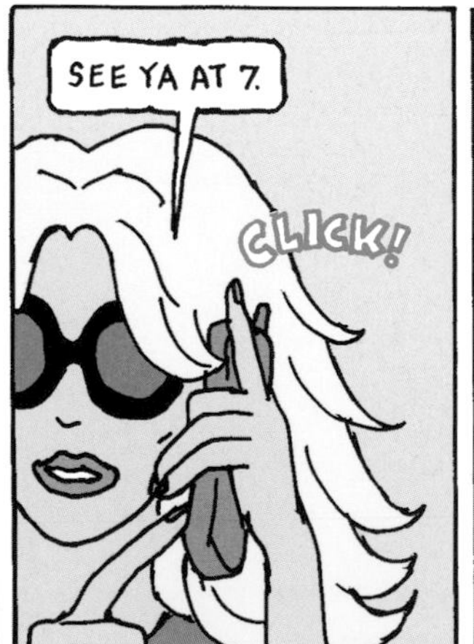
SEE YA AT 7.
CLICK!

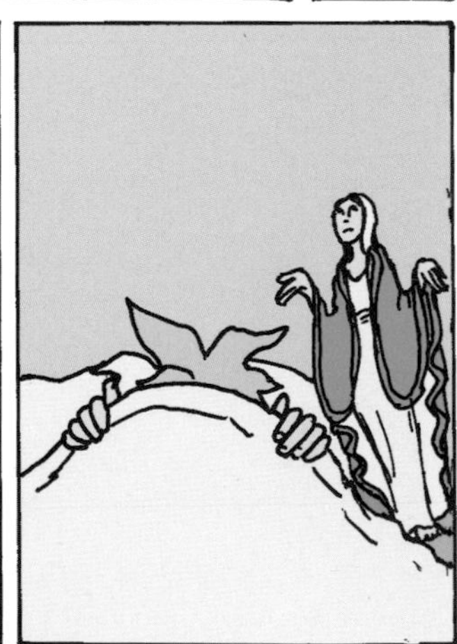

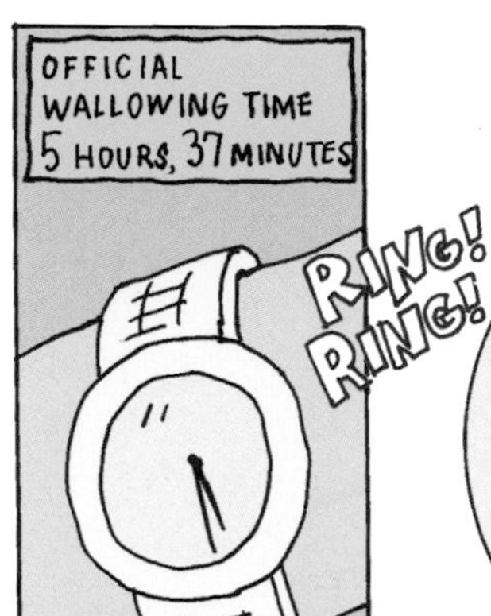
OFFICIAL WALLOWING TIME 5 HOURS, 37 MINUTES
RING! RING!

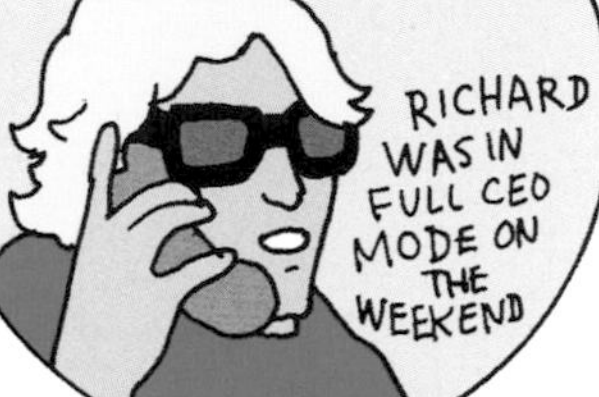
YOU HAVE TO TALK TO LINDA THALER, SHE'S A BREAST CANCER SURVIVOR AND AN INSPIRATION.
RICHARD WAS IN FULL CEO MODE ON THE WEEKEND
ONE OF MY DEAR FRIENDS JUST MARRIED AN ONCOLOGIST AT MEMORIAL SLOAN-KETTERING; AND YOU HAVE TO SEE HIM!
FASHION EXECUTRIX ANNIE CRACKING THE WHIP

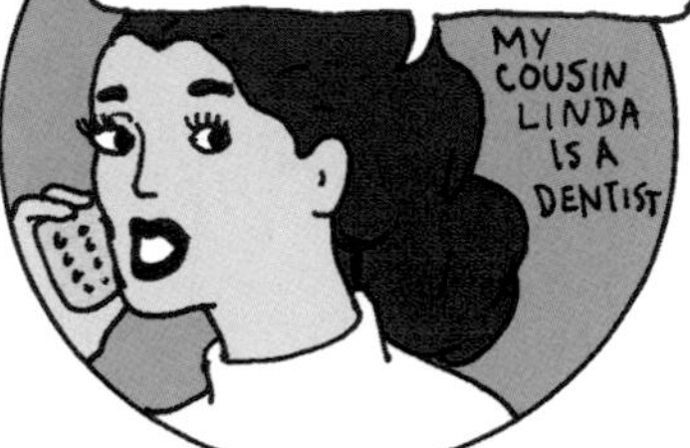
YOU HAVE TO EDUCATE YOURSELF; I'LL GO ONLINE AND SEND YOU SOME RESEARCH.
MY COUSIN LINDA IS A DENTIST
I JUST FOUND THE TOP ONCOLOGIST IN THE WORLD... YOU HAVE TO GO TO HER!
SHARON'S CLIENTS WERE THE MOST POWERFUL WOMEN IN NY

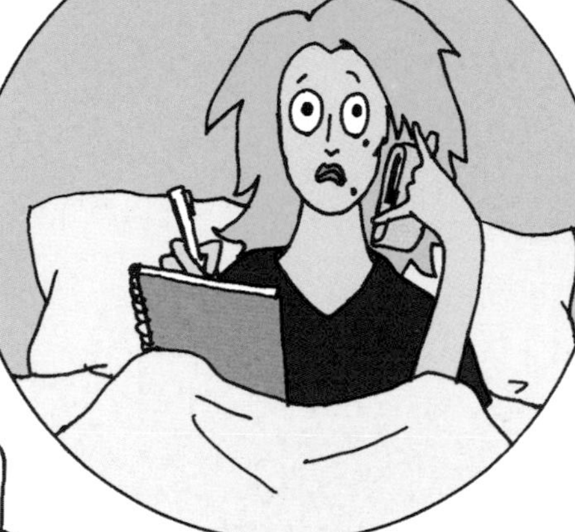

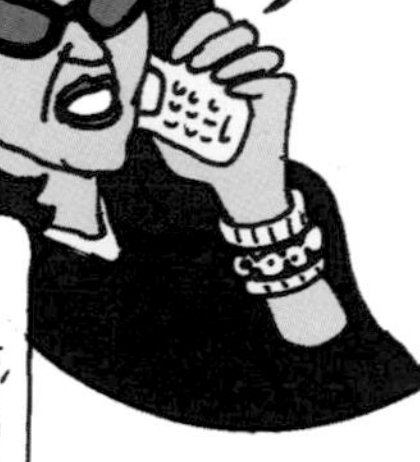
YOU HAVE TO GET A 2ND OPINION, I'D GET A 3RD, 4TH, 5TH, 6TH, 7TH, 8TH...

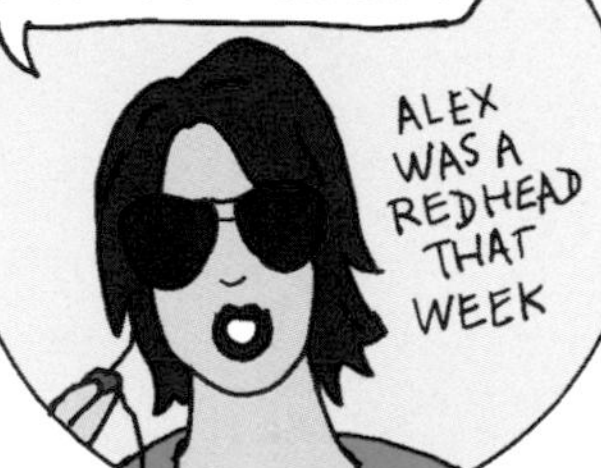
YOU HAVE TO GO TO THE HEALTH FOOD STORE AND GET MAITAKE MUSHROOM SUPPLEMENTS—IT FIGHTS TUMORS!
ALEX WAS A REDHEAD THAT WEEK
IT'S KIMBERLEY; MY UNCLE ANTHONY IS A DOCTOR AT ST. VINCENTS, YOU HAVE TO TALK TO HIM!

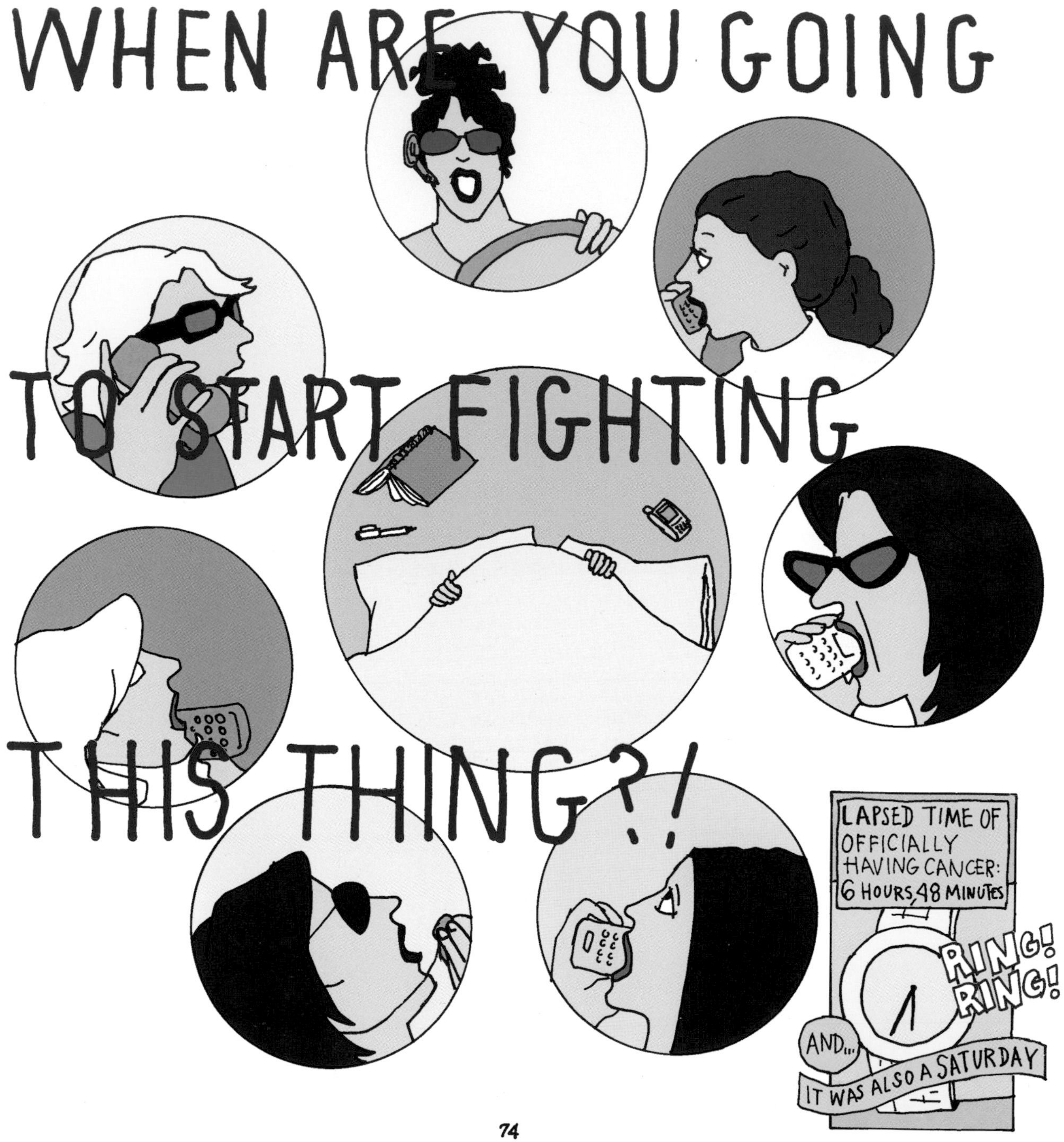

WHEN ARE YOU GOING TO START FIGHTING THIS THING?!

LAPSED TIME OF OFFICIALLY HAVING CANCER: 6 HOURS, 48 MINUTES

RING! RING!

AND...

IT WAS ALSO A SATURDAY

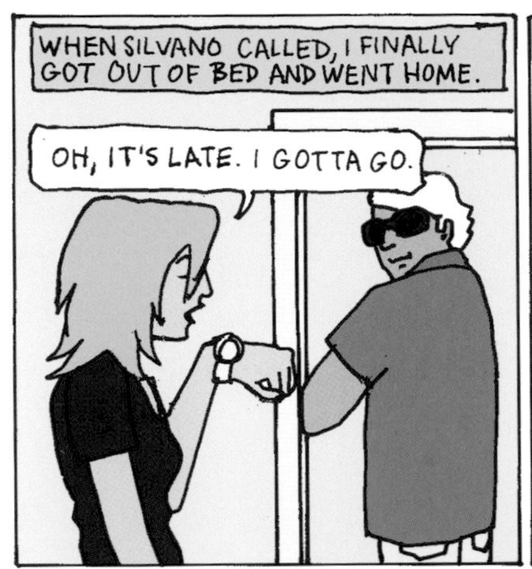
WHEN SILVANO CALLED, I FINALLY GOT OUT OF BED AND WENT HOME.
OH, IT'S LATE. I GOTTA GO.

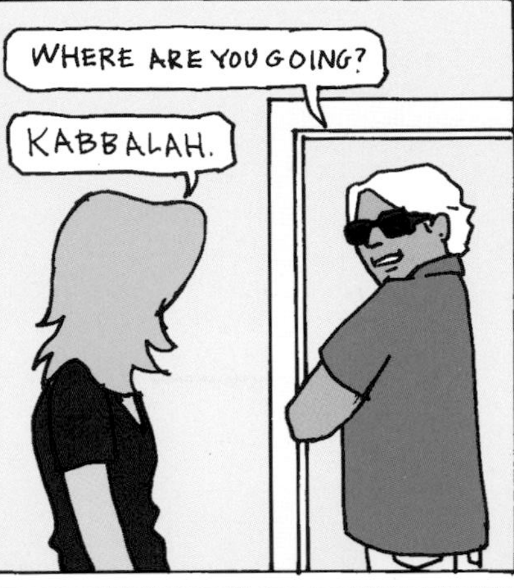
WHERE ARE YOU GOING?
KABBALAH.

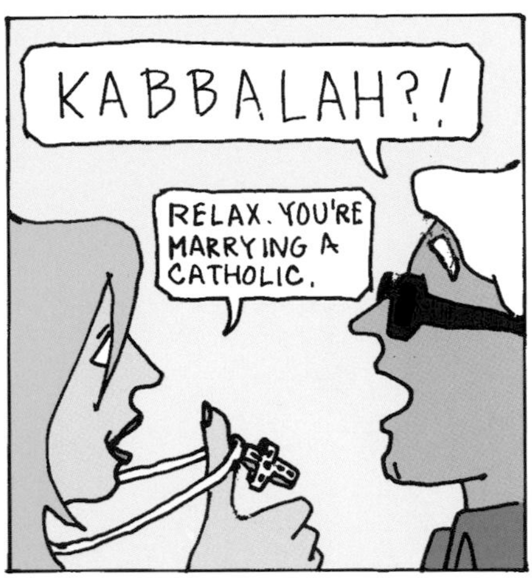
KABBALAH?!
RELAX. YOU'RE MARRYING A CATHOLIC.

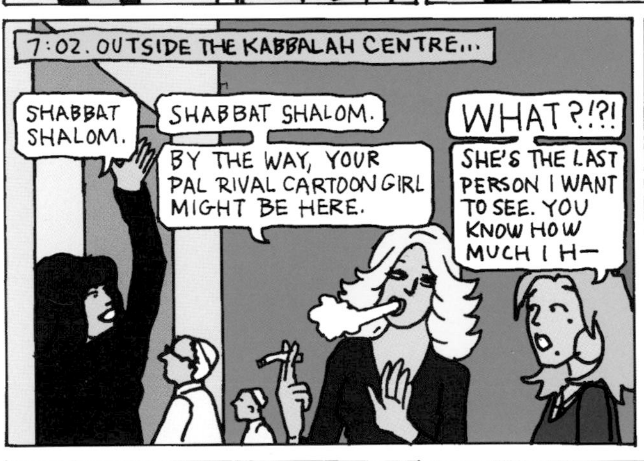
7:02. OUTSIDE THE KABBALAH CENTRE...
SHABBAT SHALOM.
SHABBAT SHALOM.
BY THE WAY, YOUR PAL RIVAL CARTOON GIRL MIGHT BE HERE.
WHAT?!?!
SHE'S THE LAST PERSON I WANT TO SEE. YOU KNOW HOW MUCH I H—

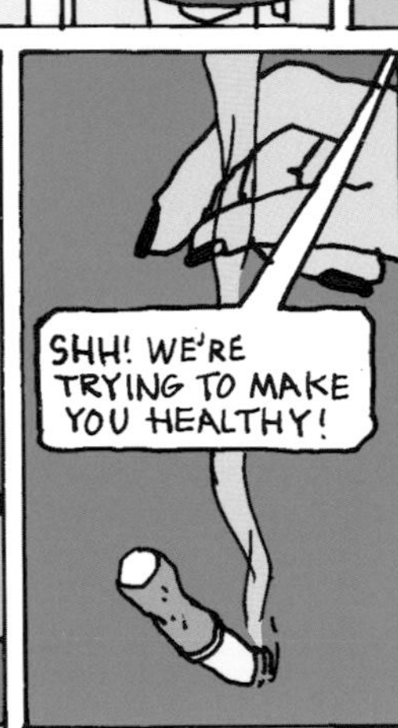
SHH! WE'RE TRYING TO MAKE YOU HEALTHY!

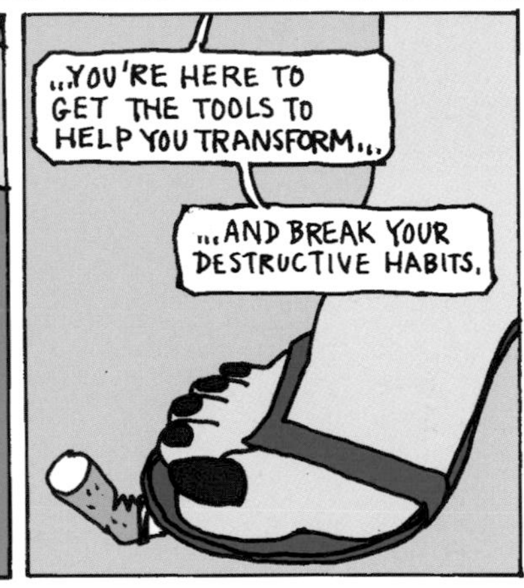
...YOU'RE HERE TO GET THE TOOLS TO HELP YOU TRANSFORM...
...AND BREAK YOUR DESTRUCTIVE HABITS.

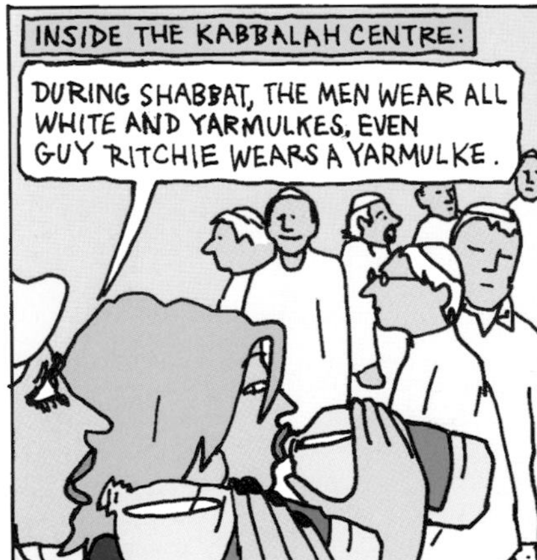
INSIDE THE KABBALAH CENTRE:
DURING SHABBAT, THE MEN WEAR ALL WHITE AND YARMULKES. EVEN GUY RITCHIE WEARS A YARMULKE.

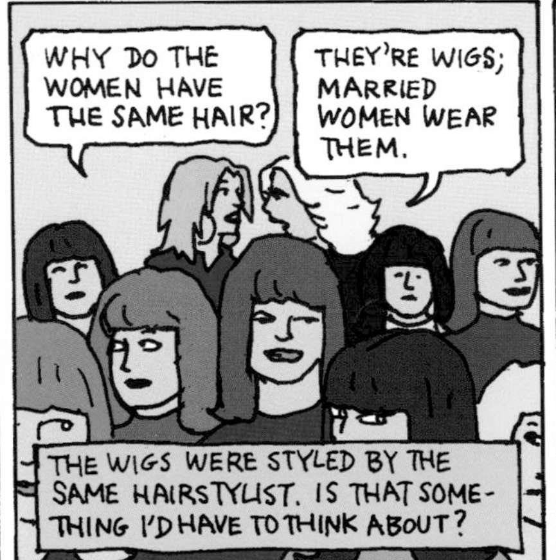
WHY DO THE WOMEN HAVE THE SAME HAIR?
THEY'RE WIGS; MARRIED WOMEN WEAR THEM.
THE WIGS WERE STYLED BY THE SAME HAIRSTYLIST. IS THAT SOMETHING I'D HAVE TO THINK ABOUT?

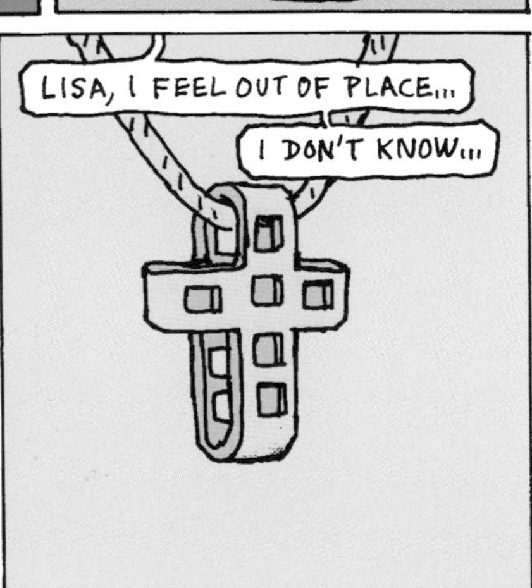
LISA, I FEEL OUT OF PLACE...
I DON'T KNOW...

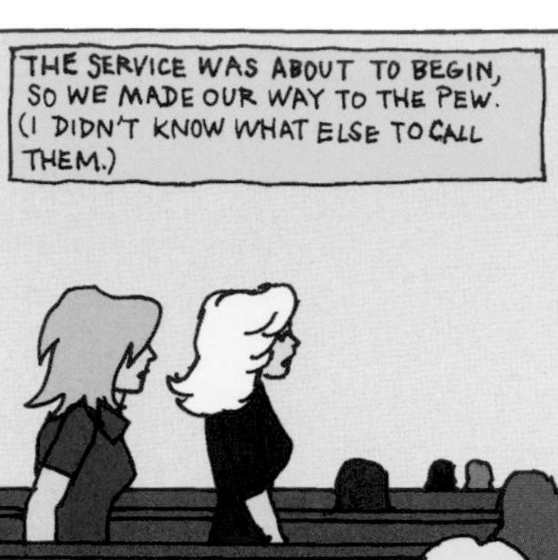

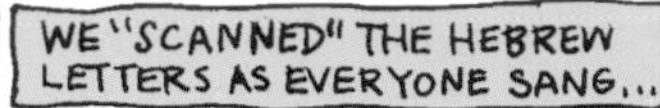

ידיד נפש אב הרחמן,

משוך עבדך אל רצונך,

retz'onecha el avdecha meshoch

ירוץ עבדך כמו איל

a'yal k'mo av'd'cha yarutz

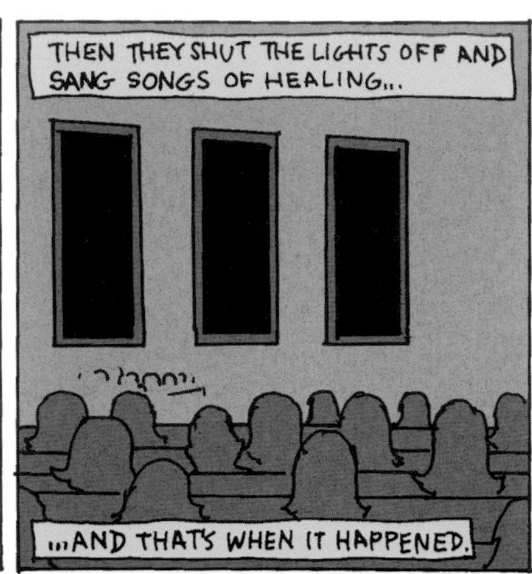

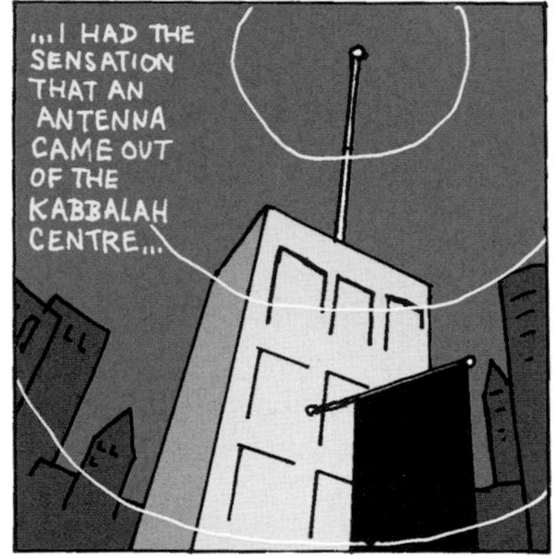

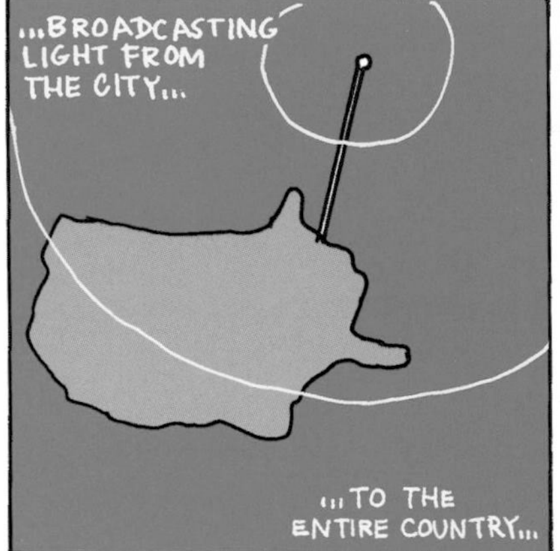

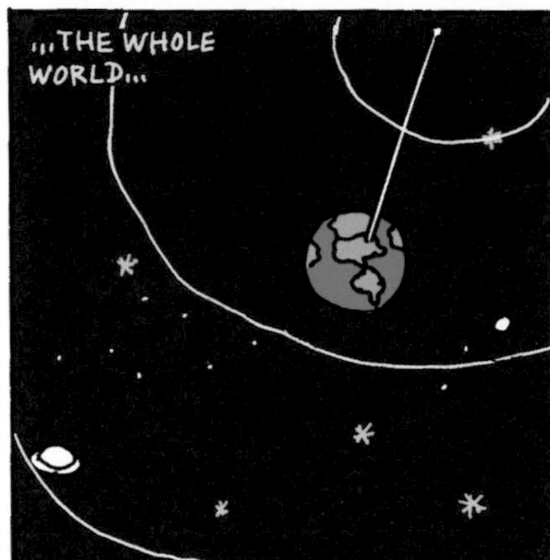

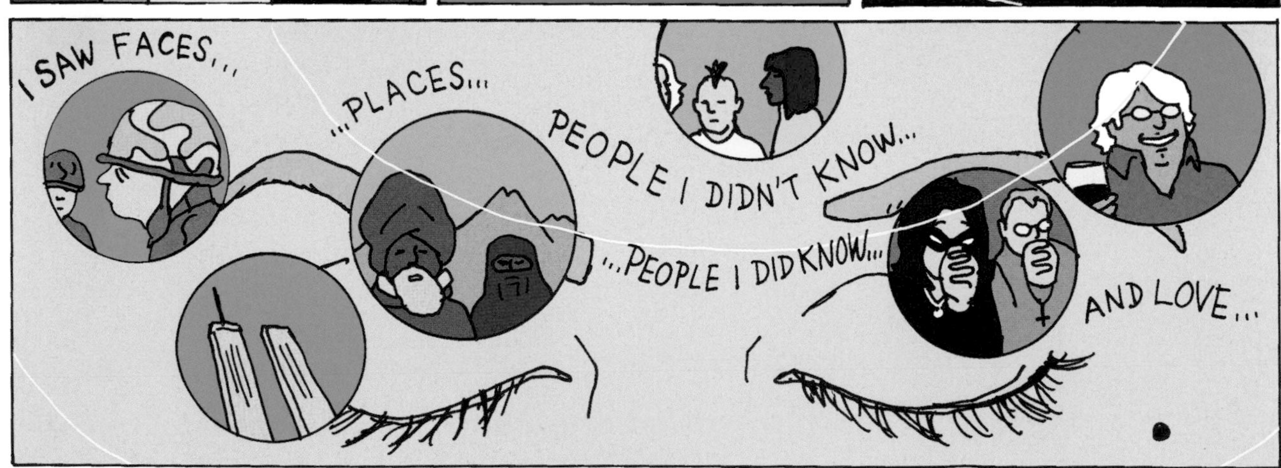

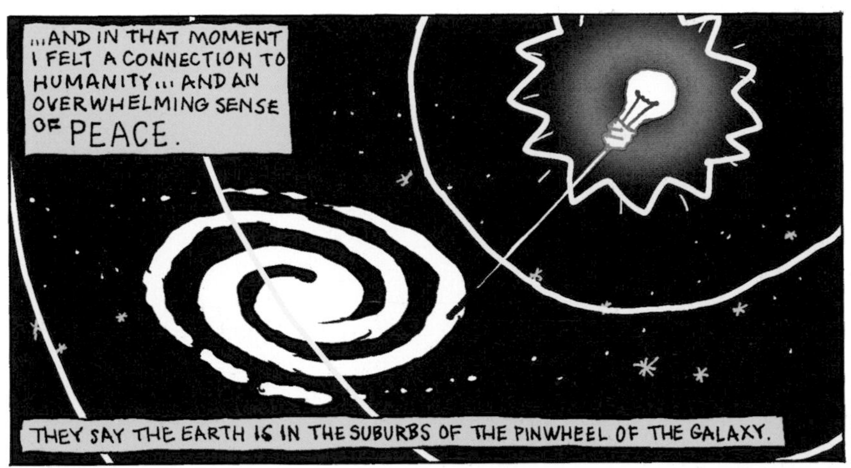
...AND IN THAT MOMENT I FELT A CONNECTION TO HUMANITY... AND AN OVERWHELMING SENSE OF PEACE.
THEY SAY THE EARTH IS IN THE SUBURBS OF THE PINWHEEL OF THE GALAXY.

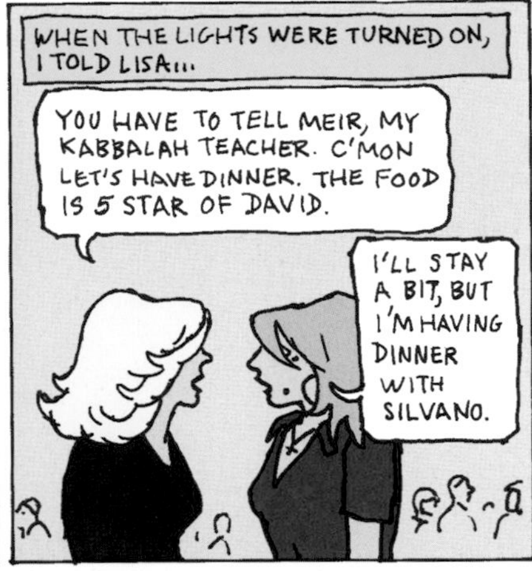
WHEN THE LIGHTS WERE TURNED ON, I TOLD LISA...
YOU HAVE TO TELL MEIR, MY KABBALAH TEACHER. C'MON LET'S HAVE DINNER. THE FOOD IS 5 STAR OF DAVID.
I'LL STAY A BIT, BUT I'M HAVING DINNER WITH SILVANO.

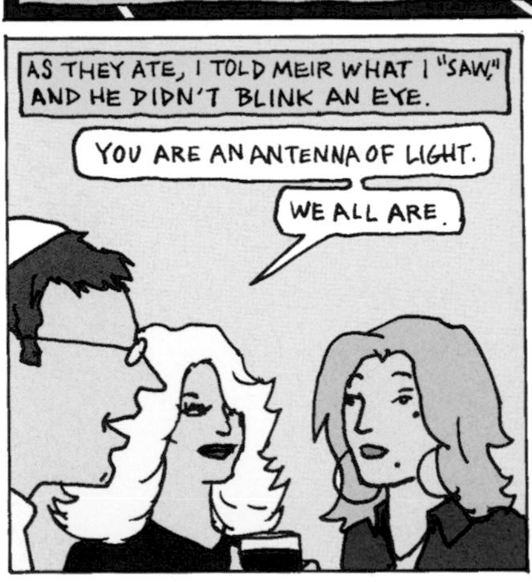
AS THEY ATE, I TOLD MEIR WHAT I "SAW," AND HE DIDN'T BLINK AN EYE.
YOU ARE AN ANTENNA OF LIGHT.
WE ALL ARE.

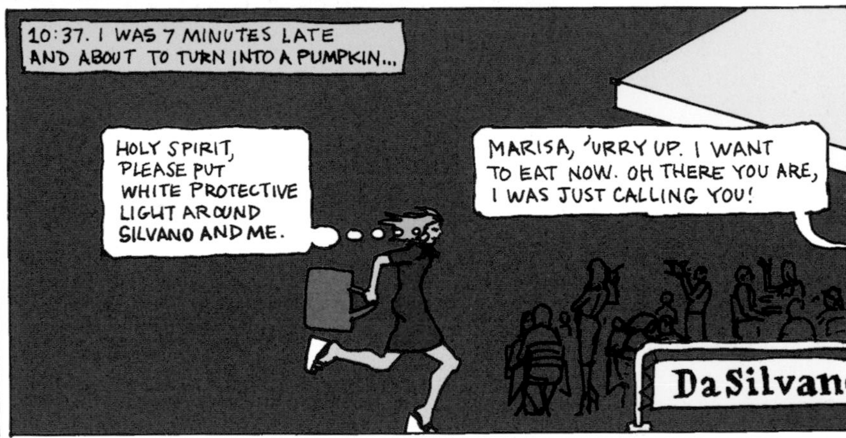
10:37. I WAS 7 MINUTES LATE AND ABOUT TO TURN INTO A PUMPKIN...
HOLY SPIRIT, PLEASE PUT WHITE PROTECTIVE LIGHT AROUND SILVANO AND ME.
MARISA, 'URRY UP. I WANT TO EAT NOW. OH THERE YOU ARE, I WAS JUST CALLING YOU!
DaSilvan

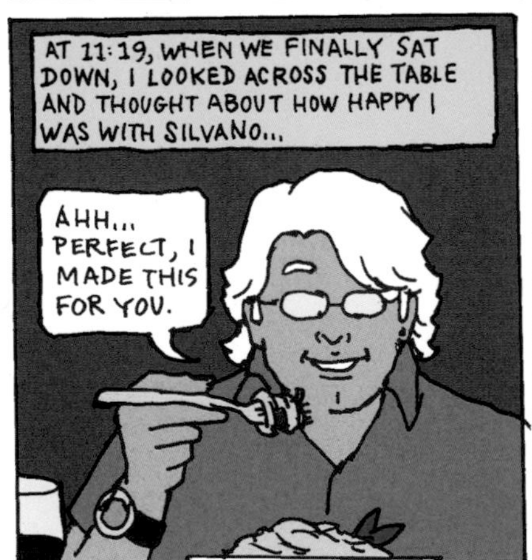
AT 11:19, WHEN WE FINALLY SAT DOWN, I LOOKED ACROSS THE TABLE AND THOUGHT ABOUT HOW HAPPY I WAS WITH SILVANO...
AHH... PERFECT, I MADE THIS FOR YOU.

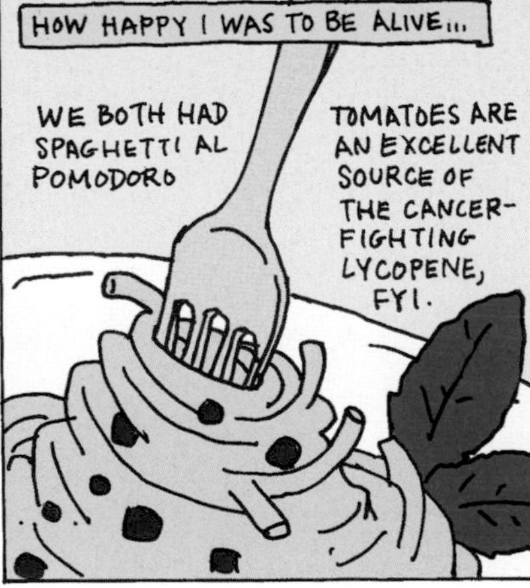
HOW HAPPY I WAS TO BE ALIVE...
WE BOTH HAD SPAGHETTI AL POMODORO
TOMATOES ARE AN EXCELLENT SOURCE OF THE CANCER-FIGHTING LYCOPENE, FYI.

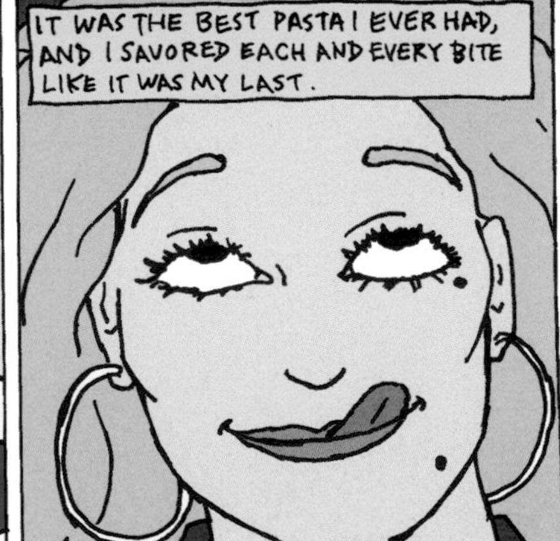
IT WAS THE BEST PASTA I EVER HAD, AND I SAVORED EACH AND EVERY BITE LIKE IT WAS MY LAST.

AS WE WERE FINISHING DINNER, CLAUDIO, SILVANO'S BFF, JOINED US. HE WAS IN FROM ITALY DOING SOME BUSINESS IN THE STATES.
CIAO, SILVANO!
CIAO, MARISA!

SILVANO TOLD ME. I'M VERY SORRY.
IT'S OK, CLAUDIO, I'M LOOKING AT IT LIKE IT'S AN OPPORTUNITY.

AN OPPORTUNITY?!!
BO.*
* "BO" MEANS "I DON'T KNOW."

WHAT I MEAN IS, INSTEAD OF SEEING THE TUMOR AS A BLACK HOLE...

...I'M LOOKING AT IT AS A WHITE PEARL OF OPPORTUNITY TO CLEAN EVERYTHING UP AND GET RID OF MY TOXIC BEHAVIOR.

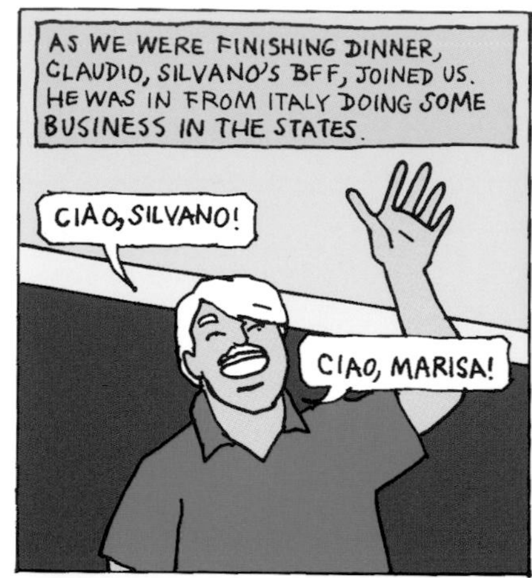

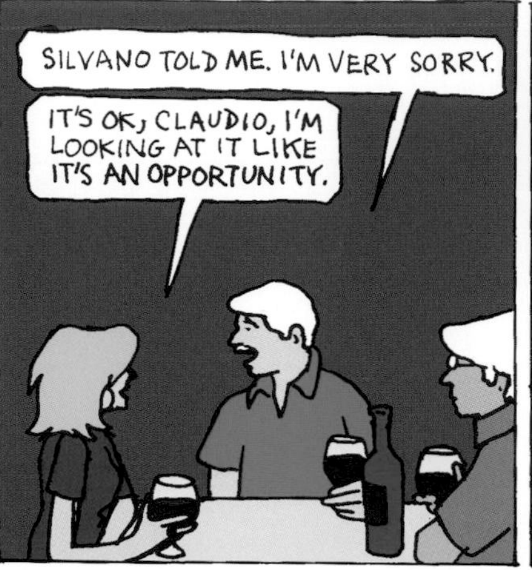

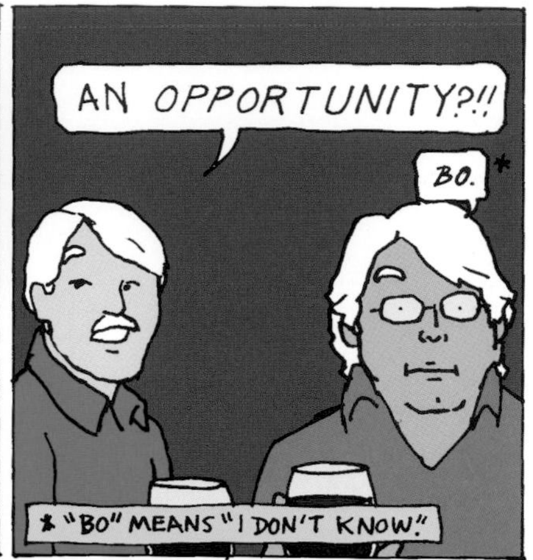

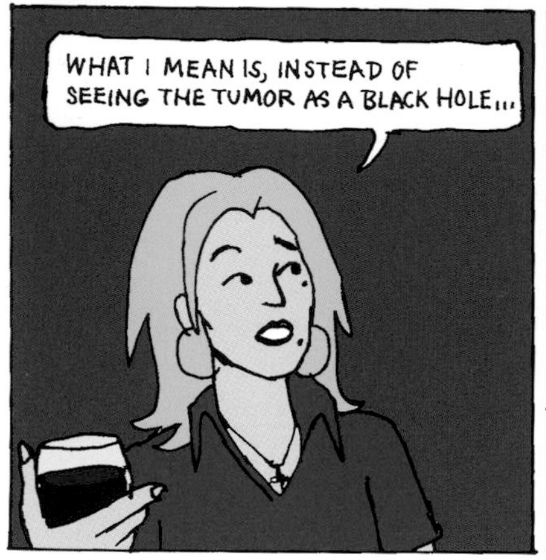

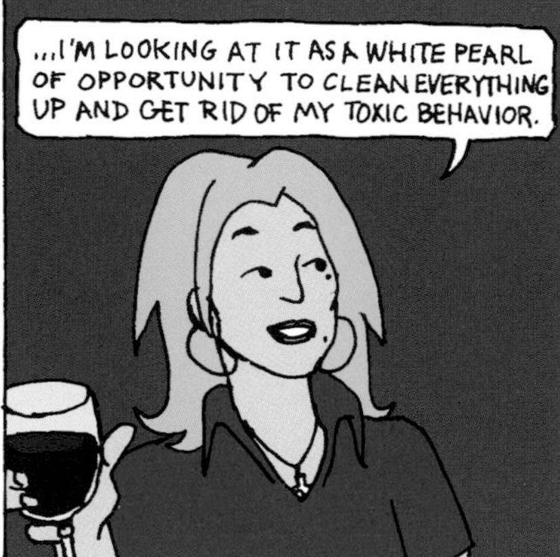

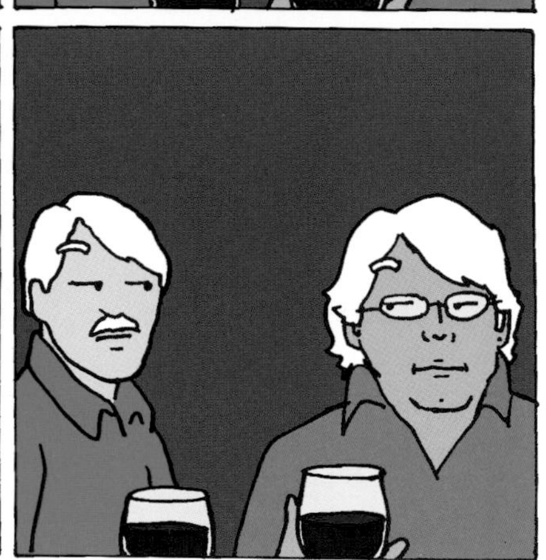

AND THAT'S ALL THAT HAPPENED ON MAY 15, 2004, THE DAY THAT WILL BE FOREVER KNOWN TO ME AS "D. DAY," AKA "DIAGNOSIS DAY"...

I'M EXHAUSTED.
ME TOO.
AN OPPORTUNITY?

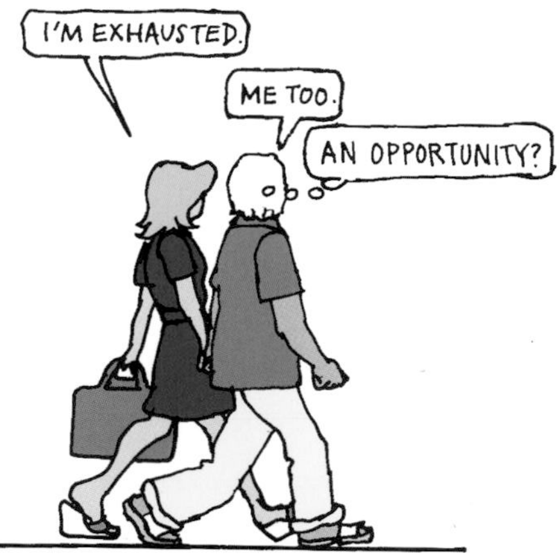

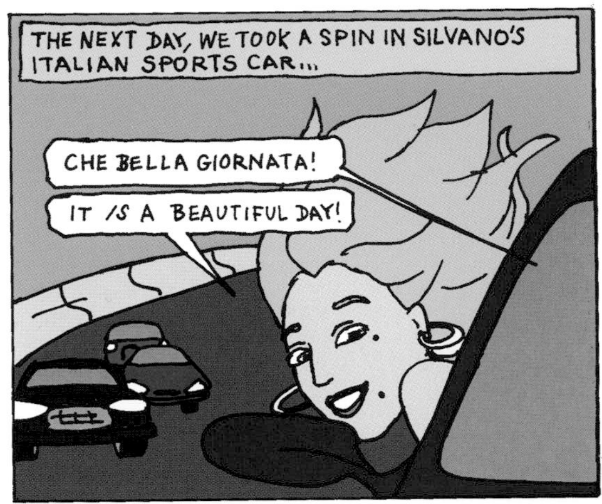
THE NEXT DAY, WE TOOK A SPIN IN SILVANO'S ITALIAN SPORTS CAR...
CHE BELLA GIORNATA!
IT IS A BEAUTIFUL DAY!

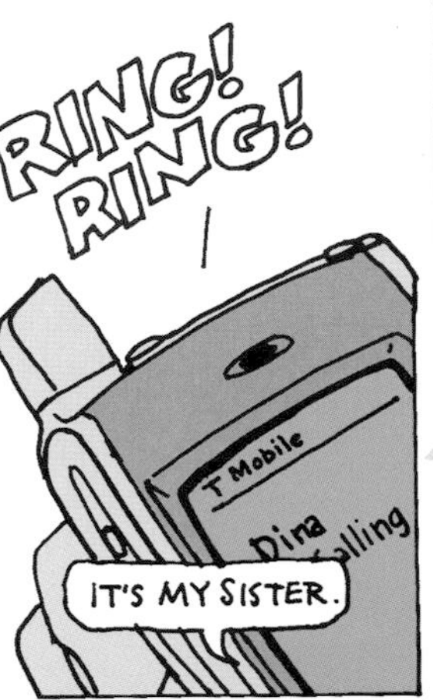
RING! RING!
T Mobile
Dina Calling
IT'S MY SISTER.

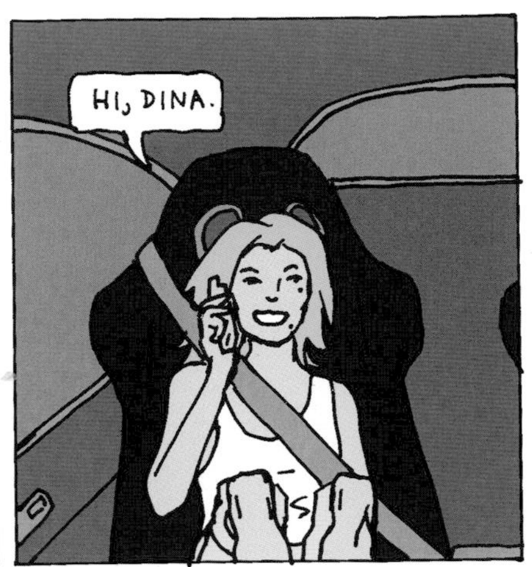
HI, DINA.

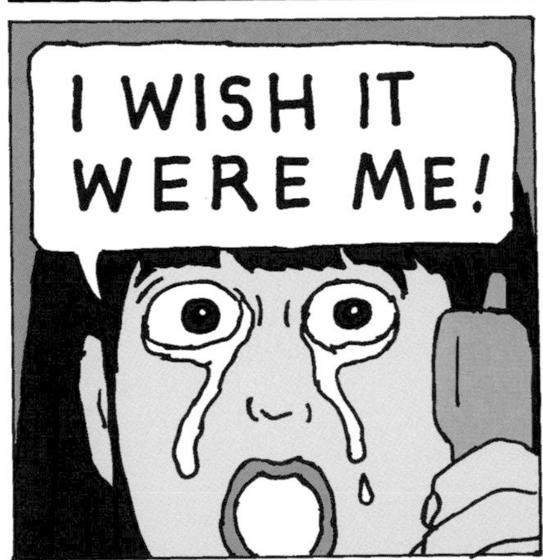
I WISH IT WERE ME!

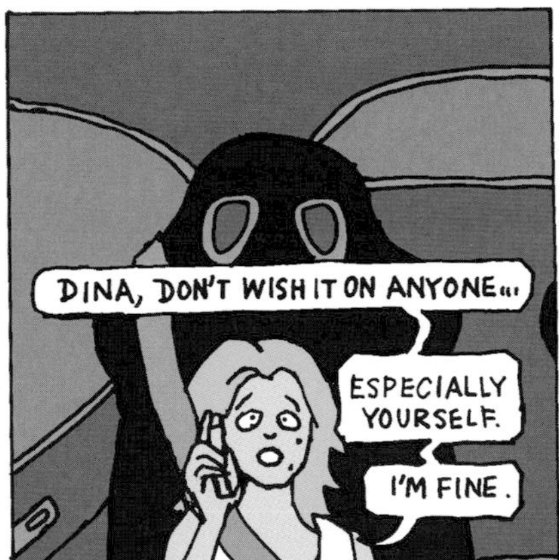
DINA, DON'T WISH IT ON ANYONE...
ESPECIALLY YOURSELF.
I'M FINE.

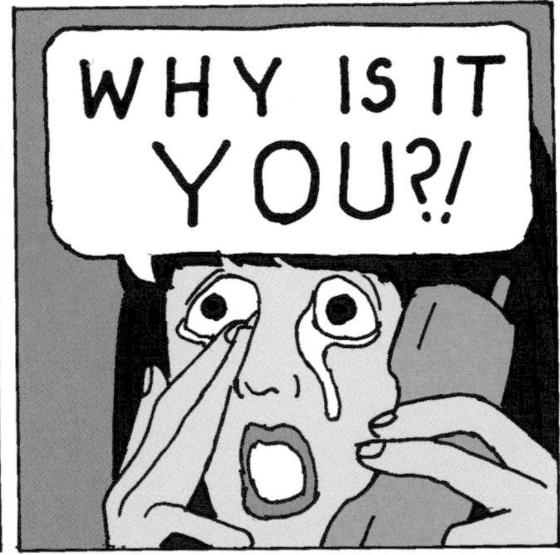
WHY IS IT YOU?!

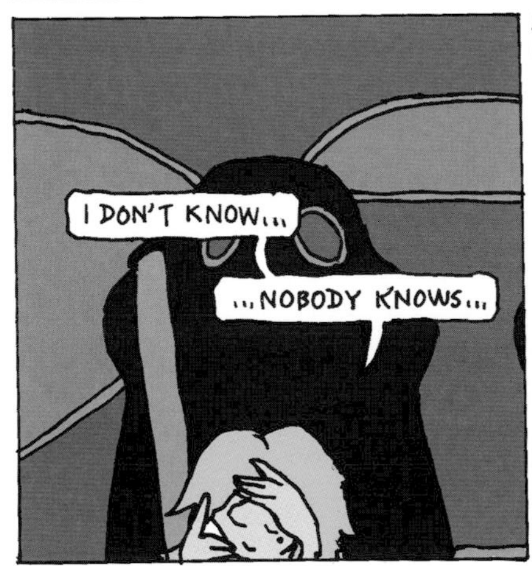
I DON'T KNOW...
...NOBODY KNOWS...

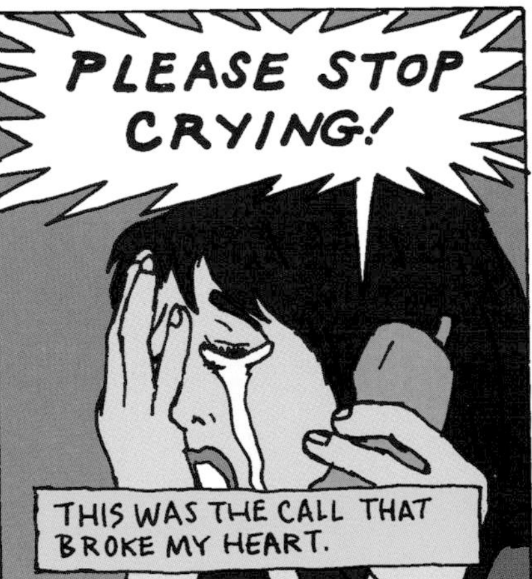
PLEASE STOP CRYING!
THIS WAS THE CALL THAT BROKE MY HEART.

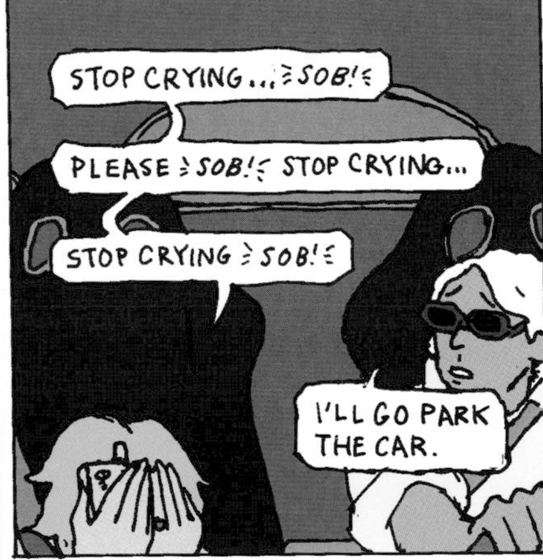
STOP CRYING... SOB!
PLEASE SOB! STOP CRYING...
STOP CRYING SOB!
I'LL GO PARK THE CAR.

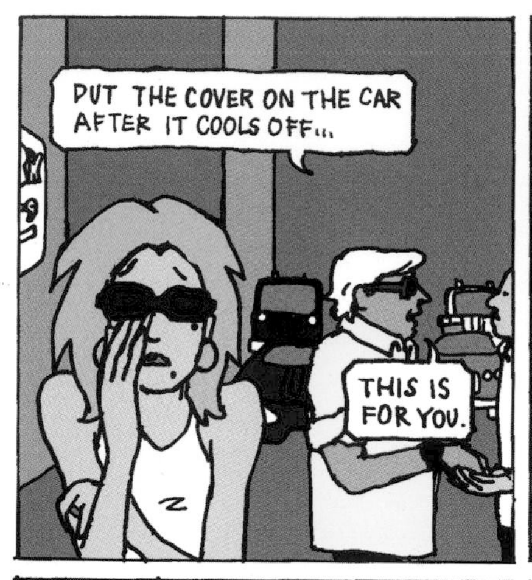
PUT THE COVER ON THE CAR AFTER IT COOLS OFF...
THIS IS FOR YOU.

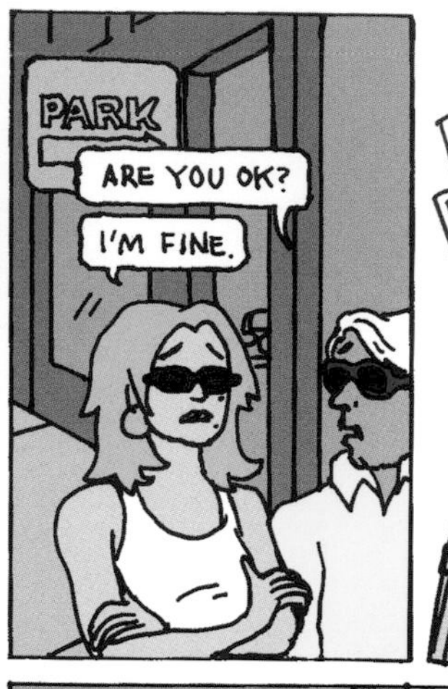
PARK
ARE YOU OK?
I'M FINE.

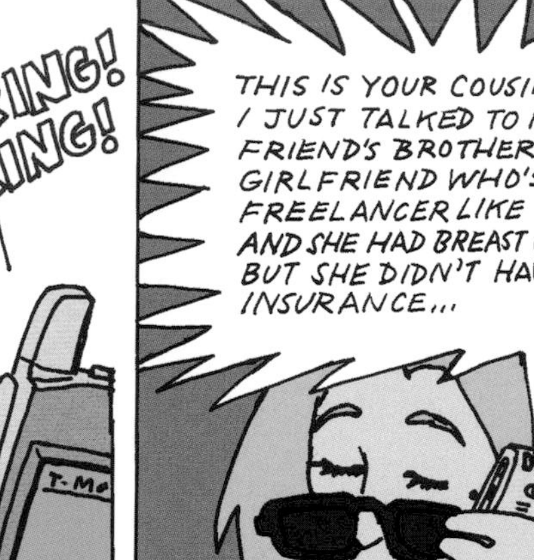
RING! RING!
T-Mo
THIS IS YOUR COUSIN; I JUST TALKED TO MY FRIEND'S BROTHER'S GIRLFRIEND WHO'S A FREELANCER LIKE YOU AND SHE HAD BREAST CANCER BUT SHE DIDN'T HAVE INSURANCE...

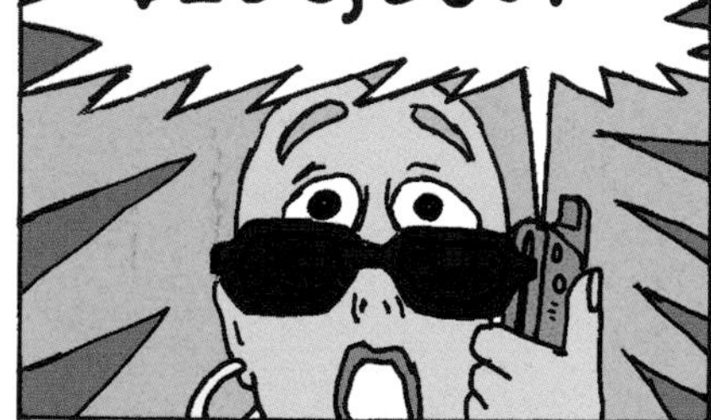
IF HER DOCTORS HAD BILLED HER, IT WOULD HAVE COST HER $200,000!

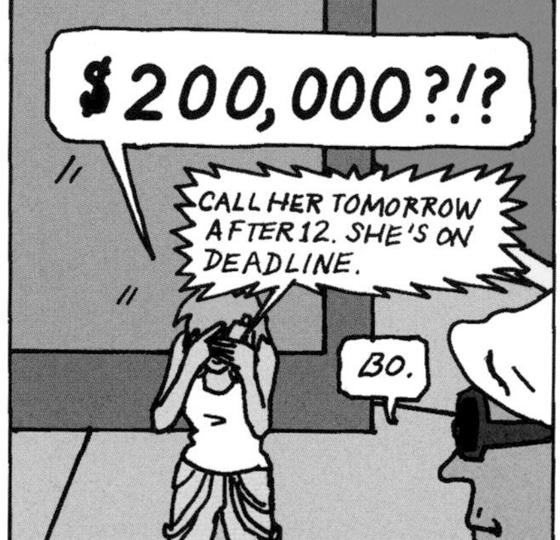
$200,000?!?
CALL HER TOMORROW AFTER 12. SHE'S ON DEADLINE.
BO.

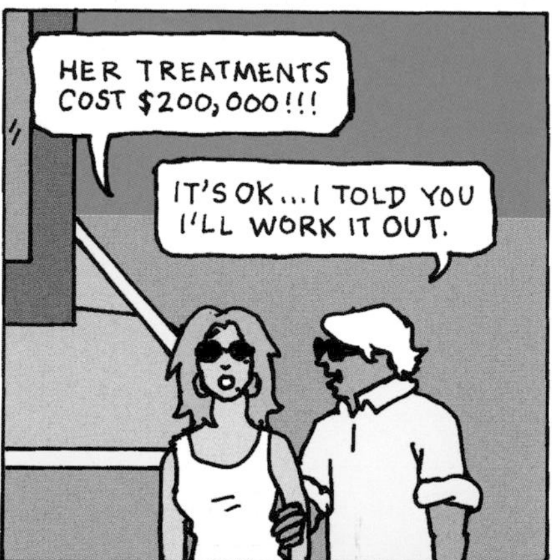
HER TREATMENTS COST $200,000!!!
IT'S OK... I TOLD YOU I'LL WORK IT OUT.

THE NEXT MORNING, I RANG BREAST SURGEON DR. MILLS, AND BEGAN THE ENDLESS PHONE CALLS OF MY NEW LIFE.
DR. MILLS'S OFFICE...
...PLEASE HANG ON WHILE I PUT YOU ON HOLD...
CLICK!

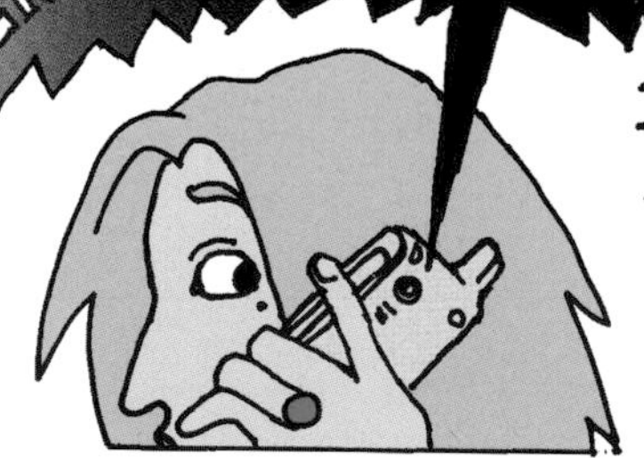
HA HA HA HA...STAYIN' ALIVE, STAYIN' ALIVE...
I'M NOT MAKING THIS TONY MANERO MOMENT UP.

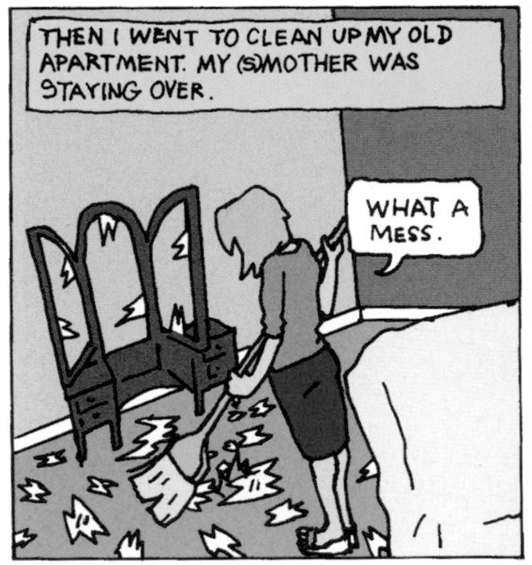
THEN I WENT TO CLEAN UP MY OLD APARTMENT. MY (S)MOTHER WAS STAYING OVER.
WHAT A MESS.

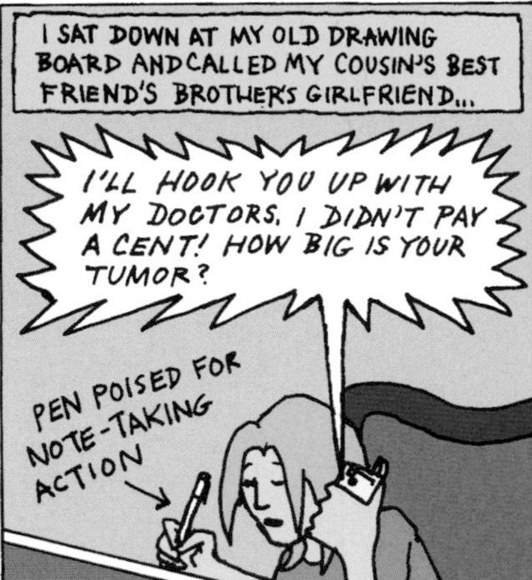
I SAT DOWN AT MY OLD DRAWING BOARD AND CALLED MY COUSIN'S BEST FRIEND'S BROTHER'S GIRLFRIEND...
I'LL HOOK YOU UP WITH MY DOCTORS. I DIDN'T PAY A CENT! HOW BIG IS YOUR TUMOR?
PEN POISED FOR NOTE-TAKING ACTION

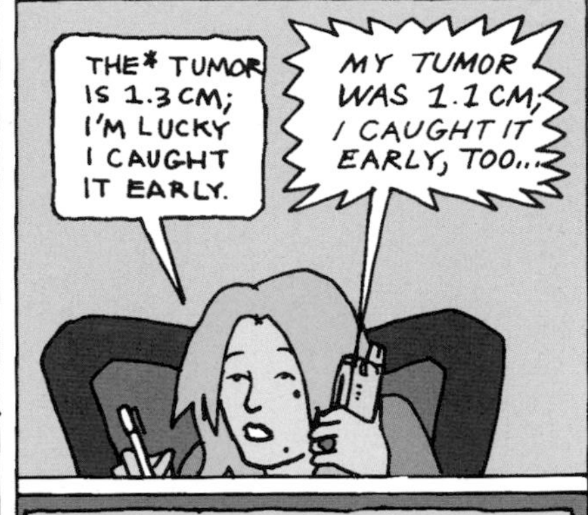
THE* TUMOR IS 1.3 CM; I'M LUCKY I CAUGHT IT EARLY.
MY TUMOR WAS 1.1 CM; I CAUGHT IT EARLY, TOO...
*I NEVER USED "MY" IN FRONT OF TUMOR I DIDN'T WANT TO OWN IT.

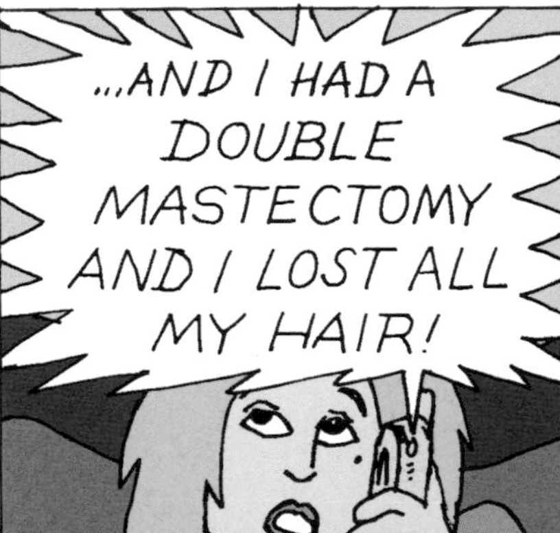
...AND I HAD A DOUBLE MASTECTOMY AND I LOST ALL MY HAIR!

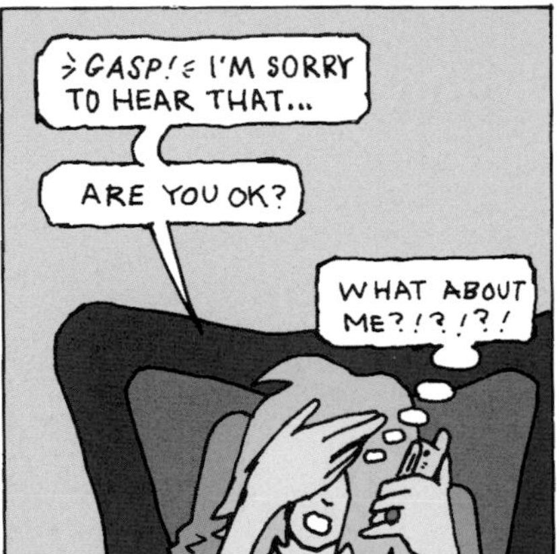
GASP! I'M SORRY TO HEAR THAT...
ARE YOU OK?
WHAT ABOUT ME?!?!?!

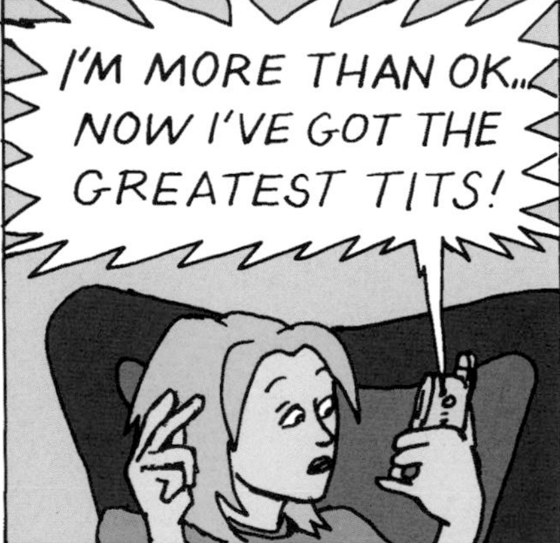
I'M MORE THAN OK... NOW I'VE GOT THE GREATEST TITS!

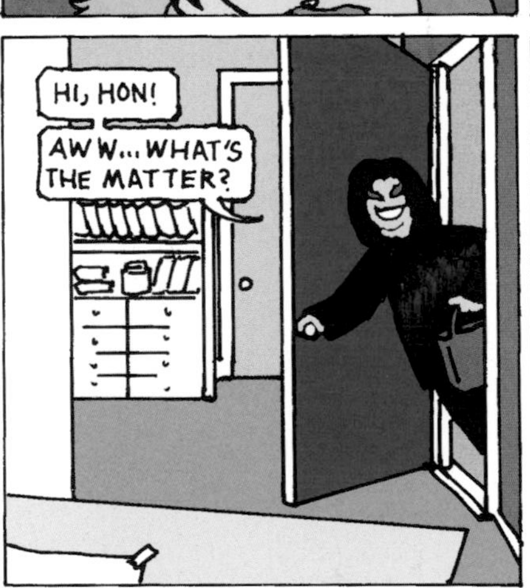
HI, HON!
AWW... WHAT'S THE MATTER?

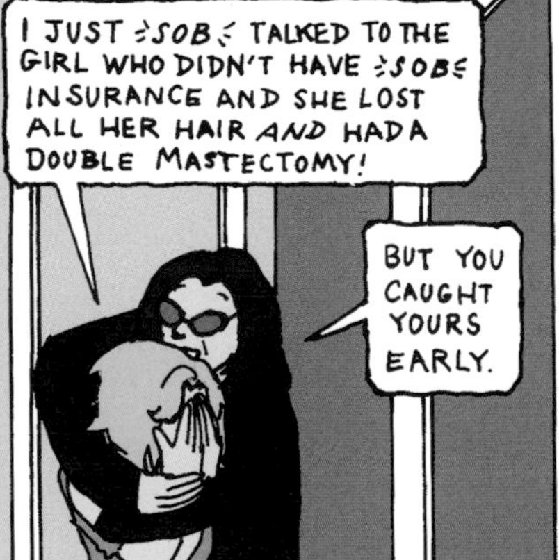
I JUST SOB TALKED TO THE GIRL WHO DIDN'T HAVE SOB INSURANCE AND SHE LOST ALL HER HAIR AND HAD A DOUBLE MASTECTOMY!
BUT YOU CAUGHT YOURS EARLY.

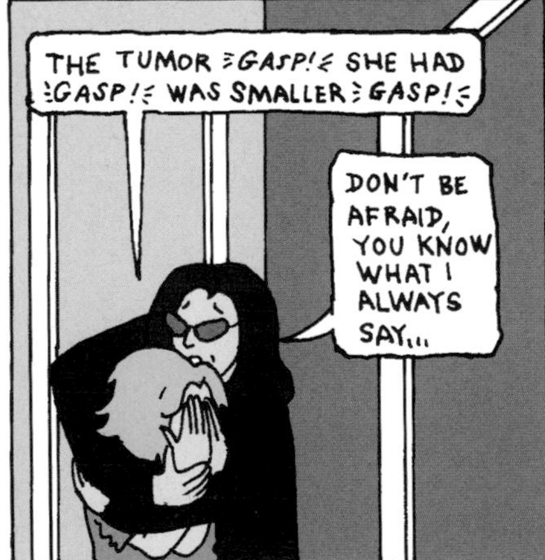
THE TUMOR GASP! SHE HAD GASP! WAS SMALLER GASP!
DON'T BE AFRAID, YOU KNOW WHAT I ALWAYS SAY...

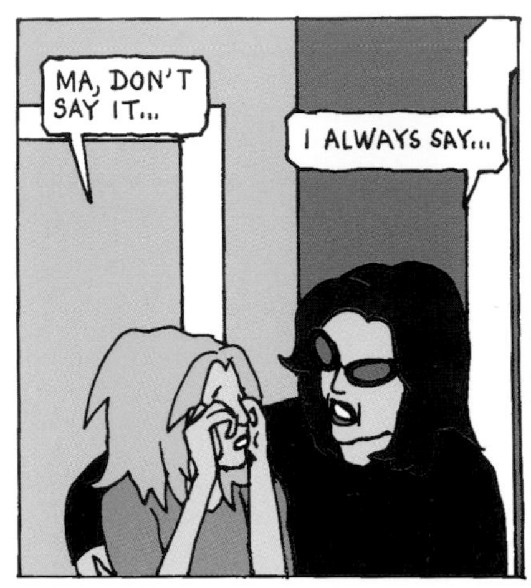
MA, DON'T SAY IT...
I ALWAYS SAY...

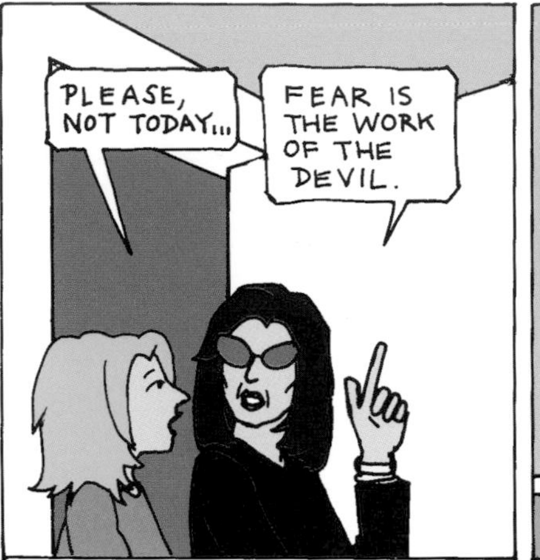
PLEASE, NOT TODAY...
FEAR IS THE WORK OF THE DEVIL.

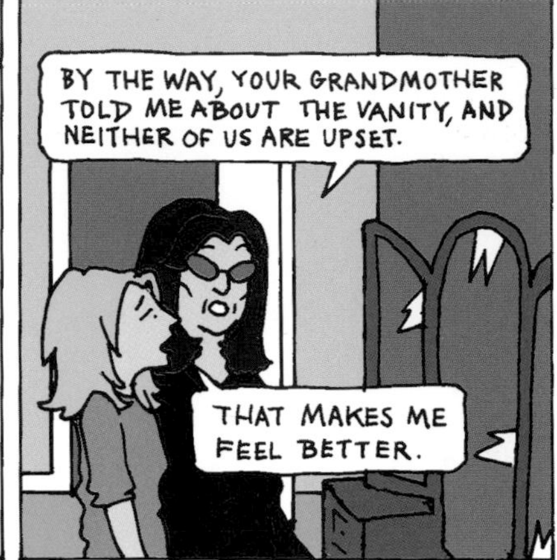
BY THE WAY, YOUR GRANDMOTHER TOLD ME ABOUT THE VANITY, AND NEITHER OF US ARE UPSET.
THAT MAKES ME FEEL BETTER.

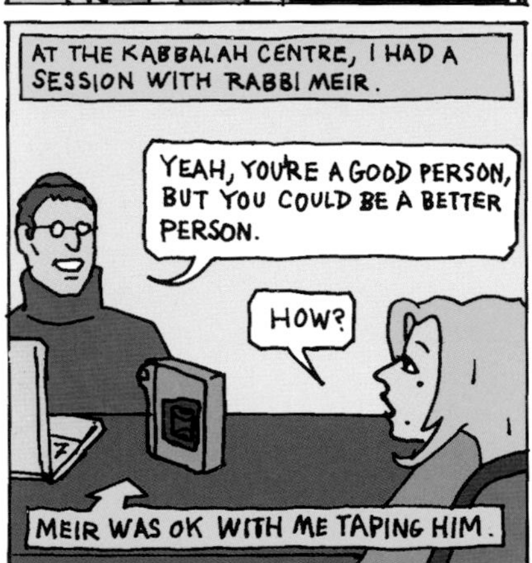
AT THE KABBALAH CENTRE, I HAD A SESSION WITH RABBI MEIR.
YEAH, YOU'RE A GOOD PERSON, BUT YOU COULD BE A BETTER PERSON.
HOW?
MEIR WAS OK WITH ME TAPING HIM.

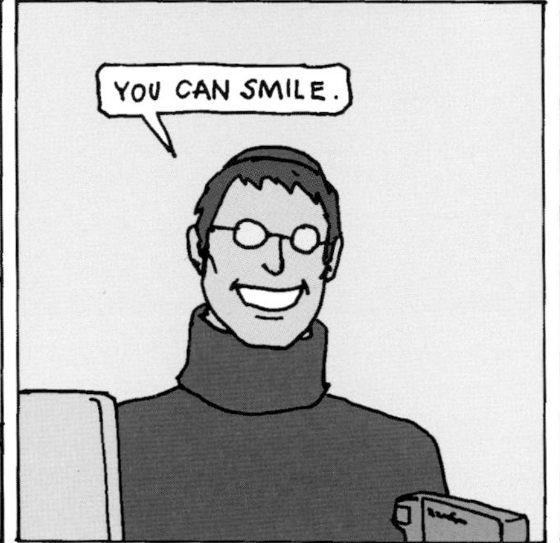
YOU CAN SMILE.

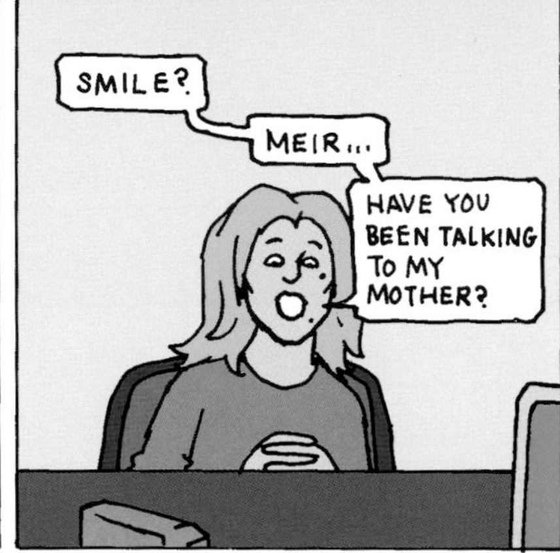
SMILE?
MEIR...
HAVE YOU BEEN TALKING TO MY MOTHER?

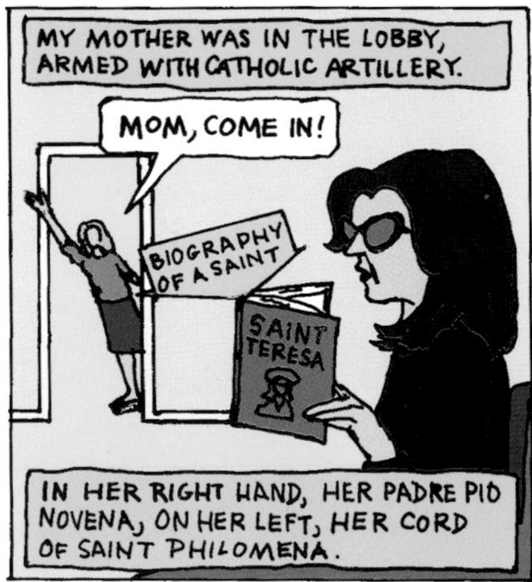
MY MOTHER WAS IN THE LOBBY, ARMED WITH CATHOLIC ARTILLERY.
MOM, COME IN!
BIOGRAPHY OF A SAINT
SAINT TERESA
IN HER RIGHT HAND, HER PADRE PIO NOVENA, ON HER LEFT, HER CORD OF SAINT PHILOMENA.

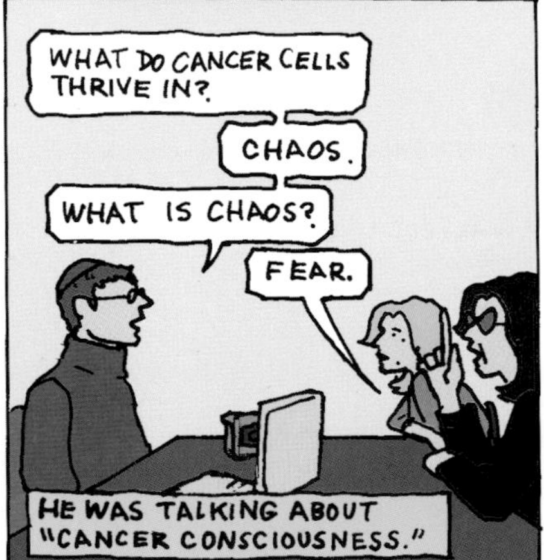
WHAT DO CANCER CELLS THRIVE IN?
CHAOS.
WHAT IS CHAOS?
FEAR.
HE WAS TALKING ABOUT "CANCER CONSCIOUSNESS."

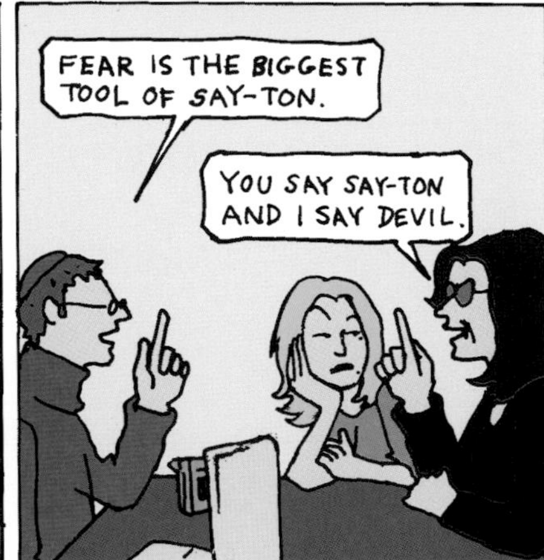
FEAR IS THE BIGGEST TOOL OF SAY-TON.
YOU SAY SAY-TON AND I SAY DEVIL.

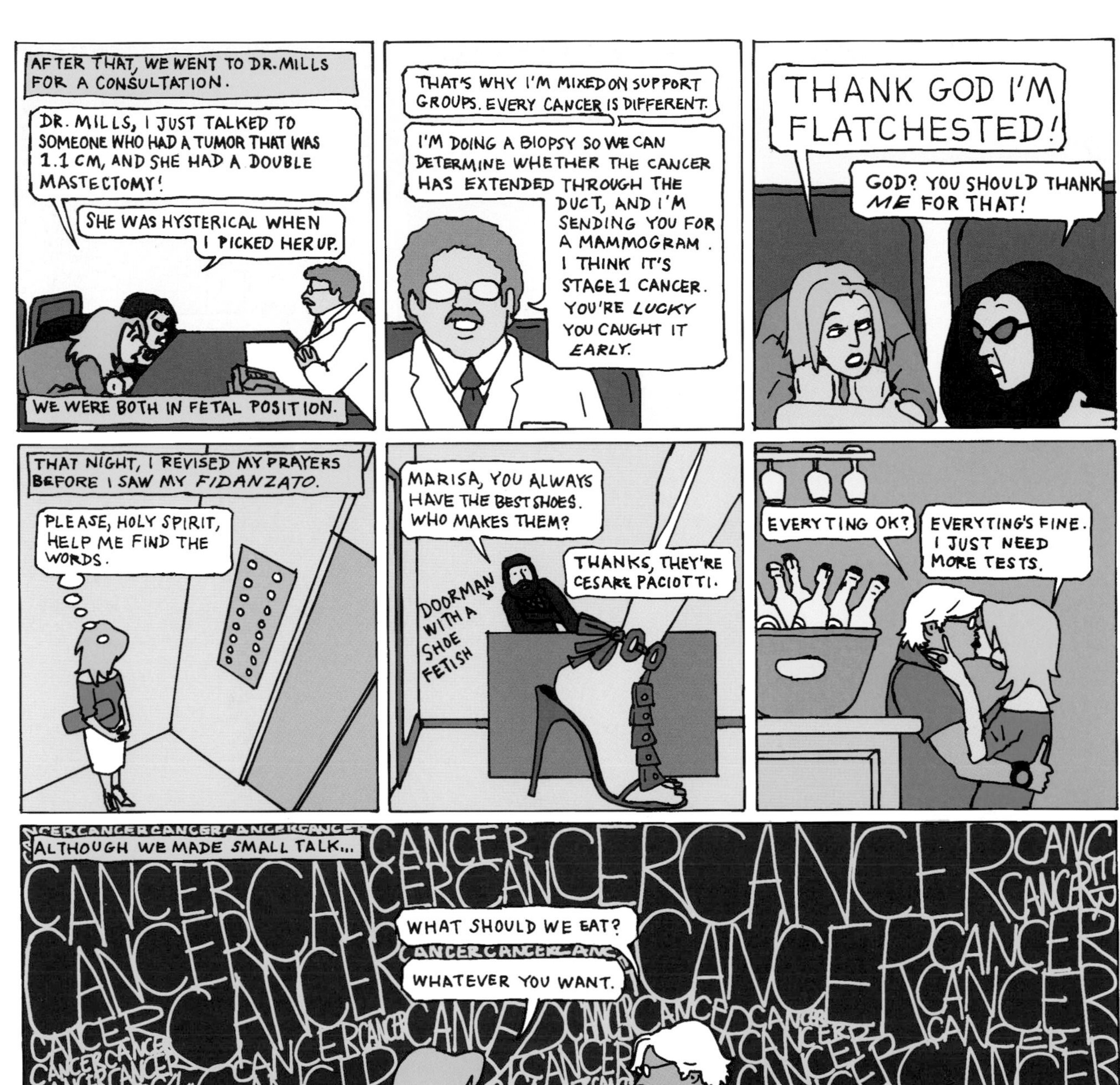
AFTER THAT, WE WENT TO DR. MILLS FOR A CONSULTATION.
DR. MILLS, I JUST TALKED TO SOMEONE WHO HAD A TUMOR THAT WAS 1.1 CM, AND SHE HAD A DOUBLE MASTECTOMY!
SHE WAS HYSTERICAL WHEN I PICKED HER UP.
WE WERE BOTH IN FETAL POSITION.
THAT'S WHY I'M MIXED ON SUPPORT GROUPS. EVERY CANCER IS DIFFERENT.
I'M DOING A BIOPSY SO WE CAN DETERMINE WHETHER THE CANCER HAS EXTENDED THROUGH THE DUCT, AND I'M SENDING YOU FOR A MAMMOGRAM. I THINK IT'S STAGE 1 CANCER. YOU'RE LUCKY YOU CAUGHT IT EARLY.
THANK GOD I'M FLATCHESTED!
GOD? YOU SHOULD THANK ME FOR THAT!
THAT NIGHT, I REVISED MY PRAYERS BEFORE I SAW MY FIDANZATO.
PLEASE, HOLY SPIRIT, HELP ME FIND THE WORDS.
MARISA, YOU ALWAYS HAVE THE BEST SHOES. WHO MAKES THEM?
THANKS, THEY'RE CESARE PACIOTTI.
DOORMAN WITH A SHOE FETISH
EVERYTING OK?
EVERYTING'S FINE. I JUST NEED MORE TESTS.
ALTHOUGH WE MADE SMALL TALK...
WHAT SHOULD WE EAT?
WHATEVER YOU WANT.

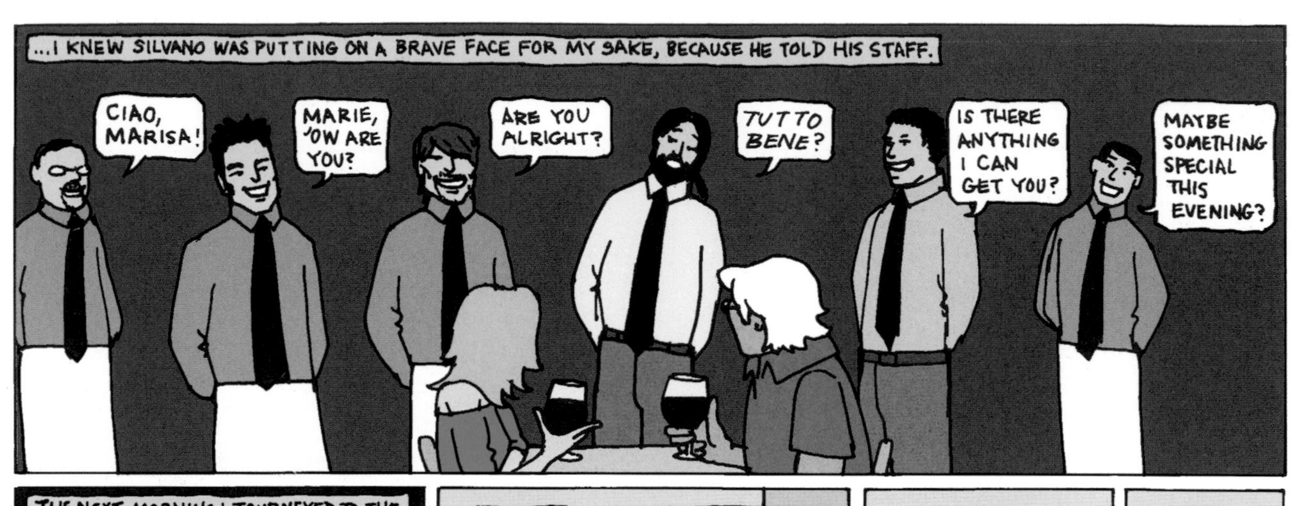
...I KNEW SILVANO WAS PUTTING ON A BRAVE FACE FOR MY SAKE, BECAUSE HE TOLD HIS STAFF.
CIAO, MARISA!
MARIE, 'OW ARE YOU?
ARE YOU ALRIGHT?
TUTTO BENE?
IS THERE ANYTHING I CAN GET YOU?
MAYBE SOMETHING SPECIAL THIS EVENING?

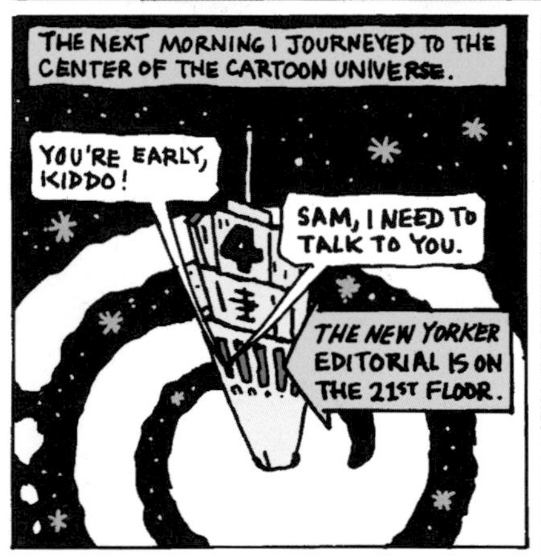
THE NEXT MORNING I JOURNEYED TO THE CENTER OF THE CARTOON UNIVERSE.
YOU'RE EARLY, KIDDO!
SAM, I NEED TO TALK TO YOU.
THE NEW YORKER EDITORIAL IS ON THE 21ST FLOOR.

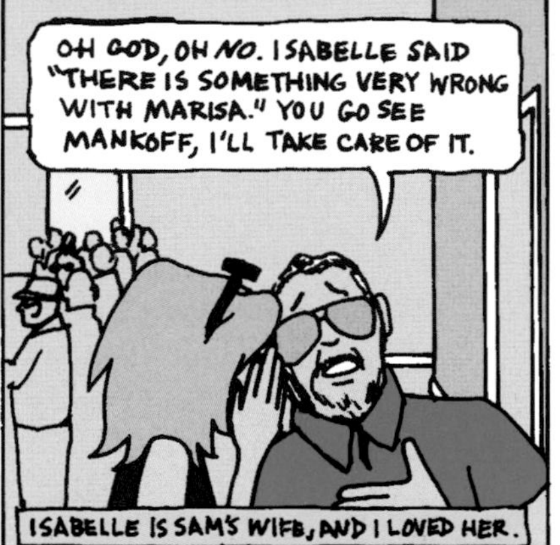
OH GOD, OH NO. ISABELLE SAID "THERE IS SOMETHING VERY WRONG WITH MARISA." YOU GO SEE MANKOFF, I'LL TAKE CARE OF IT.
ISABELLE IS SAM'S WIFE, AND I LOVED HER.

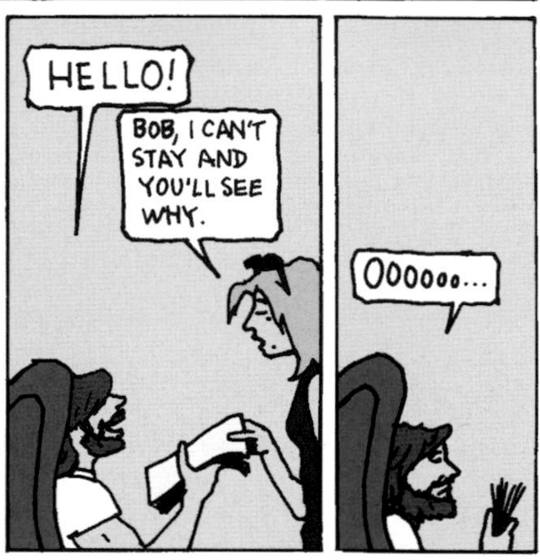
HELLO!
BOB, I CAN'T STAY AND YOU'LL SEE WHY.
OOOOOO...

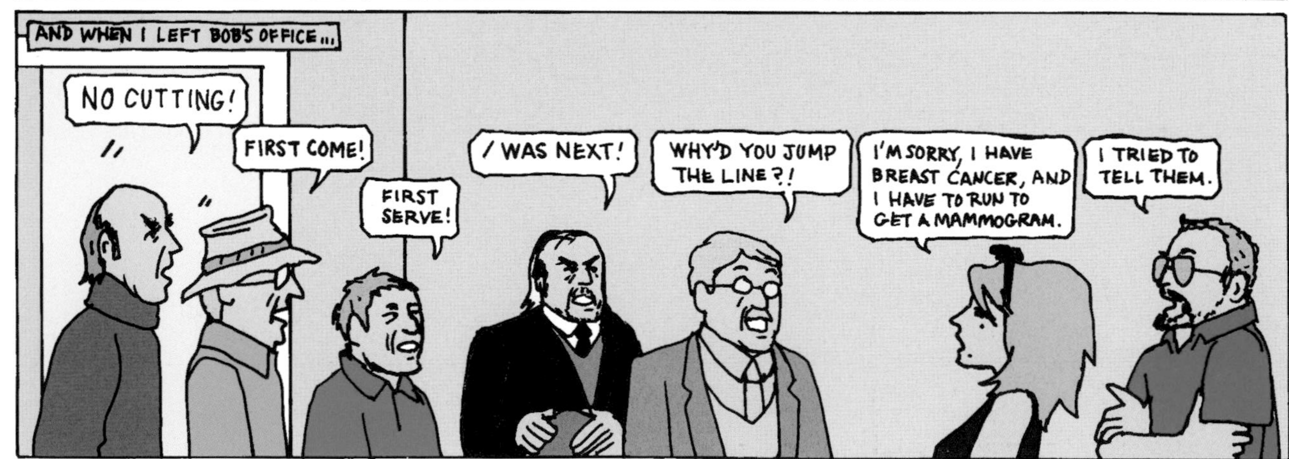
AND WHEN I LEFT BOB'S OFFICE...
NO CUTTING!
FIRST COME!
FIRST SERVE!
I WAS NEXT!
WHY'D YOU JUMP THE LINE?!
I'M SORRY, I HAVE BREAST CANCER, AND I HAVE TO RUN TO GET A MAMMOGRAM.
I TRIED TO TELL THEM.

11:45. NAZ MET ME AT THE RADIOLOGY PLACE.
YOU DON'T HAVE INSURANCE?
I'M PAYING BY CHECK.

WHY DON'T YOU HAVE INSURANCE?!
LOOK, I ALREADY FEEL BAD, DON'T MAKE ME FEEL WORSE, OK?

MARISA?
SEE YA AFTER TORTURE.

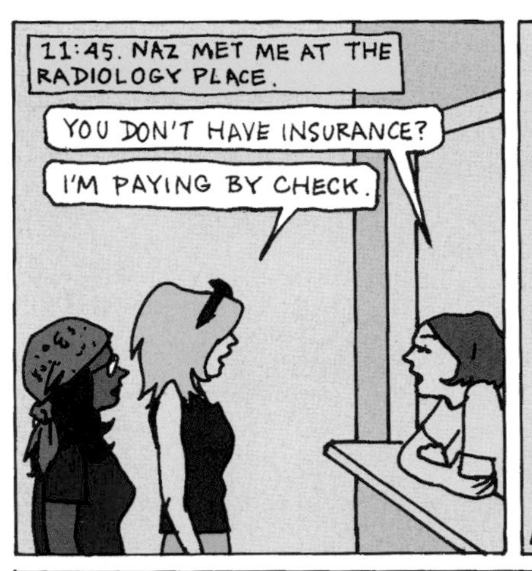

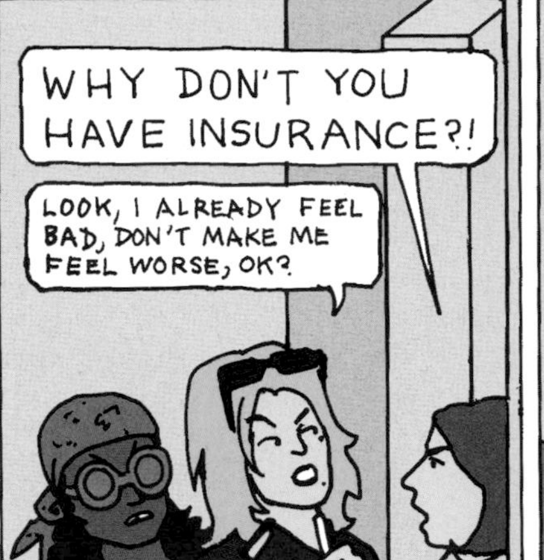

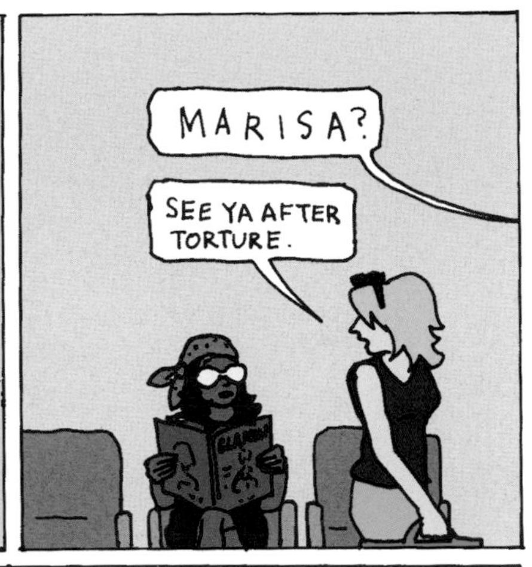

SO I HAD MY FIRST MAMMOGRAM AT 43...

AND I GOT SQUEEZED...

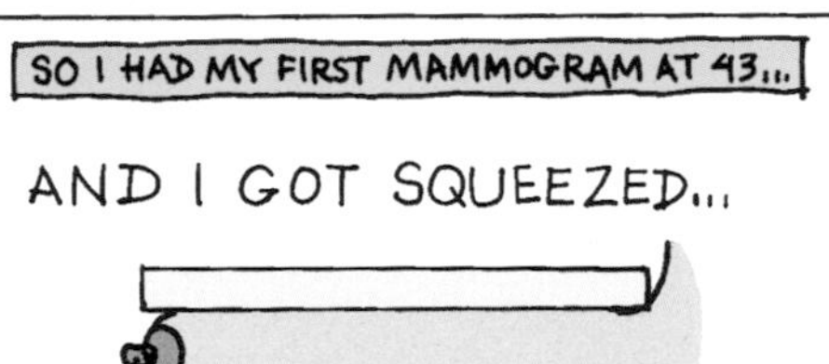

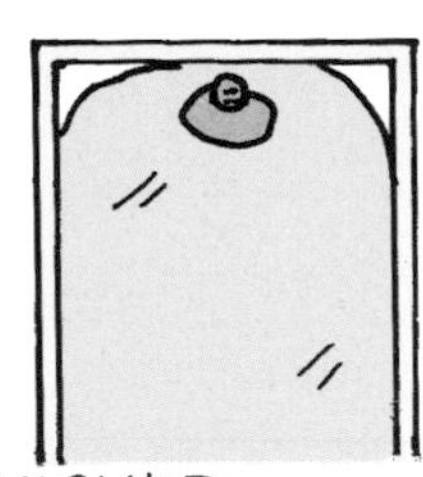

...SQUISHED...

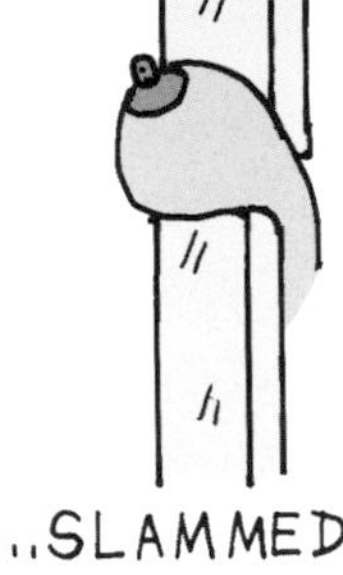

...SLAMMED...

...AND JAMMED...

WHY DON'T THEY PUT *TESTICLES* IN A VISE?!

THAT AFTERNOON, I WENT BACK TO WORK WHEN...
IT'S DR. MILLS'S OFFICE; HE WANTS YOU TO COME IN AT 9 A.M. FOR A BIOPSY.

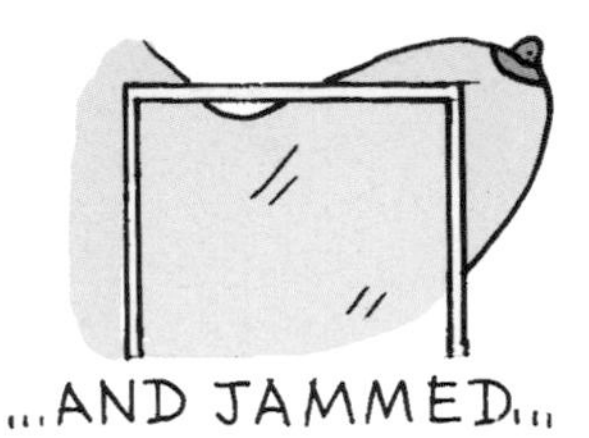

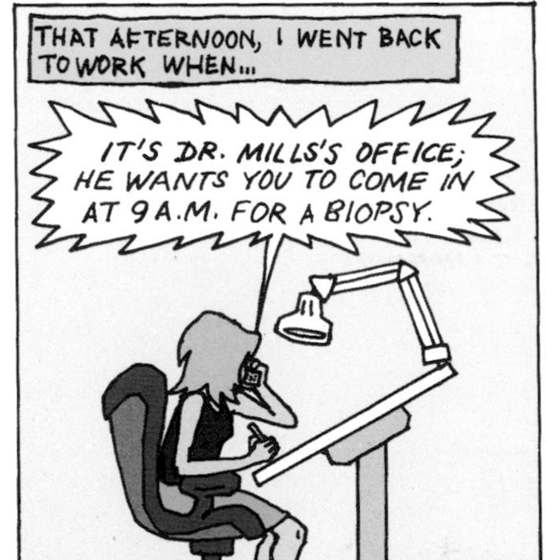

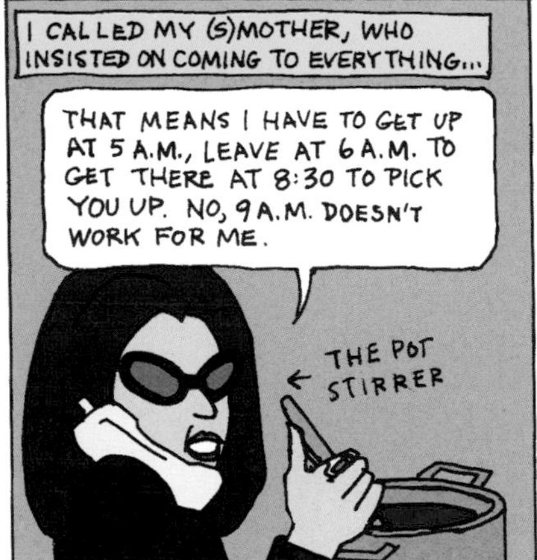

YOU WANT ME TO ASK DR. MILLS TO ARRANGE HIS HEAD OF THE HOSPITAL SURGEON'S SCHEDULE AROUND HIS PATIENT'S MOTHER?!

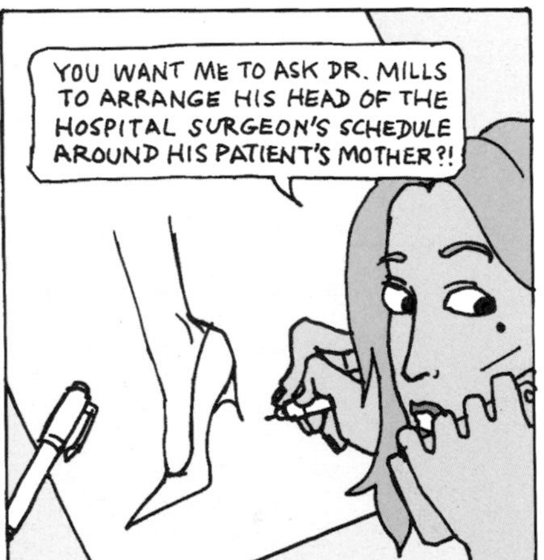

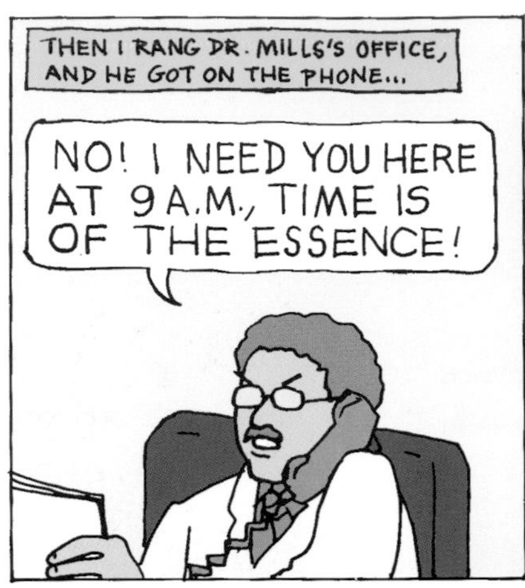
THEN I RANG DR. MILLS'S OFFICE, AND HE GOT ON THE PHONE...
NO! I NEED YOU HERE AT 9 A.M., TIME IS OF THE ESSENCE!

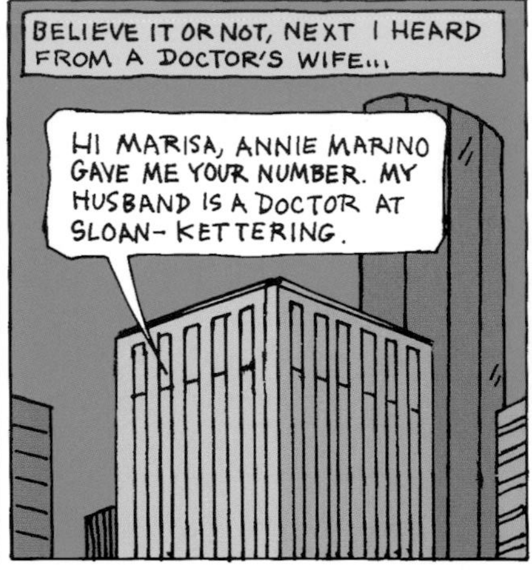
BELIEVE IT OR NOT, NEXT I HEARD FROM A DOCTOR'S WIFE...
HI MARISA, ANNIE MARINO GAVE ME YOUR NUMBER. MY HUSBAND IS A DOCTOR AT SLOAN-KETTERING.

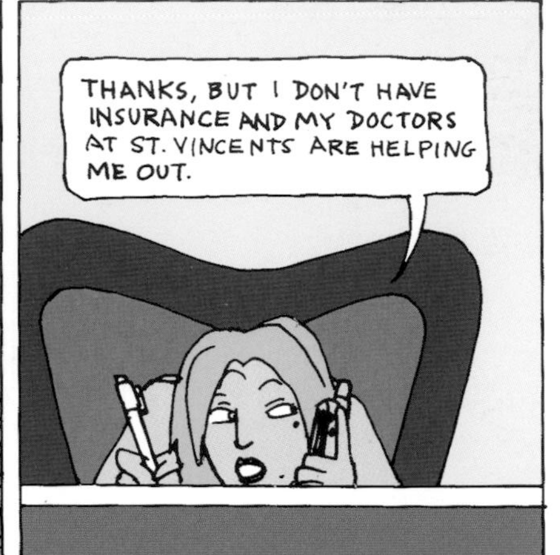
THANKS, BUT I DON'T HAVE INSURANCE AND MY DOCTORS AT ST. VINCENTS ARE HELPING ME OUT.

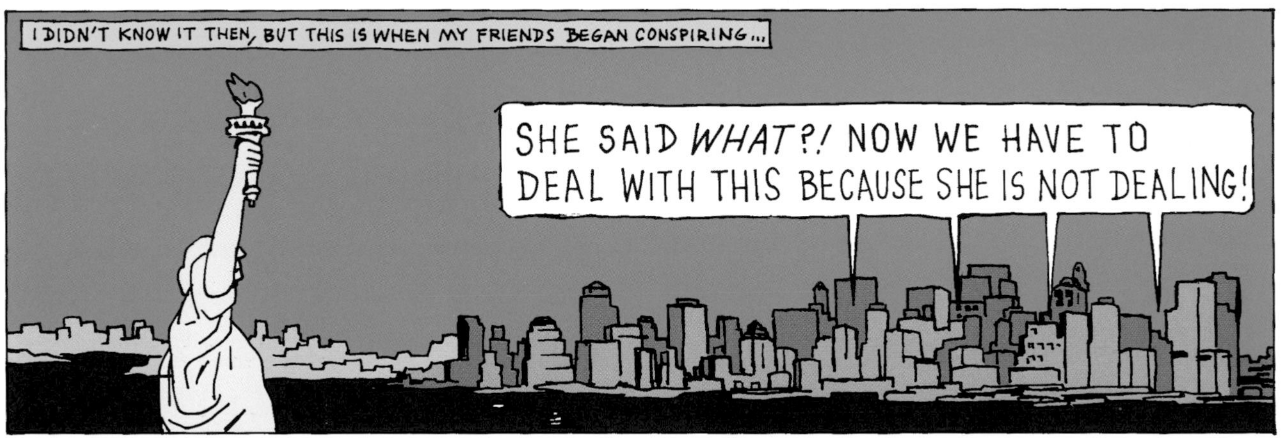
I DIDN'T KNOW IT THEN, BUT THIS IS WHEN MY FRIENDS BEGAN CONSPIRING...
SHE SAID *WHAT*?! NOW WE HAVE TO DEAL WITH THIS BECAUSE SHE IS NOT DEALING!

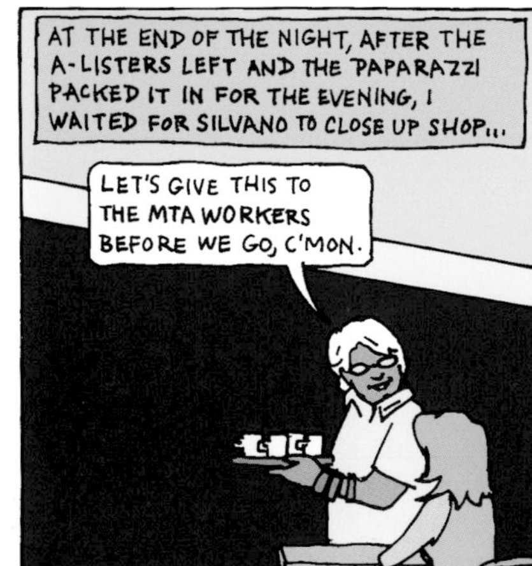
AT THE END OF THE NIGHT, AFTER THE A-LISTERS LEFT AND THE PAPARAZZI PACKED IT IN FOR THE EVENING, I WAITED FOR SILVANO TO CLOSE UP SHOP...
LET'S GIVE THIS TO THE MTA WORKERS BEFORE WE GO, C'MON.

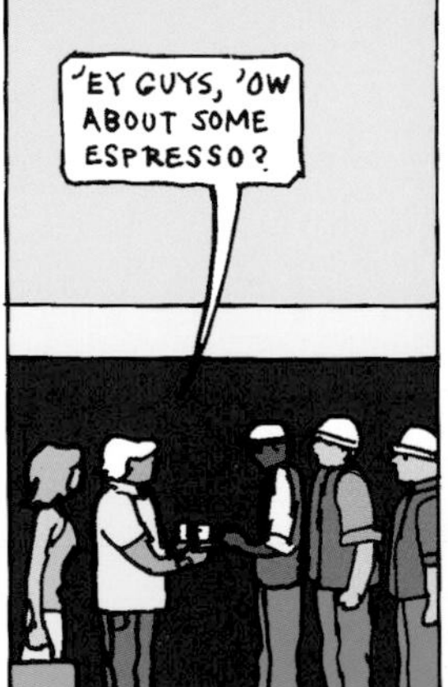
'EY GUYS, 'OW ABOUT SOME ESPRESSO?

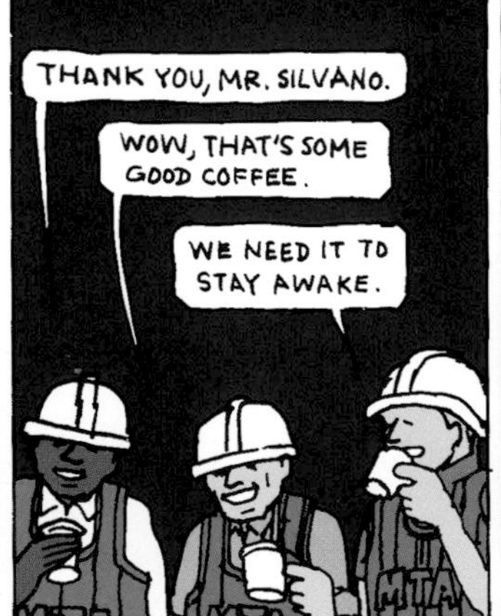
THANK YOU, MR. SILVANO.
WOW, THAT'S SOME GOOD COFFEE.
WE NEED IT TO STAY AWAKE.

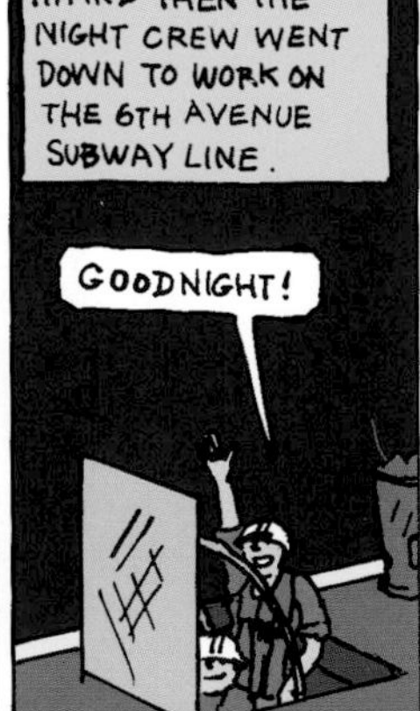
...AND THEN THE NIGHT CREW WENT DOWN TO WORK ON THE 6TH AVENUE SUBWAY LINE.
GOODNIGHT!

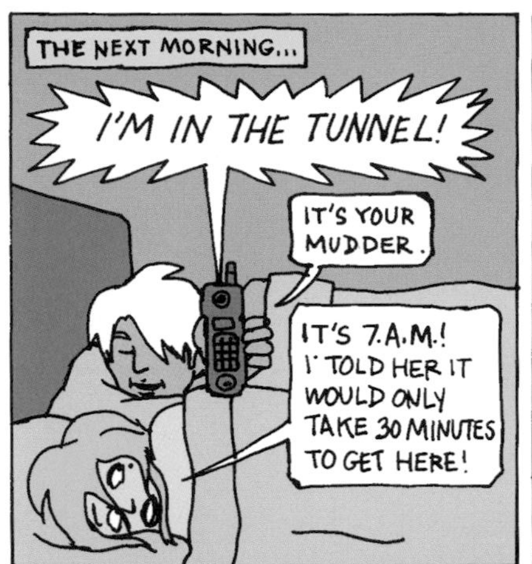
THE NEXT MORNING...
I'M IN THE TUNNEL!
IT'S YOUR MUDDER.
IT'S 7 A.M.! I TOLD HER IT WOULD ONLY TAKE 30 MINUTES TO GET HERE!

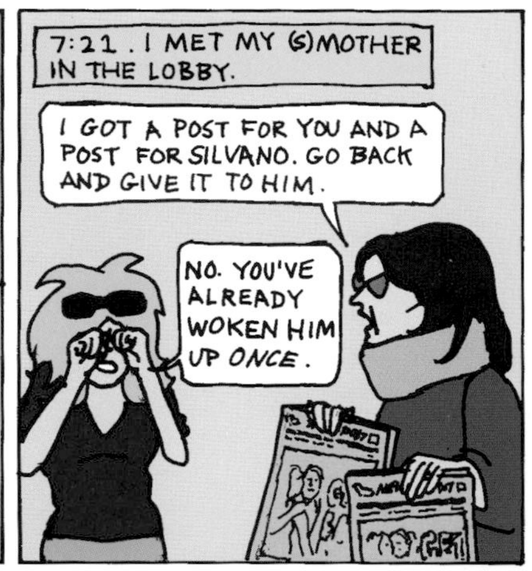
7:21. I MET MY (S)MOTHER IN THE LOBBY.
I GOT A POST FOR YOU AND A POST FOR SILVANO. GO BACK AND GIVE IT TO HIM.
NO. YOU'VE ALREADY WOKEN HIM UP ONCE.

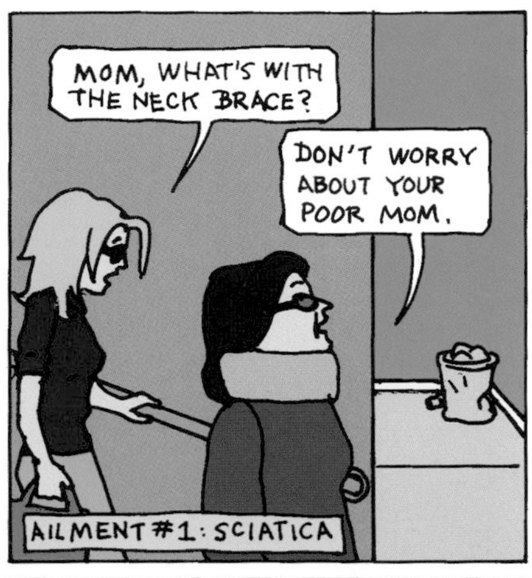
MOM, WHAT'S WITH THE NECK BRACE?
DON'T WORRY ABOUT YOUR POOR MOM.
AILMENT #1: SCIATICA

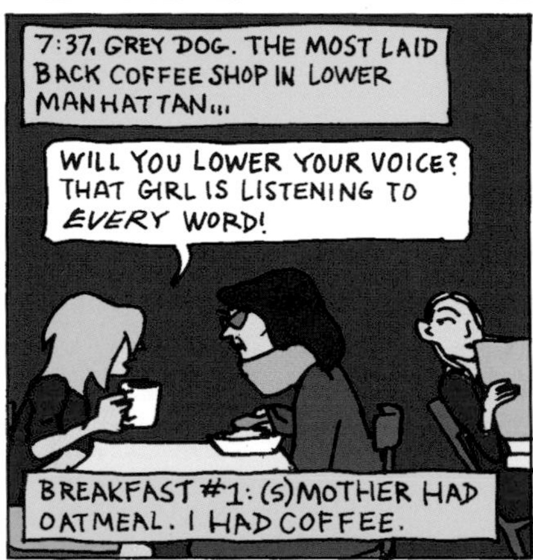
7:37. GREY DOG. THE MOST LAID BACK COFFEE SHOP IN LOWER MANHATTAN...
WILL YOU LOWER YOUR VOICE? THAT GIRL IS LISTENING TO EVERY WORD!
BREAKFAST #1: (S)MOTHER HAD OATMEAL. I HAD COFFEE.

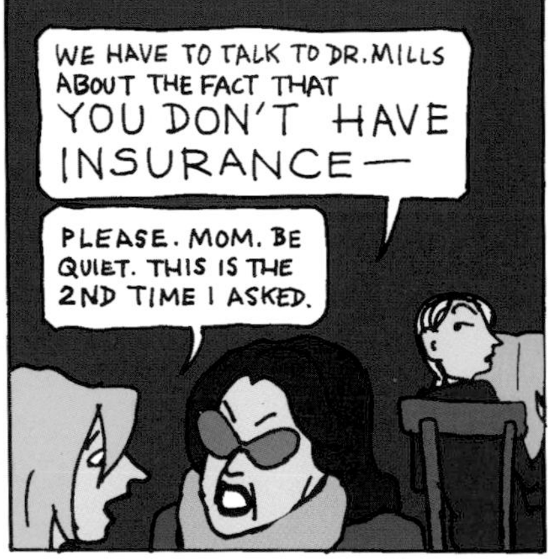
WE HAVE TO TALK TO DR. MILLS ABOUT THE FACT THAT YOU DON'T HAVE INSURANCE—
PLEASE. MOM. BE QUIET. THIS IS THE 2ND TIME I ASKED.

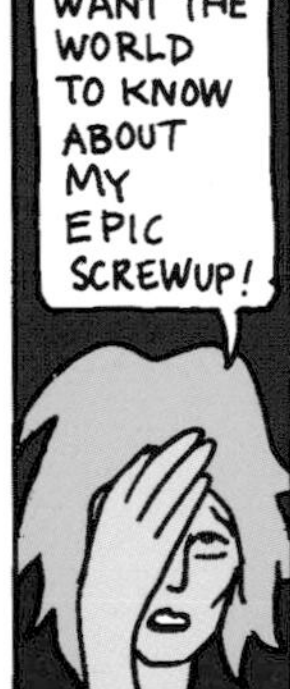
I DON'T WANT THE WORLD TO KNOW ABOUT MY EPIC SCREWUP!

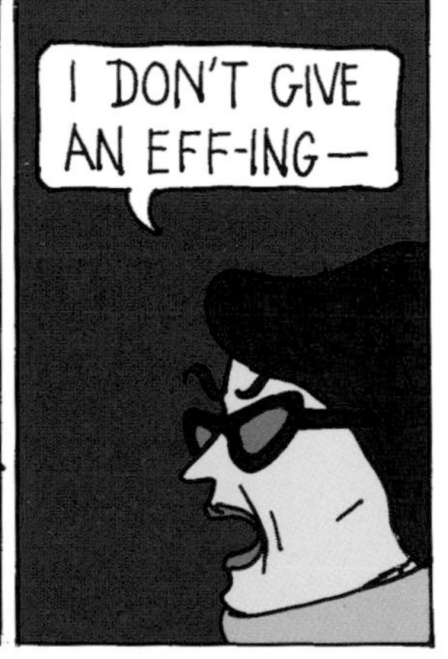
I DON'T GIVE AN EFF-ING—

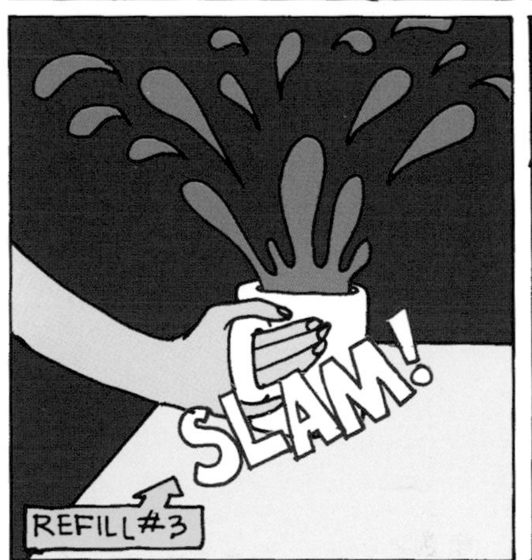
SLAM!
REFILL #3

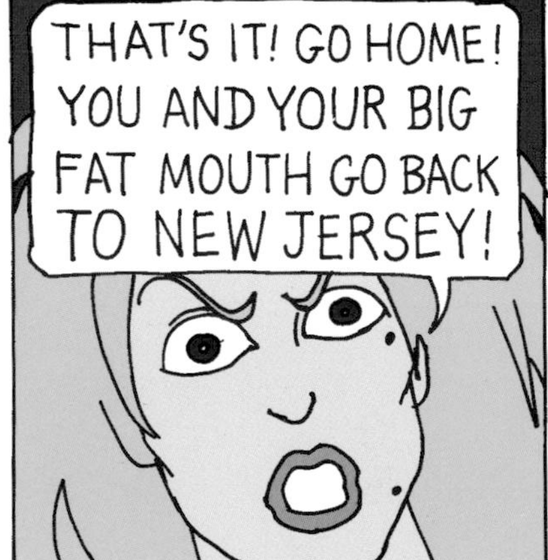
THAT'S IT! GO HOME! YOU AND YOUR BIG FAT MOUTH GO BACK TO NEW JERSEY!

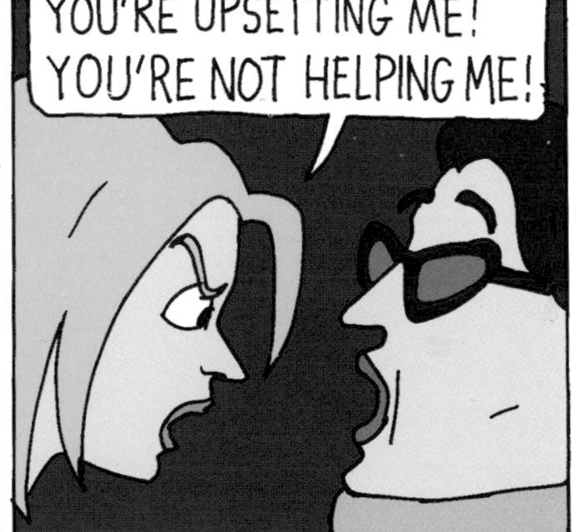
YOU'RE UPSETTING ME! YOU'RE NOT HELPING ME!

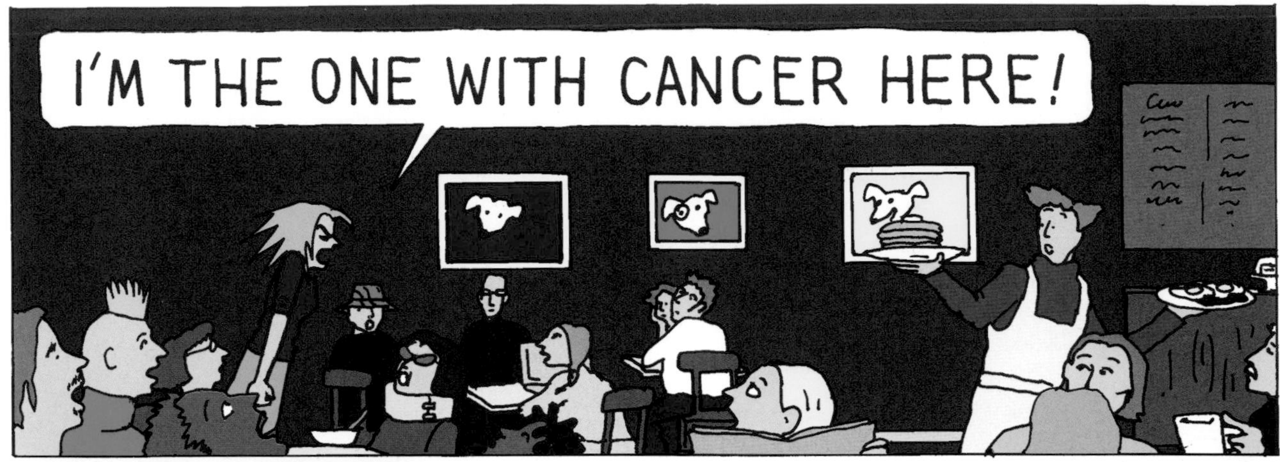
I'M THE ONE WITH CANCER HERE!

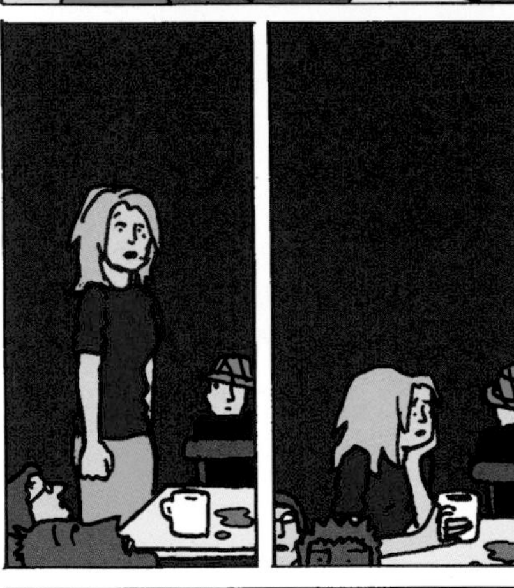

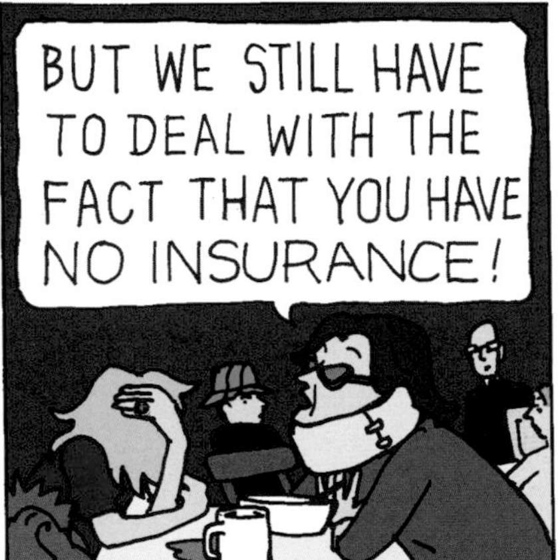
BUT WE STILL HAVE TO DEAL WITH THE FACT THAT YOU HAVE NO INSURANCE!

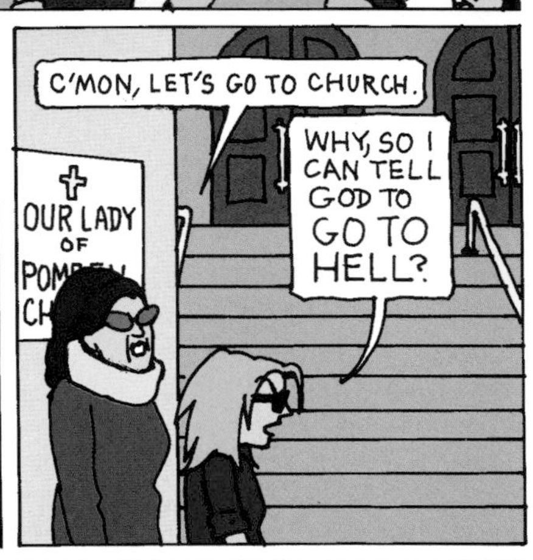
C'MON, LET'S GO TO CHURCH.
WHY, SO I CAN TELL GOD TO GO TO HELL?
OUR LADY OF

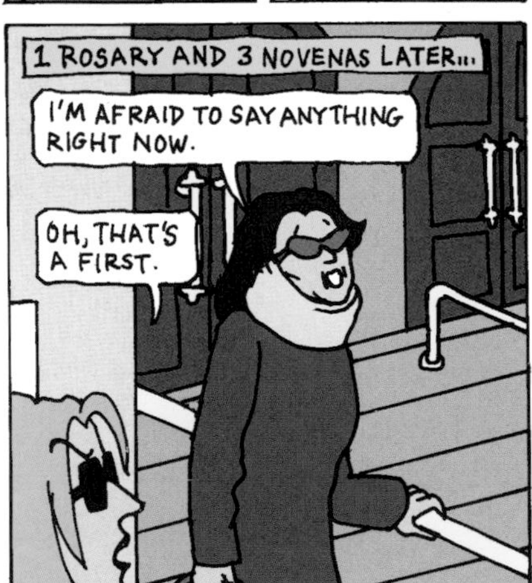
1 ROSARY AND 3 NOVENAS LATER...
I'M AFRAID TO SAY ANYTHING RIGHT NOW.
OH, THAT'S A FIRST.

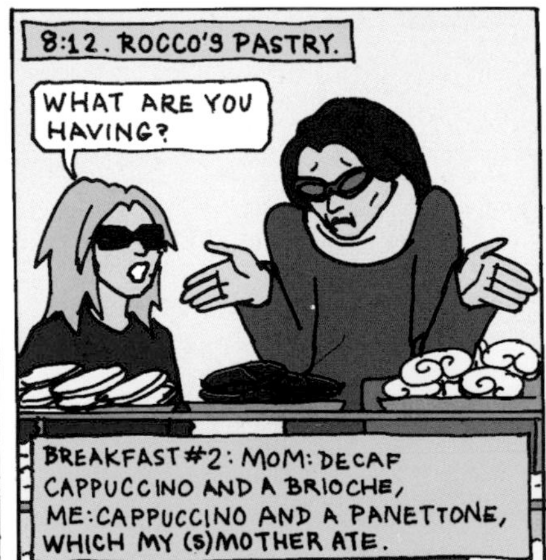
8:12. ROCCO'S PASTRY.
WHAT ARE YOU HAVING?
BREAKFAST #2: MOM: DECAF CAPPUCCINO AND A BRIOCHE, ME: CAPPUCCINO AND A PANETTONE, WHICH MY (S)MOTHER ATE.

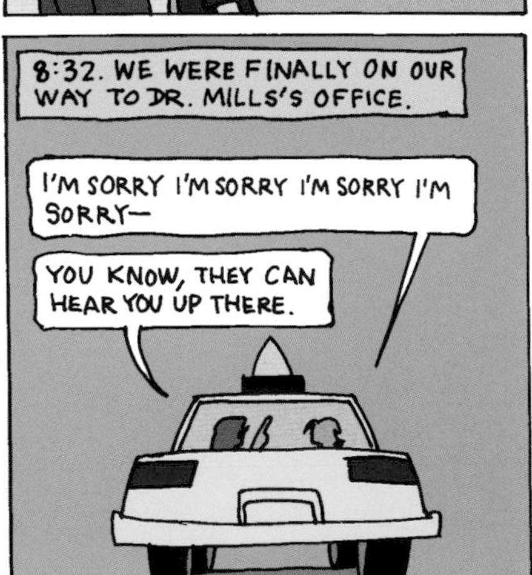
8:32. WE WERE FINALLY ON OUR WAY TO DR. MILLS'S OFFICE.
I'M SORRY I'M SORRY I'M SORRY I'M SORRY—
YOU KNOW, THEY CAN HEAR YOU UP THERE.

BEFORE THE DREADED CORE BIOPSY, DR. MILLS FILLS US IN.
CANCER LUMPECTOMY MAY NOT BE INVASIVE LYMPH NODES.
THE LAST DOCTOR'S VISIT WITHOUT A TAPE RECORDER.

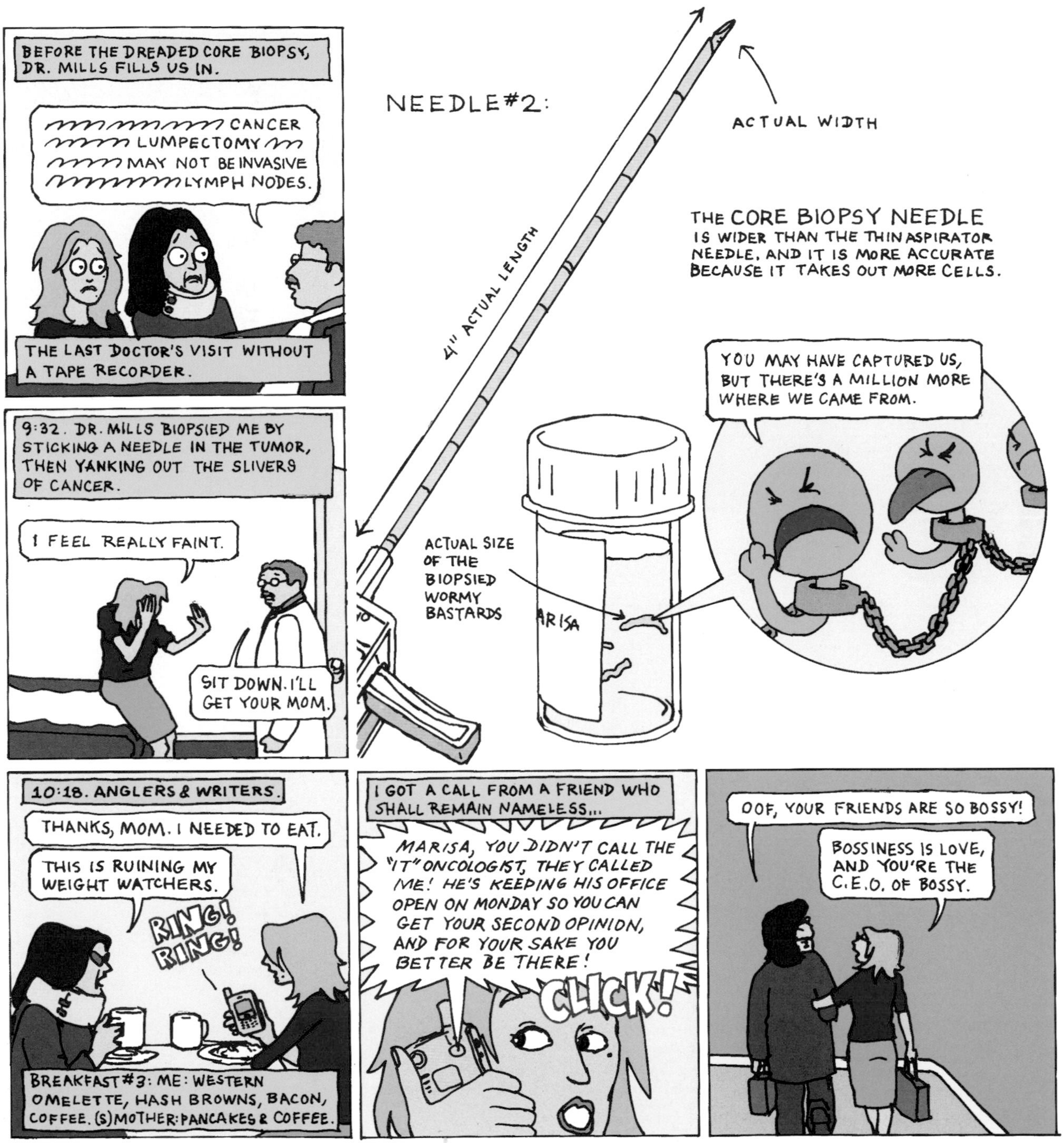

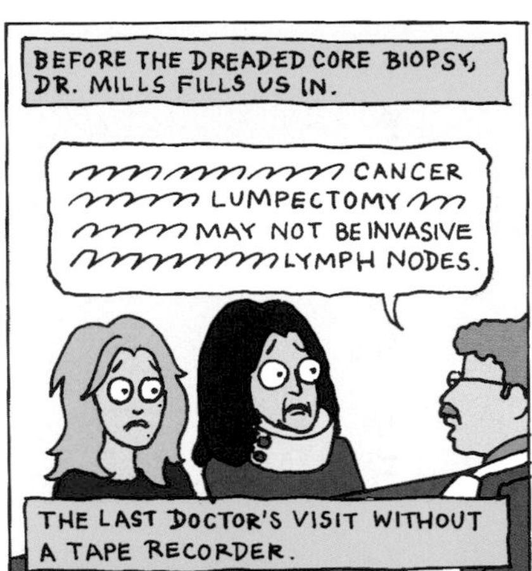

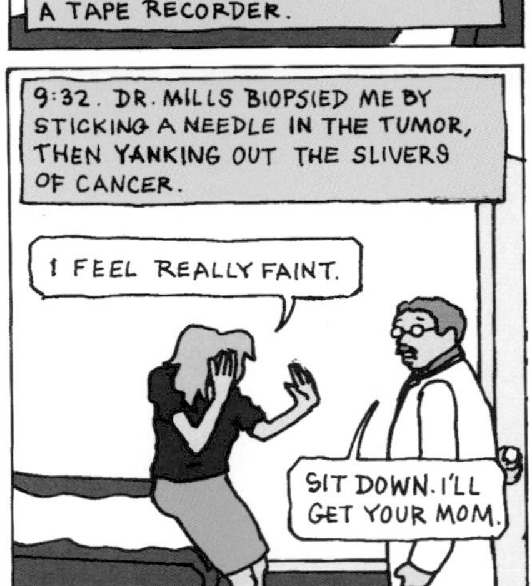

NEEDLE#2:

ACTUAL WIDTH

4" ACTUAL LENGTH

THE CORE BIOPSY NEEDLE IS WIDER THAN THE THIN ASPIRATOR NEEDLE, AND IT IS MORE ACCURATE BECAUSE IT TAKES OUT MORE CELLS.

ACTUAL SIZE OF THE BIOPSIED WORMY BASTARDS

ARISA

YOU MAY HAVE CAPTURED US, BUT THERE'S A MILLION MORE WHERE WE CAME FROM.

10:18. ANGLERS & WRITERS.
THANKS, MOM. I NEEDED TO EAT.
THIS IS RUINING MY WEIGHT WATCHERS.
RING! RING!
BREAKFAST #3: ME: WESTERN OMELETTE, HASH BROWNS, BACON, COFFEE. (S)MOTHER: PANCAKES & COFFEE.

I GOT A CALL FROM A FRIEND WHO SHALL REMAIN NAMELESS...
MARISA, YOU DIDN'T CALL THE "IT" ONCOLOGIST, THEY CALLED ME! HE'S KEEPING HIS OFFICE OPEN ON MONDAY SO YOU CAN GET YOUR SECOND OPINION, AND FOR YOUR SAKE YOU BETTER BE THERE!
CLICK!

OOF, YOUR FRIENDS ARE SO BOSSY!
BOSSINESS IS LOVE, AND YOU'RE THE C.E.O. OF BOSSY.

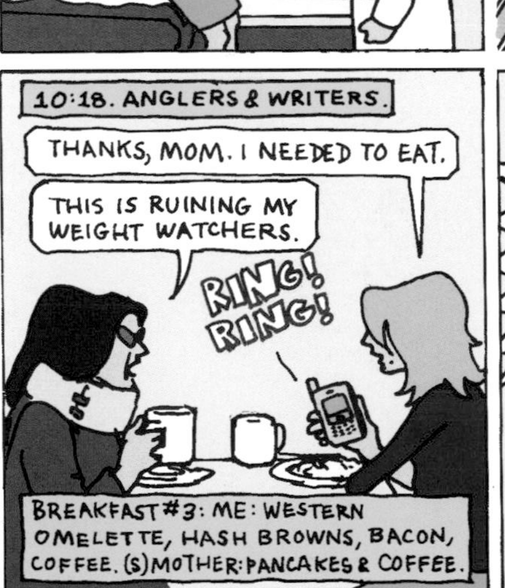

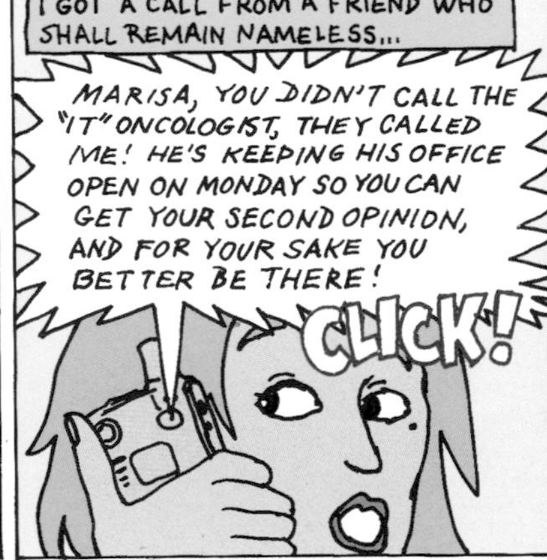

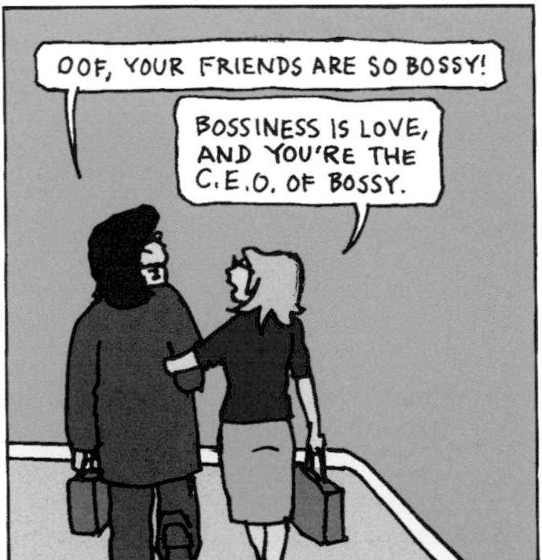

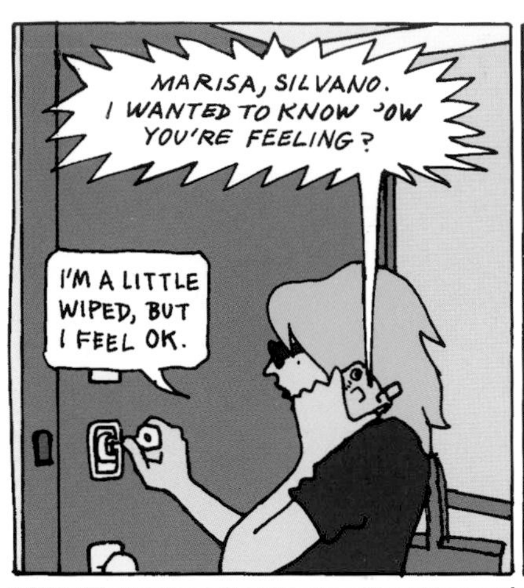
MARISA, SILVANO. I WANTED TO KNOW 'OW YOU'RE FEELING?
I'M A LITTLE WIPED, BUT I FEEL OK.

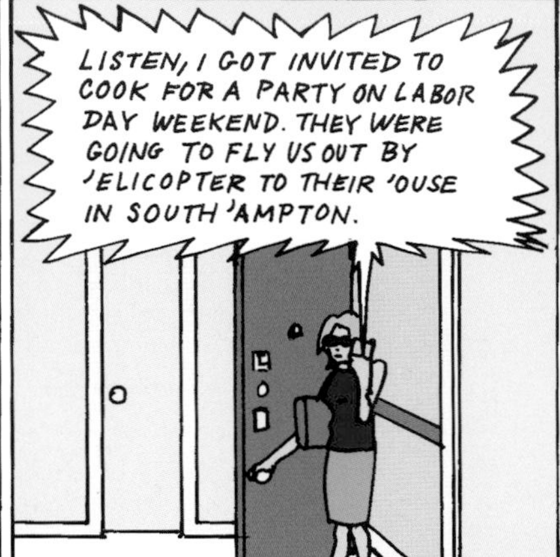
LISTEN, I GOT INVITED TO COOK FOR A PARTY ON LABOR DAY WEEKEND. THEY WERE GOING TO FLY US OUT BY 'ELICOPTER TO THEIR 'OUSE IN SOUTH'AMPTON.

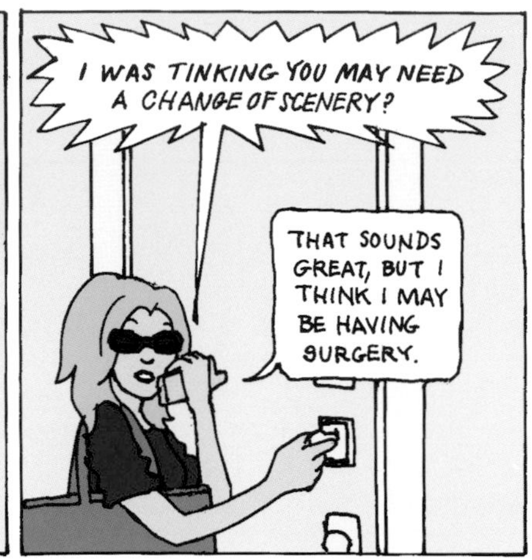
I WAS TINKING YOU MAY NEED A CHANGE OF SCENERY?
THAT SOUNDS GREAT, BUT I THINK I MAY BE HAVING SURGERY.

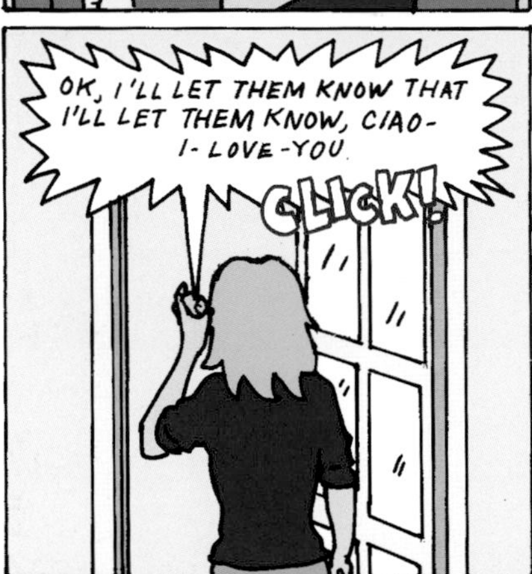
OK, I'LL LET THEM KNOW THAT I'LL LET THEM KNOW, CIAO-I-LOVE-YOU.
CLICK!

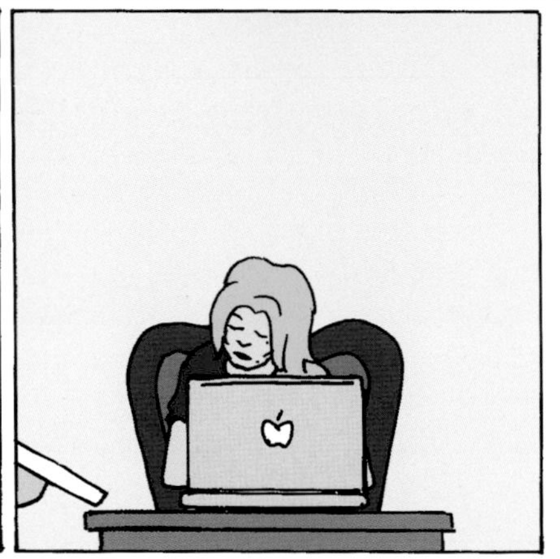

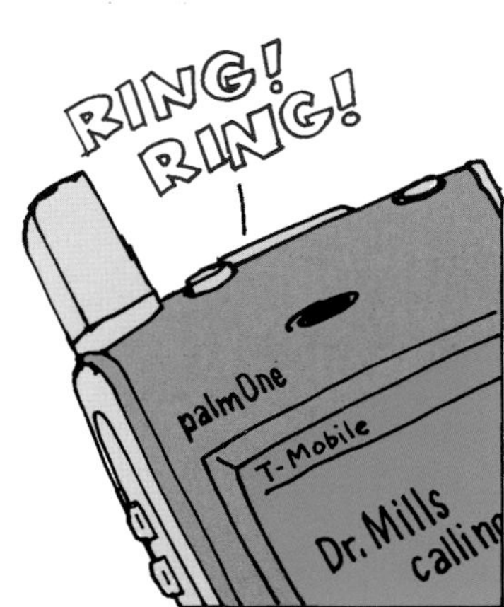
RING! RING!
palmOne
T-Mobile
Dr. Mills callin

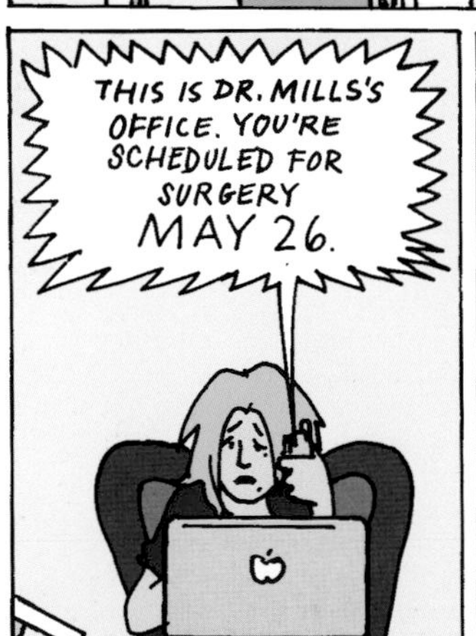
THIS IS DR. MILLS'S OFFICE. YOU'RE SCHEDULED FOR SURGERY MAY 26.

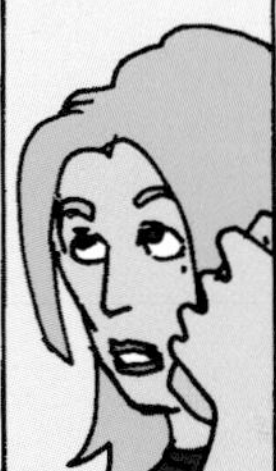
MAY 26? HANG ON, LET ME CHECK...

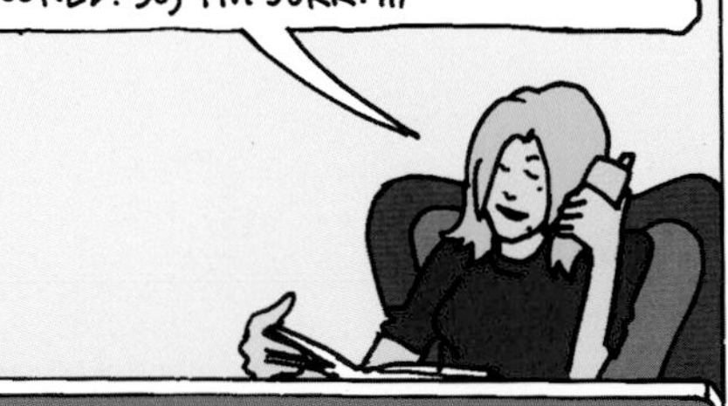
...THAT MORNING I'VE GOT A BROW WAXING FOLLOWED BY A MEETING UPTOWN, THEN LUNCH WITH AN EDITOR; IN FACT AS I LOOK AT MY CALENDAR I SEE THE WHOLE MONTH IS COMPLETELY BOOKED. SO, I'M SORRY...

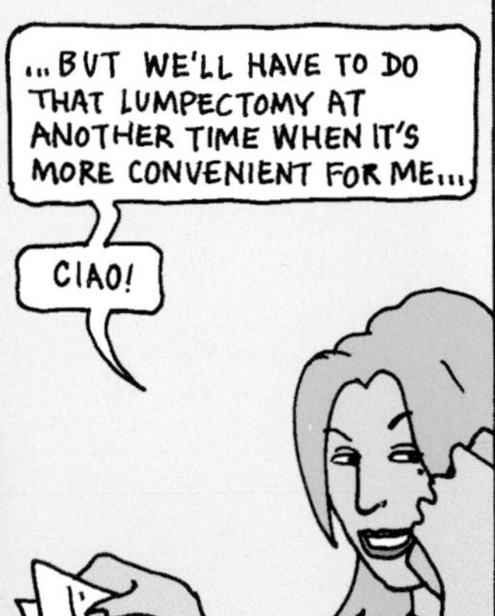
...BUT WE'LL HAVE TO DO THAT LUMPECTOMY AT ANOTHER TIME WHEN IT'S MORE CONVENIENT FOR ME...
CIAO!

IF I SAID THAT, I WOULD NEED TO GET MY HEAD EXAMINED, ON TOP OF EVERYTHING ELSE.

HERE'S WHAT I REALLY SAID...

MAY 26...?!
27, 28, 29, 30, 31
1, 2, 3, 4, 5, 6, 7,
8, 9, 10, 11=
16 DAYS...HMM...

WILL I BE OK BY JUNE 11?!
SURGERIES ARE LIKE WEDDINGS: THEY'RE ONLY REAL WHEN YOU'VE SET A DATE.

I NEED TO TAKE A NAP.

11 MINUTES LATER:
RING! RING!
I SLEPT ON MY BACK BECAUSE OF THE BIOPSY

MARISA, IT'S MATT... ARE YOU SURE YOU'RE UP FOR DOING "THE REJECTION SHOW" TONIGHT?

OF COURSE I'M UP FOR IT; BESIDES, MATT... I PROMISED YOU I'D DO IT!
OUCH!
AND I THOUGHT IT WOULD BE GOOD FOR ME.

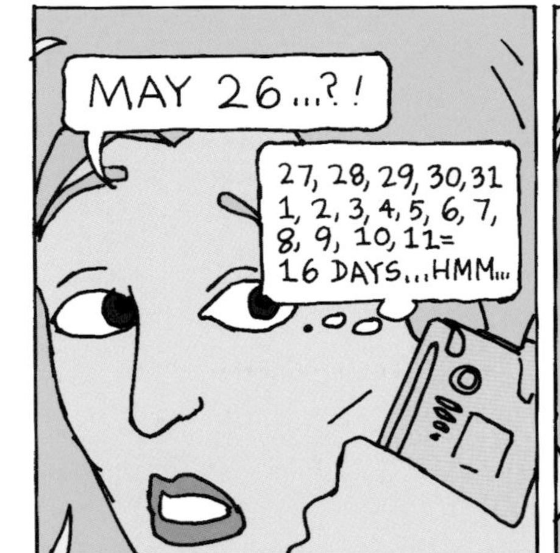

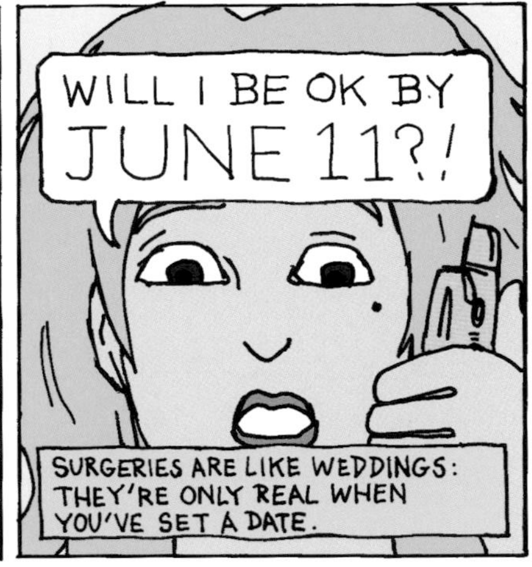

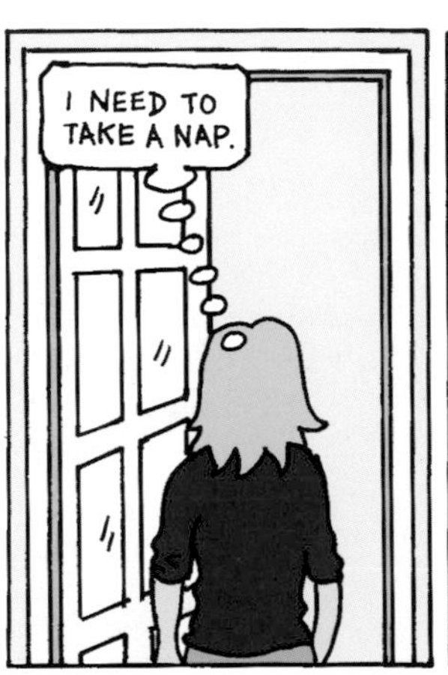

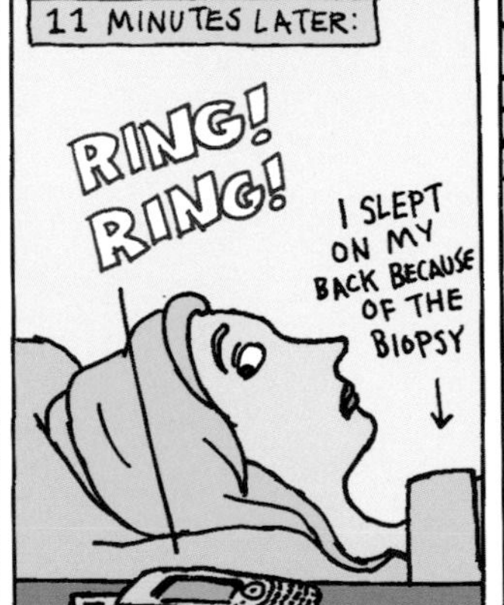

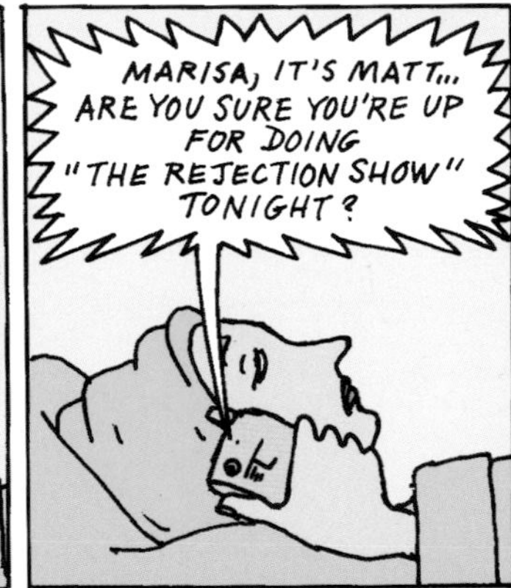

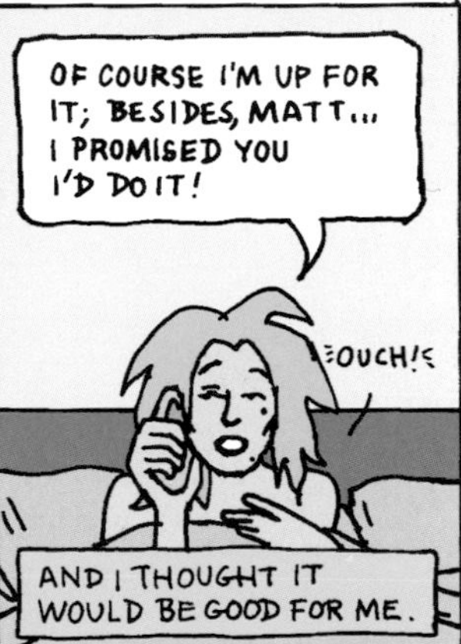

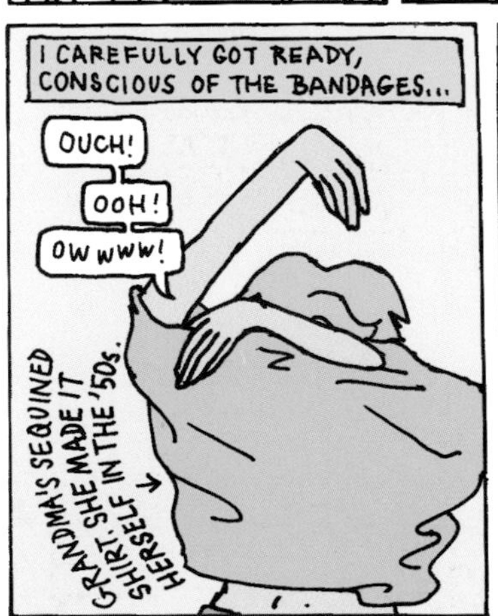

'ALLO, 'ALLO! I'M 'OME... YOU'RE GOING OUT?!
I'M DOING "THE REJECTION SHOW," REMEMBER?
CHE È "THE REJECTION SHOW"?

IT'S A SHOW WHERE WRITERS, COMEDIANS, CARTOONISTS, ANYONE PERFORMS THEIR REJECTED MATERIAL TO A LIVE AUDIENCE ONSTAGE.
AND YOU'RE DOING THIS TODAY?!

YEP. SEE YA AT 10:30. I LOVE YOU. CIAO!

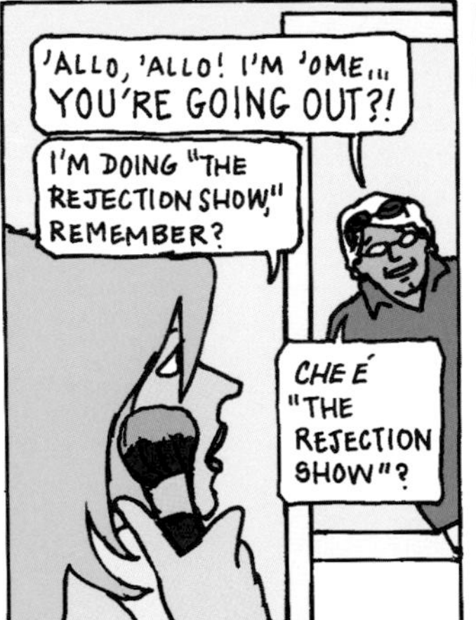

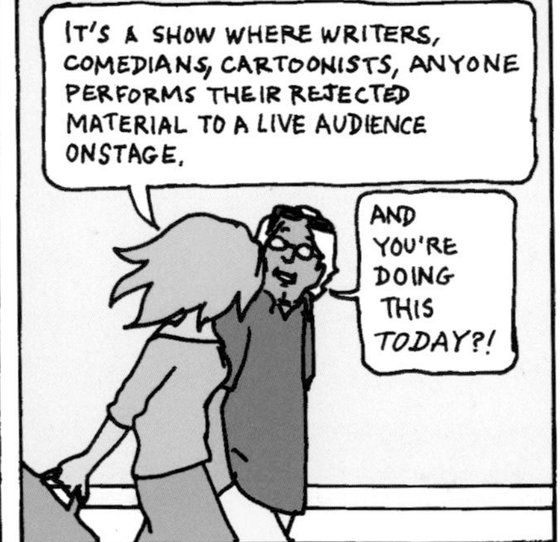

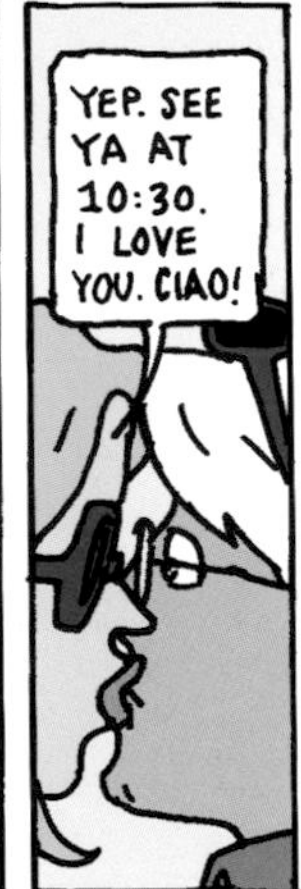

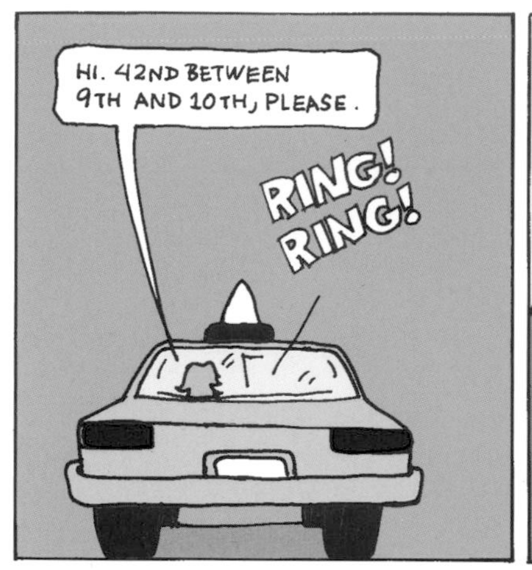
HI. 42ND BETWEEN 9TH AND 10TH, PLEASE.
RING! RING!

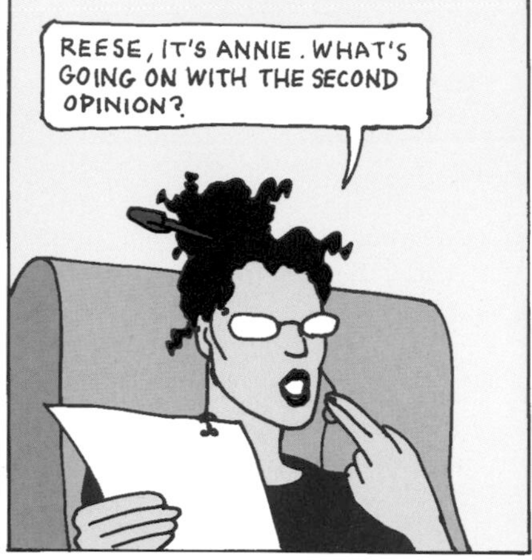
REESE, IT'S ANNIE. WHAT'S GOING ON WITH THE SECOND OPINION?

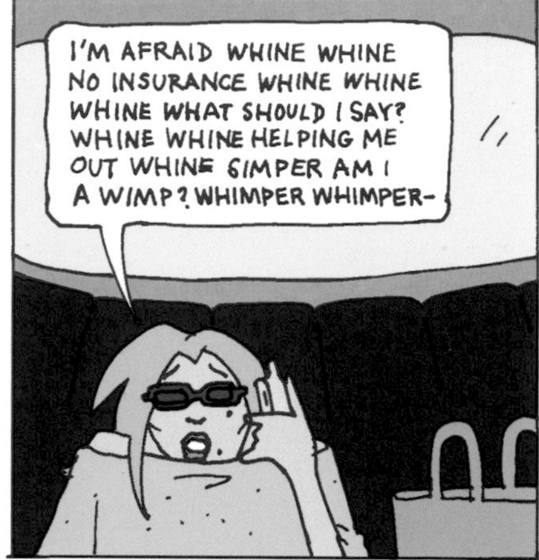
I'M AFRAID WHINE WHINE NO INSURANCE WHINE WHINE WHINE WHAT SHOULD I SAY? WHINE WHINE HELPING ME OUT WHINE SIMPER AM I A WIMP? WHIMPER WHIMPER-

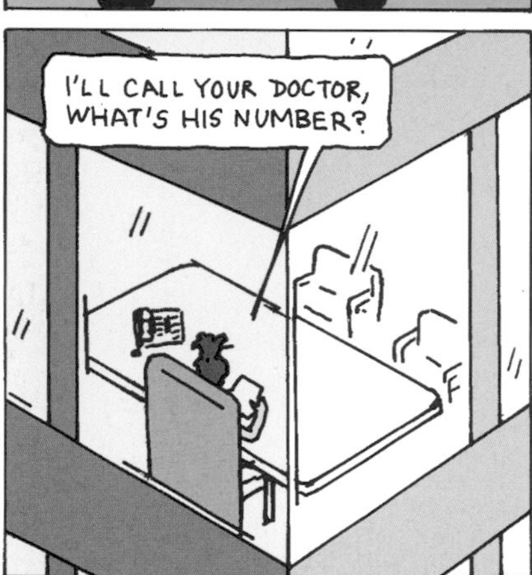
I'LL CALL YOUR DOCTOR, WHAT'S HIS NUMBER?

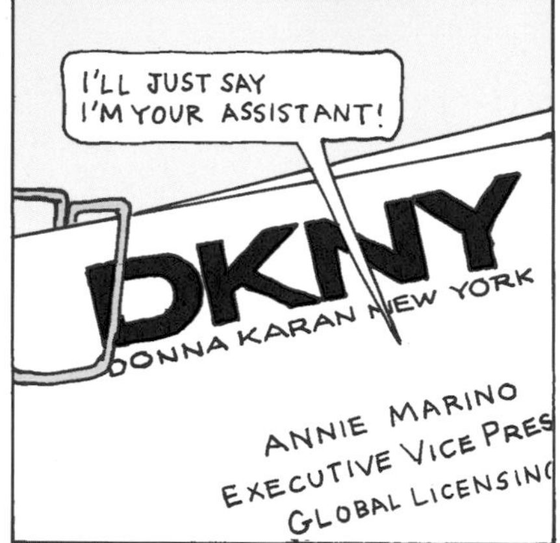
I'LL JUST SAY I'M YOUR ASSISTANT!
DKNY
DONNA KARAN NEW YORK
ANNIE MARINO
EXECUTIVE VICE PRES
GLOBAL LICENSIN

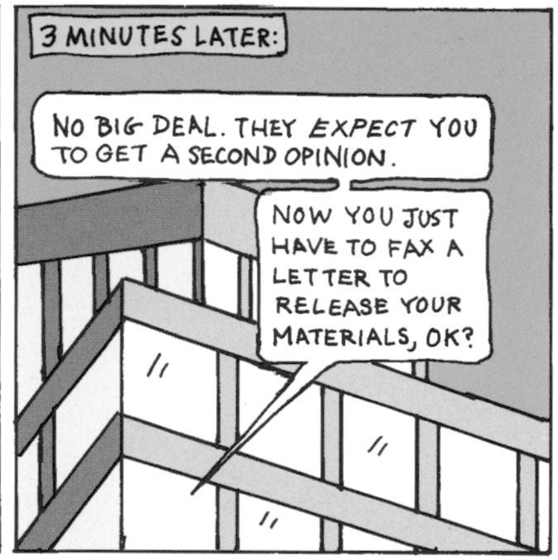
3 MINUTES LATER:
NO BIG DEAL. THEY *EXPECT* YOU TO GET A SECOND OPINION.
NOW YOU JUST HAVE TO FAX A LETTER TO RELEASE YOUR MATERIALS, OK?

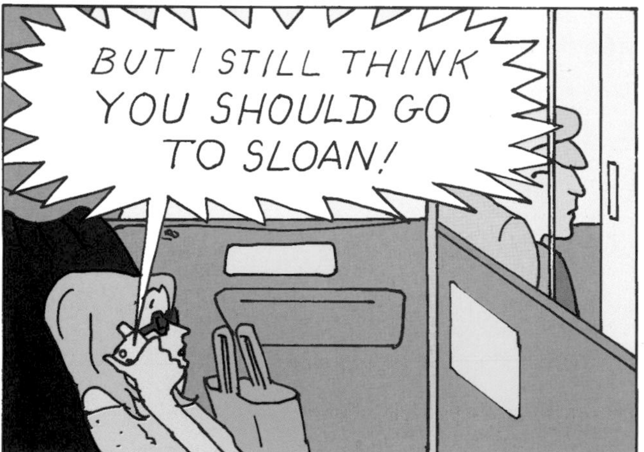
BUT I STILL THINK YOU SHOULD GO TO SLOAN!

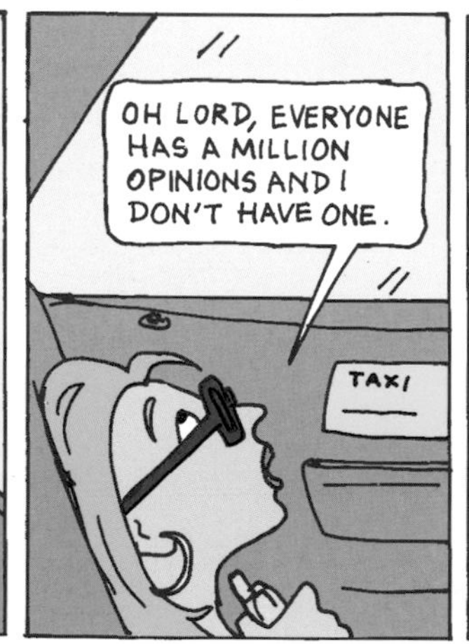
OH LORD, EVERYONE HAS A MILLION OPINIONS AND I DON'T HAVE ONE.
TAXI

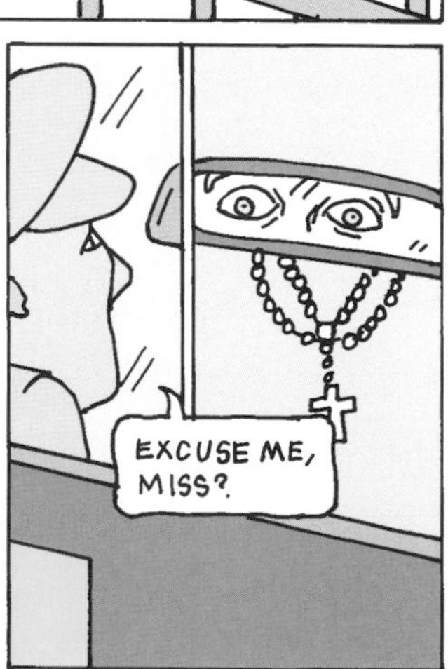
EXCUSE ME, MISS?

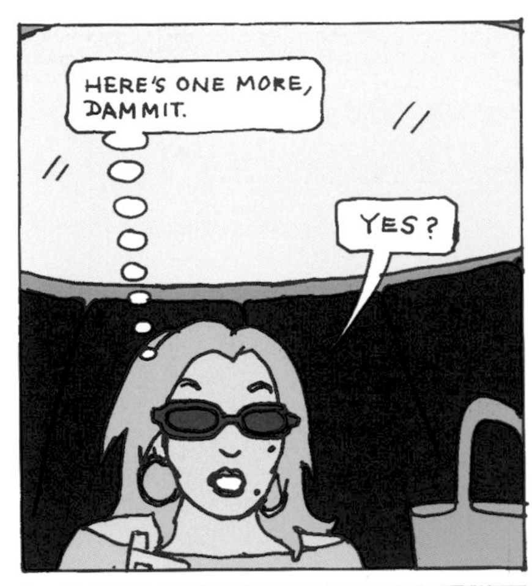
HERE'S ONE MORE, DAMMIT.
YES?

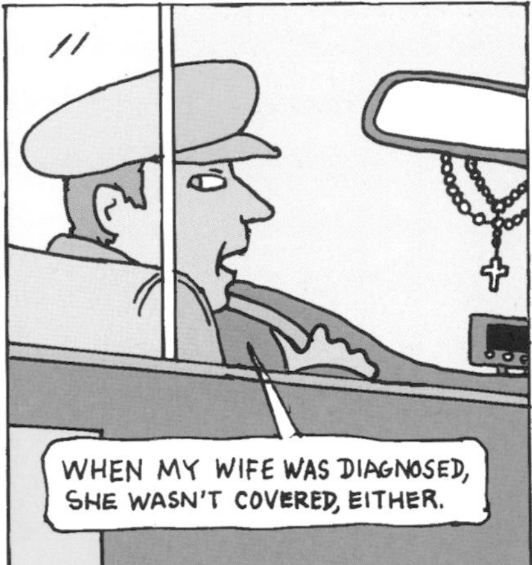
WHEN MY WIFE WAS DIAGNOSED, SHE WASN'T COVERED, EITHER.

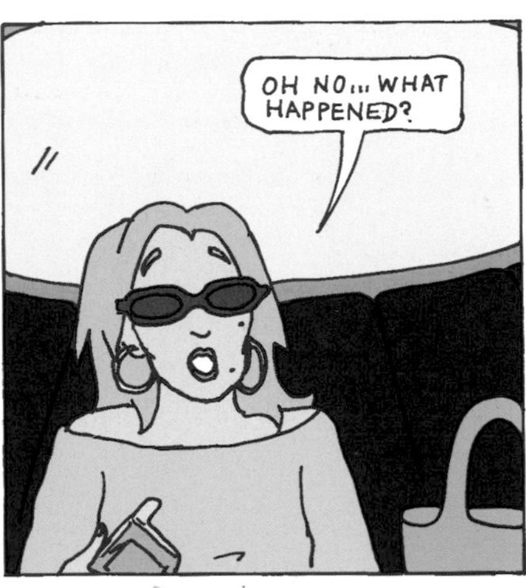
OH NO... WHAT HAPPENED?

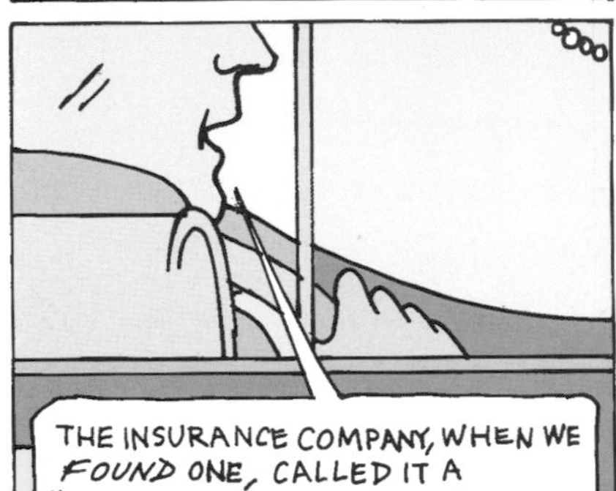
THE INSURANCE COMPANY, WHEN WE FOUND ONE, CALLED IT A "PRE-EXISTING CONDITION" AND WAITED 6 MONTHS TO GIVE IT TO HER.

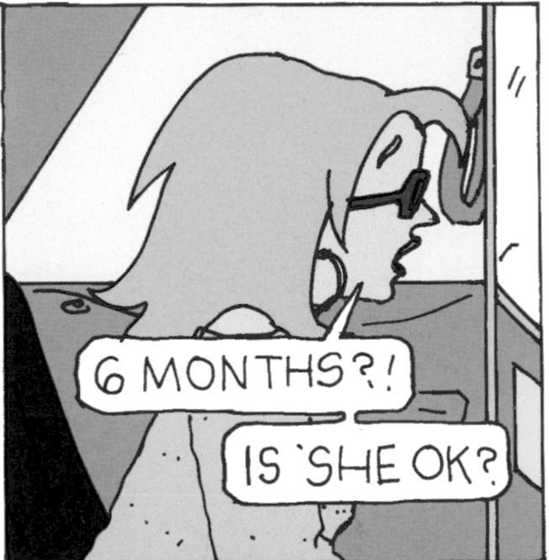
6 MONTHS?!
IS SHE OK?

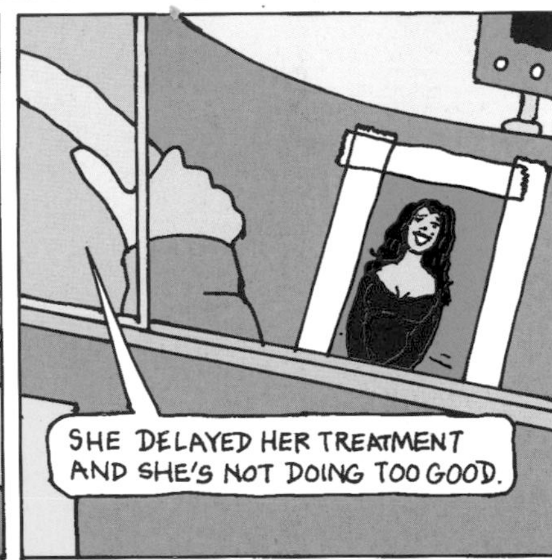
SHE DELAYED HER TREATMENT AND SHE'S NOT DOING TOO GOOD.

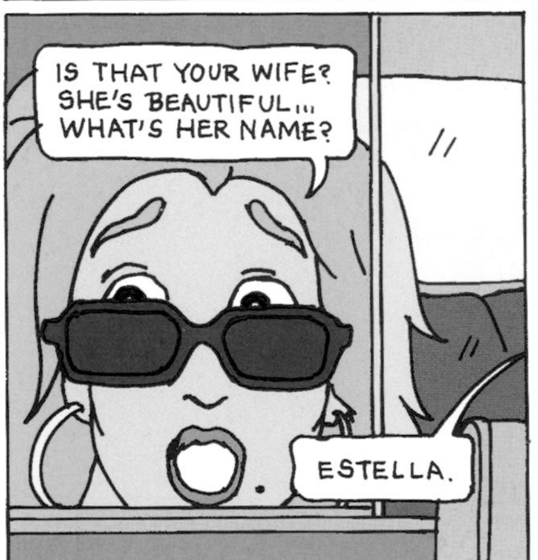
IS THAT YOUR WIFE? SHE'S BEAUTIFUL... WHAT'S HER NAME?
ESTELLA.

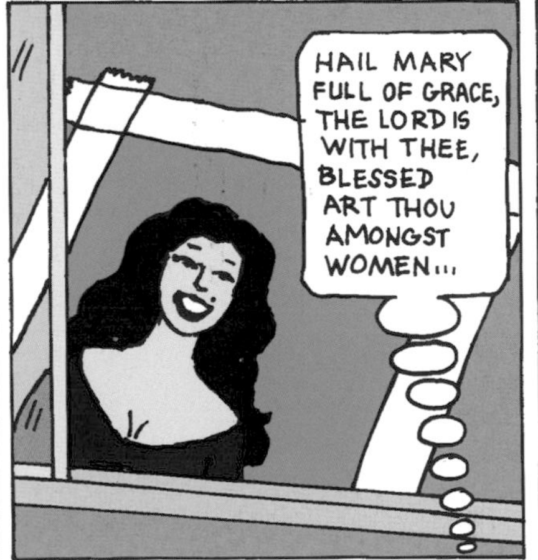
HAIL MARY FULL OF GRACE, THE LORD IS WITH THEE, BLESSED ART THOU AMONGST WOMEN...

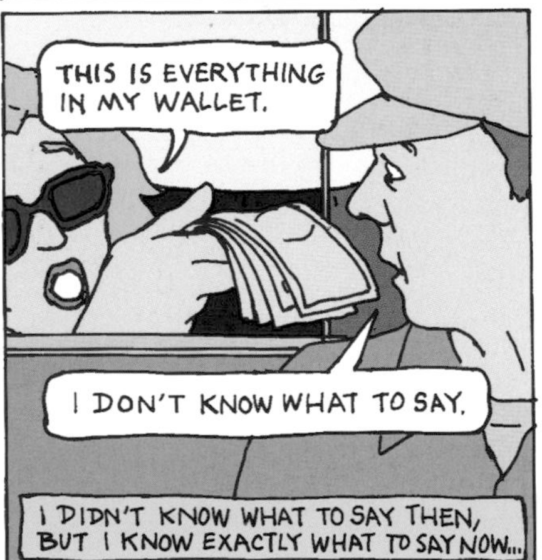
THIS IS EVERYTHING IN MY WALLET.
I DON'T KNOW WHAT TO SAY.
I DIDN'T KNOW WHAT TO SAY THEN, BUT I KNOW EXACTLY WHAT TO SAY NOW...

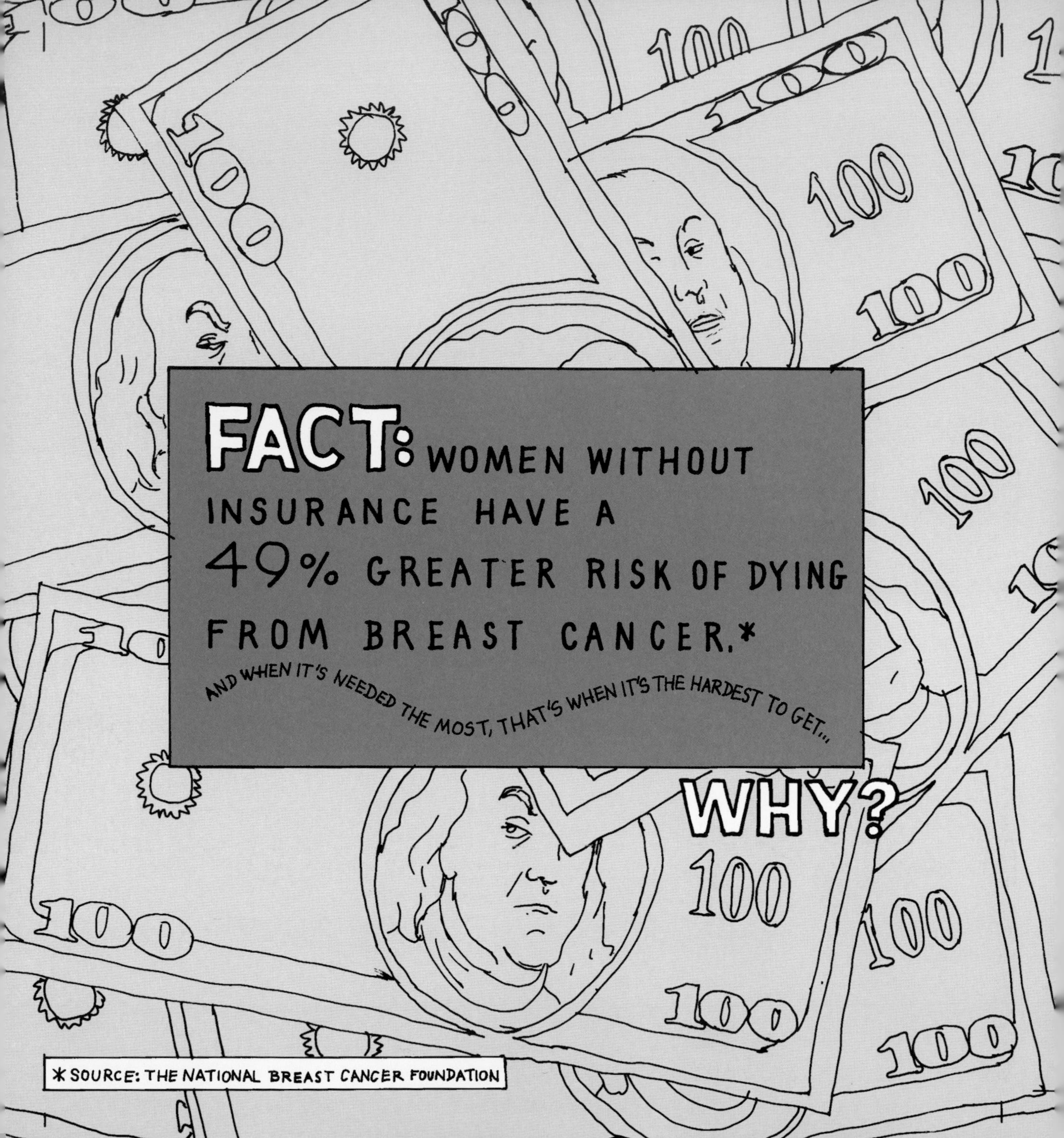
FACT: WOMEN WITHOUT INSURANCE HAVE A 49% GREATER RISK OF DYING FROM BREAST CANCER.*
AND WHEN IT'S NEEDED THE MOST, THAT'S WHEN IT'S THE HARDEST TO GET...
WHY?
100
* SOURCE: THE NATIONAL BREAST CANCER FOUNDATION

REMEMBER MY PILES OF REJECTS? WELL, *NEW YORKER* CARTOONIST MATT DIFFEE INGENIOUSLY FOUND SOMETHING FOR THE REST OF US CARTOONISTS TO DO WITH THEM...

THE REJECTION SHOW
SOLD OUT

HI, I'M THE REJECTED CARTOONIST.
NO CHARGE FOR PERFORMERS.
TICKETS $10.00

MATT COCREATED "THE REJECTION SHOW"...
LET'S GO ONSTAGE AND DO A RUN-THROUGH. I EDITED YOUR BATCH DOWN TO 10.
GREAT EDIT, BY THE WAY.

HERE'S YOUR CHANCE TO PROVE YOUR STUFF IS FUNNY, IF THE AUDIENCE LAUGHS. FIRST I'LL INTRODUCE YOU AND YOU'LL PUT A CARTOON ON THE PROJECTOR...

...THEN IT'LL BE PROJECTED ON THE SCREEN HERE, AND WE'LL TELL STORIES OF OUR LIVES AS CARTOONISTS... WE'LL TAKE TURNS.

YOU MEAN OUR LIVES OF REJECTION. YOU KNOW, SAM ONCE SAID THAT THE AVERAGE DISAPPROVAL RATING FOR A CARTOONIST IS 97%. THAT MEANS 3% OF OUR STUFF IS PRINTED.

BEFORE THE SHOW STARTED, I WAITED AT THE BAR AS MY FRIENDS CAME IN...*
JUST HAVE FUN WITH THIS THING, KIDDO.
SAM, I LOVE THAT YOU CALL ME KIDDO AT 43.
* I SENT OUT A MASS E-MAIL, AND I GOT A GOOD RETURN.

I ALSO E-MAILED MY COUSIN'S BEST FRIEND'S BROTHER'S GIRLFRIEND, SHE OF THE 1.1-CM TUMOR, DOUBLE MASTECTOMY, COMPLETE HAIR LOSS FAME...
MARISA?
HILARY, I THOUGHT THAT WAS YOU...
...BECAUSE OF YOUR TITS!
SHH!

SHE GAVE ME A LOT OF POSITIVE POINTERS.
I'M A SWIMMER AND I SWAM THROUGH ALL OF MY TREATMENTS.
I SWIM 5 TIMES A WEEK, WILL I KEEP DOING THAT?
YOU TWO, TAKE IT SOMEWHERE ELSE!

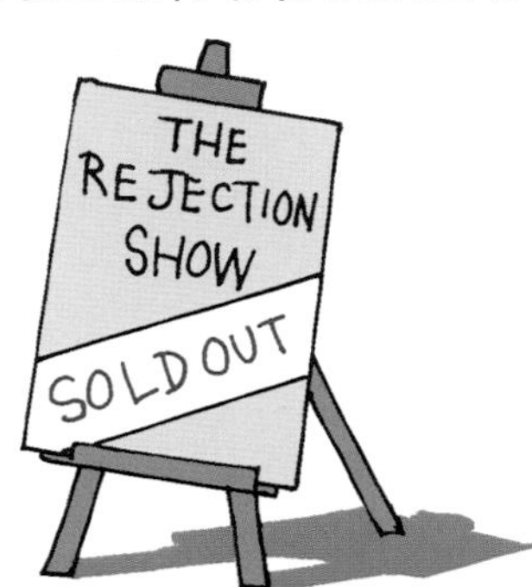

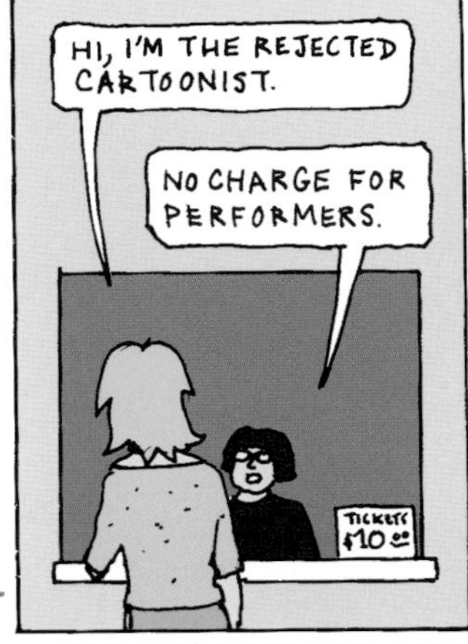

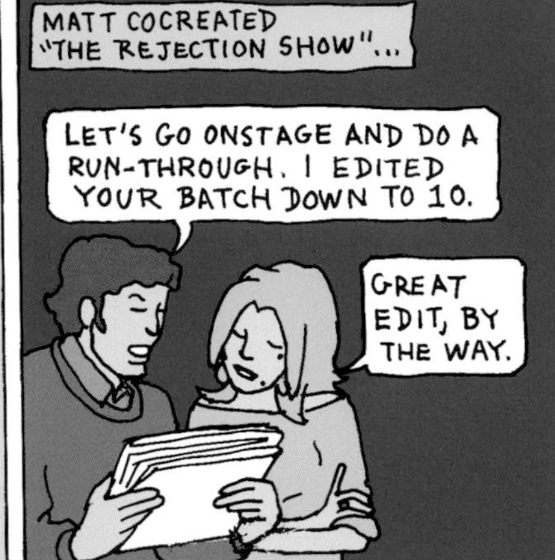

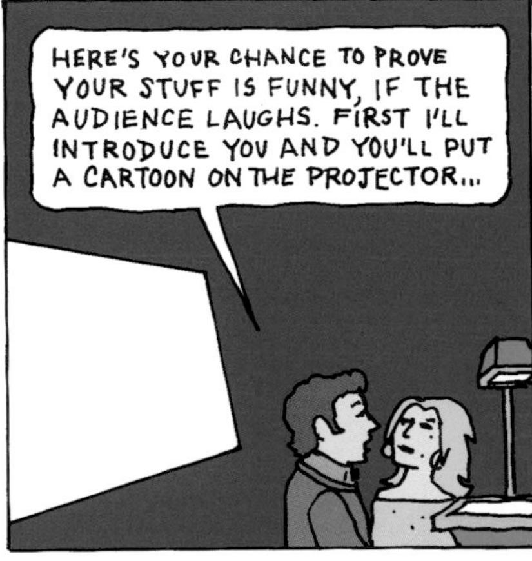

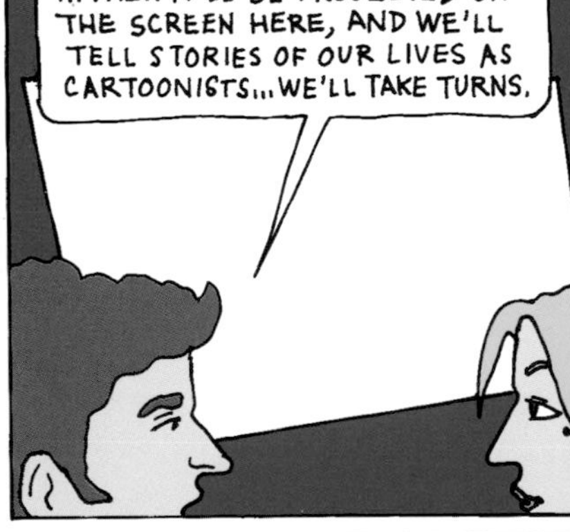

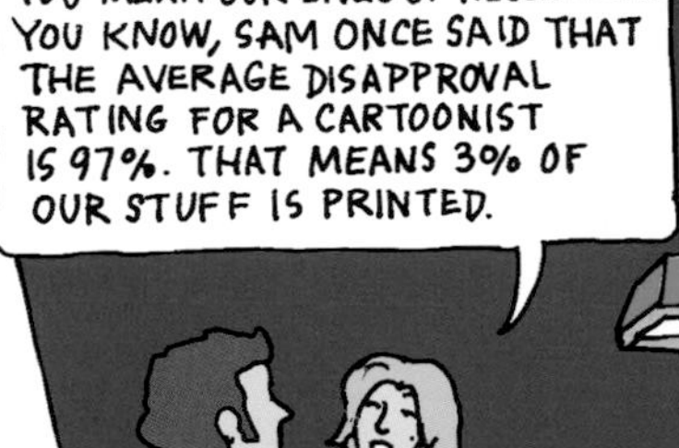

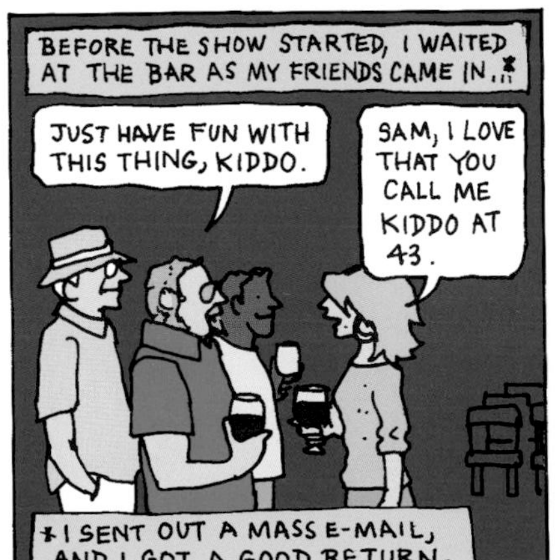

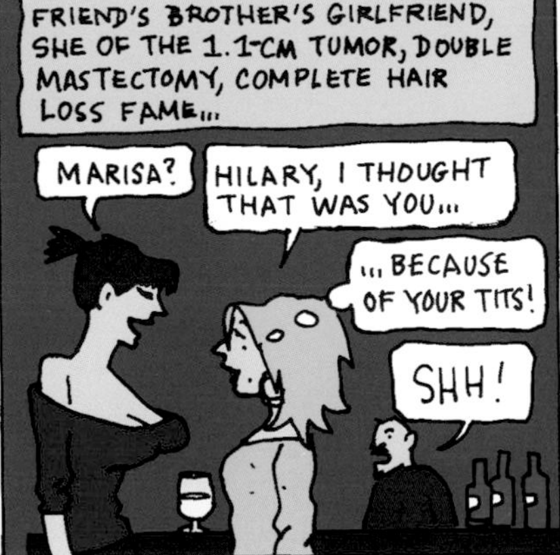

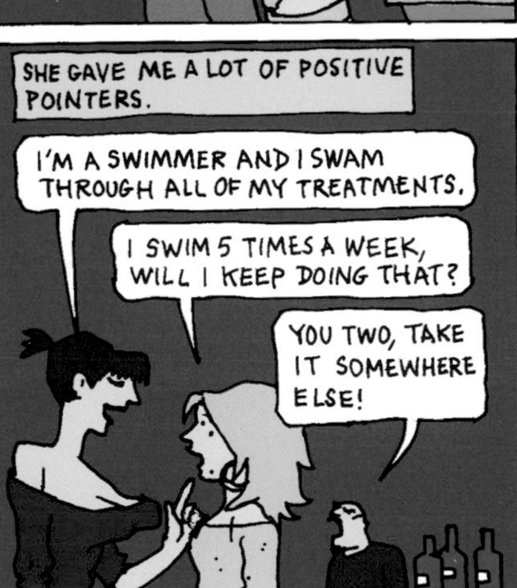

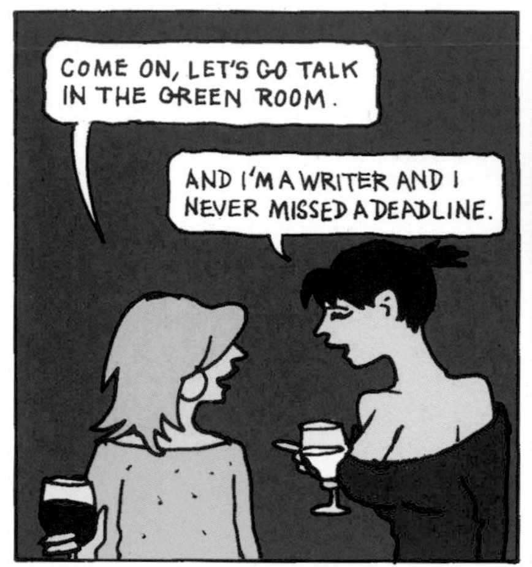
COME ON, LET'S GO TALK IN THE GREEN ROOM.
AND I'M A WRITER AND I NEVER MISSED A DEADLINE.

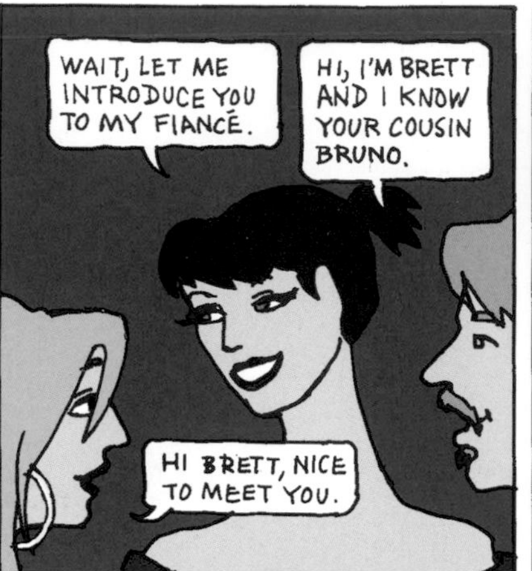
WAIT, LET ME INTRODUCE YOU TO MY FIANCÉ.
HI, I'M BRETT AND I KNOW YOUR COUSIN BRUNO.
HI BRETT, NICE TO MEET YOU.

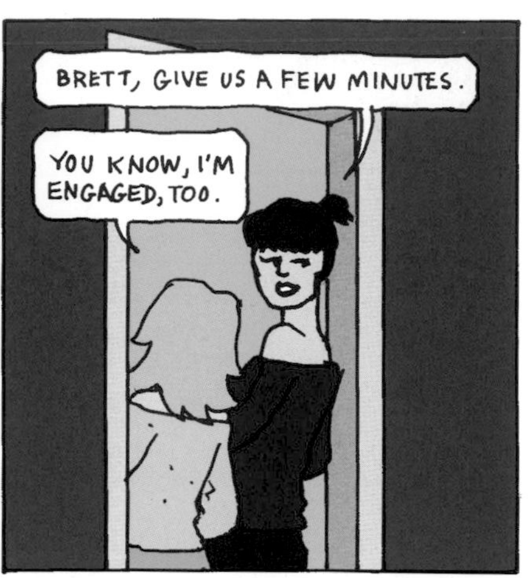
BRETT, GIVE US A FEW MINUTES.
YOU KNOW, I'M ENGAGED, TOO.

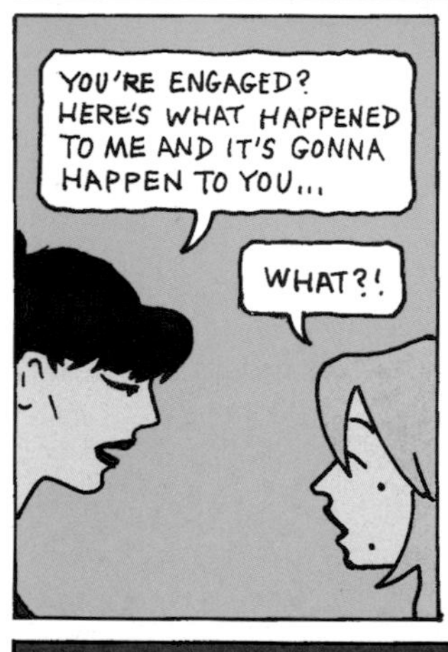
YOU'RE ENGAGED? HERE'S WHAT HAPPENED TO ME AND IT'S GONNA HAPPEN TO YOU...
WHAT?!

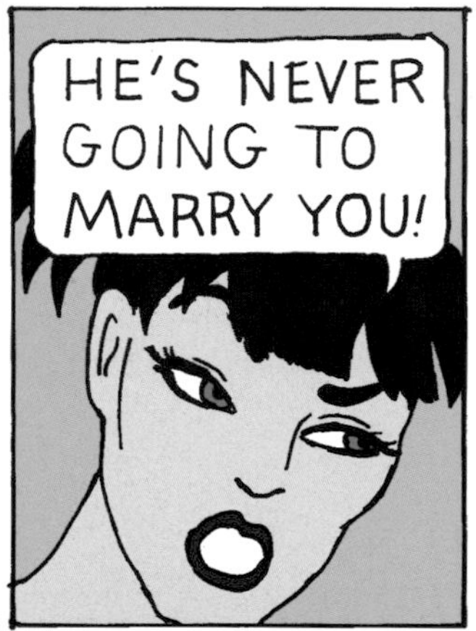
HE'S NEVER GOING TO MARRY YOU!

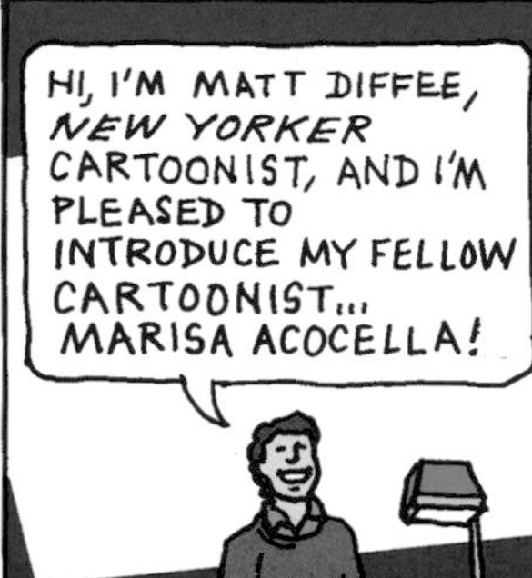
HI, I'M MATT DIFFEE, *NEW YORKER* CARTOONIST, AND I'M PLEASED TO INTRODUCE MY FELLOW CARTOONIST... MARISA ACOCELLA!

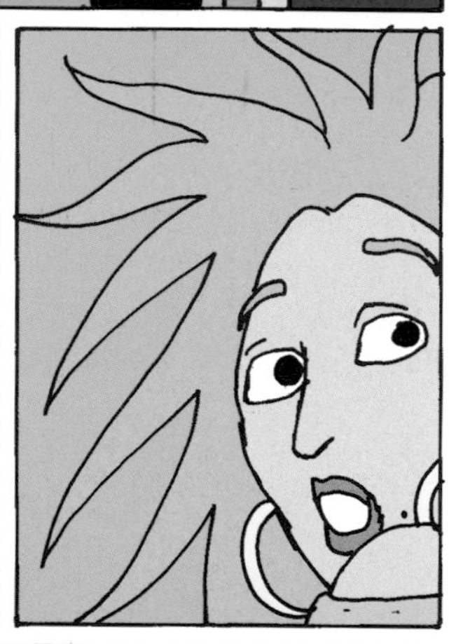

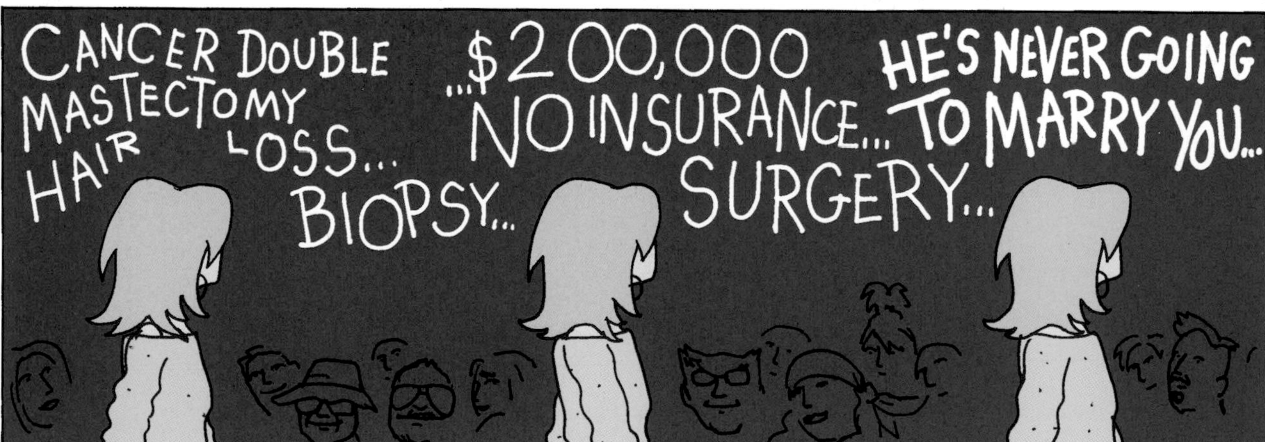
CANCER DOUBLE MASTECTOMY
HAIR LOSS...
BIOPSY...
...$200,000
NO INSURANCE...
SURGERY...
HE'S NEVER GOING TO MARRY YOU...

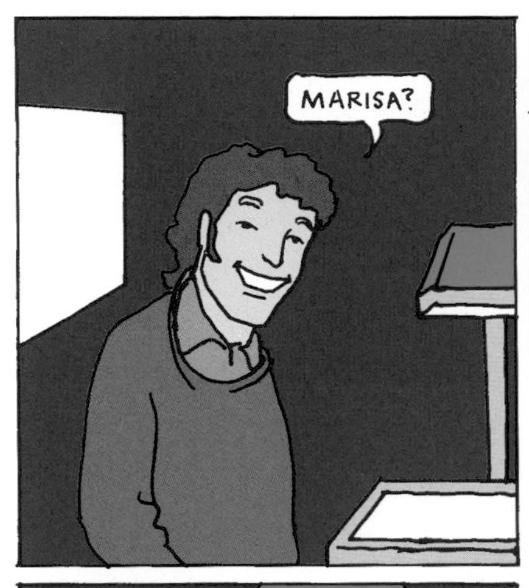
MARISA?

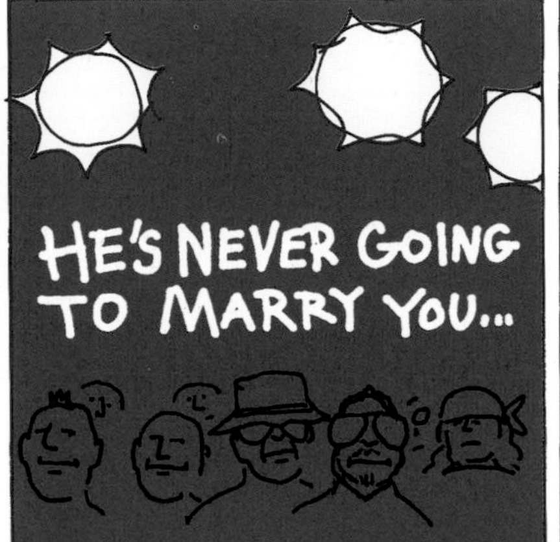
HE'S NEVER GOING TO MARRY YOU...

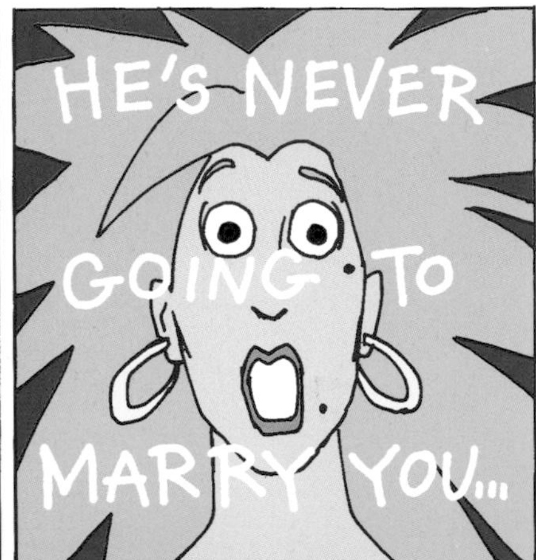
HE'S NEVER
GOING TO
MARRY YOU...

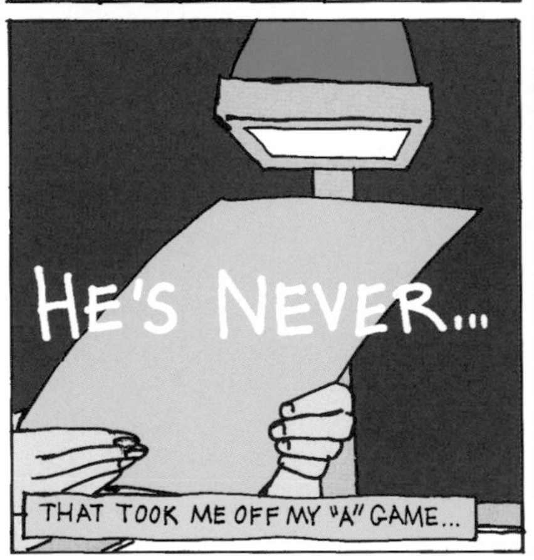
HE'S NEVER...
THAT TOOK ME OFF MY "A" GAME...

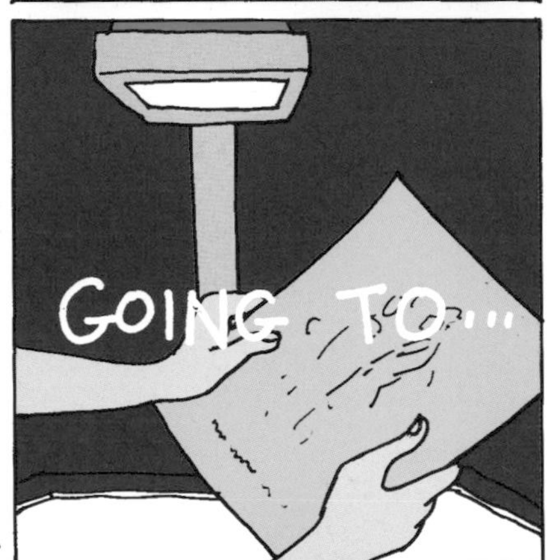
GOING TO...

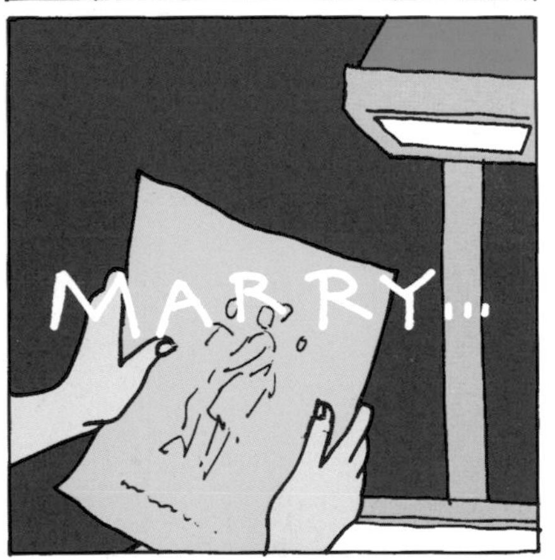
MARRY...

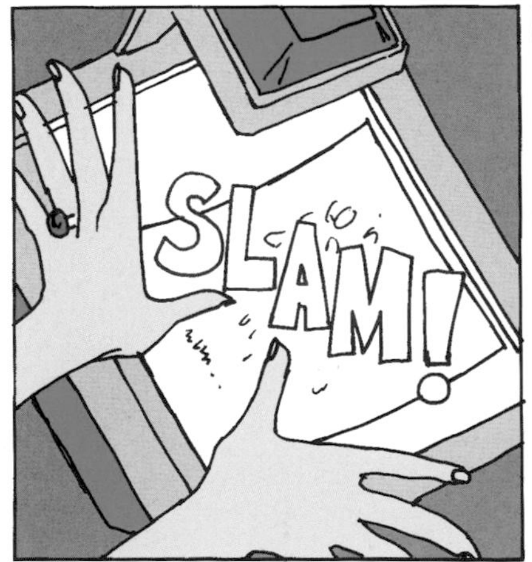
SLAM!

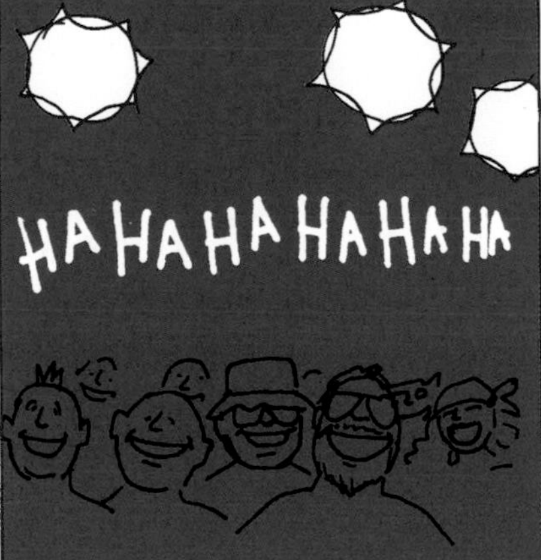
HA HA HA HA HA HA HA

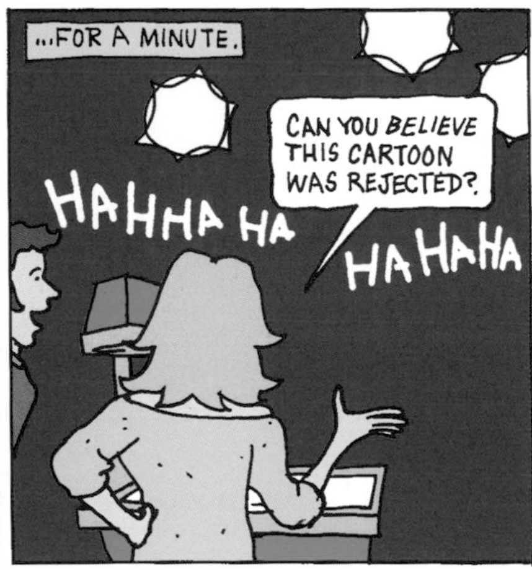
...FOR A MINUTE.
CAN YOU BELIEVE THIS CARTOON WAS REJECTED?
HA HHA HA HA
HA HAHA

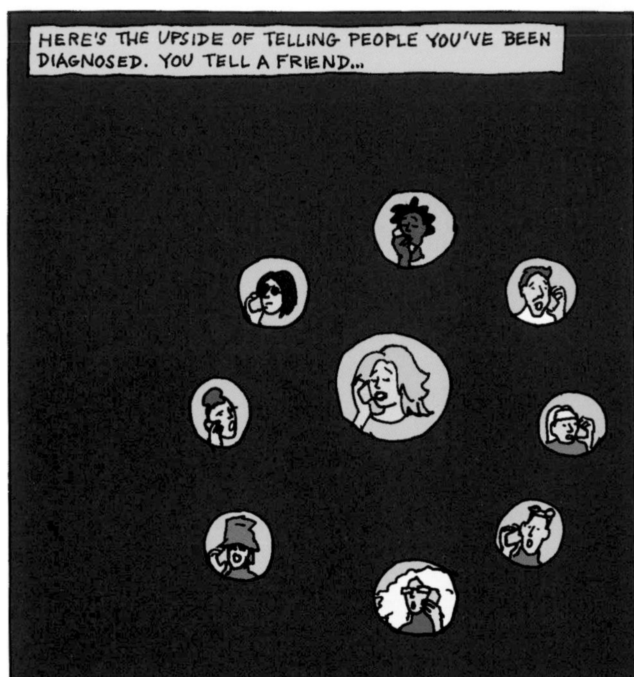
HERE'S THE UPSIDE OF TELLING PEOPLE YOU'VE BEEN DIAGNOSED. YOU TELL A FRIEND...

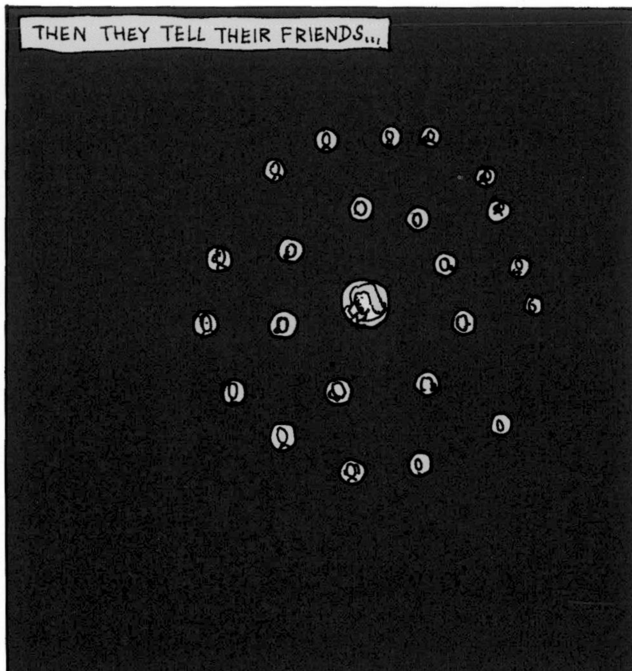
THEN THEY TELL THEIR FRIENDS...

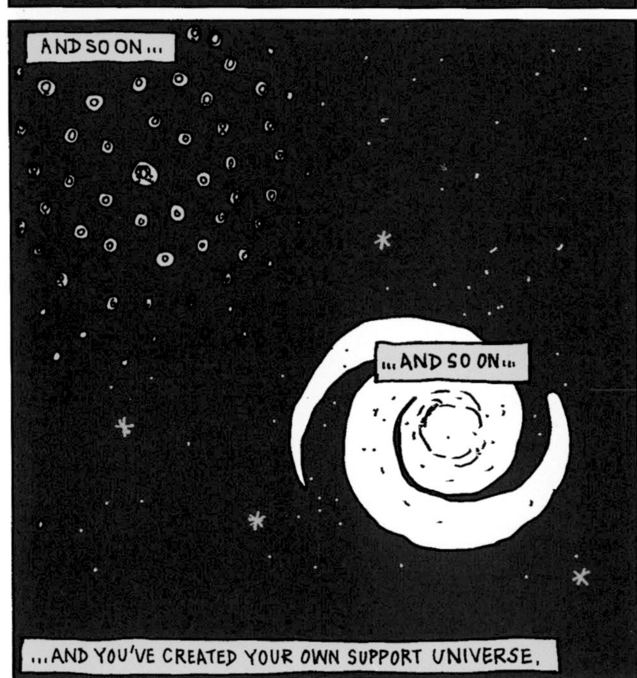
AND SO ON...
...AND SO ON...
...AND YOU'VE CREATED YOUR OWN SUPPORT UNIVERSE.

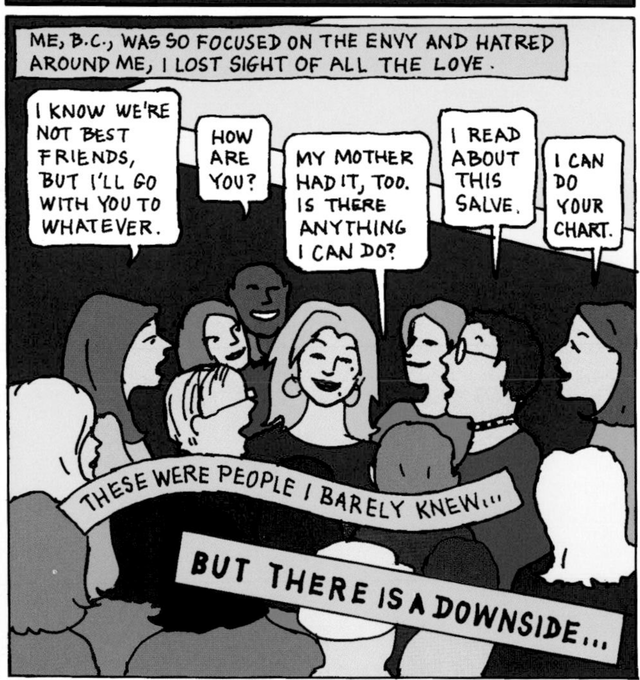
ME, B.C., WAS SO FOCUSED ON THE ENVY AND HATRED AROUND ME, I LOST SIGHT OF ALL THE LOVE.
I KNOW WE'RE NOT BEST FRIENDS, BUT I'LL GO WITH YOU TO WHATEVER.
HOW ARE YOU?
MY MOTHER HAD IT, TOO. IS THERE ANYTHING I CAN DO?
I READ ABOUT THIS SALVE.
I CAN DO YOUR CHART.
THESE WERE PEOPLE I BARELY KNEW...
BUT THERE IS A DOWNSIDE...

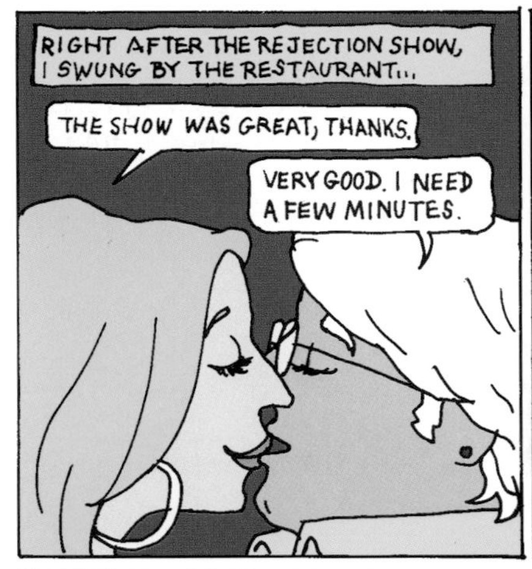
RIGHT AFTER THE REJECTION SHOW, I SWUNG BY THE RESTAURANT...
THE SHOW WAS GREAT, THANKS.
VERY GOOD. I NEED A FEW MINUTES.

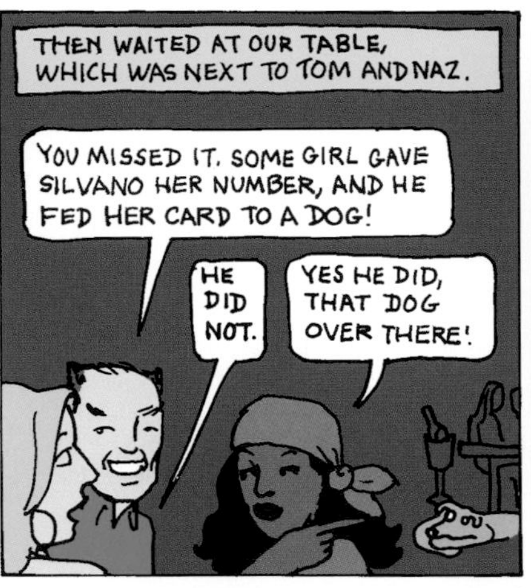
THEN WAITED AT OUR TABLE, WHICH WAS NEXT TO TOM AND NAZ.
YOU MISSED IT. SOME GIRL GAVE SILVANO HER NUMBER, AND HE FED HER CARD TO A DOG!
HE DID NOT.
YES HE DID, THAT DOG OVER THERE!

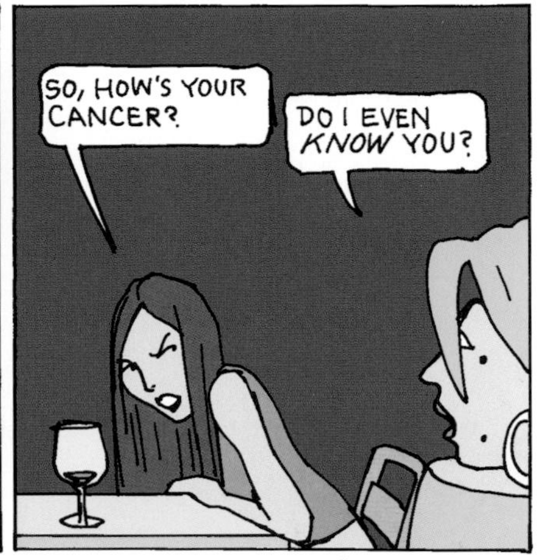
SO, HOW'S YOUR CANCER?
DO I EVEN KNOW YOU?

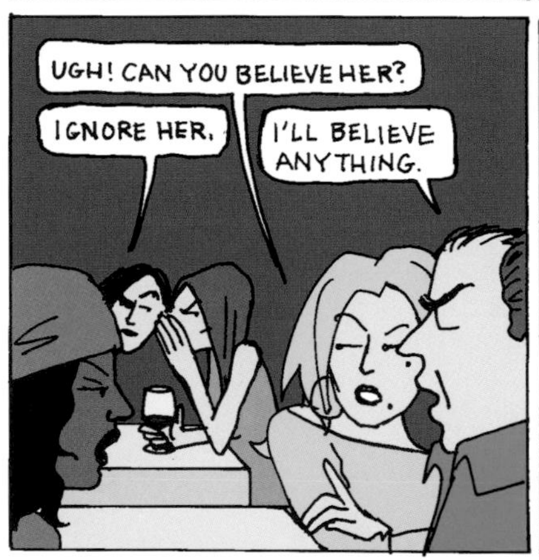
UGH! CAN YOU BELIEVE HER?
IGNORE HER.
I'LL BELIEVE ANYTHING.

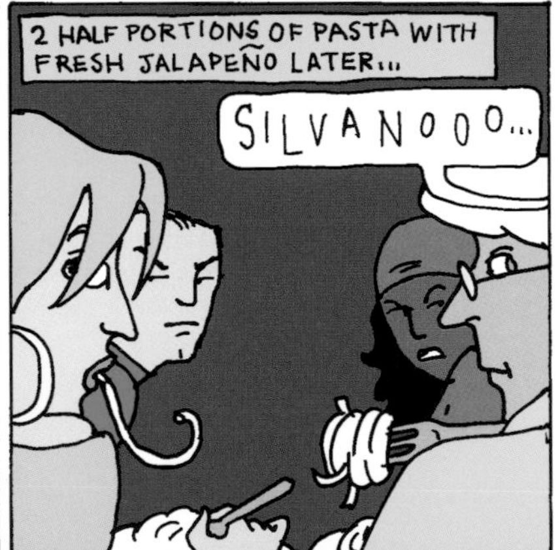
2 HALF PORTIONS OF PASTA WITH FRESH JALAPEÑO LATER...
SILVANOOO...

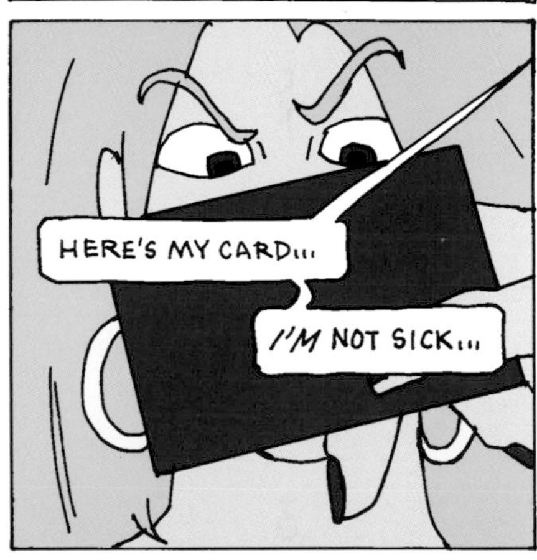
HERE'S MY CARD...
I'M NOT SICK...

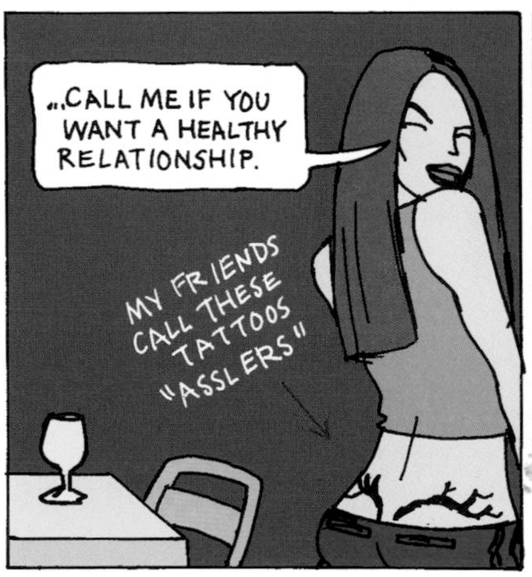
...CALL ME IF YOU WANT A HEALTHY RELATIONSHIP.
MY FRIENDS CALL THESE TATTOOS "ASSLERS"

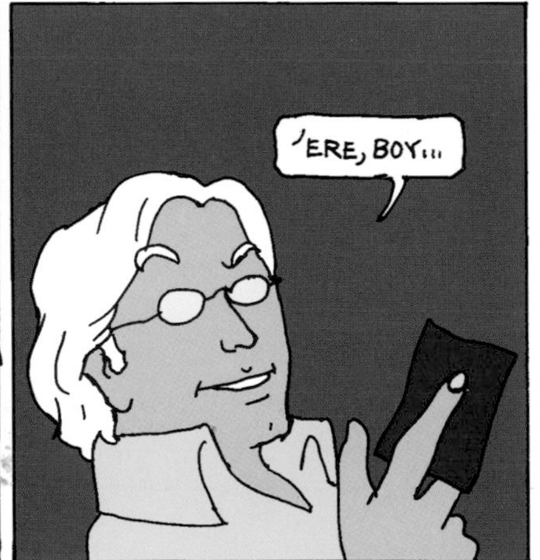
'ERE, BOY...

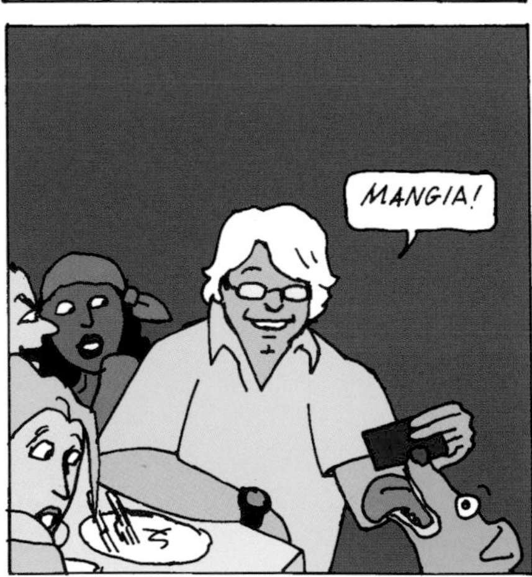
MANGIA!

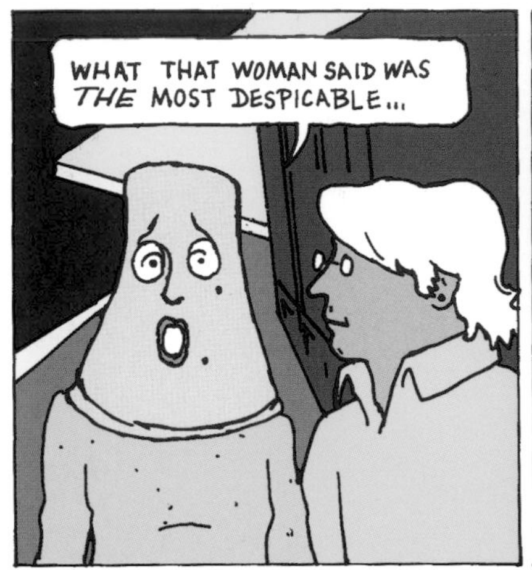
WHAT THAT WOMAN SAID WAS *THE* MOST DESPICABLE...

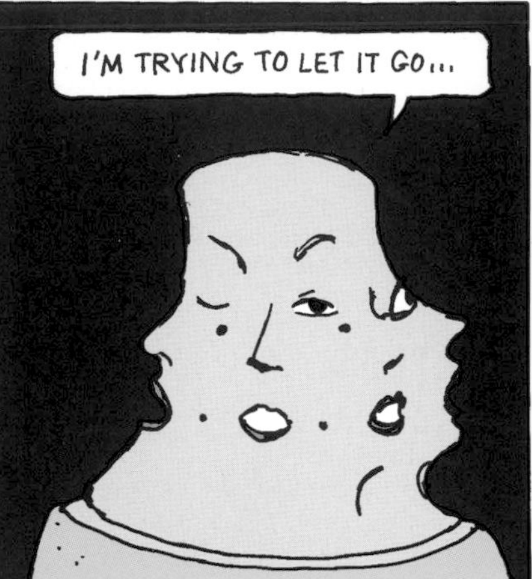
I'M TRYING TO LET IT GO...

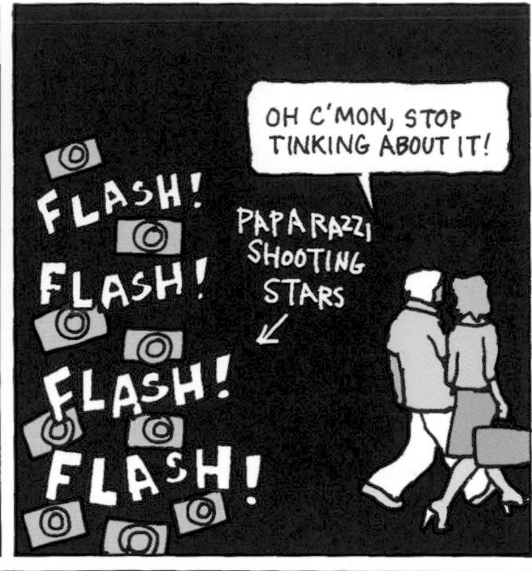
OH C'MON, STOP TINKING ABOUT IT!
FLASH!
FLASH!
FLASH!
FLASH!
PAPARAZZI SHOOTING STARS

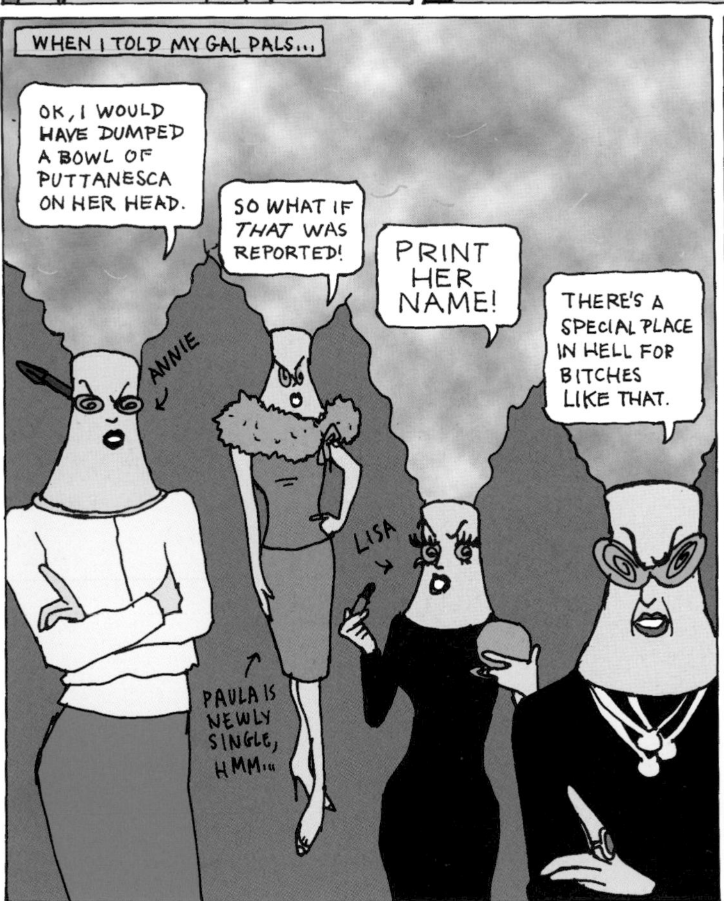
WHEN I TOLD MY GAL PALS...
OK, I WOULD HAVE DUMPED A BOWL OF PUTTANESCA ON HER HEAD.
SO WHAT IF *THAT* WAS REPORTED!
PRINT HER NAME!
THERE'S A SPECIAL PLACE IN HELL FOR BITCHES LIKE THAT.
ANNIE
LISA
PAULA IS NEWLY SINGLE, HMM...

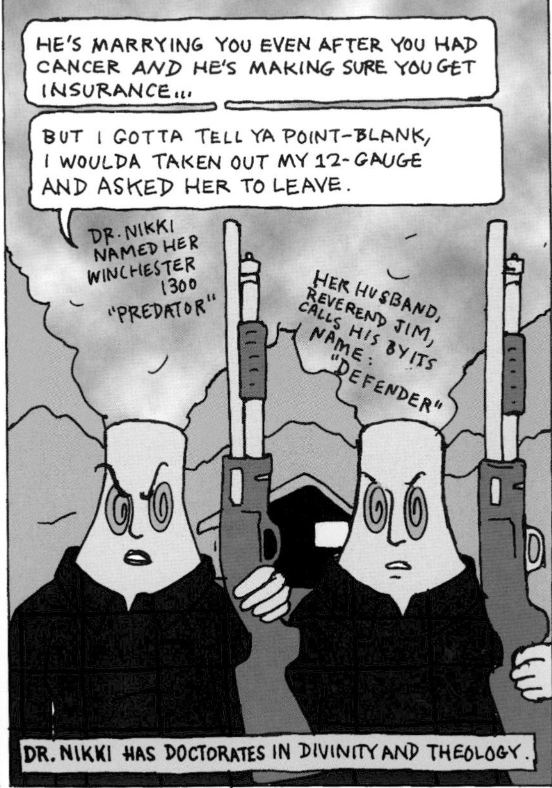
AND AFTER I GOT PAST THAT CHEESY NEW AGE MUSIC ON THE PSYCHIC HOTLINE, SOMEWHERE IN MONTANA...
HE'S MARRYING YOU EVEN AFTER YOU HAD CANCER *AND* HE'S MAKING SURE YOU GET INSURANCE...
BUT I GOTTA TELL YA POINT-BLANK, I WOULDA TAKEN OUT MY 12-GAUGE AND ASKED HER TO LEAVE.
DR. NIKKI NAMED HER WINCHESTER 1300 "PREDATOR"
HER HUSBAND, REVEREND JIM, CALLS HIS BY ITS NAME: "DEFENDER"
DR. NIKKI HAS DOCTORATES IN DIVINITY AND THEOLOGY.

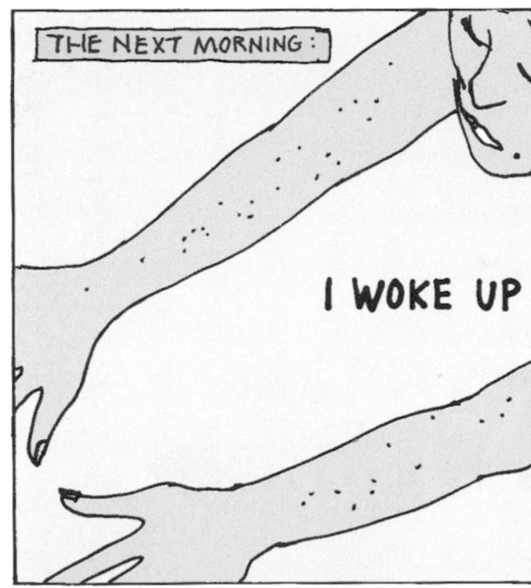
THE NEXT MORNING:
I WOKE UP

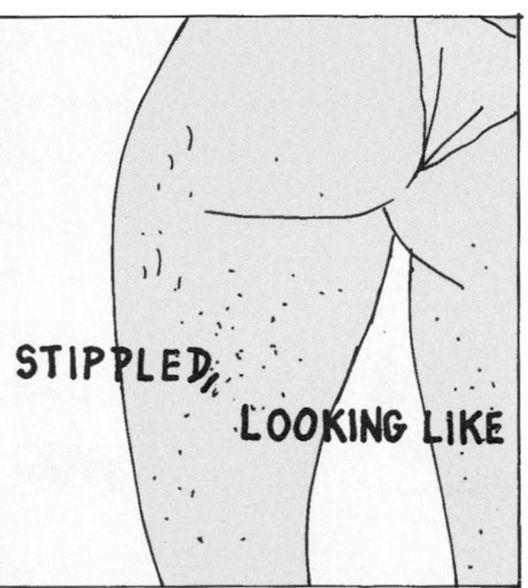
STIPPLED,
LOOKING LIKE

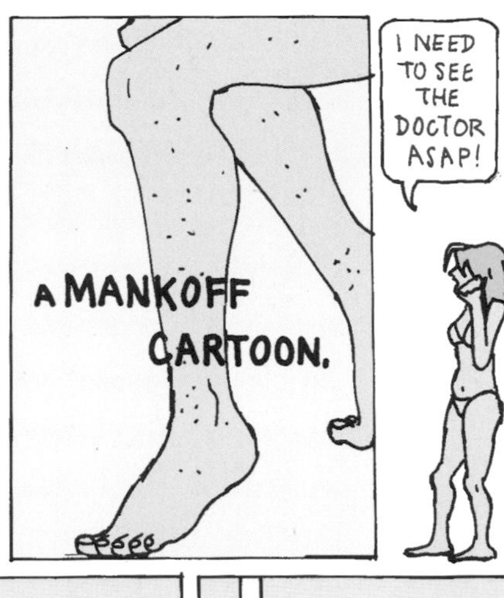
A MANKOFF CARTOON.
I NEED TO SEE THE DOCTOR ASAP!

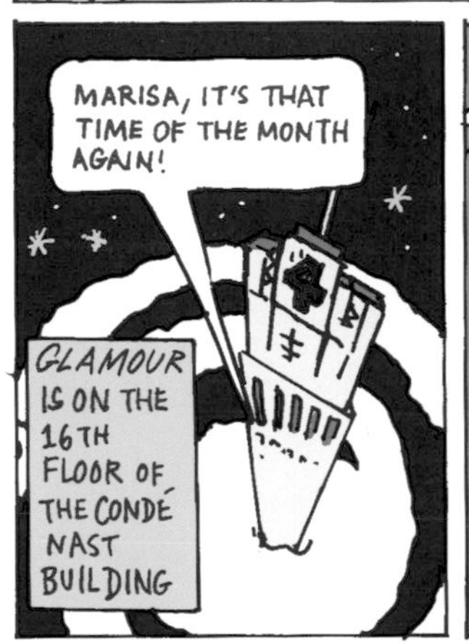
MARISA, IT'S THAT TIME OF THE MONTH AGAIN!
GLAMOUR IS ON THE 16TH FLOOR OF THE CONDÉ NAST BUILDING

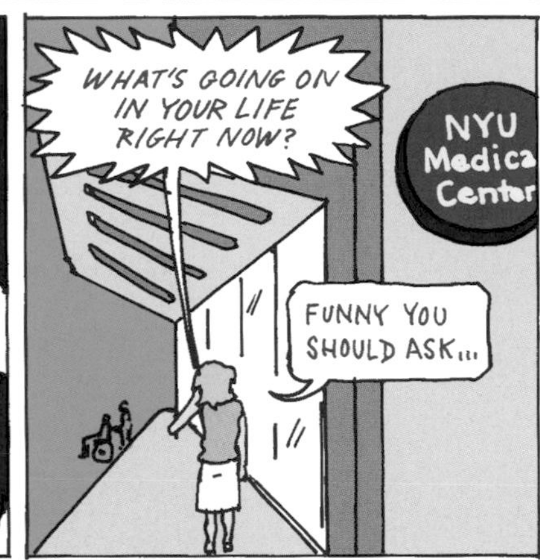
WHAT'S GOING ON IN YOUR LIFE RIGHT NOW?
NYU Medical Center
FUNNY YOU SHOULD ASK...

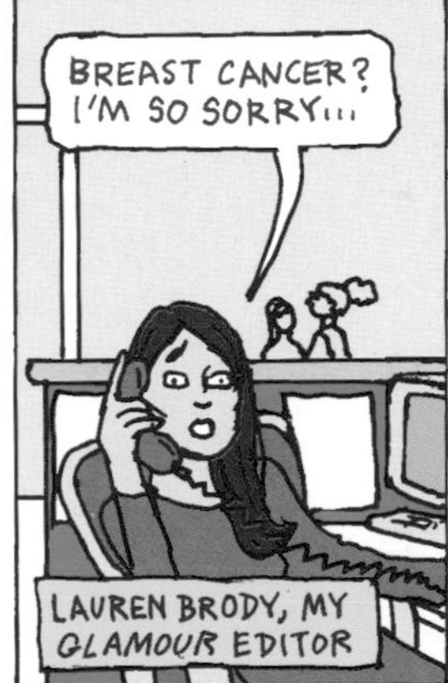
BREAST CANCER? I'M SO SORRY...
LAUREN BRODY, MY GLAMOUR EDITOR

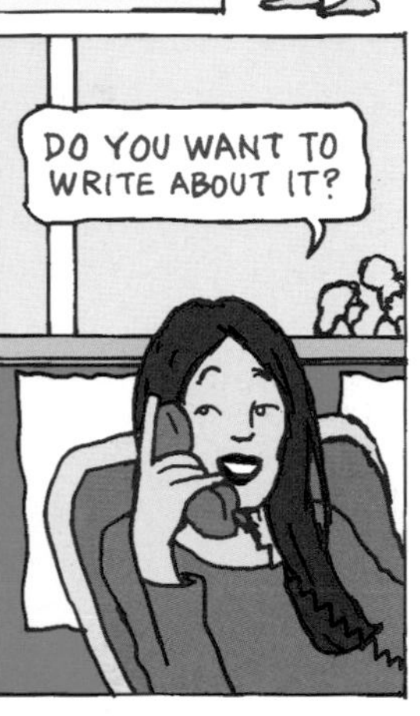
DO YOU WANT TO WRITE ABOUT IT?

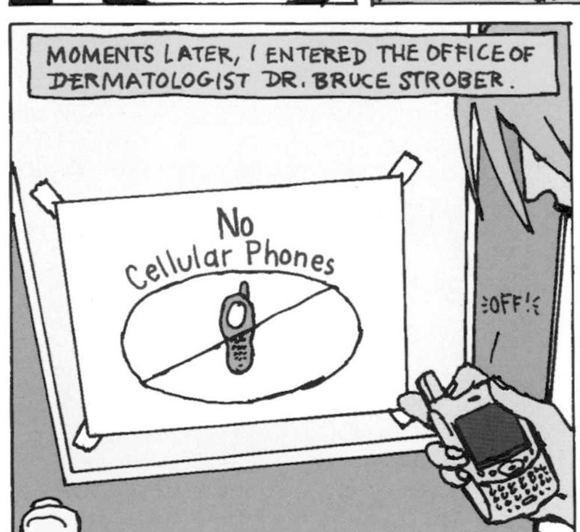
MOMENTS LATER, I ENTERED THE OFFICE OF DERMATOLOGIST DR. BRUCE STROBER.
No Cellular Phones
OFF!

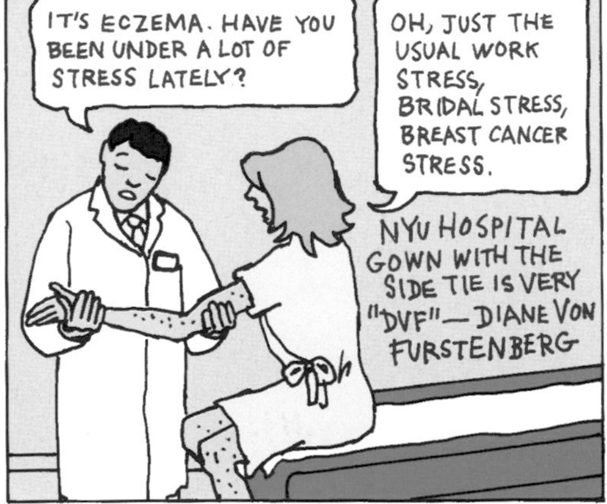
IT'S ECZEMA. HAVE YOU BEEN UNDER A LOT OF STRESS LATELY?
OH, JUST THE USUAL WORK STRESS, BRIDAL STRESS, BREAST CANCER STRESS.
NYU HOSPITAL GOWN WITH THE SIDE TIE IS VERY "DVF"—DIANE VON FURSTENBERG
I'M SORRY. MY WIFE IS A PSYCHIATRIST AT SLOAN. IF THERE'S ANYTHING I CAN DO, LET ME KNOW.
THANKS, DOCTOR.

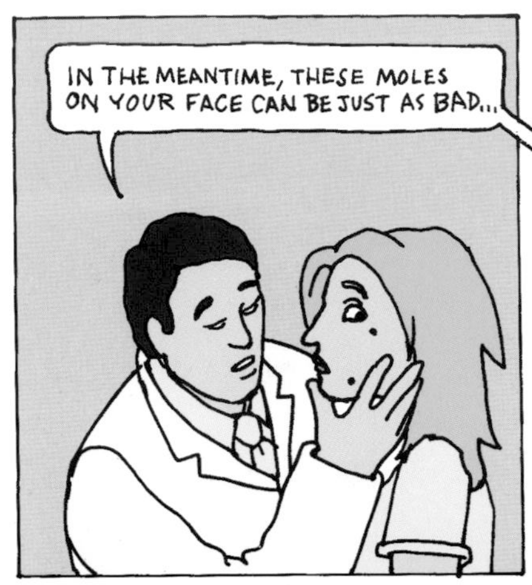
IN THE MEANTIME, THESE MOLES ON YOUR FACE CAN BE JUST AS BAD...

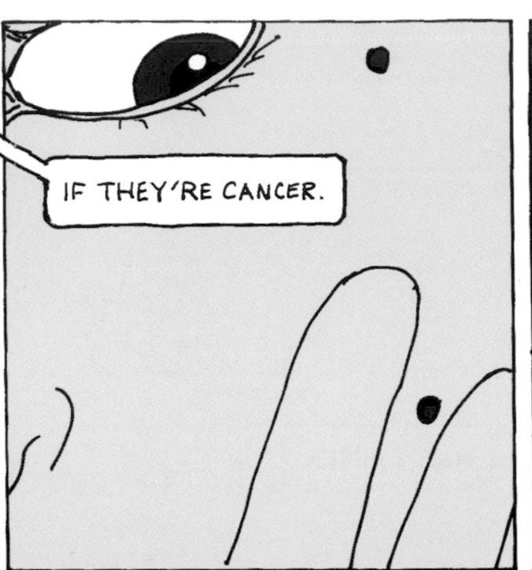
IF THEY'RE CANCER.

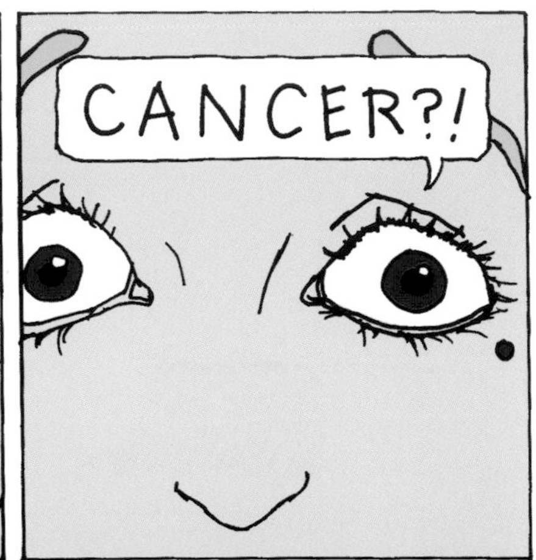
CANCER?!

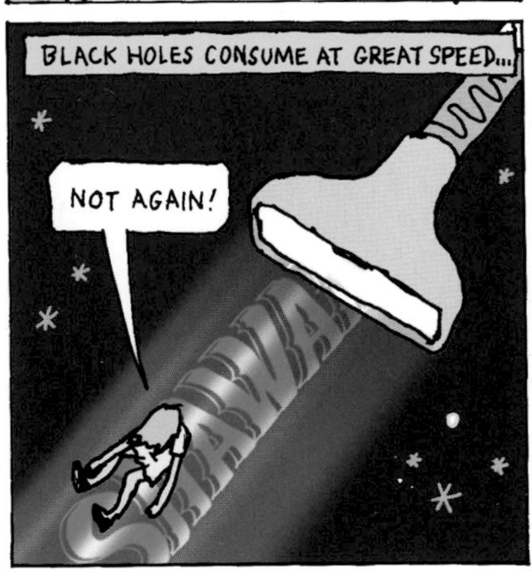
BLACK HOLES CONSUME AT GREAT SPEED...
NOT AGAIN!

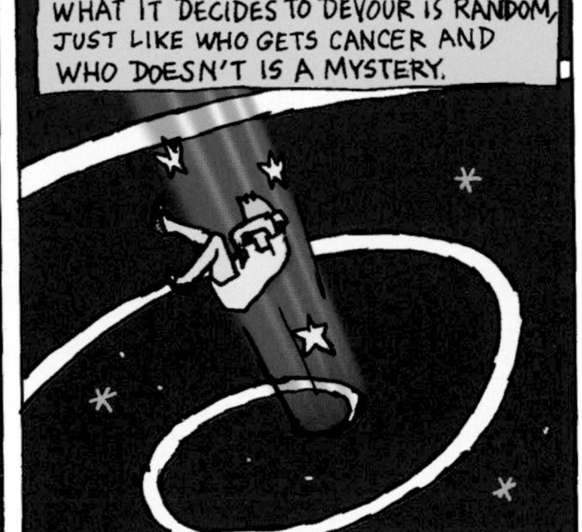
WHAT IT DECIDES TO DEVOUR IS RANDOM, JUST LIKE WHO GETS CANCER AND WHO DOESN'T IS A MYSTERY.

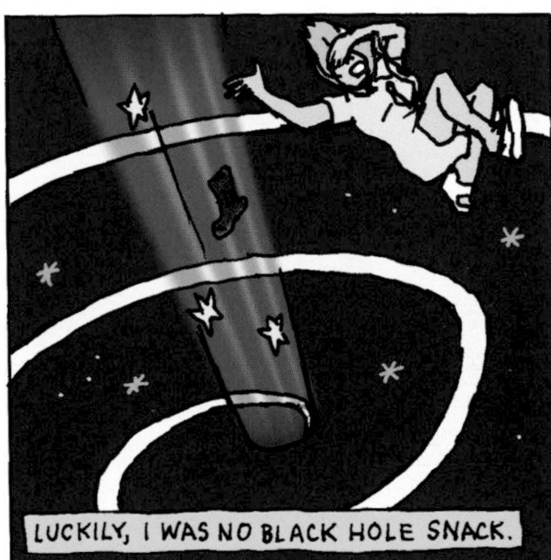
LUCKILY, I WAS NO BLACK HOLE SNACK.

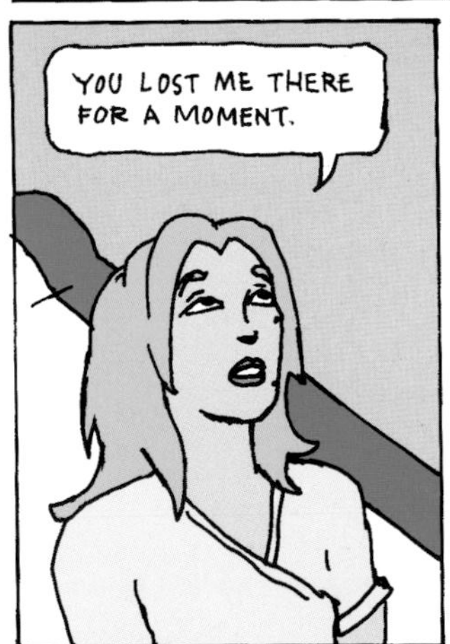
YOU LOST ME THERE FOR A MOMENT.

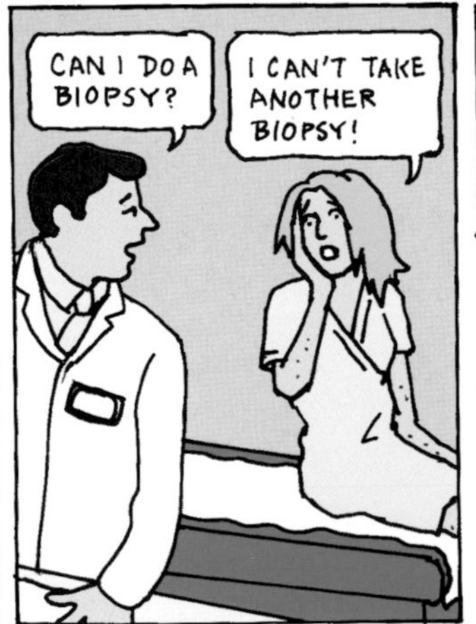
CAN I DO A BIOPSY?
I CAN'T TAKE ANOTHER BIOPSY!

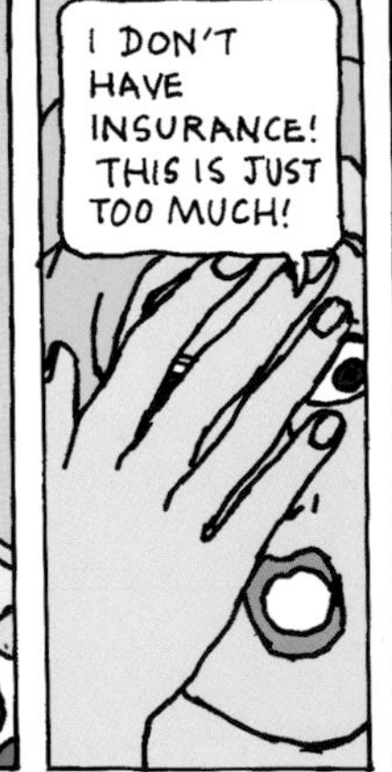
I DON'T HAVE INSURANCE! THIS IS JUST TOO MUCH!

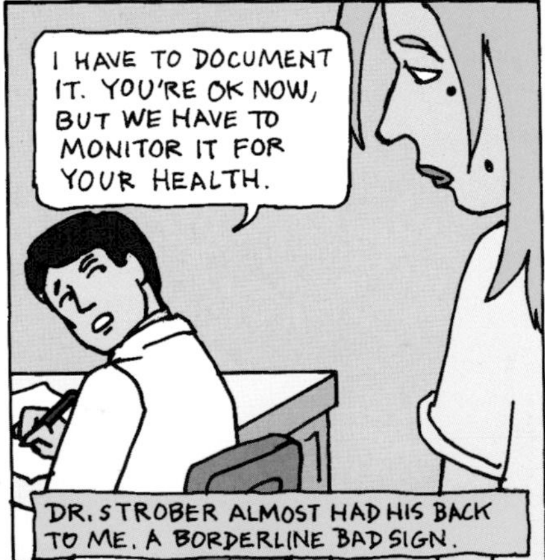
I HAVE TO DOCUMENT IT. YOU'RE OK NOW, BUT WE HAVE TO MONITOR IT FOR YOUR HEALTH.
DR. STROBER ALMOST HAD HIS BACK TO ME. A BORDERLINE BAD SIGN.

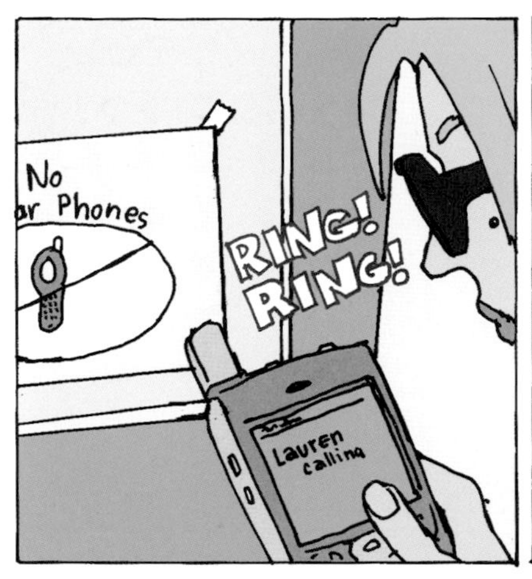
No
ar Phones
RING! RING!
Lauren calling

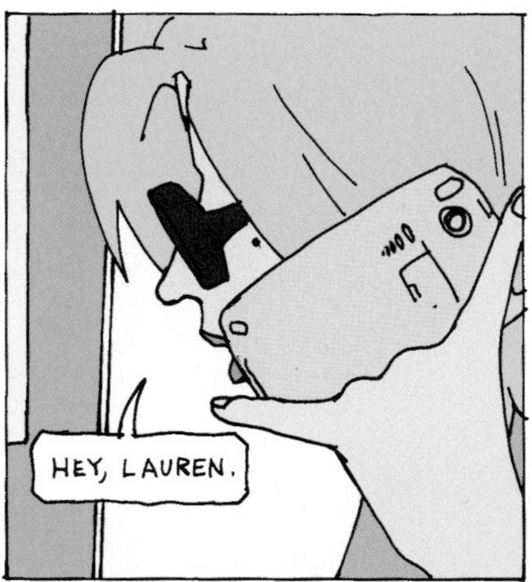
HEY, LAUREN.

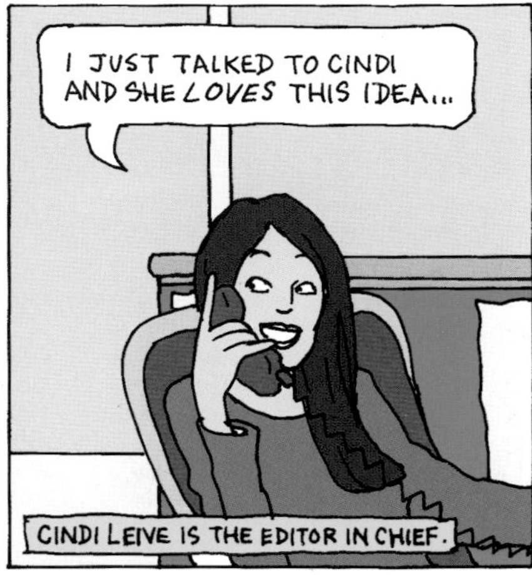
I JUST TALKED TO CINDI AND SHE LOVES THIS IDEA...
CINDI LEIVE IS THE EDITOR IN CHIEF.

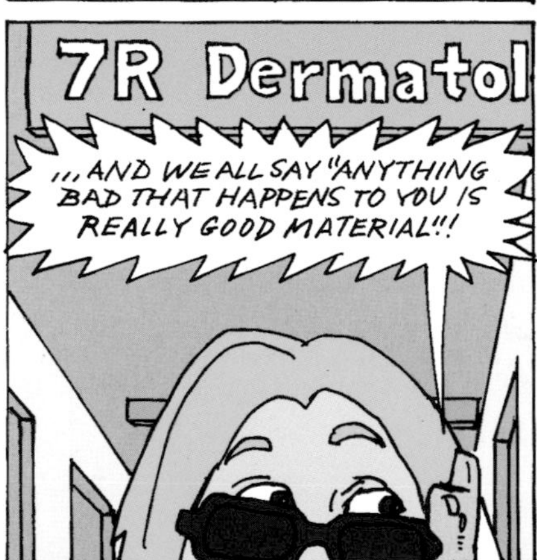
7R Dermatol
...AND WE ALL SAY "ANYTHING BAD THAT HAPPENS TO YOU IS REALLY GOOD MATERIAL"!

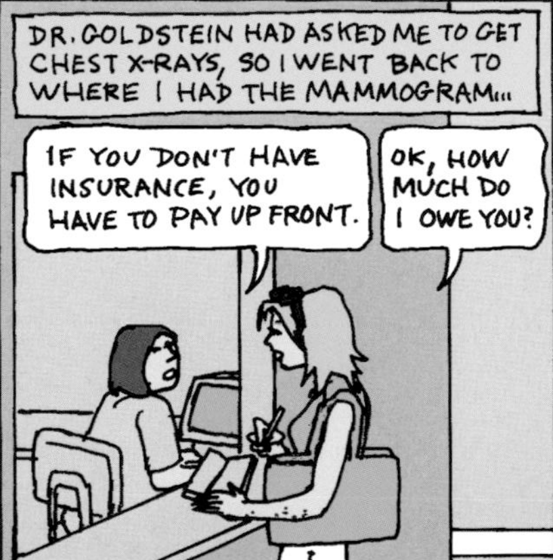
DR. GOLDSTEIN HAD ASKED ME TO GET CHEST X-RAYS, SO I WENT BACK TO WHERE I HAD THE MAMMOGRAM...
IF YOU DON'T HAVE INSURANCE, YOU HAVE TO PAY UP FRONT.
OK, HOW MUCH DO I OWE YOU?

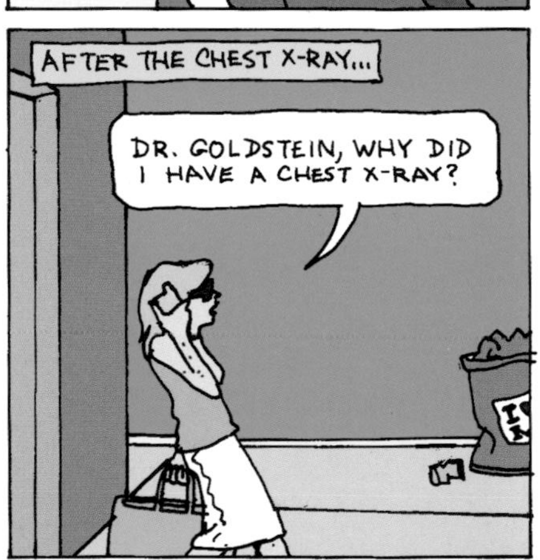
AFTER THE CHEST X-RAY...
DR. GOLDSTEIN, WHY DID I HAVE A CHEST X-RAY?

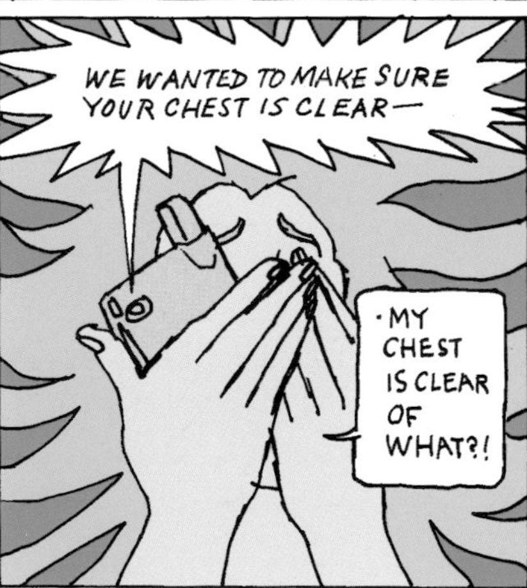
WE WANTED TO MAKE SURE YOUR CHEST IS CLEAR—
·MY CHEST IS CLEAR OF WHAT?!

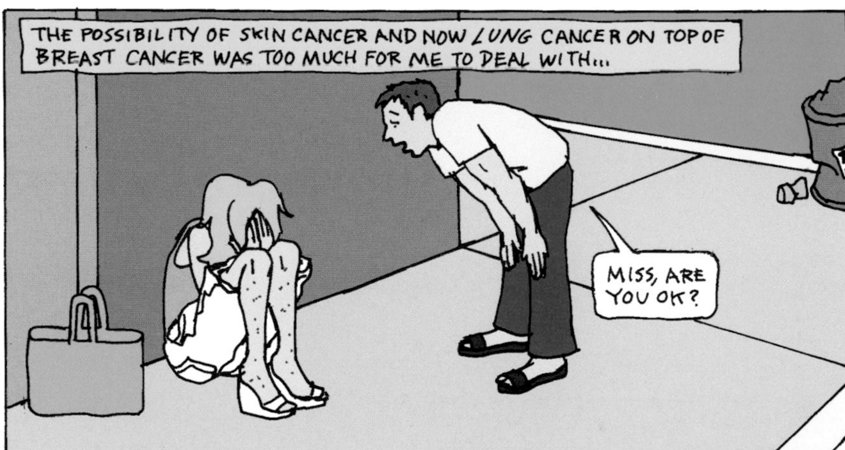
THE POSSIBILITY OF SKIN CANCER AND NOW LUNG CANCER ON TOP OF BREAST CANCER WAS TOO MUCH FOR ME TO DEAL WITH...
MISS, ARE YOU OK?

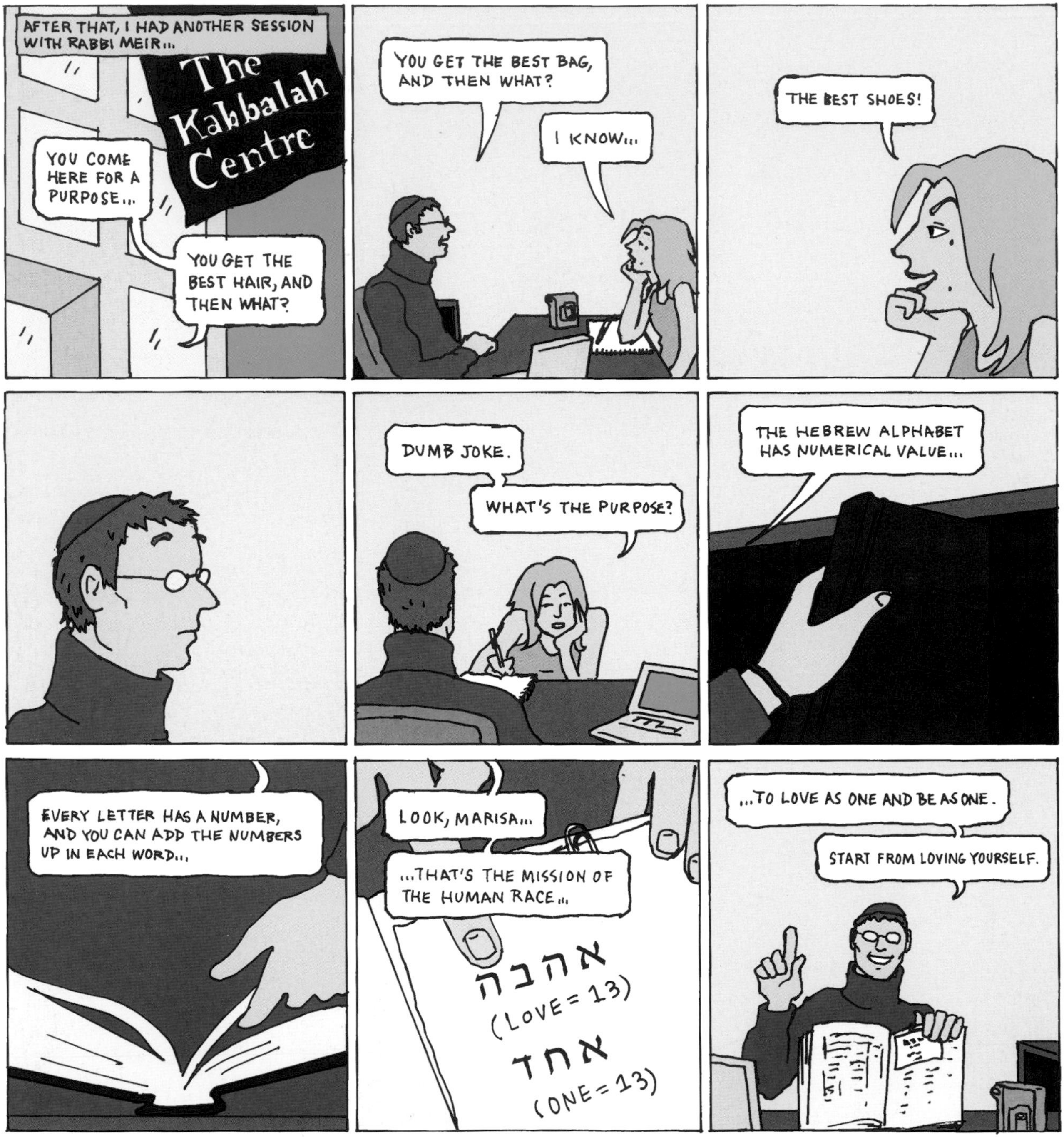

AFTER THAT, I HAD ANOTHER SESSION WITH RABBI MEIR...
The Kabbalah Centre
YOU COME HERE FOR A PURPOSE...
YOU GET THE BEST HAIR, AND THEN WHAT?

YOU GET THE BEST BAG, AND THEN WHAT?
I KNOW...

THE BEST SHOES!

DUMB JOKE.
WHAT'S THE PURPOSE?

THE HEBREW ALPHABET HAS NUMERICAL VALUE...

EVERY LETTER HAS A NUMBER, AND YOU CAN ADD THE NUMBERS UP IN EACH WORD...

LOOK, MARISA...
...THAT'S THE MISSION OF THE HUMAN RACE...
אהבה
(LOVE = 13)
אחד
(ONE = 13)

...TO LOVE AS ONE AND BE AS ONE.
START FROM LOVING YOURSELF.

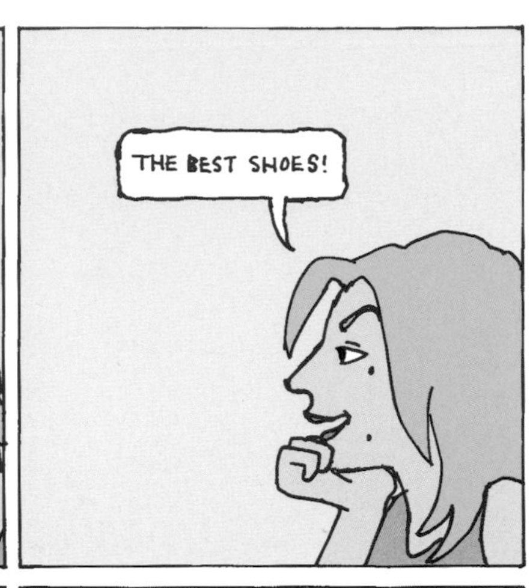

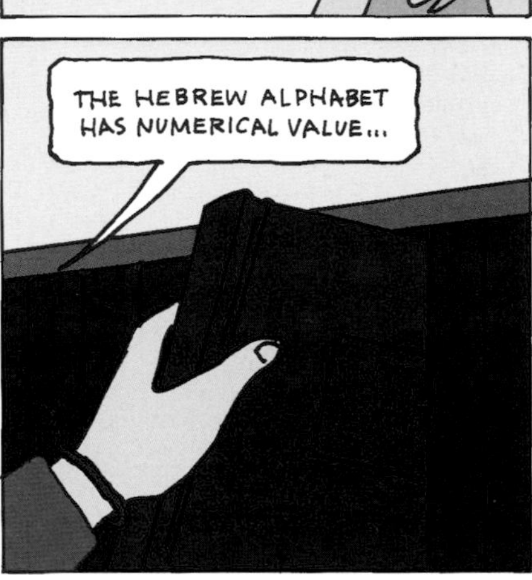

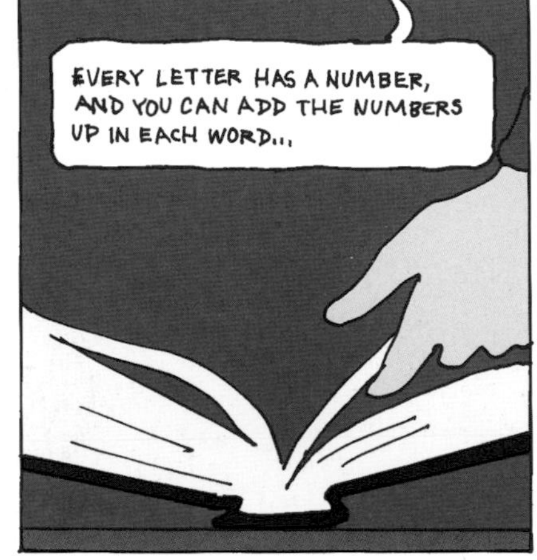

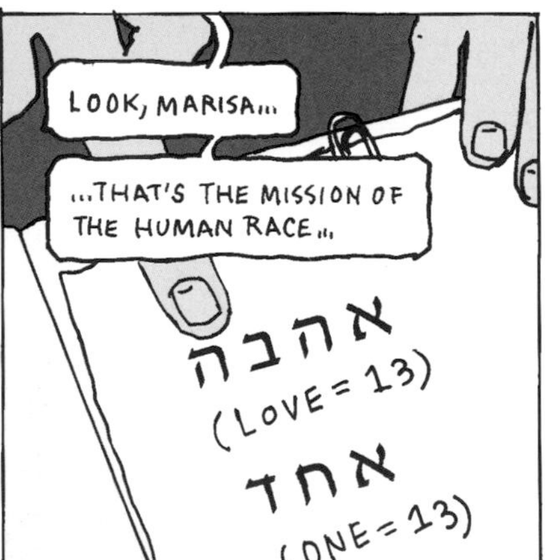

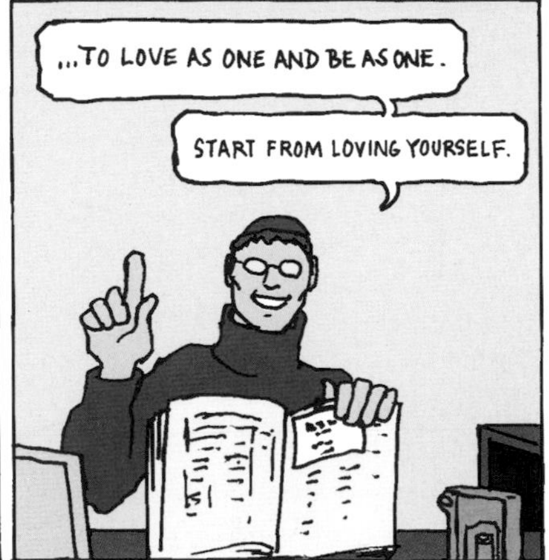

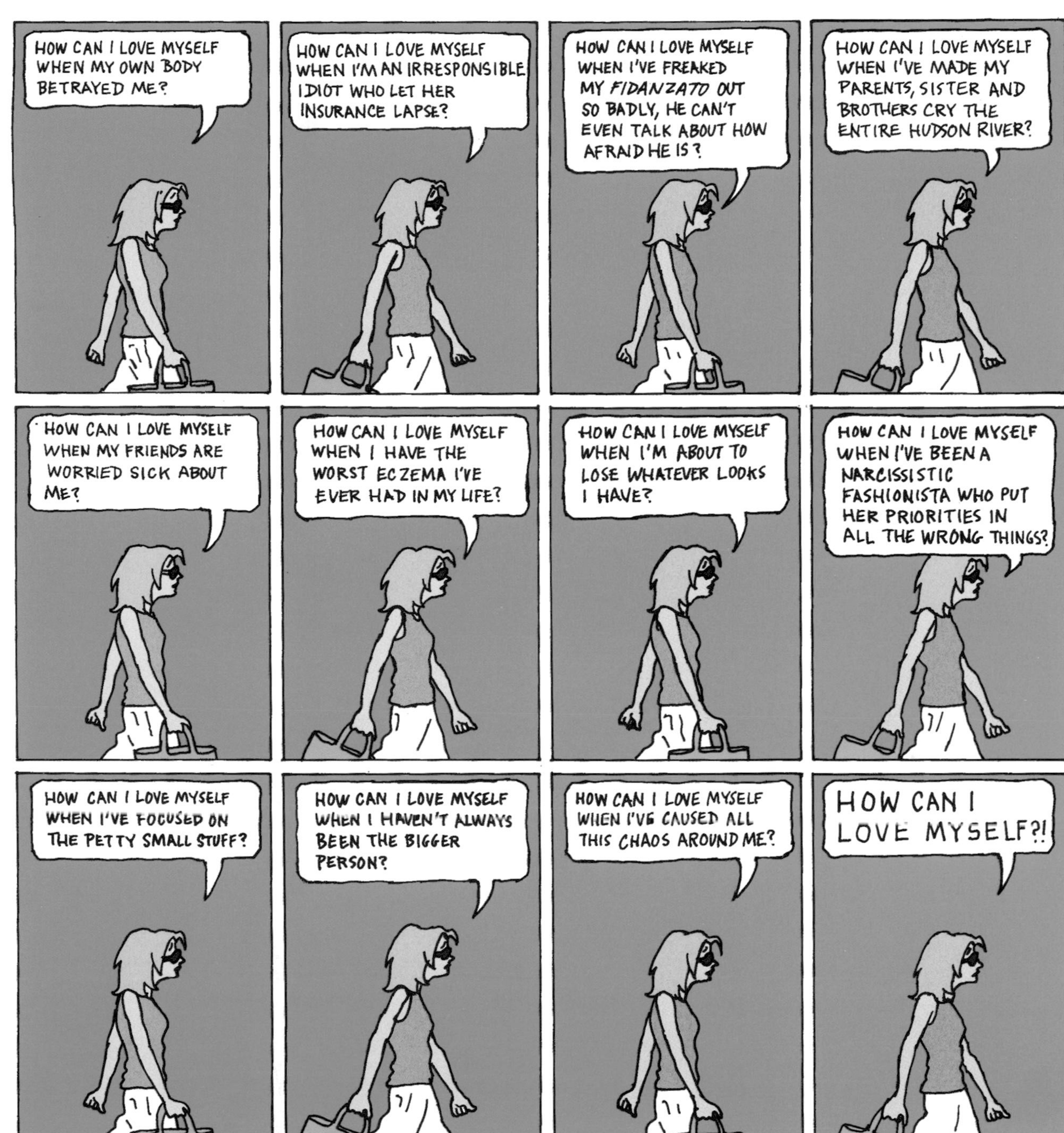
HOW CAN I LOVE MYSELF WHEN MY OWN BODY BETRAYED ME?
HOW CAN I LOVE MYSELF WHEN I'M AN IRRESPONSIBLE IDIOT WHO LET HER INSURANCE LAPSE?
HOW CAN I LOVE MYSELF WHEN I'VE FREAKED MY *FIDANZATO* OUT SO BADLY, HE CAN'T EVEN TALK ABOUT HOW AFRAID HE IS?
HOW CAN I LOVE MYSELF WHEN I'VE MADE MY PARENTS, SISTER AND BROTHERS CRY THE ENTIRE HUDSON RIVER?
HOW CAN I LOVE MYSELF WHEN MY FRIENDS ARE WORRIED SICK ABOUT ME?
HOW CAN I LOVE MYSELF WHEN I HAVE THE WORST ECZEMA I'VE EVER HAD IN MY LIFE?
HOW CAN I LOVE MYSELF WHEN I'M ABOUT TO LOSE WHATEVER LOOKS I HAVE?
HOW CAN I LOVE MYSELF WHEN I'VE BEEN A NARCISSISTIC FASHIONISTA WHO PUT HER PRIORITIES IN ALL THE WRONG THINGS?
HOW CAN I LOVE MYSELF WHEN I'VE FOCUSED ON THE PETTY SMALL STUFF?
HOW CAN I LOVE MYSELF WHEN I HAVEN'T ALWAYS BEEN THE BIGGER PERSON?
HOW CAN I LOVE MYSELF WHEN I'VE CAUSED ALL THIS CHAOS AROUND ME?
HOW CAN I LOVE MYSELF?!

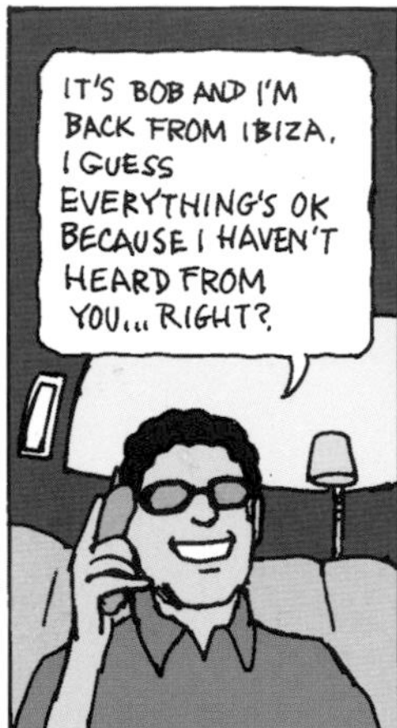
IT'S BOB AND I'M BACK FROM IBIZA. I GUESS EVERYTHING'S OK BECAUSE I HAVEN'T HEARD FROM YOU... RIGHT?

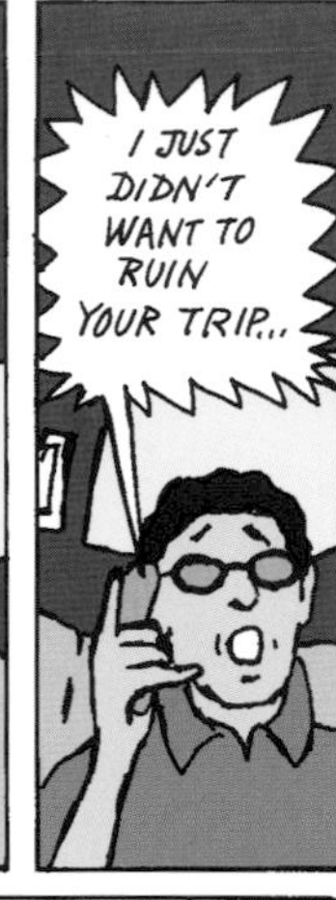
I JUST DIDN'T WANT TO RUIN YOUR TRIP...

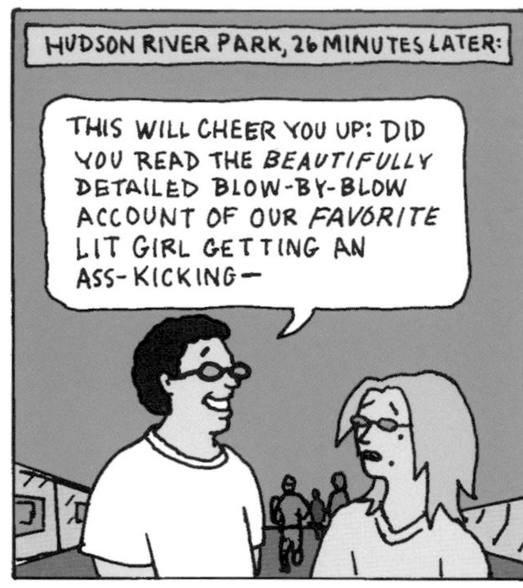
HUDSON RIVER PARK, 26 MINUTES LATER:
THIS WILL CHEER YOU UP: DID YOU READ THE BEAUTIFULLY DETAILED BLOW-BY-BLOW ACCOUNT OF OUR FAVORITE LIT GIRL GETTING AN ASS-KICKING—

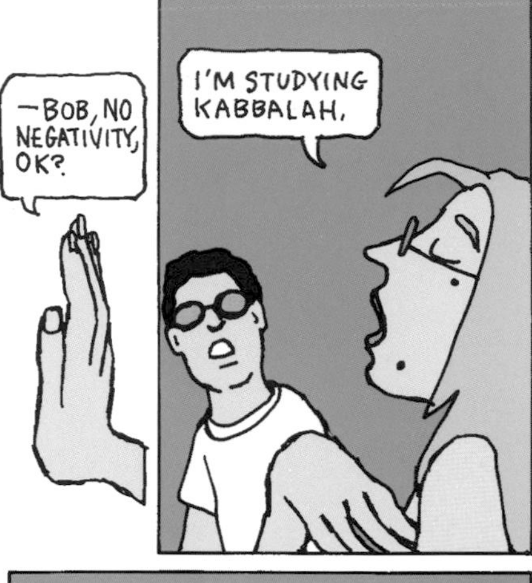
—BOB, NO NEGATIVITY, OK?
I'M STUDYING KABBALAH.

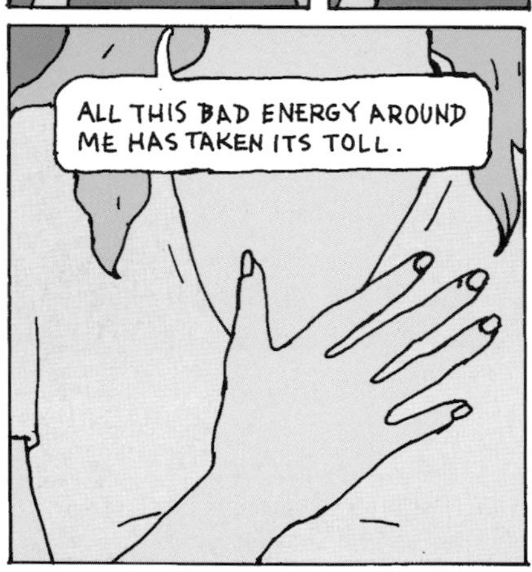
ALL THIS BAD ENERGY AROUND ME HAS TAKEN ITS TOLL.

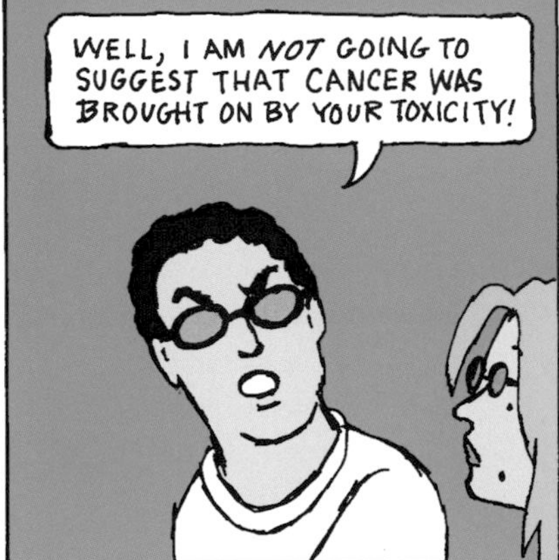
WELL, I AM NOT GOING TO SUGGEST THAT CANCER WAS BROUGHT ON BY YOUR TOXICITY!

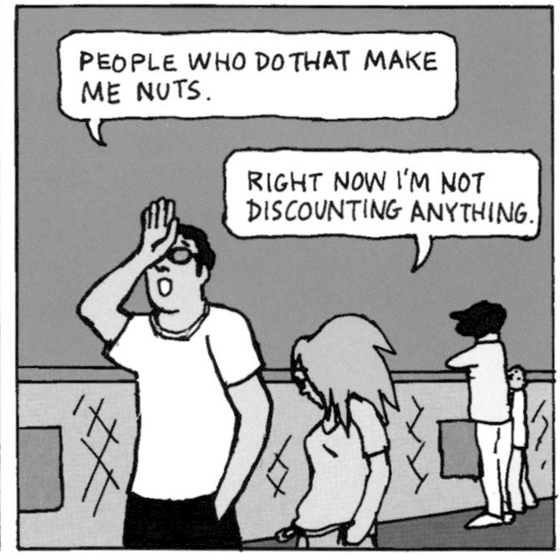
PEOPLE WHO DO THAT MAKE ME NUTS.
RIGHT NOW I'M NOT DISCOUNTING ANYTHING.

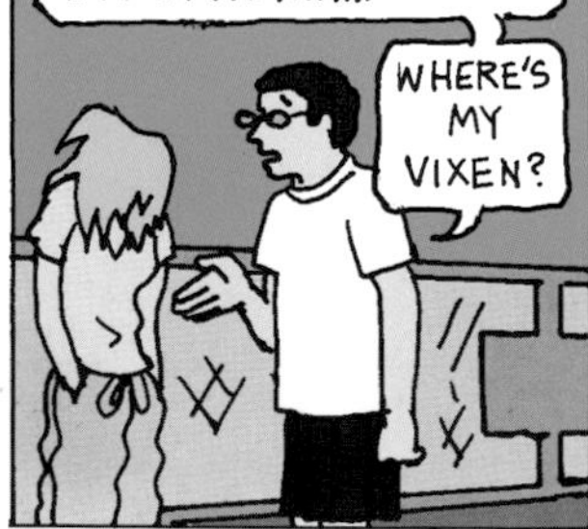
INSTEAD OF CHANGING YOUR MINDSET, CHANGE THAT OUTFIT! SWEATPANTS? SNEAKERS? YOU'RE THE DAUGHTER OF A SHOE DESIGNER! YOU LOOK LIKE A VICTIM...
WHERE'S MY VIXEN?

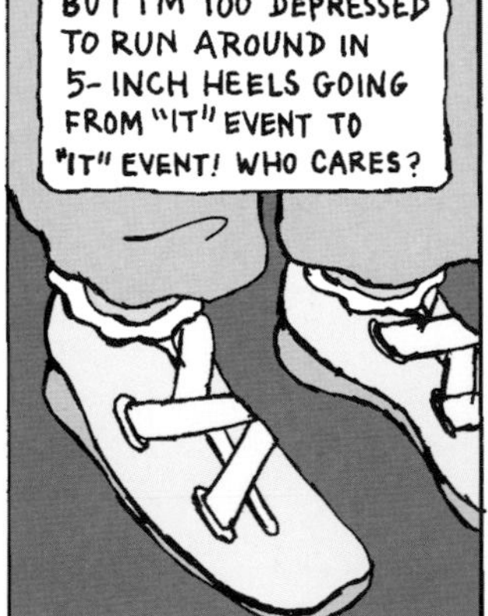
BUT I'M TOO DEPRESSED TO RUN AROUND IN 5-INCH HEELS GOING FROM "IT" EVENT TO "IT" EVENT! WHO CARES?

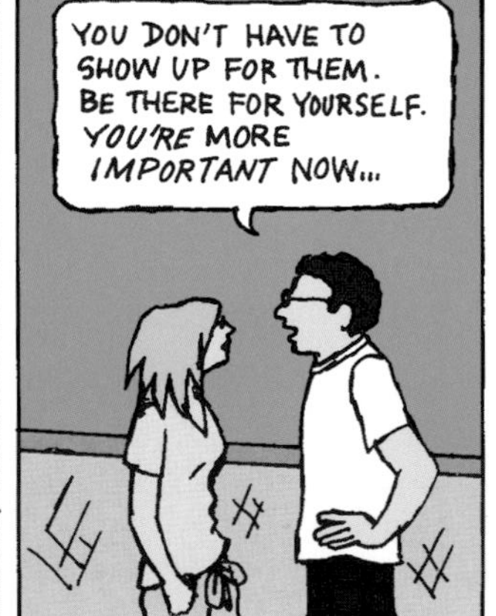
YOU DON'T HAVE TO SHOW UP FOR THEM. BE THERE FOR YOURSELF. YOU'RE MORE IMPORTANT NOW...

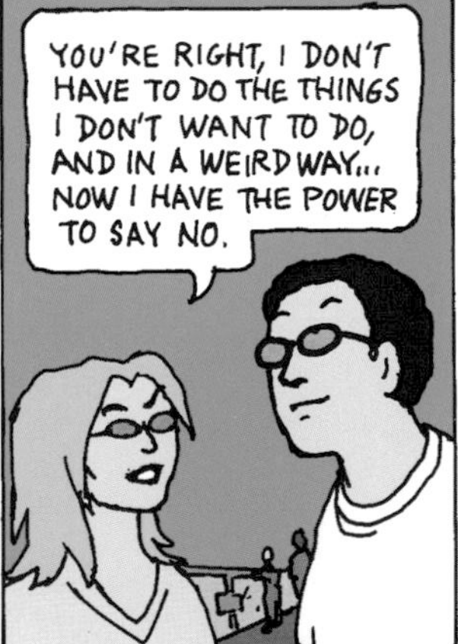
YOU'RE RIGHT, I DON'T HAVE TO DO THE THINGS I DON'T WANT TO DO, AND IN A WEIRD WAY... NOW I HAVE THE POWER TO SAY NO.

INTRODUCING THE CANCER CARD

WHEN YOU CARRY THE CANCER CARD, IT GETS YOU OUT OF DINNERS, LUNCHES, BREAKFASTS, BRUNCHES, SOCIAL OBLIGATIONS, FAMILY FUNCTIONS, CONCERTS, SHOWS, SPORTING EVENTS, PARTIES, MOVIES AND MORE!

I'M SORRY, I CAN'T MAKE IT!
THE CANCER CARD

LADY, WE SAID GO IN ALREADY!
AS IF I LOOK LIKE A TERRORIST!
SECURITY

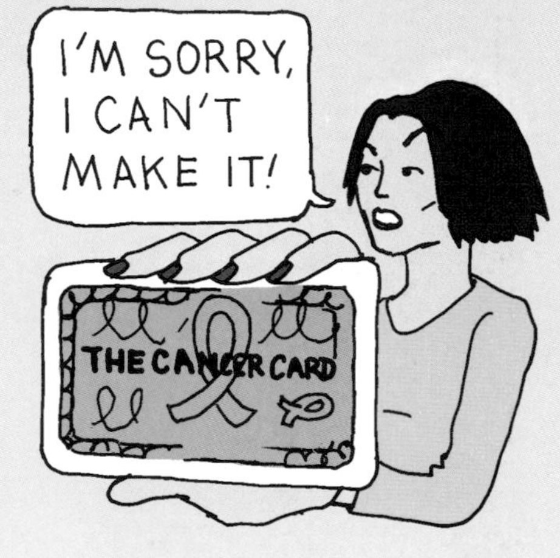

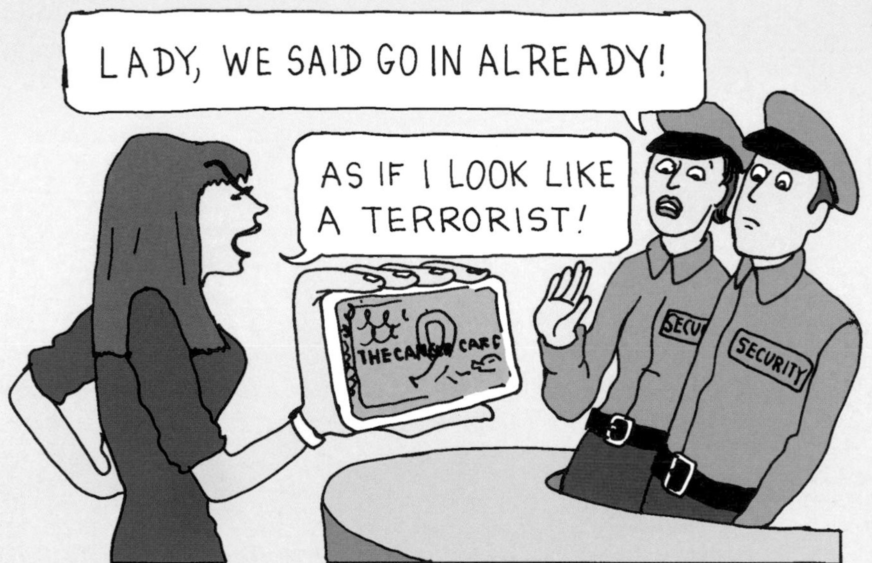

ENJOY THE CANCER CARD EASY-ACCESS BENEFITS!
NO LICENSE?
NO PHOTO I.D.?
NO PROBLEM!

NO PRESET SPENDING LIMIT—YOUR CARD IS THERE WHEN YOU NEED IT! INSTANT APPROVAL! UNIVERSAL SURVIVOR NETWORK—NOW THAT YOU'RE A MEMBER, HOTLINE OTHER SURVIVORS WHO CAN ASSIST YOU ON PHYSICIANS, MEDICATIONS AND MORE!

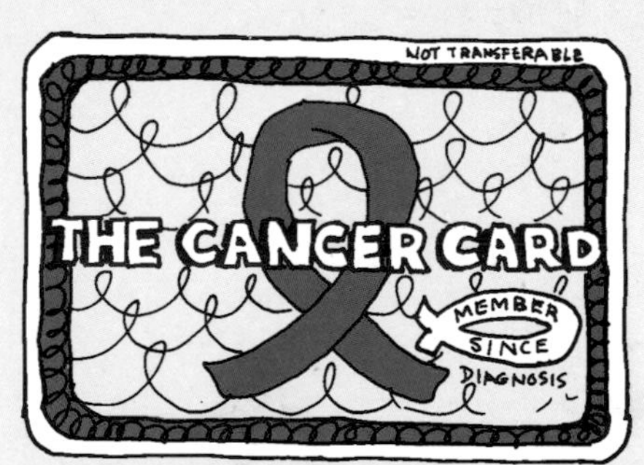

A SPECIAL KIND OF MEMBERSHIP.

MAY 24. 1 P.M. MY (S)MOTHER AND I WENT UPTOWN TO "IT" ONCOLOGIST, DR. NATURAL, THAT MY NAMELESS FRIEND INSISTED I SEE...

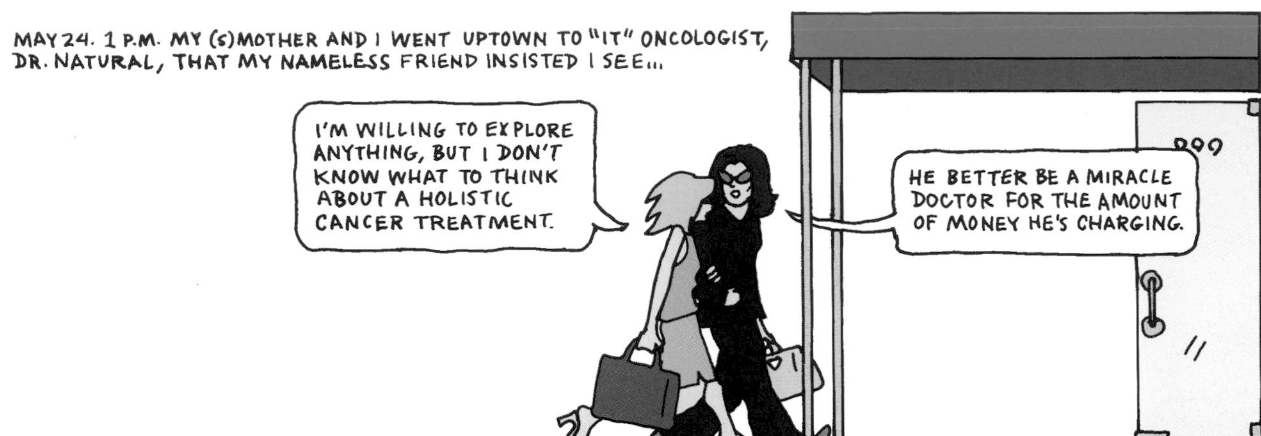

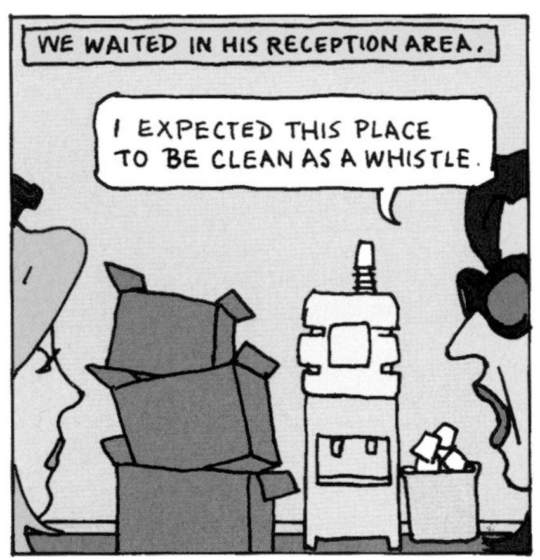

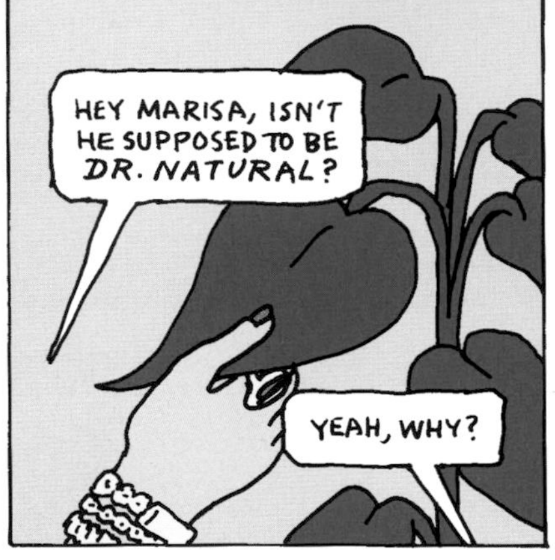

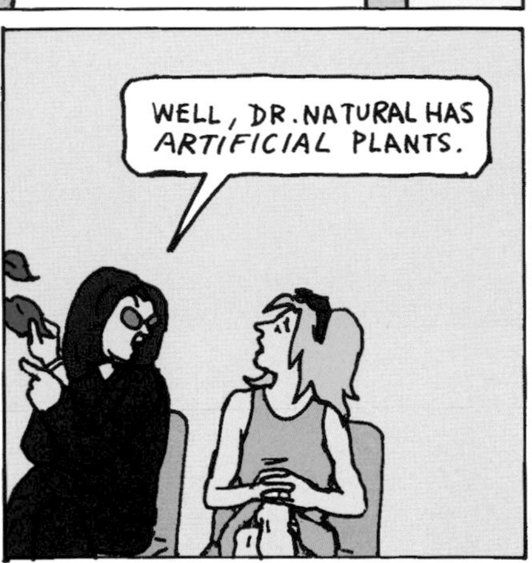

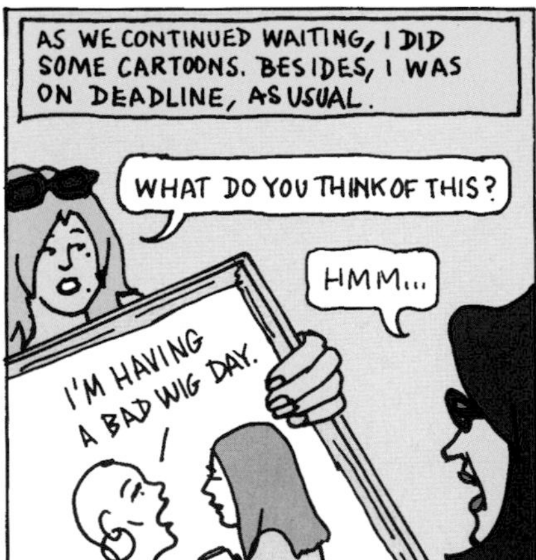

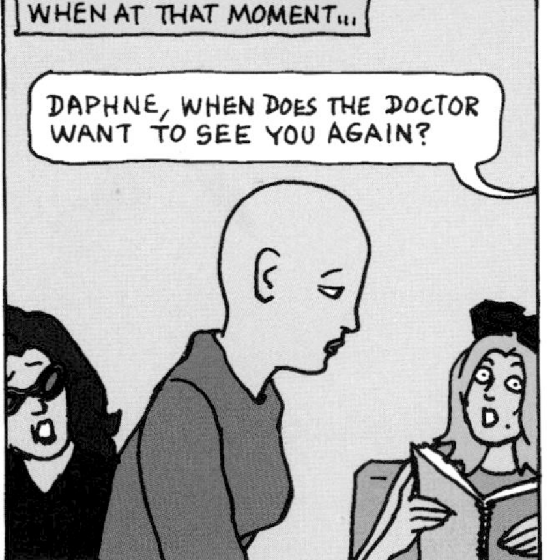

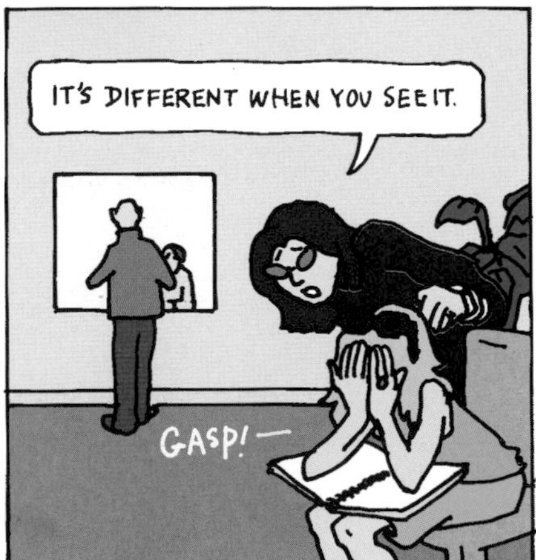

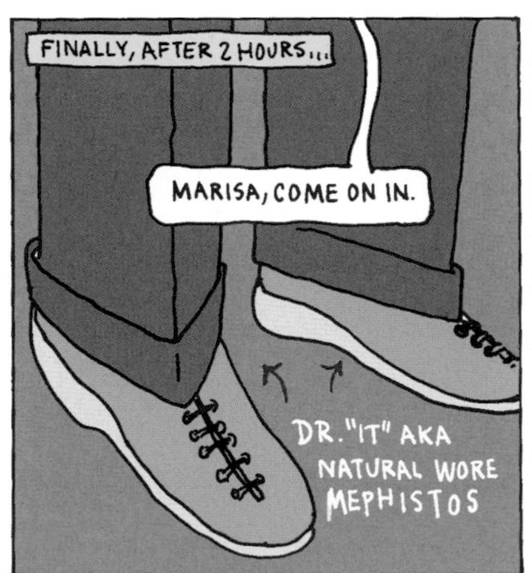

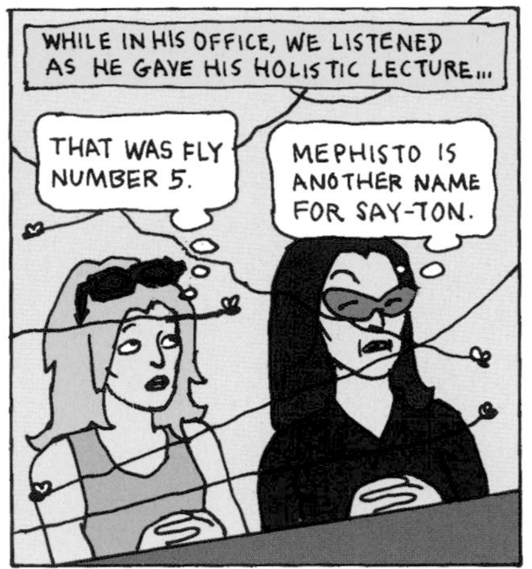

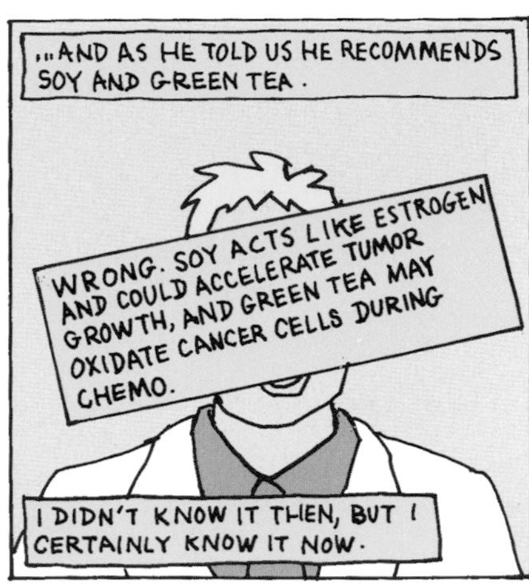

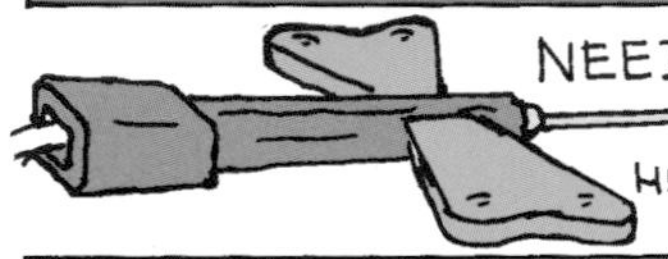

NEEDLE#3

HE TOOK ME INTO HIS EXAMINING ROOM WHERE HE DREW BLOOD, AND THEN...

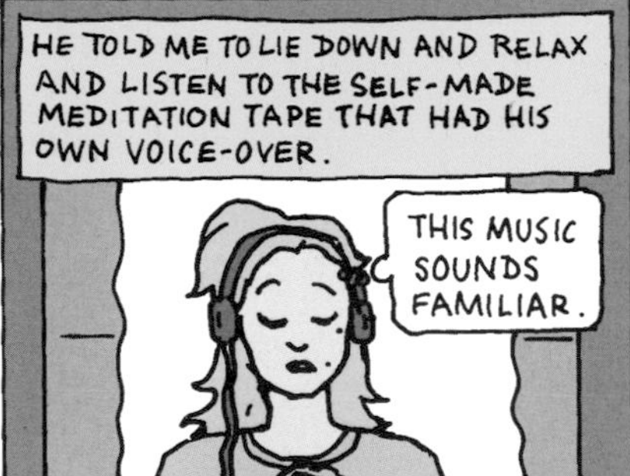

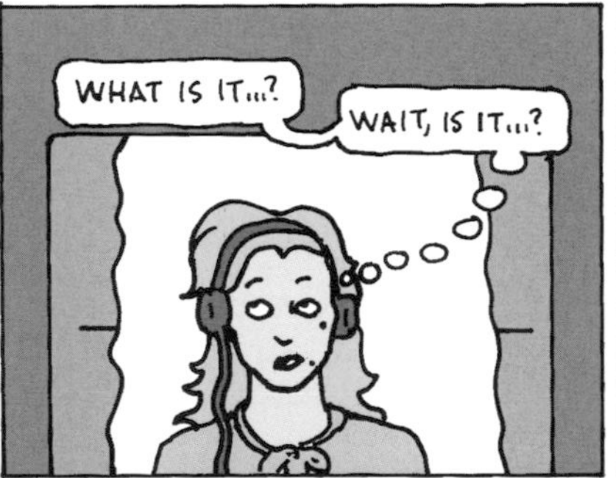

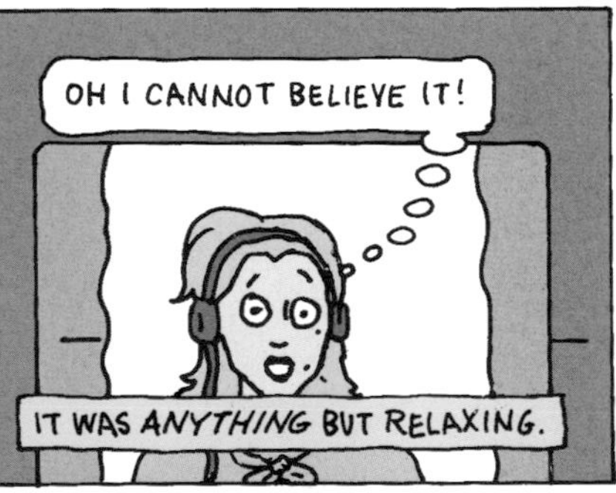

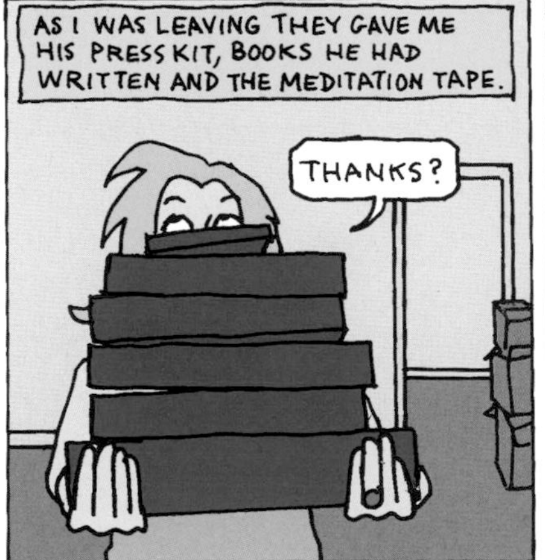

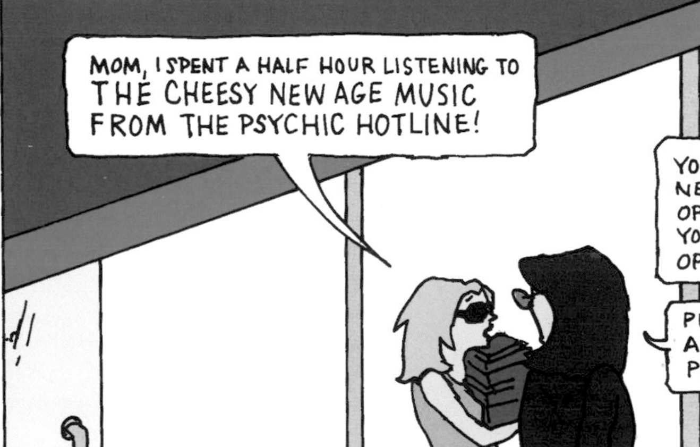

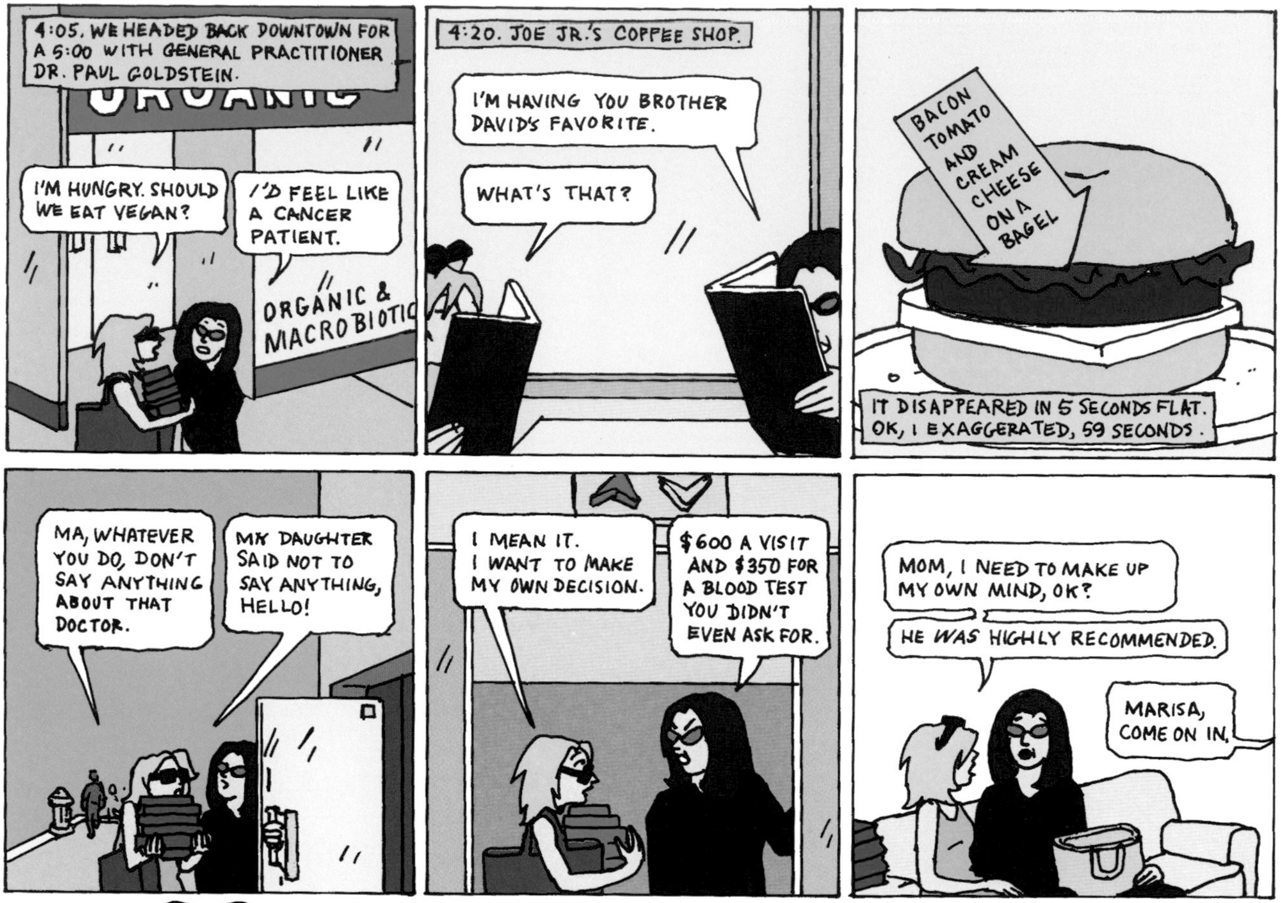

4:05. WE HEADED BACK DOWNTOWN FOR A 5:00 WITH GENERAL PRACTITIONER DR. PAUL GOLDSTEIN.

ORGANIC

I'M HUNGRY. SHOULD WE EAT VEGAN?

I'D FEEL LIKE A CANCER PATIENT.

ORGANIC & MACROBIOTIC

4:20. JOE JR.'S COFFEE SHOP.

I'M HAVING YOU BROTHER DAVID'S FAVORITE.

WHAT'S THAT?

BACON TOMATO AND CREAM CHEESE ON A BAGEL

IT DISAPPEARED IN 5 SECONDS FLAT. OK, I EXAGGERATED, 59 SECONDS.

MA, WHATEVER YOU DO, DON'T SAY ANYTHING ABOUT THAT DOCTOR.

MY DAUGHTER SAID NOT TO SAY ANYTHING, HELLO!

I MEAN IT. I WANT TO MAKE MY OWN DECISION.

$600 A VISIT AND $350 FOR A BLOOD TEST YOU DIDN'T EVEN ASK FOR.

MOM, I NEED TO MAKE UP MY OWN MIND, OK?

HE *WAS* HIGHLY RECOMMENDED.

MARISA, COME ON IN.

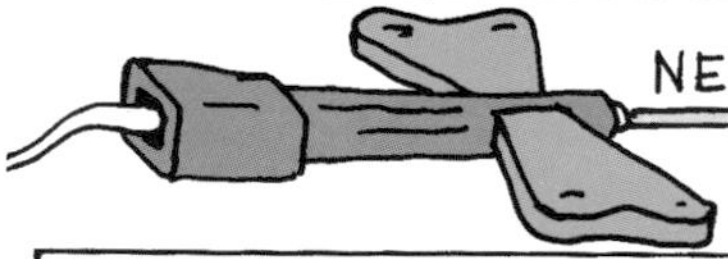

NEEDLE #4

THE BLOOD-DRAWING NEEDLE #2 THAT SAME DAY.

SPEAKING OF DRAWING...
MAYBE I CAN SKETCH WITH MY FEET TONIGHT?

HELLO, DOCTOR. I'M MARISA'S MOM.
OH, SHE LOOKS LIKE YOUR SISTER!

YOUR CHEST X-RAYS ARE CLEAR.*
EXCUSE ME, MAY I SAY SOMETHING?
*THAT'S GOOD NEWS, I DON'T HAVE *LUNG* CANCER.

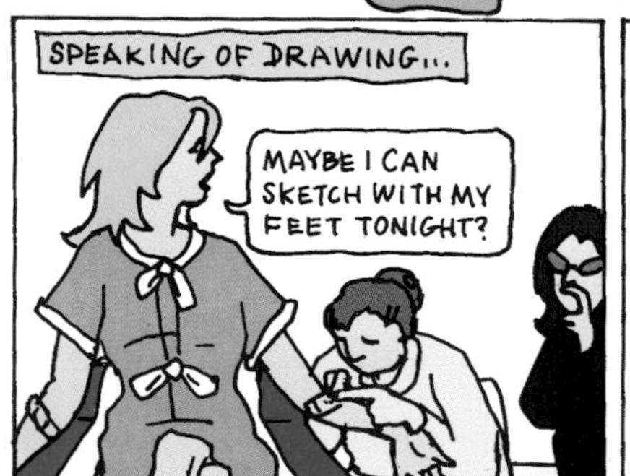

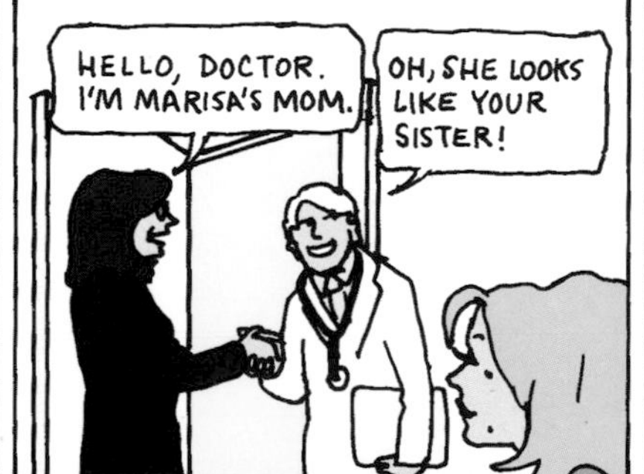

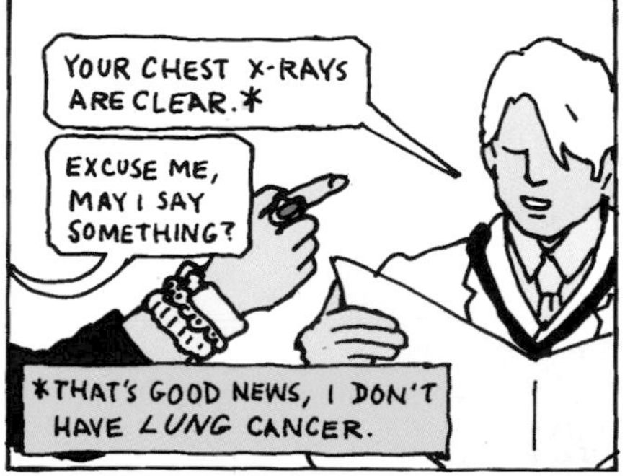

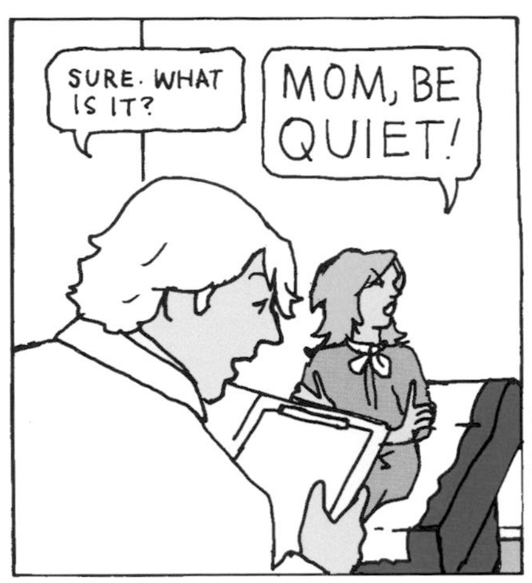
SURE. WHAT IS IT?
MOM, BE QUIET!

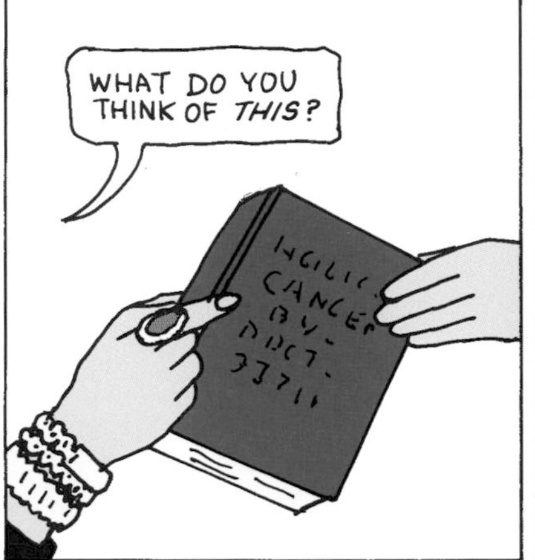
WHAT DO YOU THINK OF THIS?

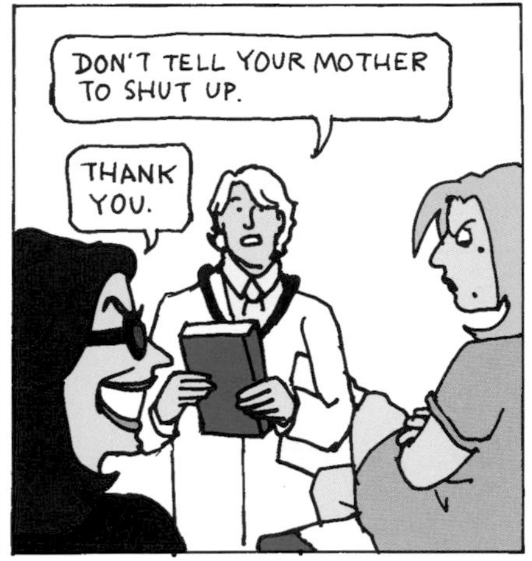
DON'T TELL YOUR MOTHER TO SHUT UP.
THANK YOU.

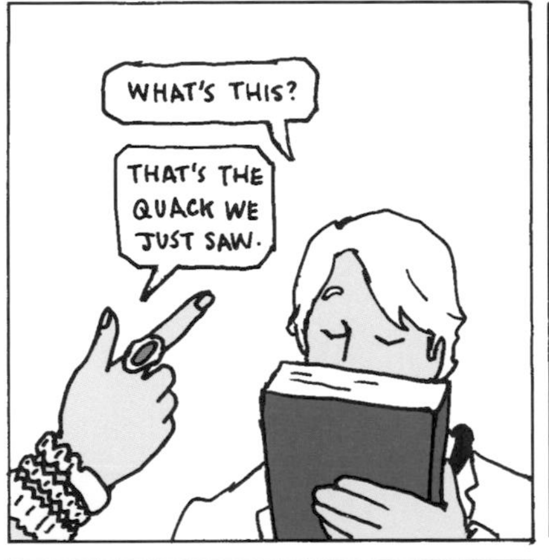
WHAT'S THIS?
THAT'S THE QUACK WE JUST SAW.

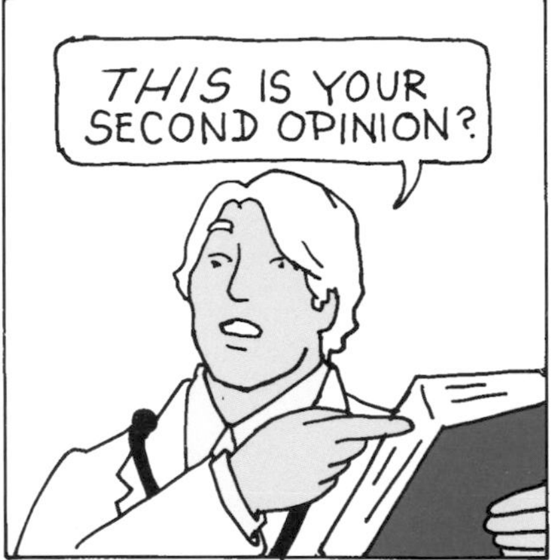
THIS IS YOUR SECOND OPINION?

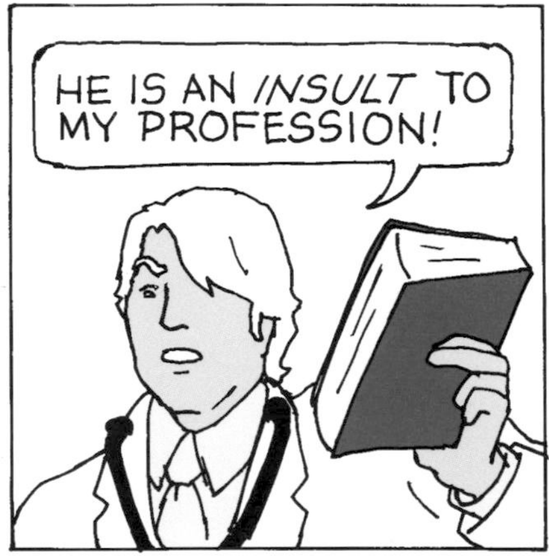
HE IS AN INSULT TO MY PROFESSION!

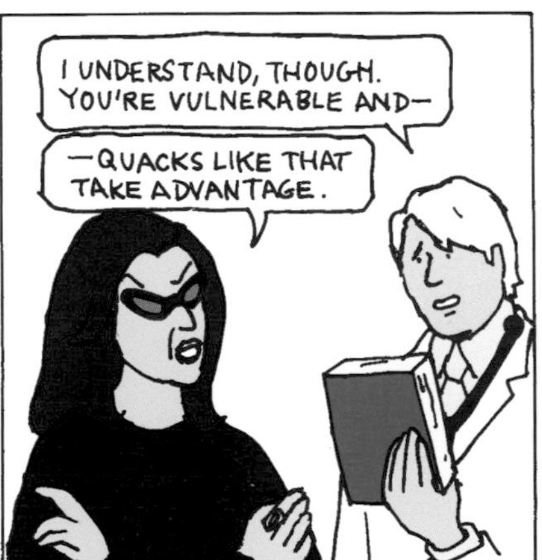
I UNDERSTAND, THOUGH. YOU'RE VULNERABLE AND—
—QUACKS LIKE THAT TAKE ADVANTAGE.

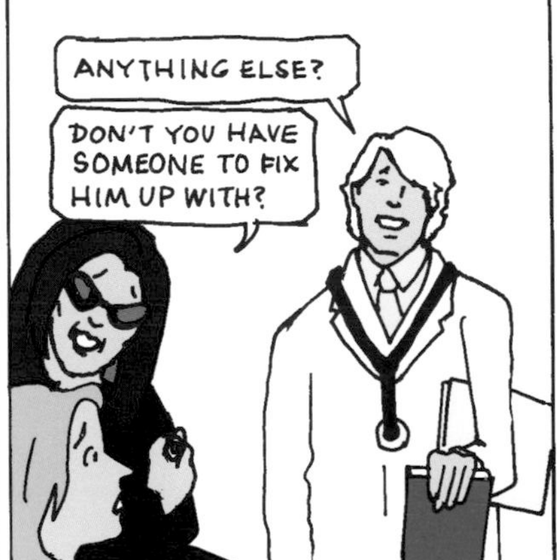
ANYTHING ELSE?
DON'T YOU HAVE SOMEONE TO FIX HIM UP WITH?

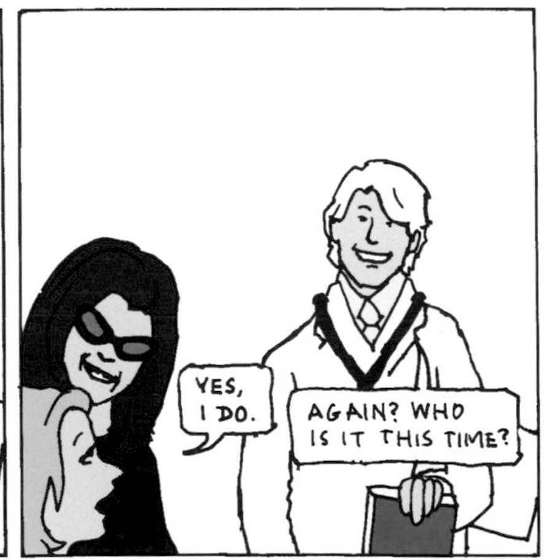
YES, I DO.
AGAIN? WHO IS IT THIS TIME?

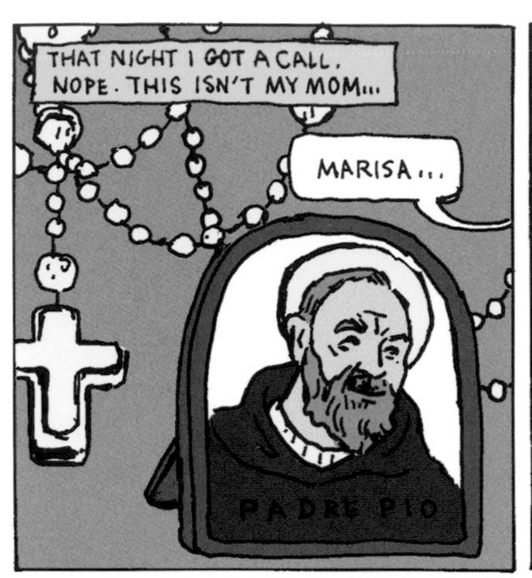
THAT NIGHT I GOT A CALL. NOPE. THIS ISN'T MY MOM...
MARISA...
PADRE PIO

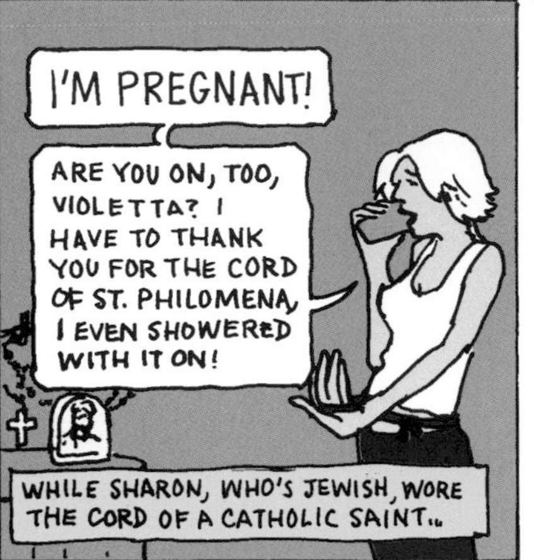
I'M PREGNANT!
ARE YOU ON, TOO, VIOLETTA? I HAVE TO THANK YOU FOR THE CORD OF ST. PHILOMENA, I EVEN SHOWERED WITH IT ON!
WHILE SHARON, WHO'S JEWISH, WORE THE CORD OF A CATHOLIC SAINT..

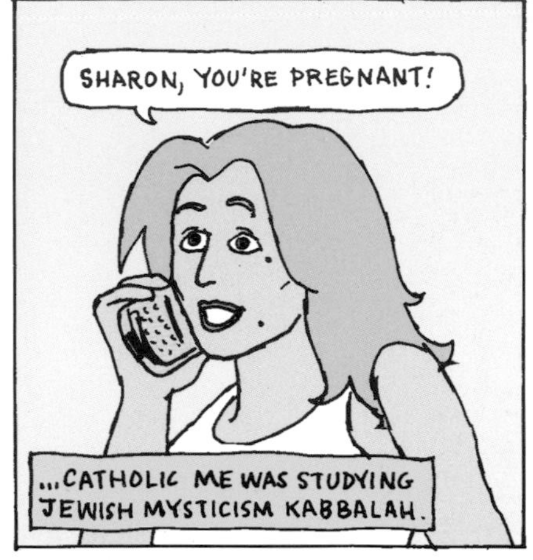
SHARON, YOU'RE PREGNANT!
...CATHOLIC ME WAS STUDYING JEWISH MYSTICISM KABBALAH.

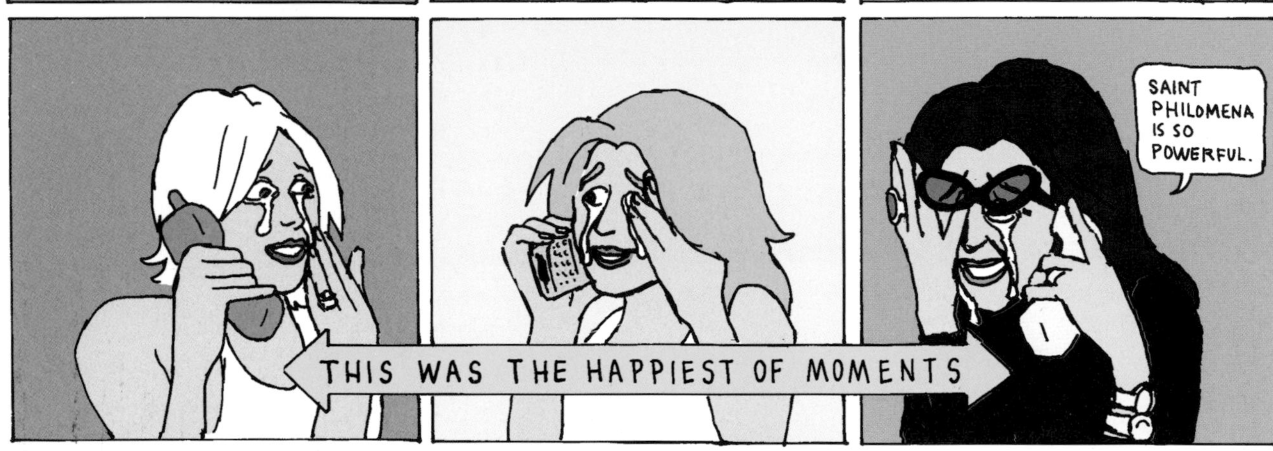
SAINT PHILOMENA IS SO POWERFUL.
THIS WAS THE HAPPIEST OF MOMENTS

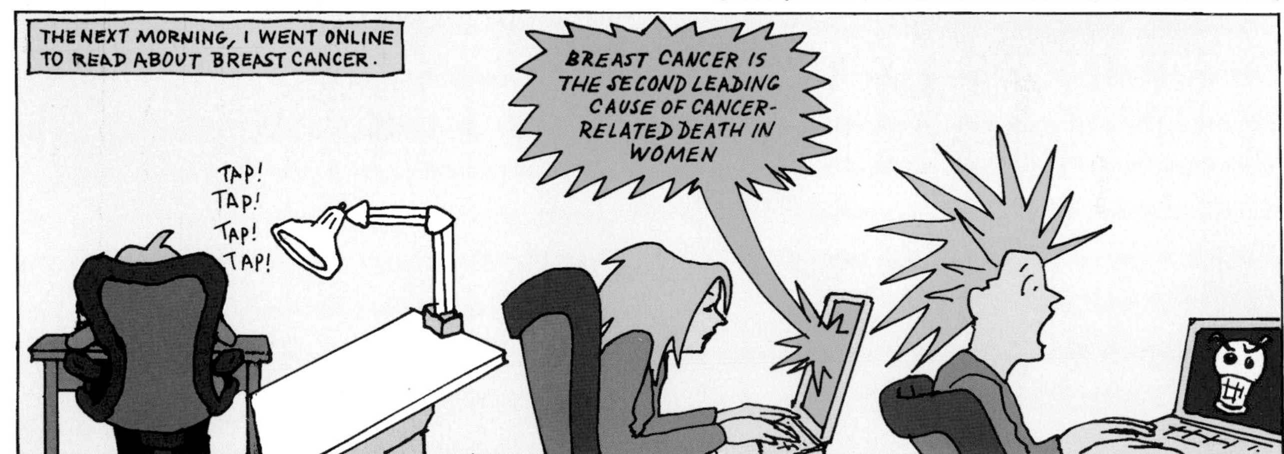
THE NEXT MORNING, I WENT ONLINE TO READ ABOUT BREAST CANCER.
BREAST CANCER IS THE SECOND LEADING CAUSE OF CANCER-RELATED DEATH IN WOMEN
TAP! TAP! TAP! TAP!

AFTER THAT, I WENT TO MY THERAPIST. I WAS GOING UNDER THE KNIFE IN LESS THAN 24 HOURS!
YOU'RE WHAT'S IMPORTANT...

YOU NEED TO FEEL ENTITLED TO YOUR NEEDS...

WHAT WERE YOU JUST THINKING OF?

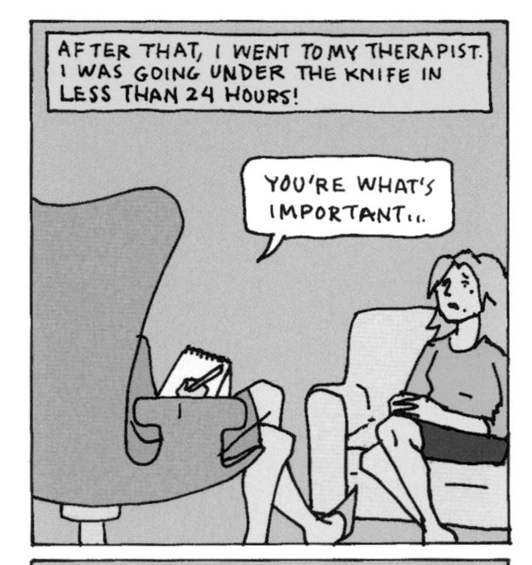

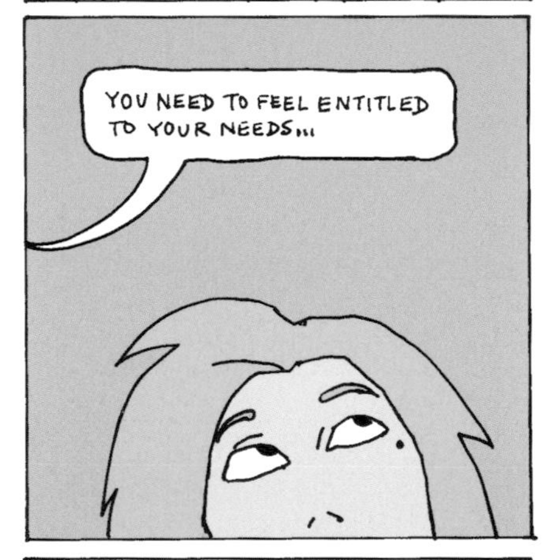

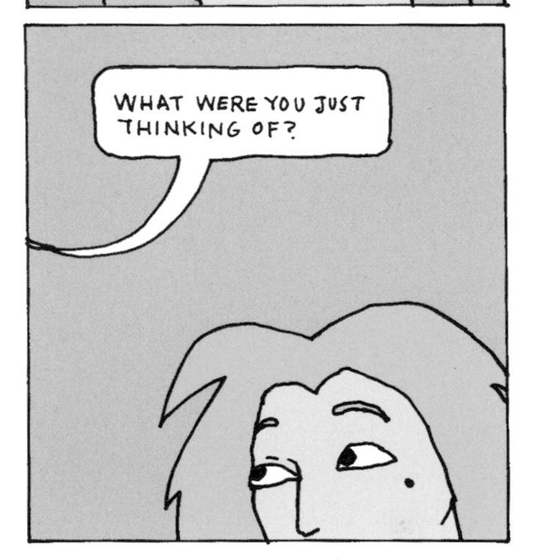

THIS IS WHAT I WAS THINKING OF, AND IT WAS THE MOST SATISFYING CHEESEBURGER DELUXE I EVER HAD.

IT WAS MY FAVORITE MEAL AS A KID. MAYBE I WAS CRAVING A TIME WHEN I WAS COMPLETELY CAREFREE?

JOHNNY ROCKETS
THE ORIGINAL HAMBURGER
42nd East 8th St
New York, New York 10003

05/25/2004
2:17 PM

Server: Kadir
2/1 #10066
Guests: 1

2.09
0.69

American Fries
Original
Add Cheddar-Tillamook

7.07
0.61

Sub Total 7.86
Tax

Total 7.68

Balance Due

FREE HAMBURGER w/ purchase of
hamburger, starter and drink.

Survey Validation Code: ________
Redeem one per 3 month period

4:00. DR. MILLS'S OFFICE. I HAD MY Qs READY.

How long will I be in the hospital?
What kind of anesthesia am I getting?
How will my normal routine be restricted?
How much discomfort will I have?
What kind of bandages will I have after surgery?
How should I care for the bandages after surgery?
When do I get the bandages off?
Will I have a scar?

THE CORE BIOPSY SHOWS AN INVASIVE COMPONENT, WHICH MEANS IT MAY BE IN THE LYMPH NODES.
SO, AS WE'RE DOING THE LUMPECTOMY, WE'RE GOING TO DO A SENTINEL NODE BIOPSY; IF THE CANCER HAS JUMPED IT WOULD BE THERE FIRST.
IF THE SENTINEL NODE IS POSITIVE?
RadioShack
RECORDER
THEN WE WILL REMOVE ADDITIONAL LYMPH NODES.

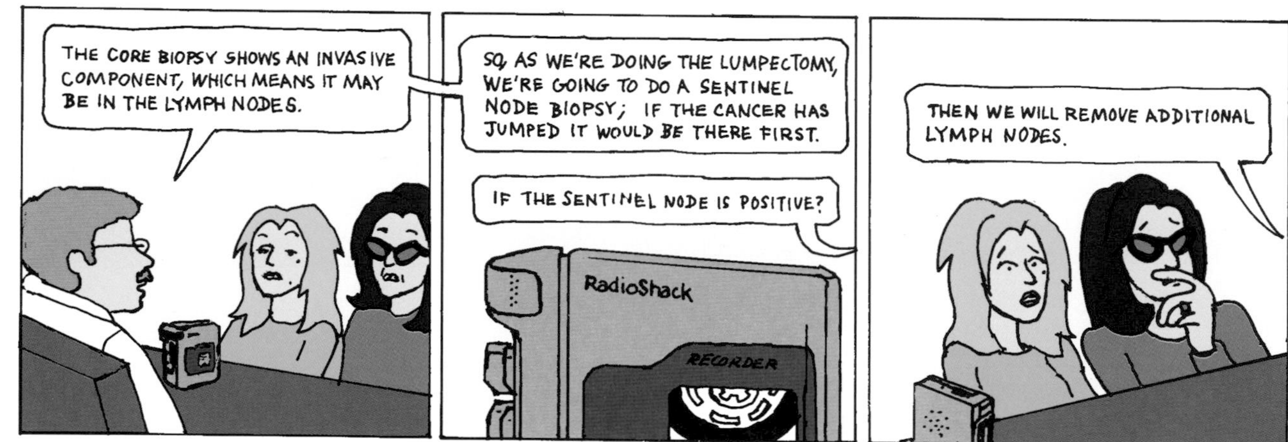

How many lymph nodes are you taking out?
What are my chances of developing lymphedema?
Are there any side effects from surgery?
When should I come back for a follow-up visit?
What kind of care will I need after surgery?
How soon can I go back to my regular schedule?
Does Saint Vincents take Amex?
Or can I write a check?

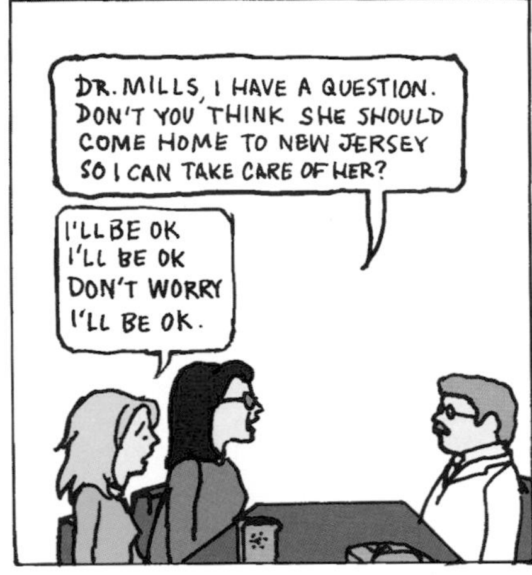
DR. MILLS, I HAVE A QUESTION. DON'T YOU THINK SHE SHOULD COME HOME TO NEW JERSEY SO I CAN TAKE CARE OF HER?
I'LL BE OK
I'LL BE OK
DON'T WORRY
I'LL BE OK.

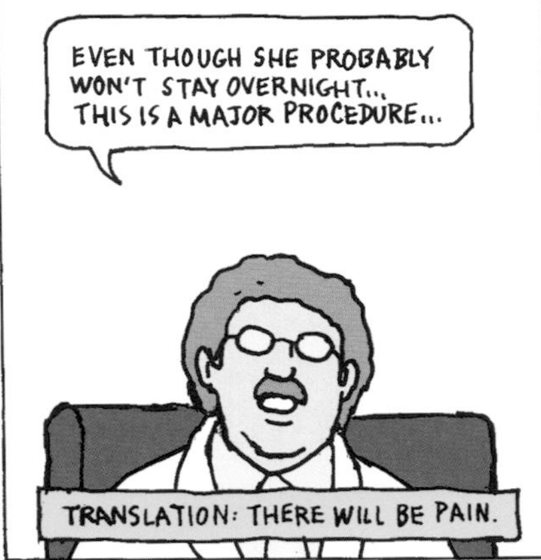
EVEN THOUGH SHE PROBABLY WON'T STAY OVERNIGHT... THIS IS A MAJOR PROCEDURE...
TRANSLATION: THERE WILL BE PAIN.

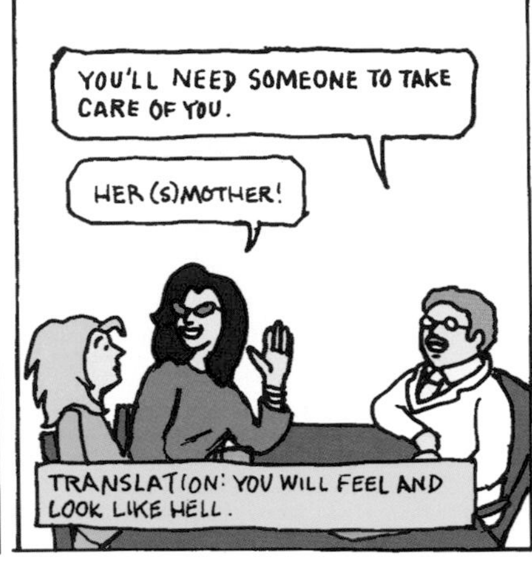
YOU'LL NEED SOMEONE TO TAKE CARE OF YOU.
HER (S)MOTHER!
TRANSLATION: YOU WILL FEEL AND LOOK LIKE HELL.

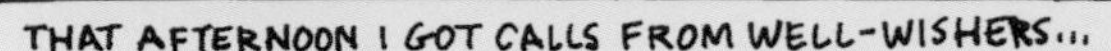
THAT AFTERNOON I GOT CALLS FROM WELL-WISHERS...

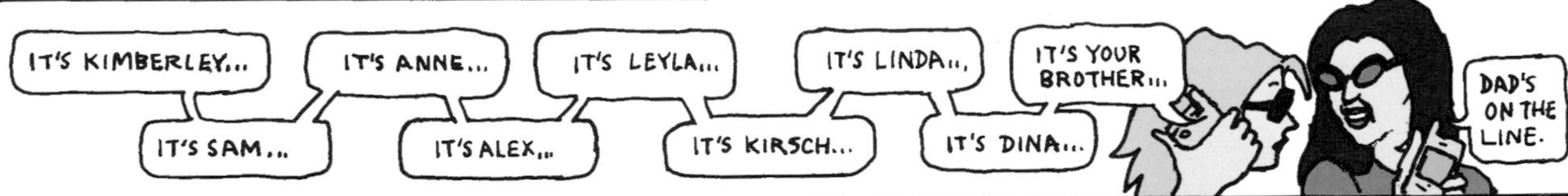
IT'S KIMBERLEY...
IT'S SAM...
IT'S ANNE...
IT'S ALEX...
IT'S LEYLA...
IT'S KIRSCH...
IT'S LINDA...
IT'S DINA...
IT'S YOUR BROTHER...
DAD'S ON THE LINE.

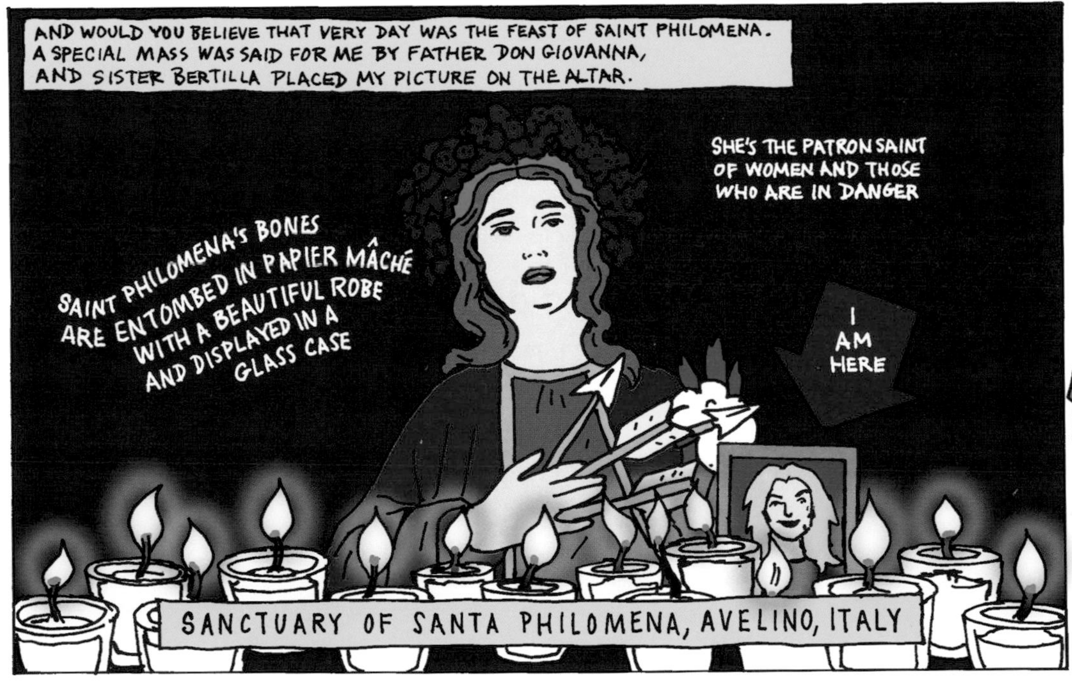
AND WOULD YOU BELIEVE THAT VERY DAY WAS THE FEAST OF SAINT PHILOMENA. A SPECIAL MASS WAS SAID FOR ME BY FATHER DON GIOVANNA, AND SISTER BERTILLA PLACED MY PICTURE ON THE ALTAR.
SHE'S THE PATRON SAINT OF WOMEN AND THOSE WHO ARE IN DANGER
SAINT PHILOMENA'S BONES ARE ENTOMBED IN PAPIER MÂCHÉ WITH A BEAUTIFUL ROBE AND DISPLAYED IN A GLASS CASE
I AM HERE
SANCTUARY OF SANTA PHILOMENA, AVELINO, ITALY

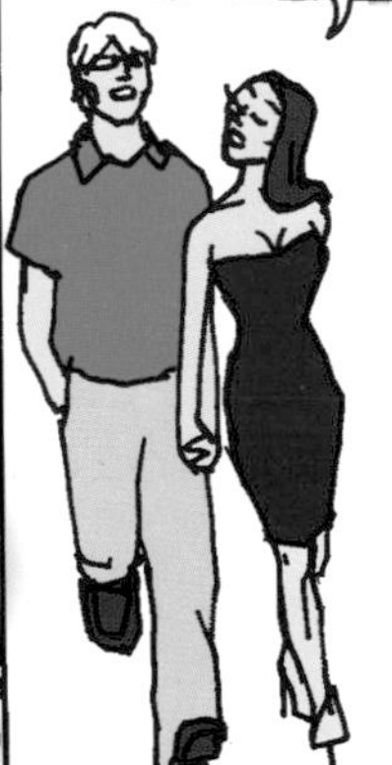
I'M AN ATHEIST AND I'M PRAYING FOR YOU.
THAT'S NOT TRUE, RICHARD. YOU'RE A PROTESTANT!

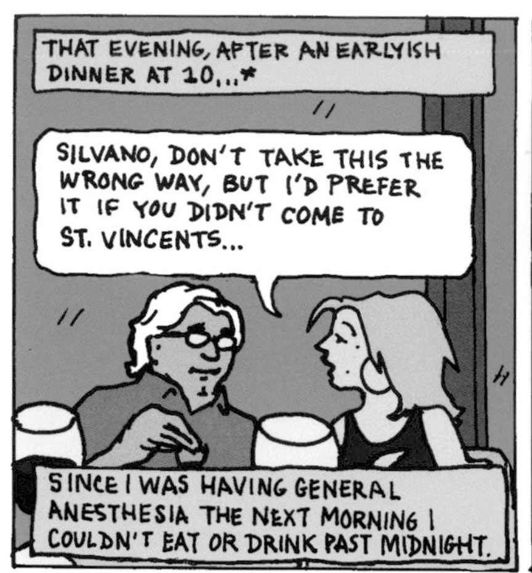
THAT EVENING, AFTER AN EARLYISH DINNER AT 10,...*
SILVANO, DON'T TAKE THIS THE WRONG WAY, BUT I'D PREFER IT IF YOU DIDN'T COME TO ST. VINCENTS...
SINCE I WAS HAVING GENERAL ANESTHESIA THE NEXT MORNING I COULDN'T EAT OR DRINK PAST MIDNIGHT.

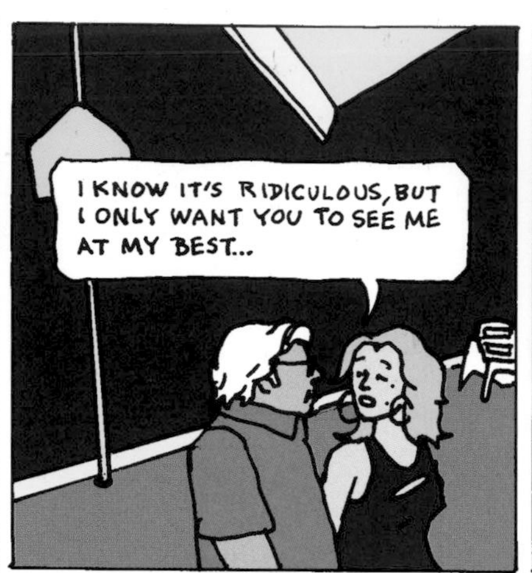
I KNOW IT'S RIDICULOUS, BUT I ONLY WANT YOU TO SEE ME AT MY BEST...

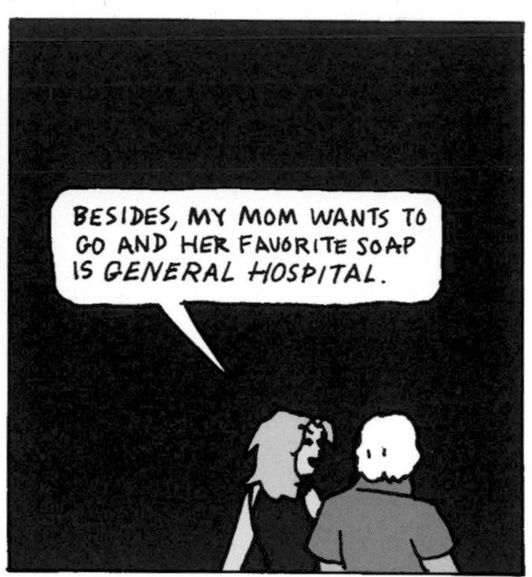
BESIDES, MY MOM WANTS TO GO AND HER FAVORITE SOAP IS *GENERAL HOSPITAL*.

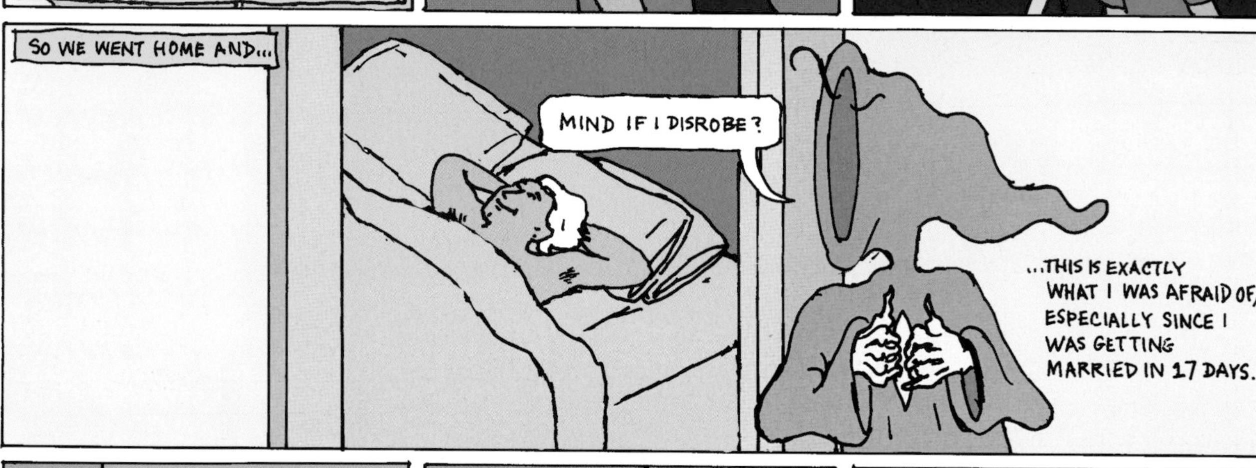
SO WE WENT HOME AND...
MIND IF I DISROBE?
...THIS IS EXACTLY WHAT I WAS AFRAID OF, ESPECIALLY SINCE I WAS GETTING MARRIED IN 17 DAYS.

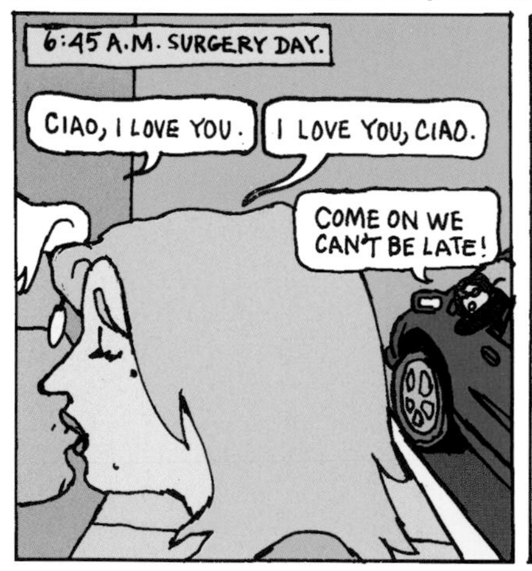
6:45 A.M. SURGERY DAY.
CIAO, I LOVE YOU.
I LOVE YOU, CIAO.
COME ON WE CAN'T BE LATE!

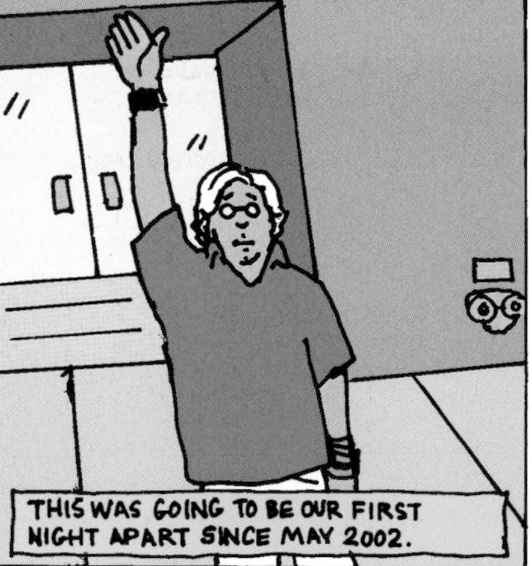
THIS WAS GOING TO BE OUR FIRST NIGHT APART SINCE MAY 2002.

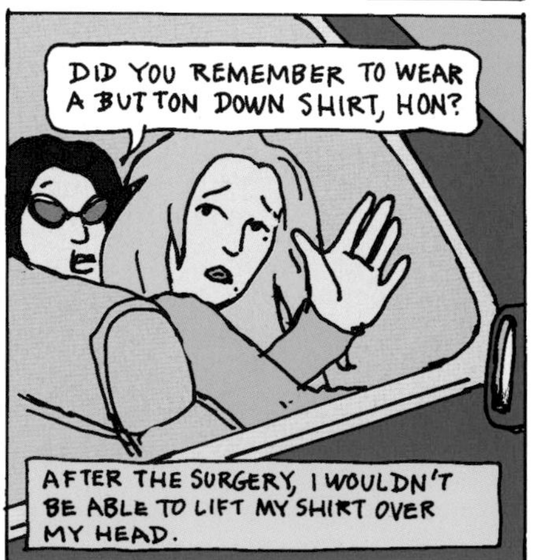
DID YOU REMEMBER TO WEAR A BUTTON DOWN SHIRT, HON?
AFTER THE SURGERY, I WOULDN'T BE ABLE TO LIFT MY SHIRT OVER MY HEAD.

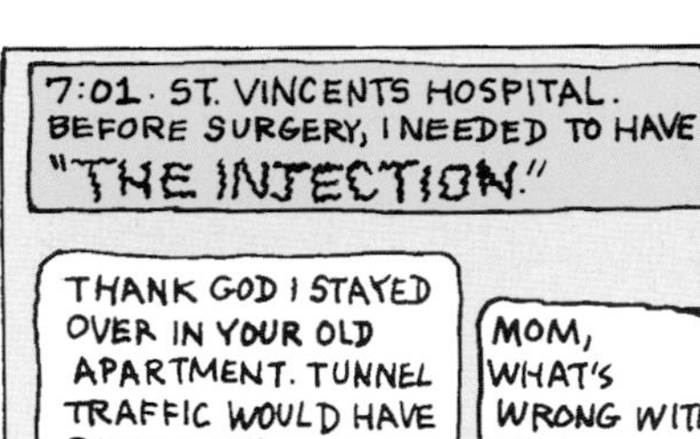

AILMENT #2: CARPAL TUNNEL SYNDROME.

7:23, THEY GAVE ME A ROBE, SLIPPERS, MY VERY OWN GARMENT BAG AND A FEW OTHER GOODIES...
THE BEDPAN IS THERE IN CASE YOU VOMIT.
I'LL HOLD YOUR HEAD IF YOU THROW UP.

I FORGOT MY LENS CASE, SO I PUT MY CONTACTS IN THE CONTAINERS THEY USE FOR URINE SAMPLES.

SIT UP STRAIGHT, I'LL GO GET THE PAPER.

MISS ACOCELLA!

BEFORE YOU GO IN, I'M TYING THE CORD OF ST. PHILOMENA ON YOU.
AND DON'T LOSE THIS ONE!

THEN I GOT BRIEFED BY DR. KODE EDIALE.
YOU'RE FROM NEW JERSEY? WELL, TO GO INTO NEW YORK, BEFORE YOU GO INTO THE TUNNEL, YOU HAVE TO PAY THE TOLL...

THE TOLL IS THE SENTINEL NODE.
HOLLAND TUNNEL
...IF THE CANCER CELLS ARE IN THE LYMPH NODES, THEY WOULD REACH THE SENTINEL NODE FIRST.

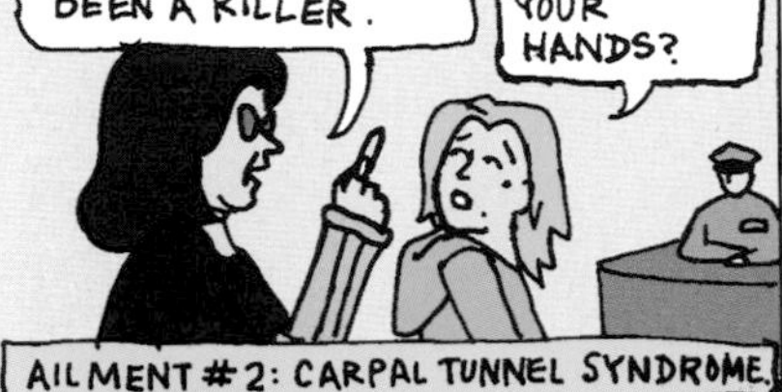

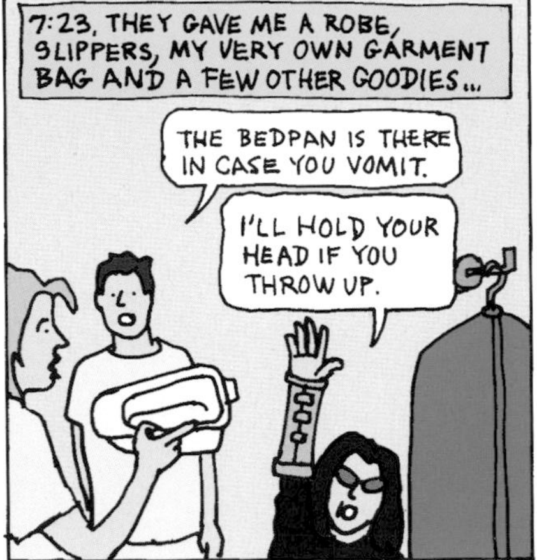

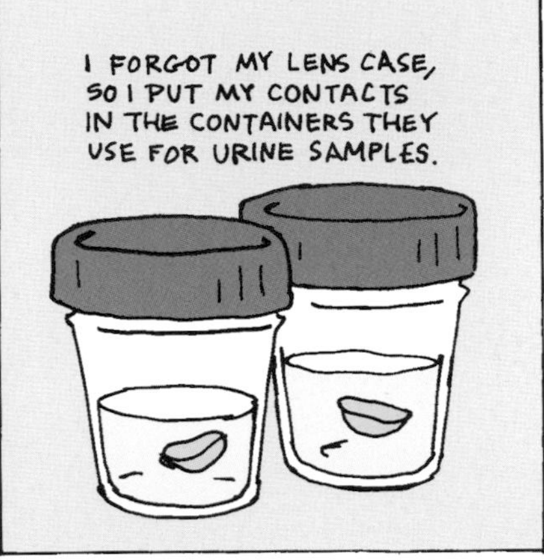

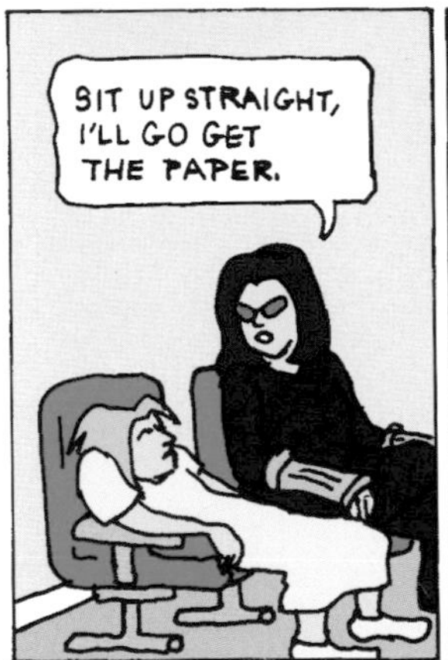

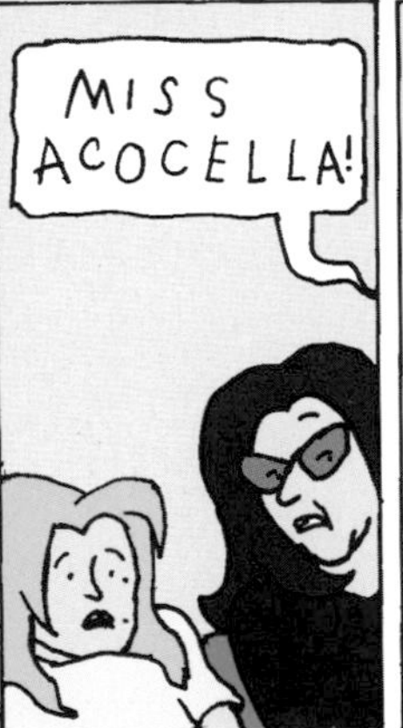

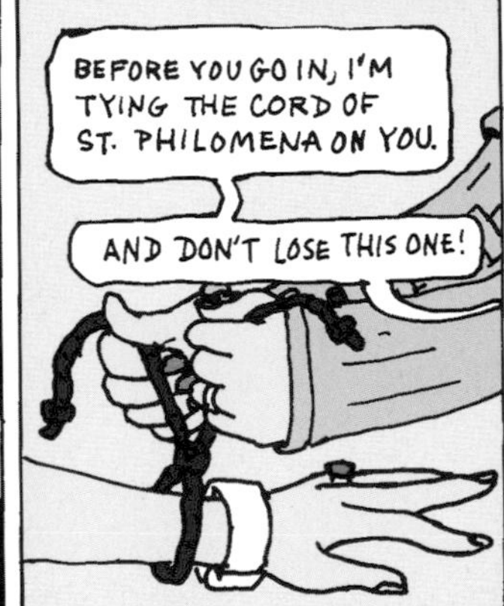

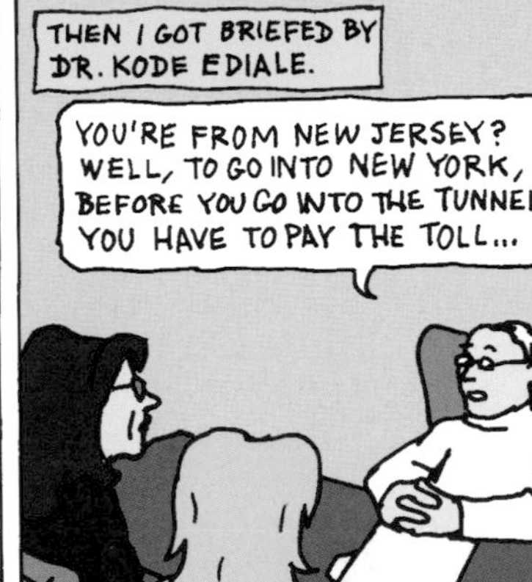

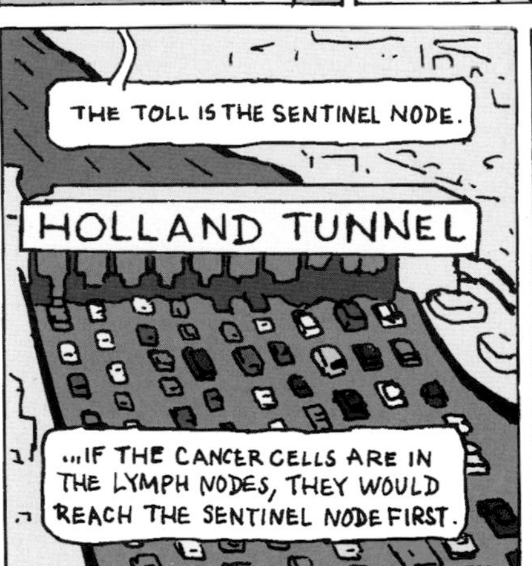

TO FIND THE SENTINEL NODE, WE INJECT A RADIOACTIVE TRACE AND A BLUE DYE INTO THE BREAST. THIS WILL TRAVEL TO THE SENTINEL NODE IN THE ARMPIT AND HELP IDENTIFY IT. A GEIGER COUNTER WILL LOCATE THE SENTINEL NODE.

BTW, DR. EDIALE LOOKED LIKE MY GRANDFATHER

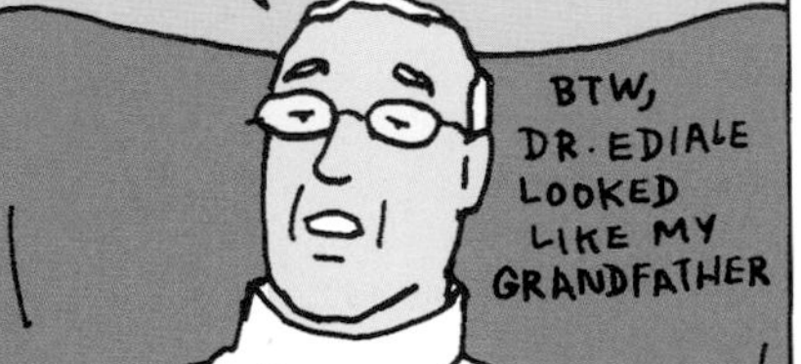

AFTER WE DO THE LUMPECTOMY WE'LL REMOVE THE SENTINEL NODE AND DO A "FROZEN SECTION" TO SEE IF IT'S POSITIVE OR NEGATIVE.

ARE WE THERE YET?

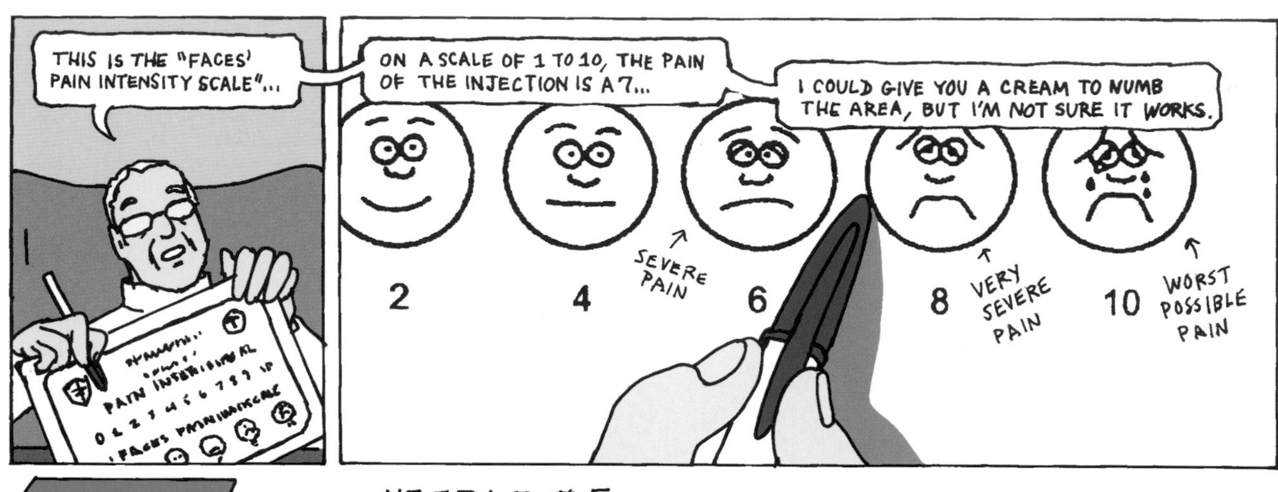
THIS IS THE "FACES' PAIN INTENSITY SCALE"...
ON A SCALE OF 1 TO 10, THE PAIN OF THE INJECTION IS A 7...
I COULD GIVE YOU A CREAM TO NUMB THE AREA, BUT I'M NOT SURE IT WORKS.
2
4
SEVERE PAIN
6
8
VERY SEVERE PAIN
10
WORST POSSIBLE PAIN

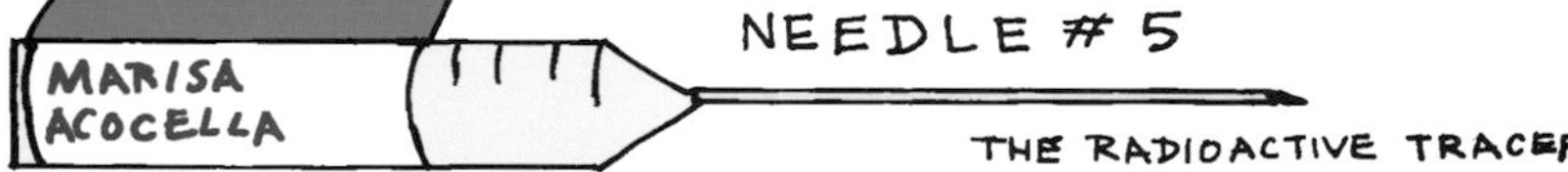
MARISA ACOCELLA
NEEDLE #5
THE RADIOACTIVE TRACER

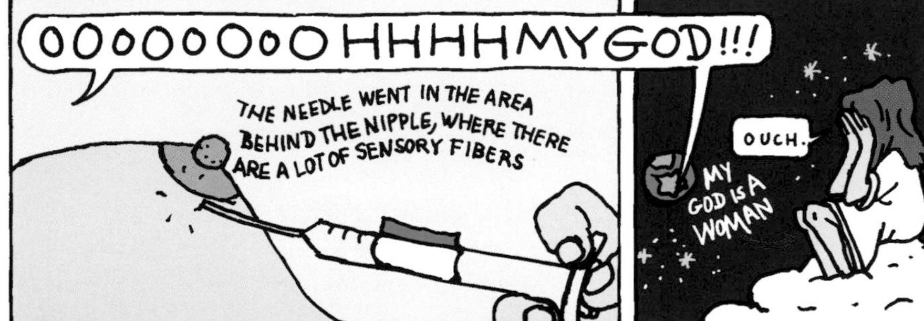
OOOOOOOOHHHHMYGOD!!!
THE NEEDLE WENT IN THE AREA BEHIND THE NIPPLE, WHERE THERE ARE A LOT OF SENSORY FIBERS
OUCH.
MY GOD IS A WOMAN

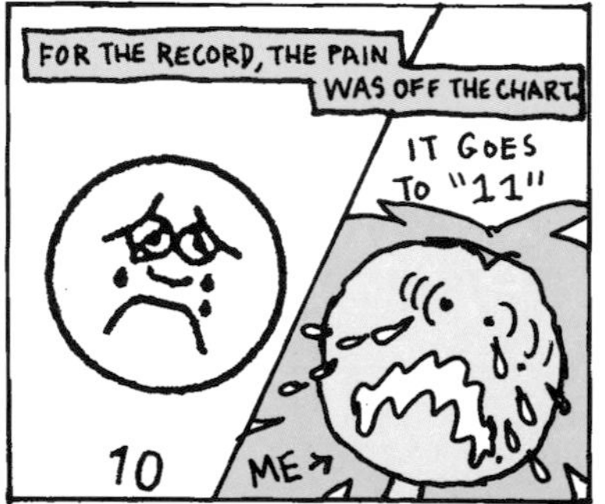
FOR THE RECORD, THE PAIN WAS OFF THE CHART.
IT GOES TO "11"
10
ME

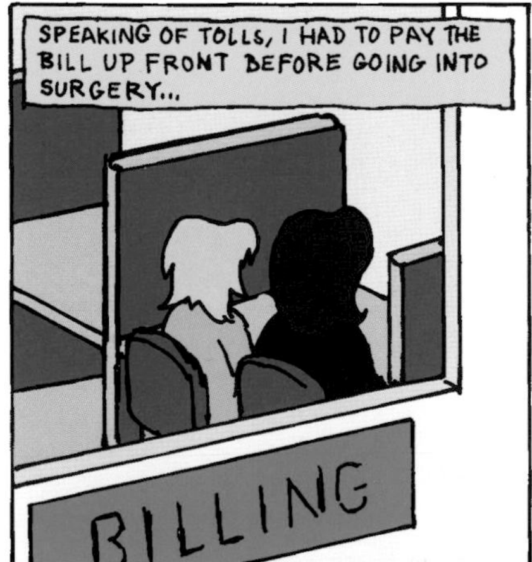
SPEAKING OF TOLLS, I HAD TO PAY THE BILL UP FRONT BEFORE GOING INTO SURGERY...
BILLING

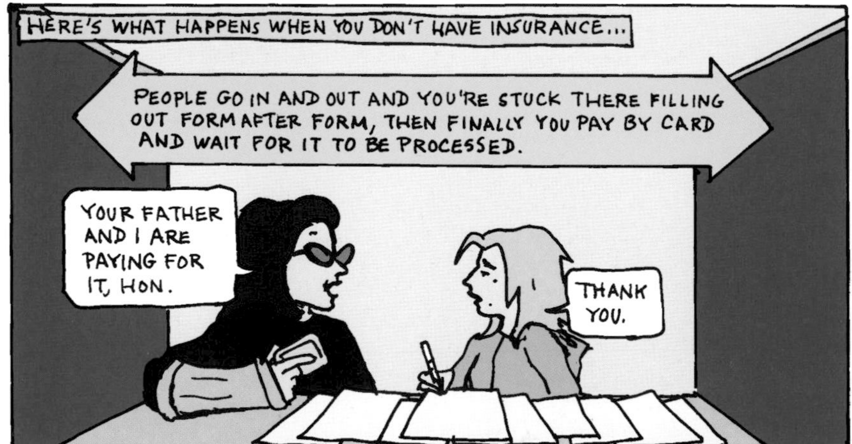
HERE'S WHAT HAPPENS WHEN YOU DON'T HAVE INSURANCE...
PEOPLE GO IN AND OUT AND YOU'RE STUCK THERE FILLING OUT FORM AFTER FORM, THEN FINALLY YOU PAY BY CARD AND WAIT FOR IT TO BE PROCESSED.
YOUR FATHER AND I ARE PAYING FOR IT, HON.
THANK YOU.

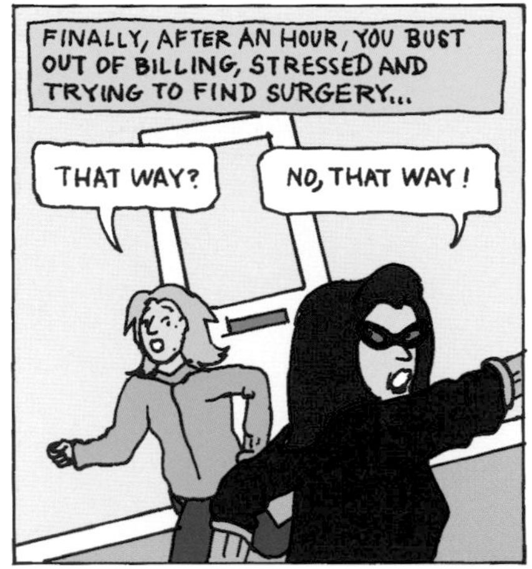
FINALLY, AFTER AN HOUR, YOU BUST OUT OF BILLING, STRESSED AND TRYING TO FIND SURGERY...
THAT WAY?
NO, THAT WAY!

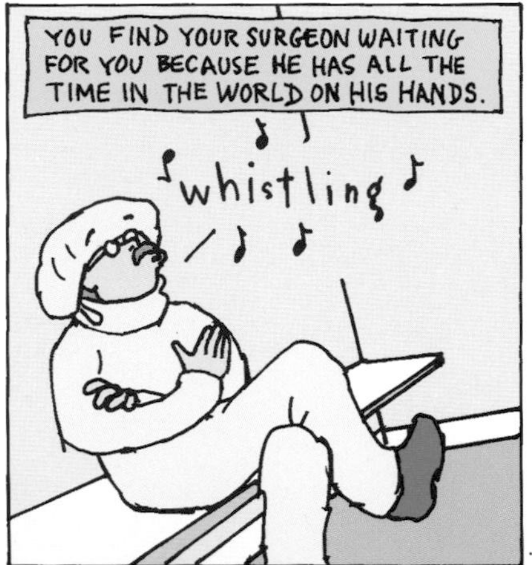
YOU FIND YOUR SURGEON WAITING FOR YOU BECAUSE HE HAS ALL THE TIME IN THE WORLD ON HIS HANDS.
whistling

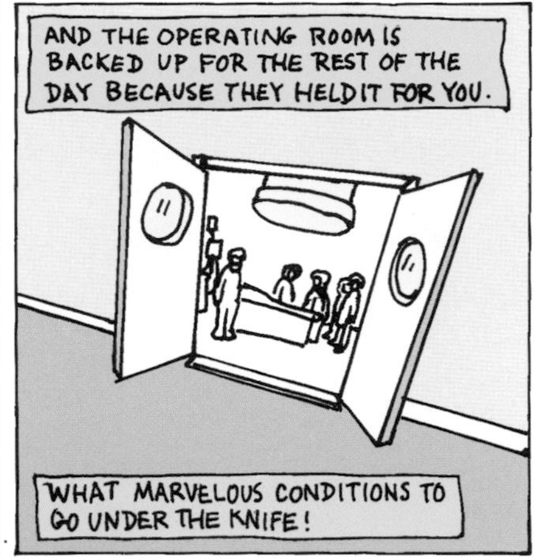
AND THE OPERATING ROOM IS BACKED UP FOR THE REST OF THE DAY BECAUSE THEY HELD IT FOR YOU.
WHAT MARVELOUS CONDITIONS TO GO UNDER THE KNIFE!

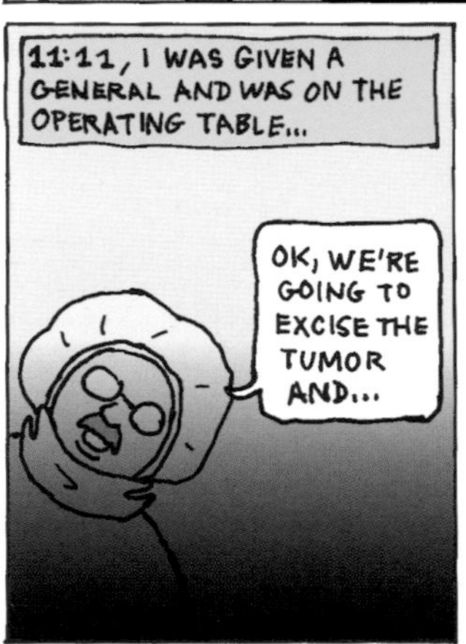
11:11, I WAS GIVEN A GENERAL AND WAS ON THE OPERATING TABLE...
OK, WE'RE GOING TO EXCISE THE TUMOR AND...

...I WAS OUT.

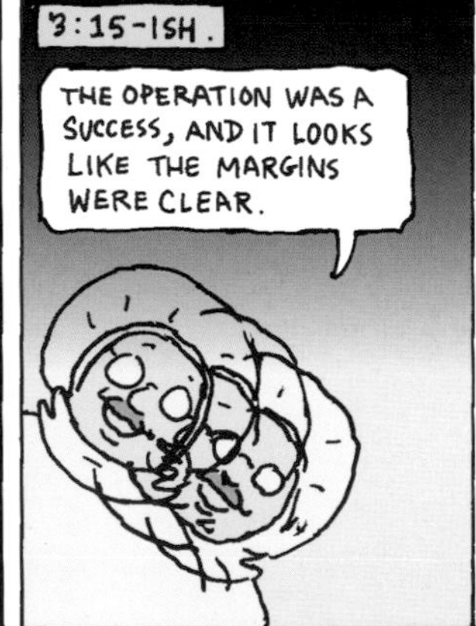
3:15-ISH.
THE OPERATION WAS A SUCCESS, AND IT LOOKS LIKE THE MARGINS WERE CLEAR.

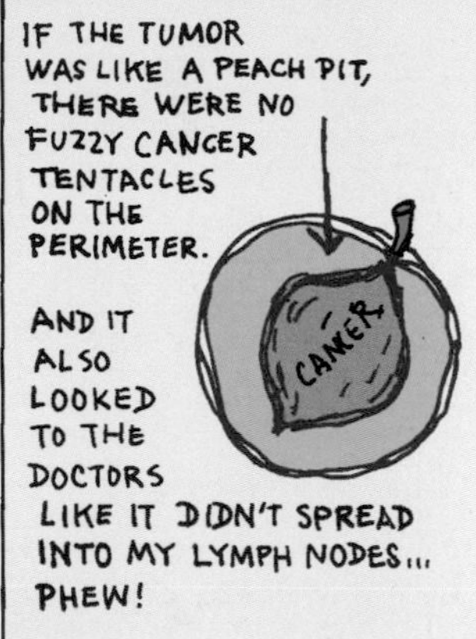
IF THE TUMOR WAS LIKE A PEACH PIT, THERE WERE NO FUZZY CANCER TENTACLES ON THE PERIMETER.
AND IT ALSO LOOKED TO THE DOCTORS LIKE IT DIDN'T SPREAD INTO MY LYMPH NODES... PHEW!
CANCER

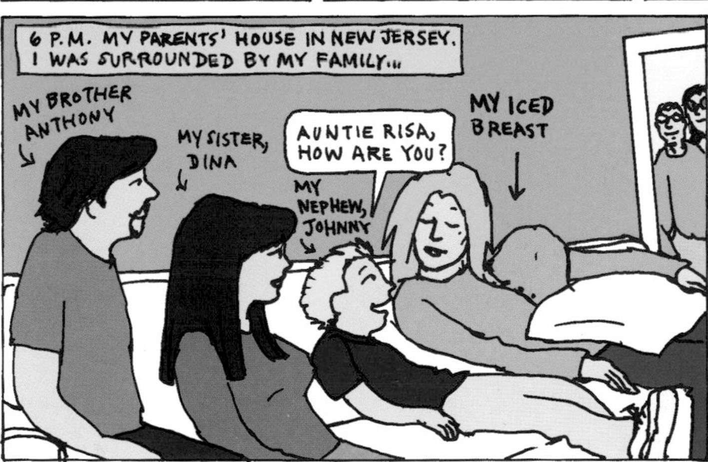
6 P.M. MY PARENTS' HOUSE IN NEW JERSEY. I WAS SURROUNDED BY MY FAMILY...
MY BROTHER ANTHONY
MY SISTER, DINA
MY NEPHEW, JOHNNY
AUNTIE RISA, HOW ARE YOU?
MY ICED BREAST

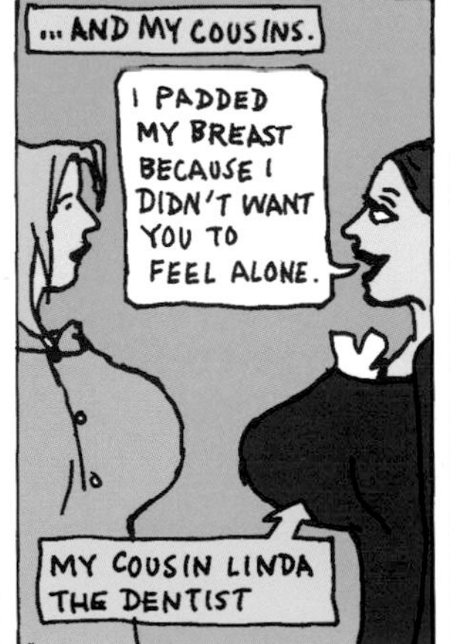
...AND MY COUSINS.
I PADDED MY BREAST BECAUSE I DIDN'T WANT YOU TO FEEL ALONE.
MY COUSIN LINDA THE DENTIST

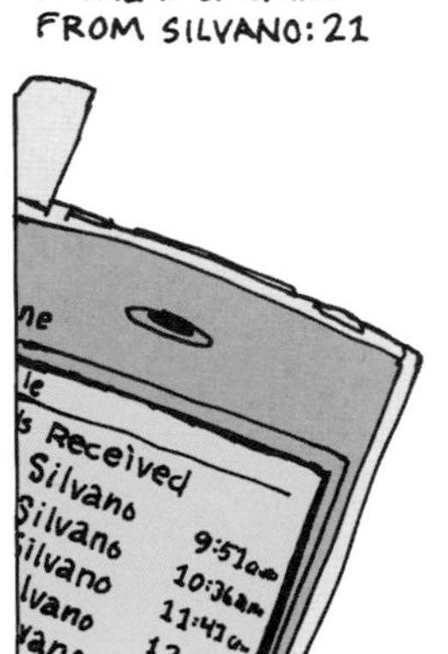
TOTAL # OF CALLS: 27
TOTAL # OF CALLS FROM SILVANO: 21
Received
Silvano
Silvano

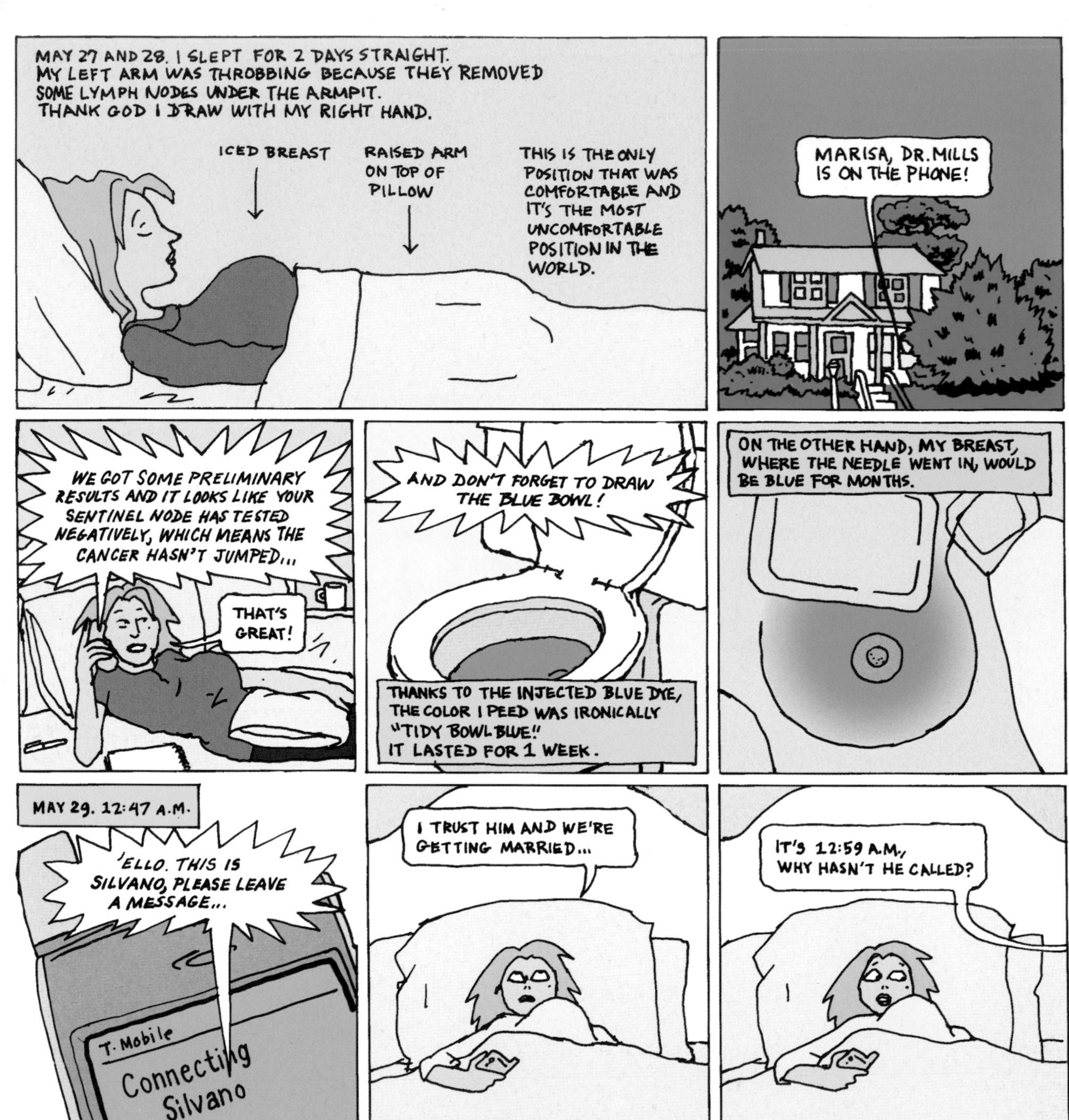
MAY 27 AND 28. I SLEPT FOR 2 DAYS STRAIGHT.
MY LEFT ARM WAS THROBBING BECAUSE THEY REMOVED
SOME LYMPH NODES UNDER THE ARMPIT.
THANK GOD I DRAW WITH MY RIGHT HAND.
ICED BREAST
RAISED ARM ON TOP OF PILLOW
THIS IS THE ONLY POSITION THAT WAS COMFORTABLE AND IT'S THE MOST UNCOMFORTABLE POSITION IN THE WORLD.
MARISA, DR. MILLS IS ON THE PHONE!
WE GOT SOME PRELIMINARY RESULTS AND IT LOOKS LIKE YOUR SENTINEL NODE HAS TESTED NEGATIVELY, WHICH MEANS THE CANCER HASN'T JUMPED...
THAT'S GREAT!
AND DON'T FORGET TO DRAW THE BLUE BOWL!
THANKS TO THE INJECTED BLUE DYE, THE COLOR I PEED WAS IRONICALLY "TIDY BOWL BLUE!" IT LASTED FOR 1 WEEK.
ON THE OTHER HAND, MY BREAST, WHERE THE NEEDLE WENT IN, WOULD BE BLUE FOR MONTHS.
MAY 29. 12:47 A.M.
'ELLO. THIS IS SILVANO, PLEASE LEAVE A MESSAGE...
T. Mobile
Connecting Silvano
I TRUST HIM AND WE'RE GETTING MARRIED...
IT'S 12:59 A.M., WHY HASN'T HE CALLED?

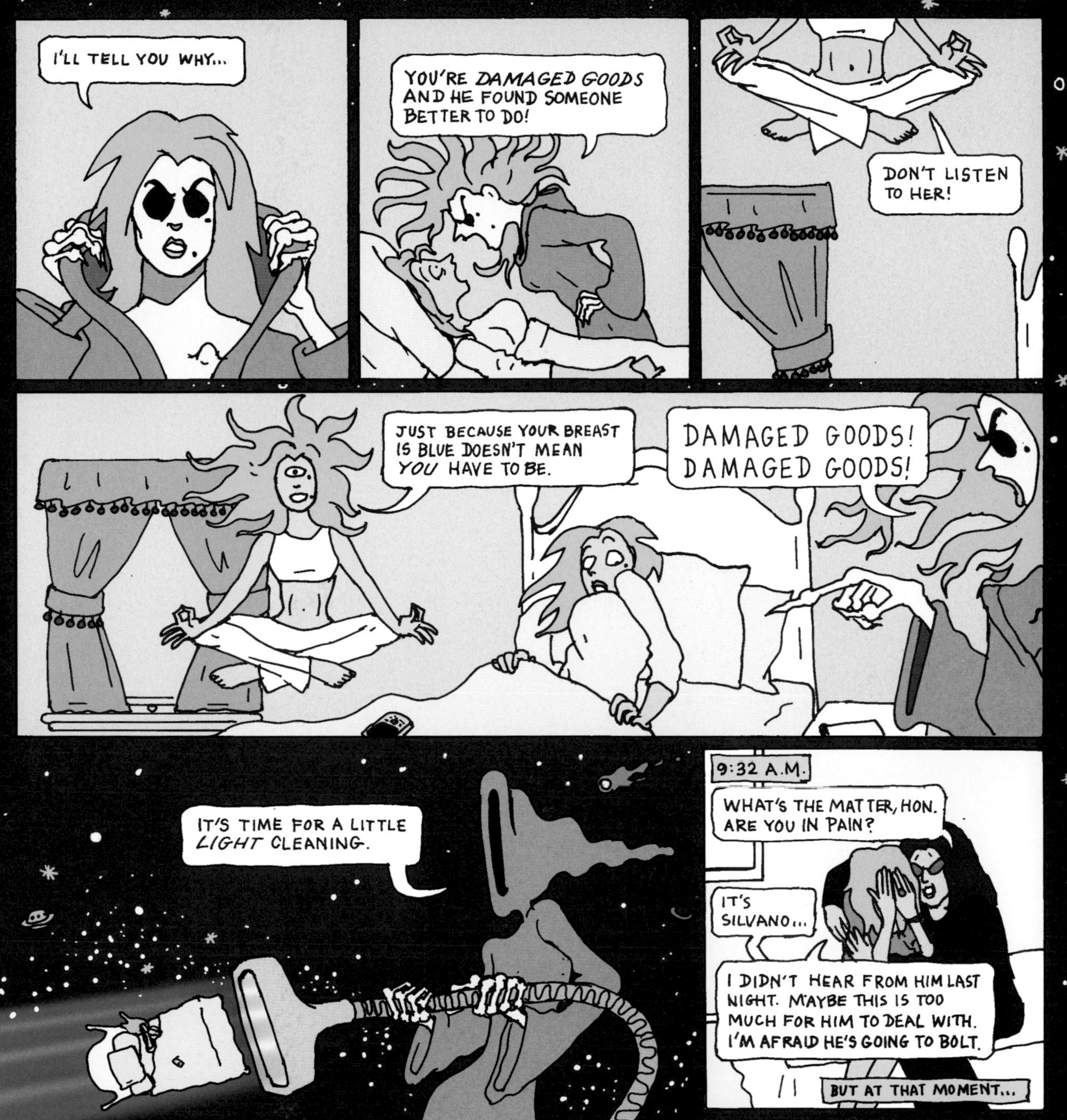
I'LL TELL YOU WHY...
YOU'RE DAMAGED GOODS AND HE FOUND SOMEONE BETTER TO DO!
DON'T LISTEN TO HER!
JUST BECAUSE YOUR BREAST IS BLUE DOESN'T MEAN YOU HAVE TO BE.
DAMAGED GOODS! DAMAGED GOODS!
IT'S TIME FOR A LITTLE LIGHT CLEANING.
9:32 A.M.
WHAT'S THE MATTER, HON. ARE YOU IN PAIN?
IT'S SILVANO...
I DIDN'T HEAR FROM HIM LAST NIGHT. MAYBE THIS IS TOO MUCH FOR HIM TO DEAL WITH. I'M AFRAID HE'S GOING TO BOLT.
BUT AT THAT MOMENT...

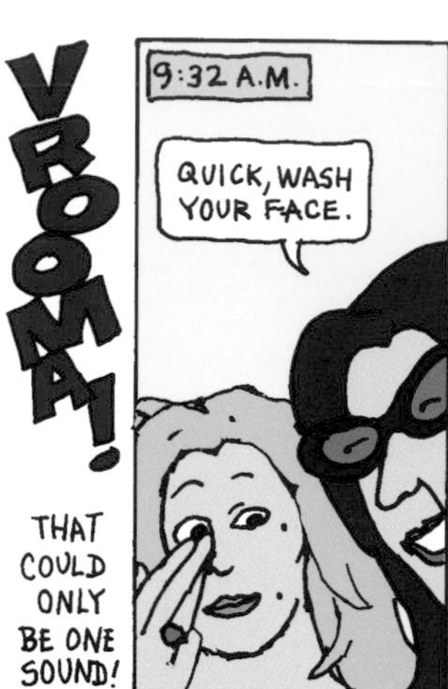
VROOMA!
THAT COULD ONLY BE ONE SOUND!
9:32 A.M.
QUICK, WASH YOUR FACE.

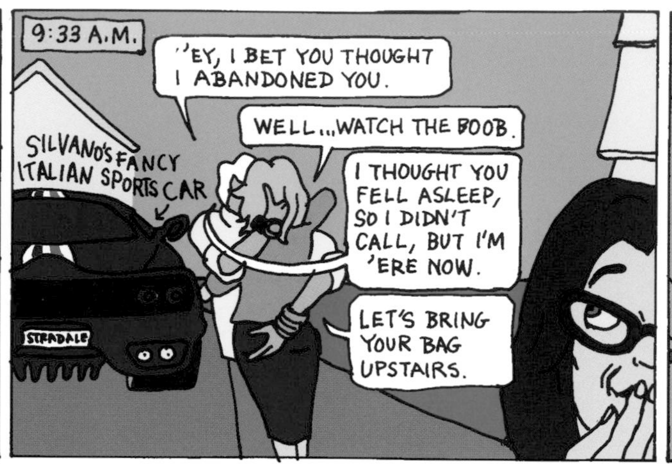
9:33 A.M.
''EY, I BET YOU THOUGHT I ABANDONED YOU.
WELL... WATCH THE BOOB.
SILVANO'S FANCY ITALIAN SPORTS CAR
STRADALE
I THOUGHT YOU FELL ASLEEP, SO I DIDN'T CALL, BUT I'M 'ERE NOW.
LET'S BRING YOUR BAG UPSTAIRS.

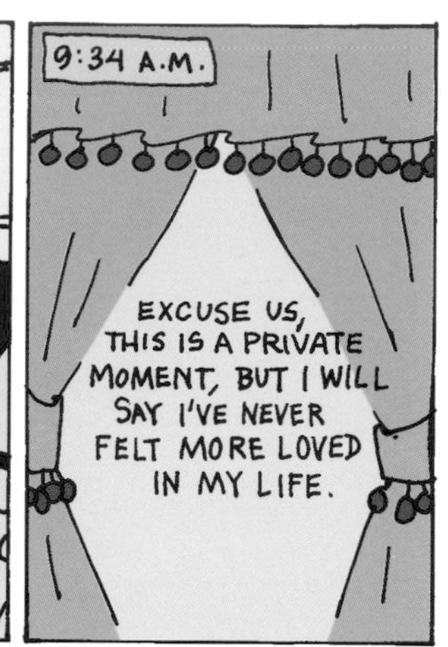
9:34 A.M.
EXCUSE US, THIS IS A PRIVATE MOMENT, BUT I WILL SAY I'VE NEVER FELT MORE LOVED IN MY LIFE.

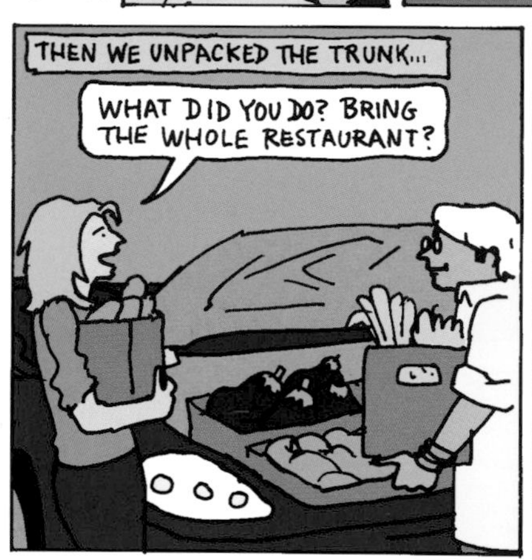
THEN WE UNPACKED THE TRUNK...
WHAT DID YOU DO? BRING THE WHOLE RESTAURANT?

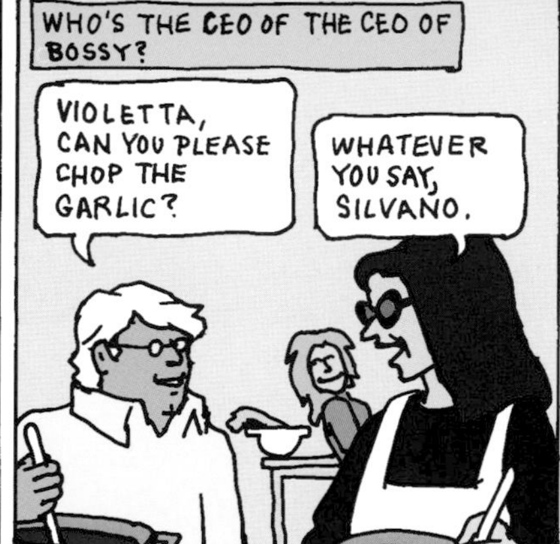
WHO'S THE CEO OF THE CEO OF BOSSY?
VIOLETTA, CAN YOU PLEASE CHOP THE GARLIC?
WHATEVER YOU SAY, SILVANO.

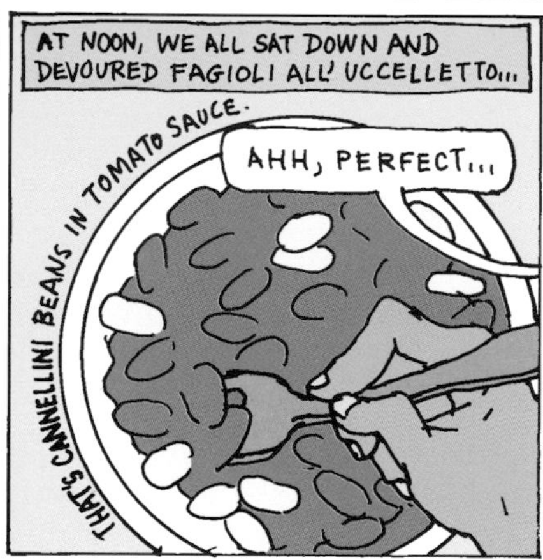
AT NOON, WE ALL SAT DOWN AND DEVOURED FAGIOLI ALL' UCCELLETTO...
THAT'S CANNELLINI BEANS IN TOMATO SAUCE.
AHH, PERFECT...

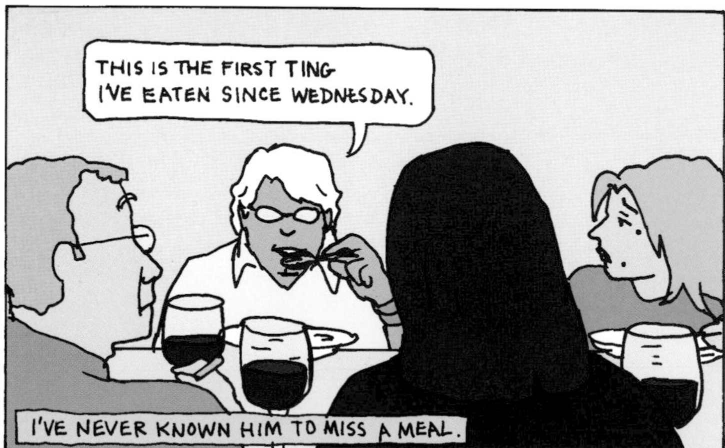
THIS IS THE FIRST TING I'VE EATEN SINCE WEDNESDAY.
I'VE NEVER KNOWN HIM TO MISS A MEAL.

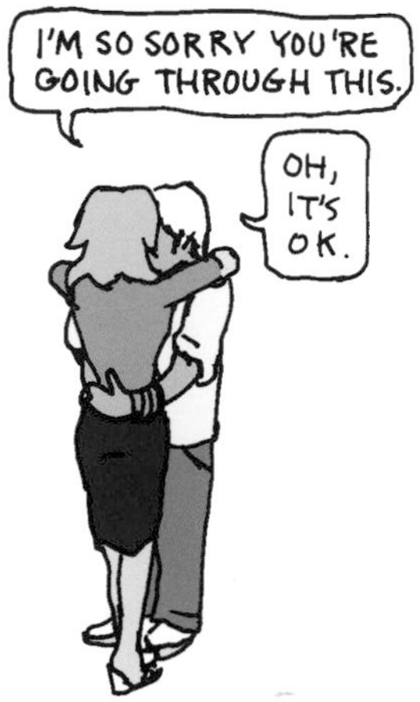
I'M SO SORRY YOU'RE GOING THROUGH THIS.
OH, IT'S OK.

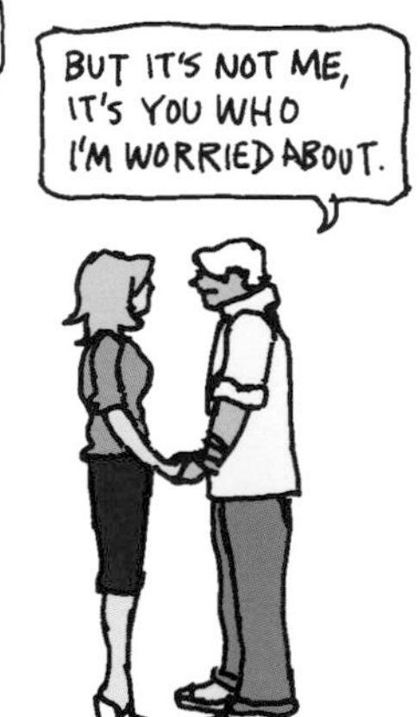
BUT IT'S NOT ME, IT'S YOU WHO I'M WORRIED ABOUT.

JUNE 3. (8 DAYS FROM OUR WEDDING!)
I HAD MY FIRST POST-OP VISIT WITH DR. MILLS,
WHERE WE DISCUSSED MY NEXT STEPS...

SAINT VINCENT CATHOLIC MEDICAL CENTERS
ST. VINCENT'S MANHATTAN LABORATORIES
DEPARTMENT OF PATHOLOGY
...EST 11 STREET, NY, NY 10011
212-604-8393 FAX: 212-604-3263

Chris Mills
5/30/04

Patient: **ACOCELLA, MARISA**
Med Rec: **V1191439**

Location: CANCER CENTER
Physician: CHRISTOPHER MILLS, MD

Case: **VVS-04-7184**
Reg #: V000440830719
Procedure Date: 05/26/2004
Date Received: 05/26/2004
Date Reported: 05/29/2004

SURGICAL PATHOLOGY REPORT

SPECIMEN: A: BREAST, WITH MARGINS, left, lumpectomy. **B:** LYMPH NODE, SENTINEL, left axillary, #1 hot and blue. **C:** LYMPH NODE, SENTINEL, left axillary adjacent node.

FINAL DIAGNOSIS:

PERFORMED AT SAINT VINCENTS COMPREHENSIVE CANCER CENTER
325 WEST 15TH STREET, NEW YORK, NY 10011

A- LEFT BREAST LUMPECTOMY:

- **INFILTRATING MODERATELY DIFFERENTIATED DUCTAL ADENOCARCINOMA, NOS, 1.3X1.1 CM,** WITH PROMINENT DESMOPLASTIC REACTION
- THE INVASIVE CARCINOMA SHOWS HIGH HISTOLOGIC GRADE (3/3), INTERMEDIATE NUCLEAR GRADE (2/3), AND INTERMEDIATE MITOTIC COUNT (2/3). SBR SCORE: 7/9, GRADE II
- **RARE FOCI OF DUCTAL CARCINOMA IN SITU (DCIS)**, SOLID TYPE, NON-COMEDO WITH CENTRAL NECROSIS, INTERMEDIATE NUCLEAR GRADE (2/3) INVOLVING ISOLATED DUCTS WITHIN THE INVASIVE TUMOR
- **ONE FOCUS** ...

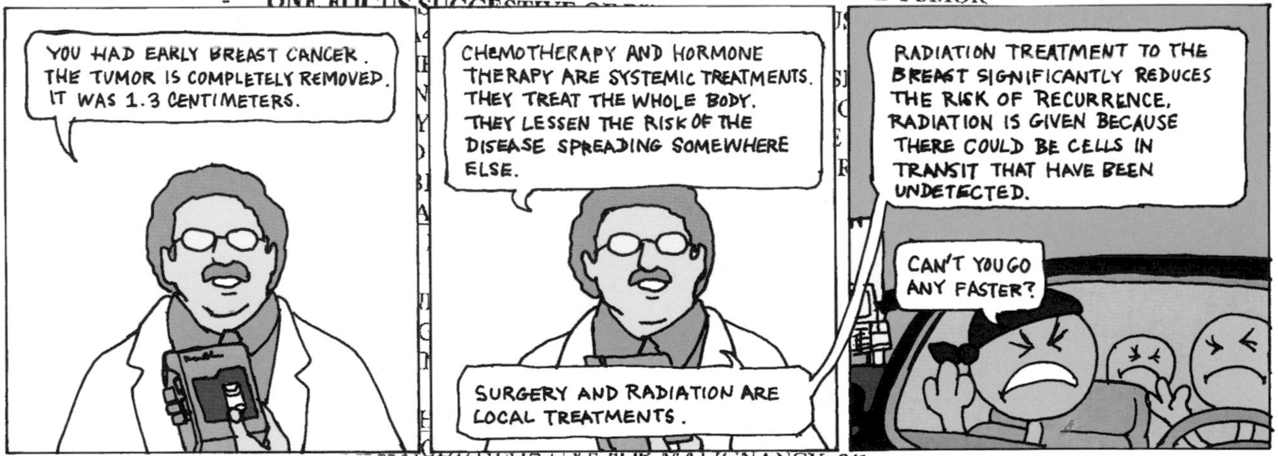

YOU HAD EARLY BREAST CANCER. THE TUMOR IS COMPLETELY REMOVED. IT WAS 1.3 CENTIMETERS.

CHEMOTHERAPY AND HORMONE THERAPY ARE SYSTEMIC TREATMENTS. THEY TREAT THE WHOLE BODY. THEY LESSEN THE RISK OF THE DISEASE SPREADING SOMEWHERE ELSE.

SURGERY AND RADIATION ARE LOCAL TREATMENTS.

RADIATION TREATMENT TO THE BREAST SIGNIFICANTLY REDUCES THE RISK OF RECURRENCE. RADIATION IS GIVEN BECAUSE THERE COULD BE CELLS IN TRANSIT THAT HAVE BEEN UNDETECTED.

CAN'T YOU GO ANY FASTER?

... NODE NEGATIVE FOR MALIGNANCY, **0/1**
- CYTOKERATIN STAIN AE-1/AE-3 IS NEGATIVE FOR MALIGNANT CELLS

C- LEFT AXILLA ADJACENT ...

When can I get the bandages off?

Can I use my arm?

What kind of exercises should I be doing?

What kind of exercise should I not be doing?

What stage of cancer did I have?

How would you define it?

Did the cancer jump anywhere else in my body?

Is there a chance that some cells are wandering in my body that haven't been detected?

What are my next steps?

Why do I need chemo?

WHEN A TUMOR IS OVER 1 CENTIMETER, WE GENERALLY RECOMMEND CHEMOTHERAPY.
WILL I LOSE MY HAIR?

SO, I HAD TO DO THE CHEMO THING.
ALL THOSE COMPLAINTS ABOUT BAD HAIR DAYS...
...I JUST SHOULD HAVE BEEN THANKFUL I HAD IT.

HEY, YOU UP THERE... HOW COULD YOU MAKE ME A BALD, UNHEALTHY BAGGAGE-RIDDEN BRIDE?!
MAYBE YOU AND I SHOULD TAKE A BREAK.

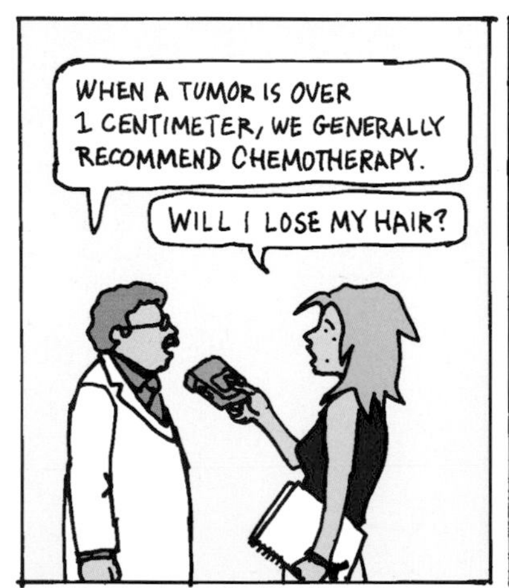

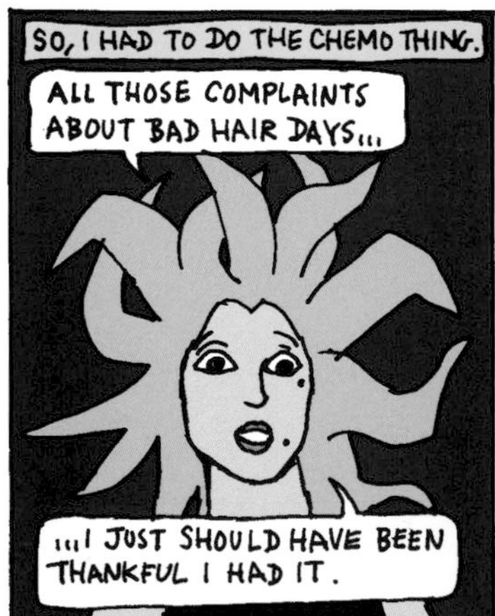

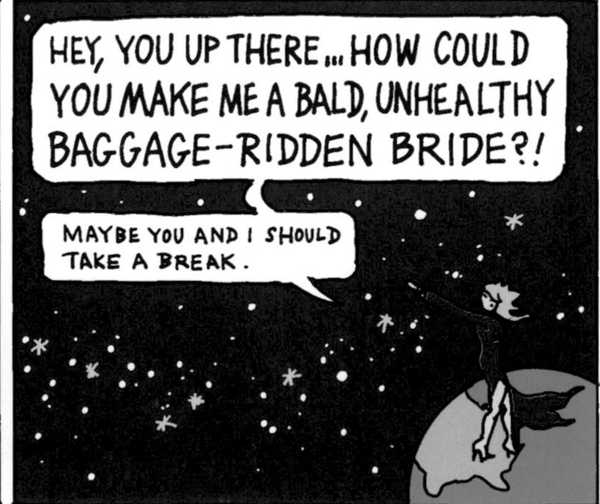

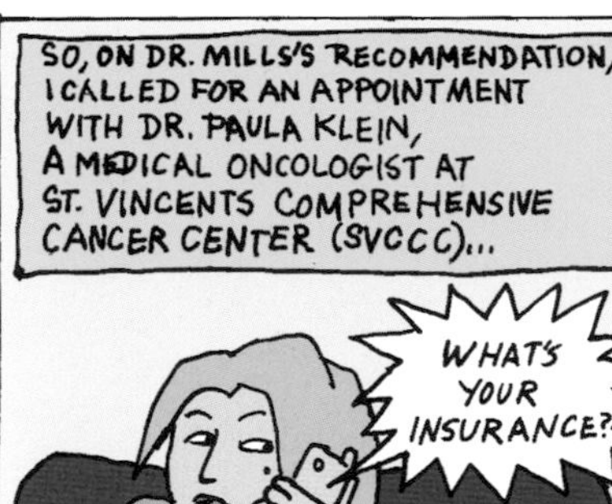
SO, ON DR. MILLS'S RECOMMENDATION, I CALLED FOR AN APPOINTMENT WITH DR. PAULA KLEIN, A MEDICAL ONCOLOGIST AT ST. VINCENTS COMPREHENSIVE CANCER CENTER (SVCCC)...
WHAT'S YOUR INSURANCE?
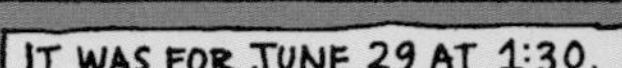
IT WAS FOR JUNE 29 AT 1:30.
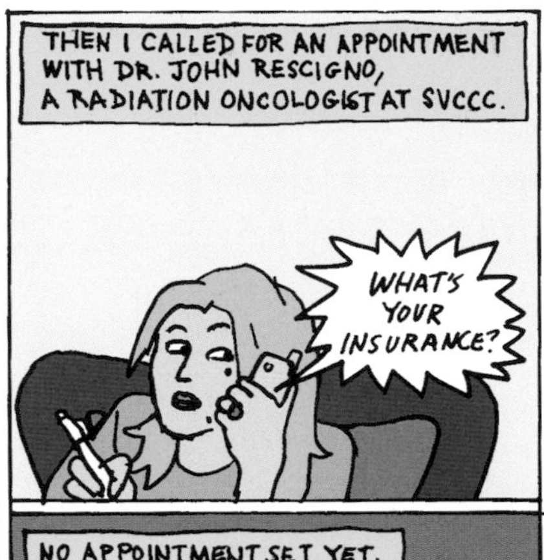
THEN I CALLED FOR AN APPOINTMENT WITH DR. JOHN RESCIGNO, A RADIATION ONCOLOGIST AT SVCCC.
WHAT'S YOUR INSURANCE?
NO APPOINTMENT SET YET.
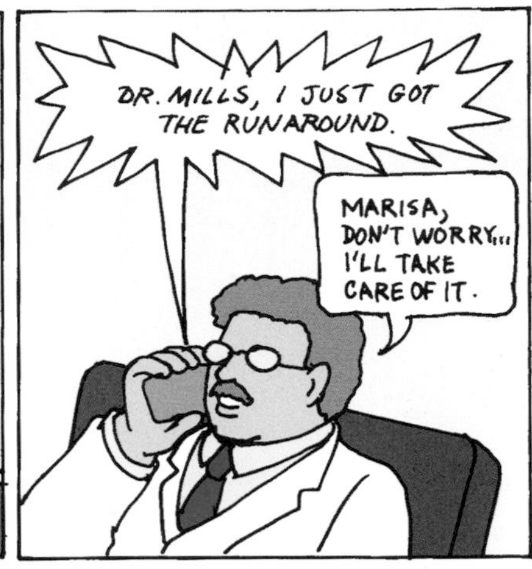
DR. MILLS, I JUST GOT THE RUNAROUND.
MARISA, DON'T WORRY... I'LL TAKE CARE OF IT.
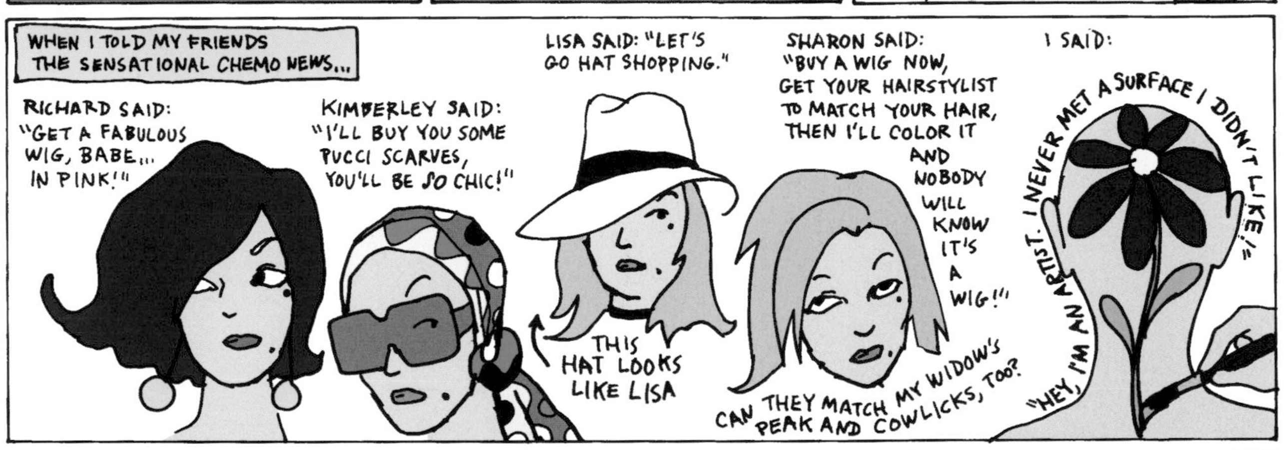
WHEN I TOLD MY FRIENDS THE SENSATIONAL CHEMO NEWS...
RICHARD SAID: "GET A FABULOUS WIG, BABE... IN PINK!"
KIMBERLEY SAID: "I'LL BUY YOU SOME PUCCI SCARVES, YOU'LL BE SO CHIC!"
LISA SAID: "LET'S GO HAT SHOPPING."
THIS HAT LOOKS LIKE LISA
SHARON SAID: "BUY A WIG NOW, GET YOUR HAIRSTYLIST TO MATCH YOUR HAIR, THEN I'LL COLOR IT AND NOBODY WILL KNOW IT'S A WIG!"
CAN THEY MATCH MY WIDOW'S PEAK AND COWLICKS, TOO?
I SAID:
"HEY, I'M AN ARTIST. I NEVER MET A SURFACE I DIDN'T LIKE!"
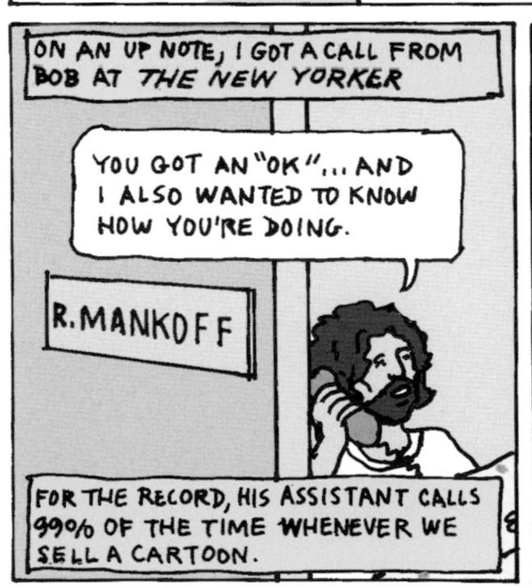
ON AN UP NOTE, I GOT A CALL FROM BOB AT *THE NEW YORKER*
YOU GOT AN "OK"... AND I ALSO WANTED TO KNOW HOW YOU'RE DOING.
R. MANKOFF
FOR THE RECORD, HIS ASSISTANT CALLS 99% OF THE TIME WHENEVER WE SELL A CARTOON.
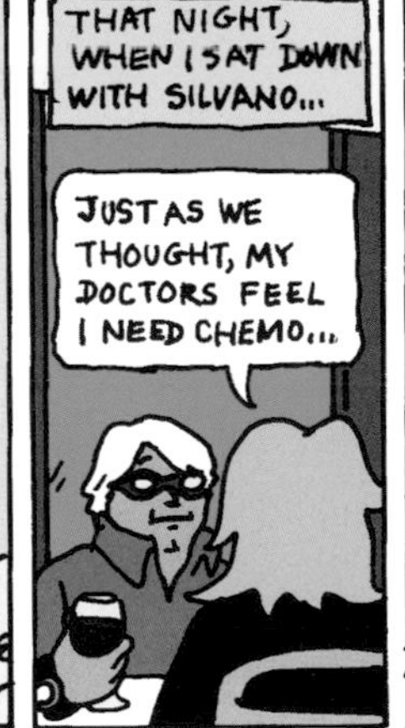
THAT NIGHT, WHEN I SAT DOWN WITH SILVANO...
JUST AS WE THOUGHT, MY DOCTORS FEEL I NEED CHEMO...
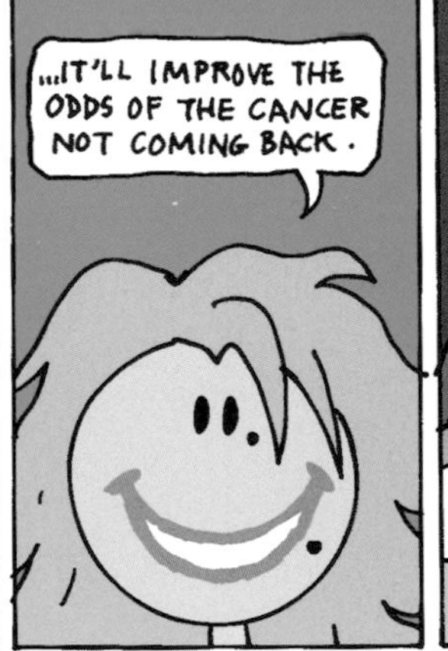
...IT'LL IMPROVE THE ODDS OF THE CANCER NOT COMING BACK.
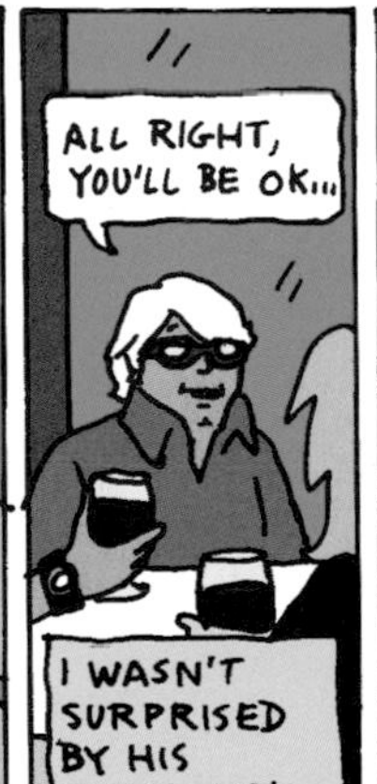
ALL RIGHT, YOU'LL BE OK...
I WASN'T SURPRISED BY HIS REACTION...
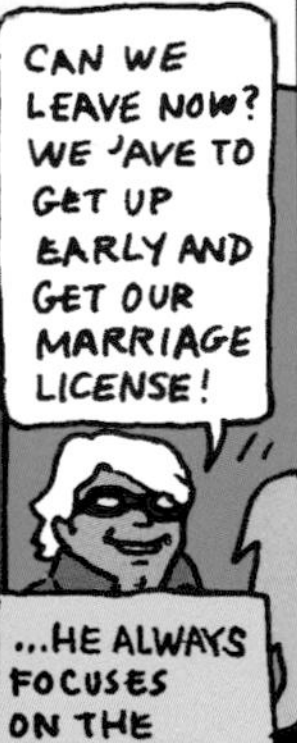
CAN WE LEAVE NOW? WE 'AVE TO GET UP EARLY AND GET OUR MARRIAGE LICENSE!
...HE ALWAYS FOCUSES ON THE POSITIVE.

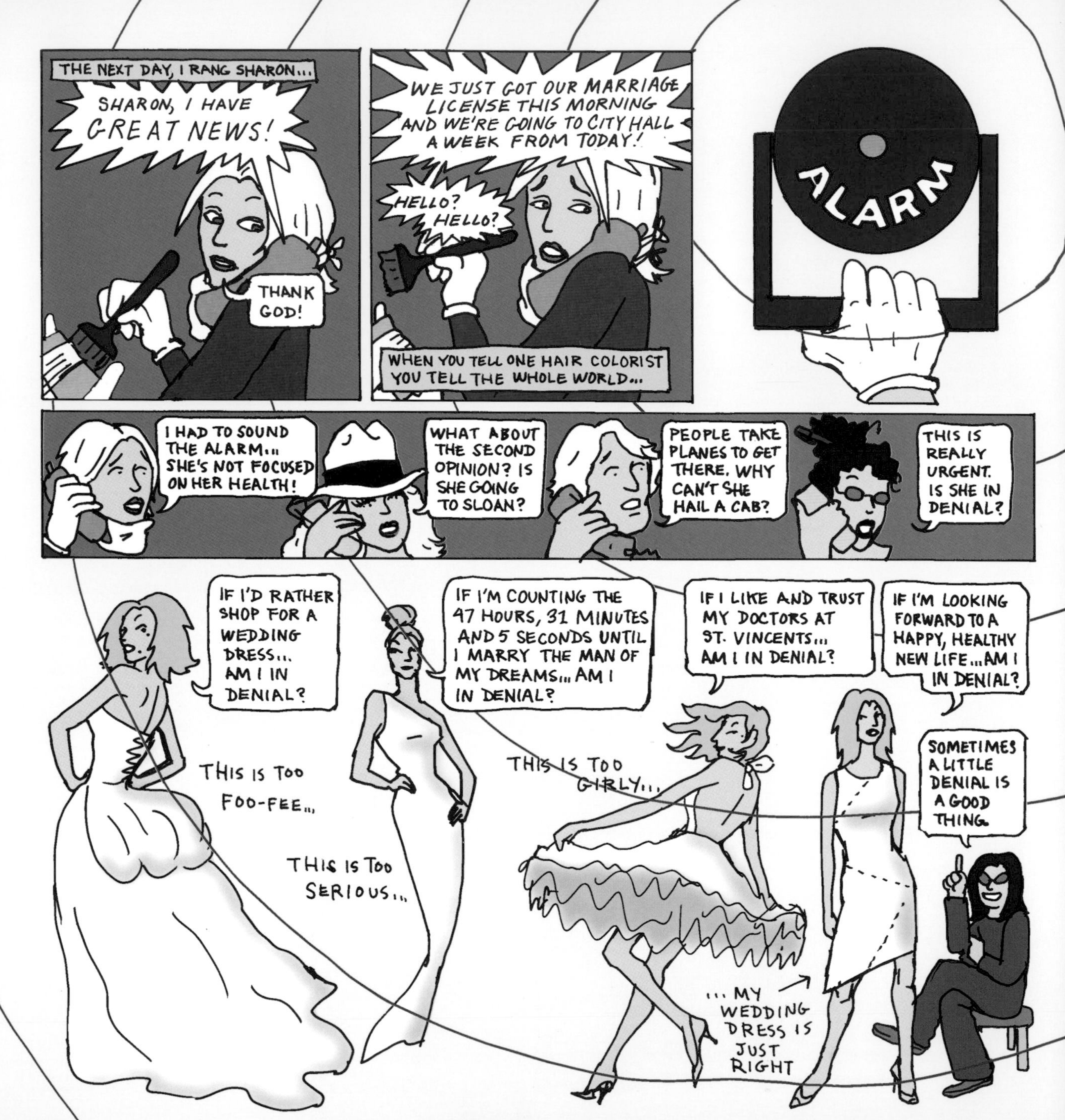
THE NEXT DAY, I RANG SHARON...
SHARON, I HAVE GREAT NEWS!
THANK GOD!
WE JUST GOT OUR MARRIAGE LICENSE THIS MORNING AND WE'RE GOING TO CITY HALL A WEEK FROM TODAY!
HELLO? HELLO?
WHEN YOU TELL ONE HAIR COLORIST YOU TELL THE WHOLE WORLD...
ALARM
I HAD TO SOUND THE ALARM... SHE'S NOT FOCUSED ON HER HEALTH!
WHAT ABOUT THE SECOND OPINION? IS SHE GOING TO SLOAN?
PEOPLE TAKE PLANES TO GET THERE. WHY CAN'T SHE HAIL A CAB?
THIS IS REALLY URGENT. IS SHE IN DENIAL?
IF I'D RATHER SHOP FOR A WEDDING DRESS... AM I IN DENIAL?
IF I'M COUNTING THE 47 HOURS, 31 MINUTES AND 5 SECONDS UNTIL I MARRY THE MAN OF MY DREAMS... AM I IN DENIAL?
IF I LIKE AND TRUST MY DOCTORS AT ST. VINCENTS... AM I IN DENIAL?
IF I'M LOOKING FORWARD TO A HAPPY, HEALTHY NEW LIFE... AM I IN DENIAL?
THIS IS TOO FOO-FEE...
THIS IS TOO SERIOUS...
THIS IS TOO GIRLY...
...MY WEDDING DRESS IS JUST RIGHT
SOMETIMES A LITTLE DENIAL IS A GOOD THING.

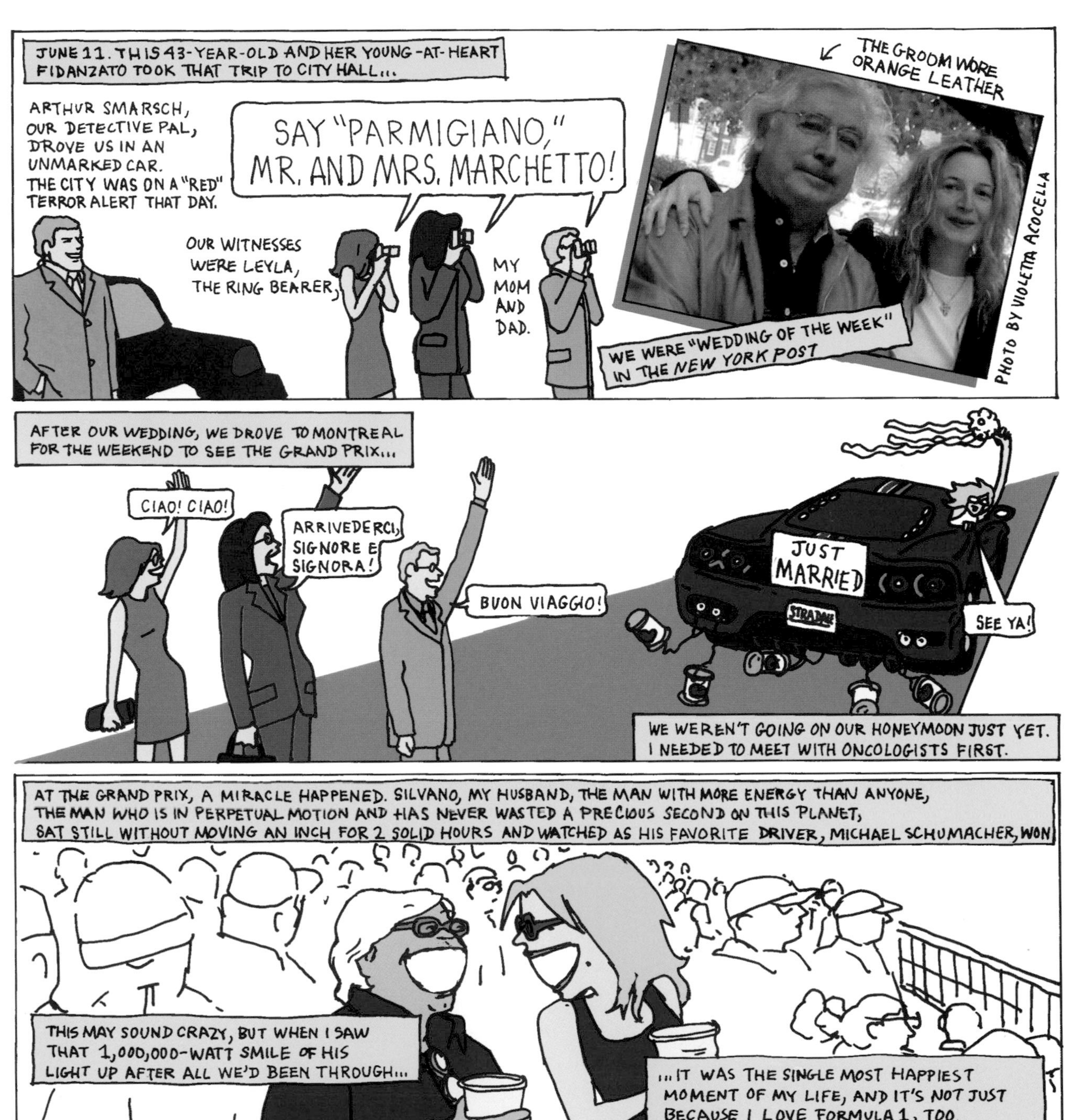
JUNE 11. THIS 43-YEAR-OLD AND HER YOUNG-AT-HEART FIDANZATO TOOK THAT TRIP TO CITY HALL...
ARTHUR SMARSCH, OUR DETECTIVE PAL, DROVE US IN AN UNMARKED CAR. THE CITY WAS ON A "RED" TERROR ALERT THAT DAY.
SAY "PARMIGIANO," MR. AND MRS. MARCHETTO!
OUR WITNESSES WERE LEYLA, THE RING BEARER,
MY MOM AND DAD.
THE GROOM WORE ORANGE LEATHER
WE WERE "WEDDING OF THE WEEK" IN THE NEW YORK POST
PHOTO BY VIOLETTA ACOCELLA
AFTER OUR WEDDING, WE DROVE TO MONTREAL FOR THE WEEKEND TO SEE THE GRAND PRIX...
CIAO! CIAO!
ARRIVEDERCI, SIGNORE E SIGNORA!
BUON VIAGGIO!
JUST MARRIED
STRADALE
SEE YA!
WE WEREN'T GOING ON OUR HONEYMOON JUST YET. I NEEDED TO MEET WITH ONCOLOGISTS FIRST.
AT THE GRAND PRIX, A MIRACLE HAPPENED. SILVANO, MY HUSBAND, THE MAN WITH MORE ENERGY THAN ANYONE, THE MAN WHO IS IN PERPETUAL MOTION AND HAS NEVER WASTED A PRECIOUS SECOND ON THIS PLANET, SAT STILL WITHOUT MOVING AN INCH FOR 2 SOLID HOURS AND WATCHED AS HIS FAVORITE DRIVER, MICHAEL SCHUMACHER, WON
THIS MAY SOUND CRAZY, BUT WHEN I SAW THAT 1,000,000-WATT SMILE OF HIS LIGHT UP AFTER ALL WE'D BEEN THROUGH...
...IT WAS THE SINGLE MOST HAPPIEST MOMENT OF MY LIFE, AND IT'S NOT JUST BECAUSE I LOVE FORMULA 1, TOO.

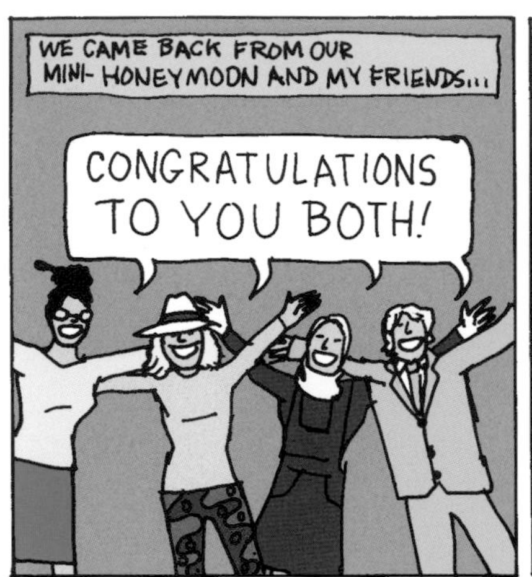
WE CAME BACK FROM OUR MINI-HONEYMOON AND MY FRIENDS...
CONGRATULATIONS TO YOU BOTH!

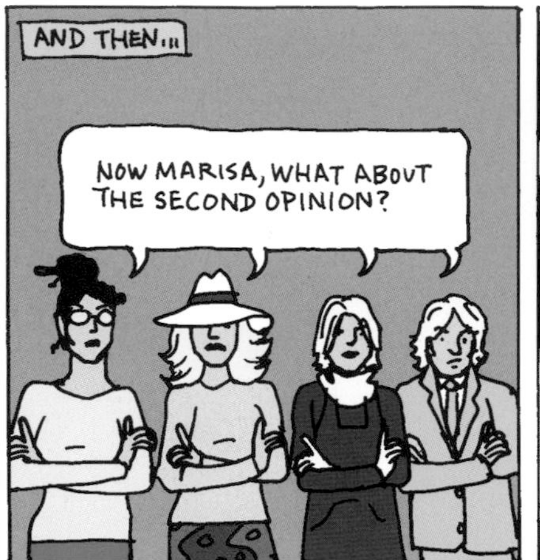
AND THEN...
NOW MARISA, WHAT ABOUT THE SECOND OPINION?

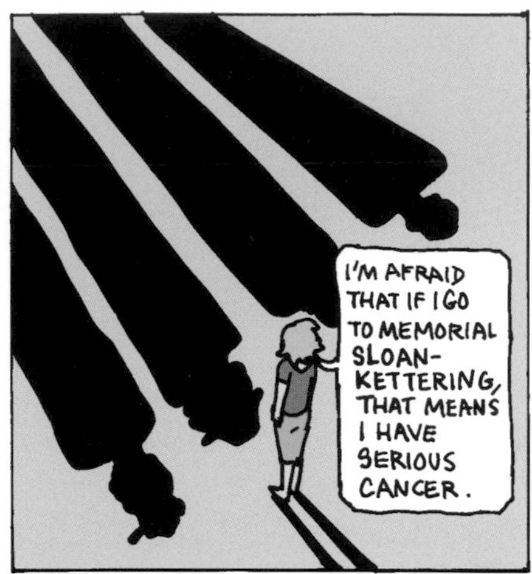
I'M AFRAID THAT IF I GO TO MEMORIAL SLOAN-KETTERING, THAT MEANS I HAVE SERIOUS CANCER.

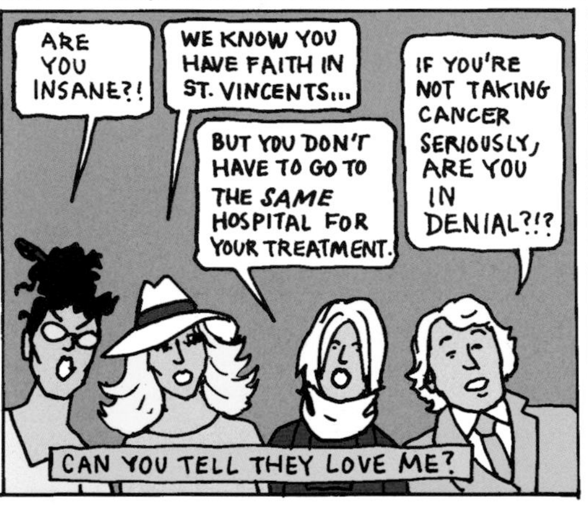
ARE YOU INSANE?!
WE KNOW YOU HAVE FAITH IN ST. VINCENTS...
BUT YOU DON'T HAVE TO GO TO THE SAME HOSPITAL FOR YOUR TREATMENT.
IF YOU'RE NOT TAKING CANCER SERIOUSLY, ARE YOU IN DENIAL?!?
CAN YOU TELL THEY LOVE ME?

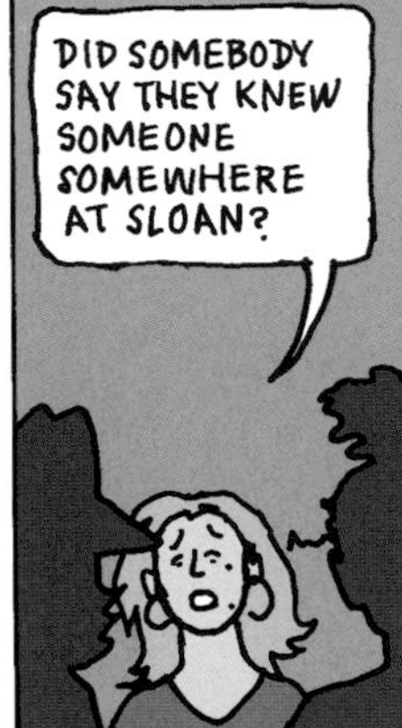
DID SOMEBODY SAY THEY KNEW SOMEONE SOMEWHERE AT SLOAN?

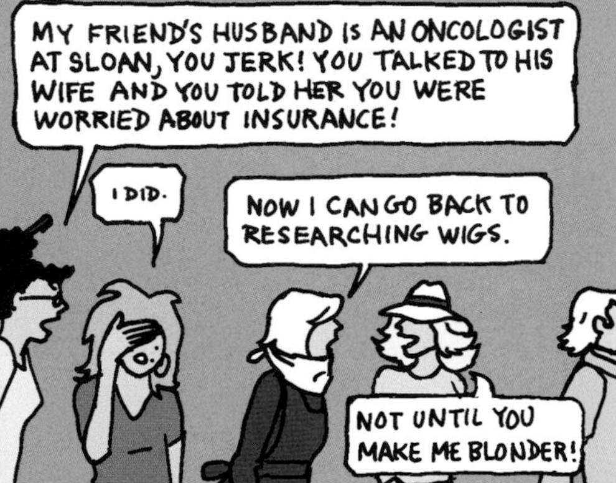
MY FRIEND'S HUSBAND IS AN ONCOLOGIST AT SLOAN, YOU JERK! YOU TALKED TO HIS WIFE AND YOU TOLD HER YOU WERE WORRIED ABOUT INSURANCE!
I DID.
NOW I CAN GO BACK TO RESEARCHING WIGS.
NOT UNTIL YOU MAKE ME BLONDER!

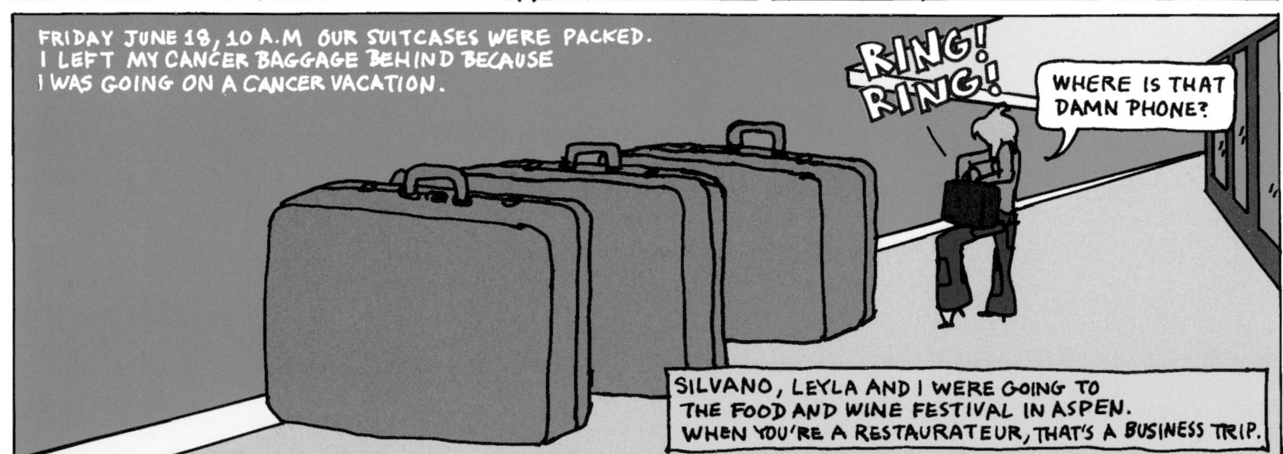
FRIDAY JUNE 18, 10 A.M OUR SUITCASES WERE PACKED. I LEFT MY CANCER BAGGAGE BEHIND BECAUSE I WAS GOING ON A CANCER VACATION.
RING! RING!
WHERE IS THAT DAMN PHONE?
SILVANO, LEYLA AND I WERE GOING TO THE FOOD AND WINE FESTIVAL IN ASPEN. WHEN YOU'RE A RESTAURATEUR, THAT'S A BUSINESS TRIP.

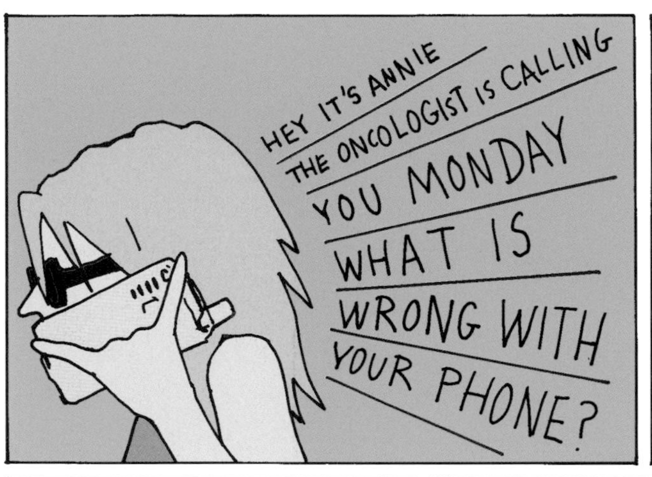
HEY IT'S ANNIE
THE ONCOLOGIST IS CALLING
YOU MONDAY
WHAT IS
WRONG WITH
YOUR PHONE?

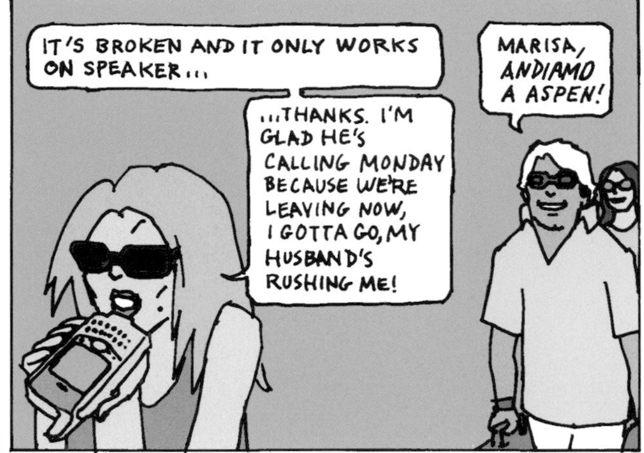
IT'S BROKEN AND IT ONLY WORKS ON SPEAKER...
...THANKS. I'M GLAD HE'S CALLING MONDAY BECAUSE WE'RE LEAVING NOW, I GOTTA GO, MY HUSBAND'S RUSHING ME!
MARISA, ANDIAMO A ASPEN!

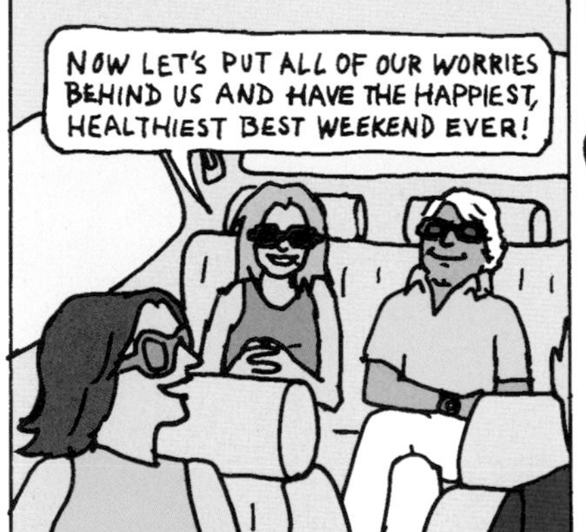
NOW LET'S PUT ALL OF OUR WORRIES BEHIND US AND HAVE THE HAPPIEST, HEALTHIEST BEST WEEKEND EVER!

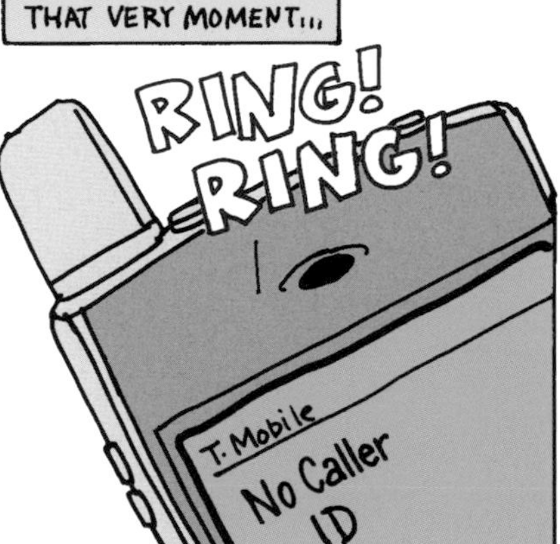
THAT VERY MOMENT...
RING! RING!
T. Mobile
No Caller ID

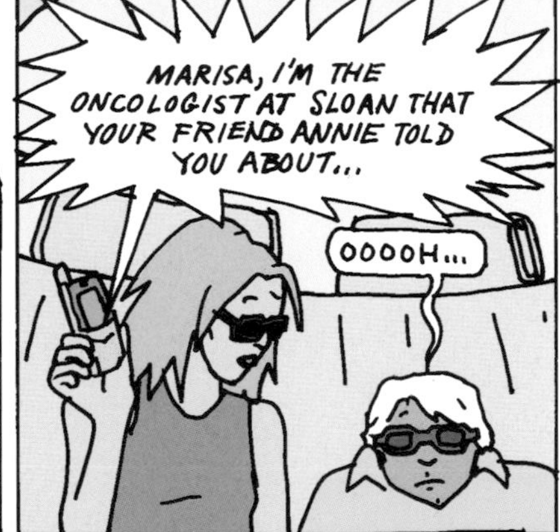
MARISA, I'M THE ONCOLOGIST AT SLOAN THAT YOUR FRIEND ANNIE TOLD YOU ABOUT...
OOOOH...

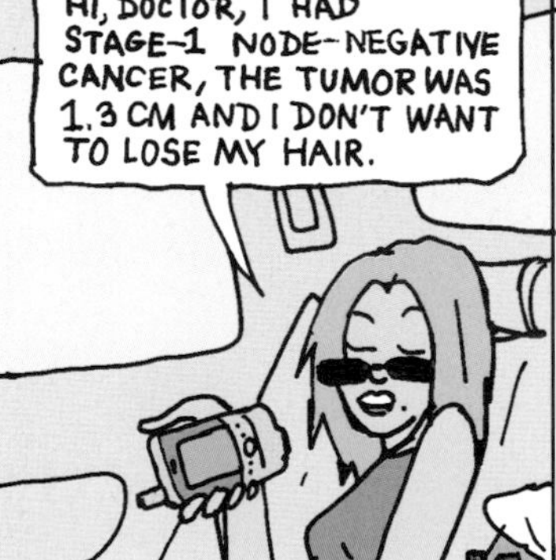
HI, DOCTOR, I HAD STAGE-1 NODE-NEGATIVE CANCER, THE TUMOR WAS 1.3 CM AND I DON'T WANT TO LOSE MY HAIR.

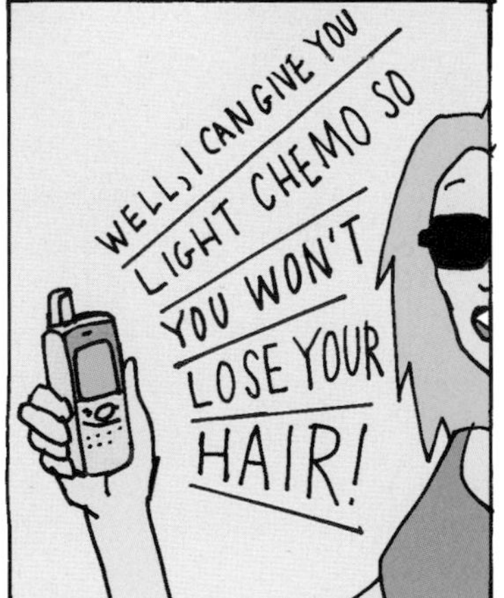
WELL, I CAN GIVE YOU
LIGHT CHEMO SO
YOU WON'T
LOSE YOUR
HAIR!

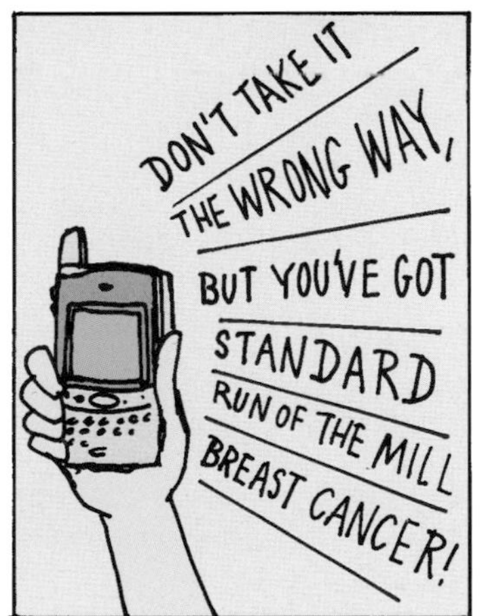
DON'T TAKE IT
THE WRONG WAY,
BUT YOU'VE GOT
STANDARD
RUN OF THE MILL
BREAST CANCER!

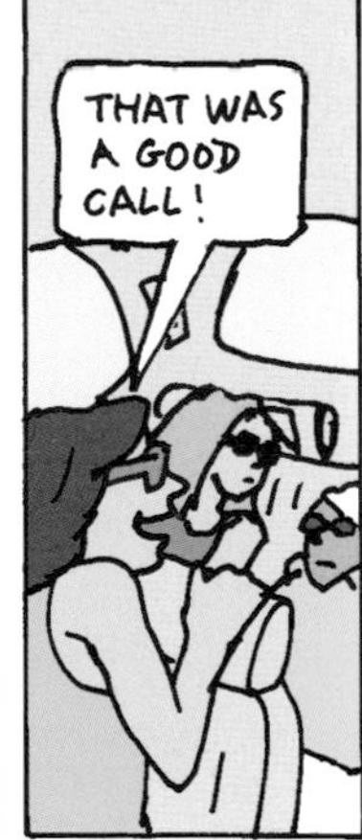
THAT WAS A GOOD CALL!

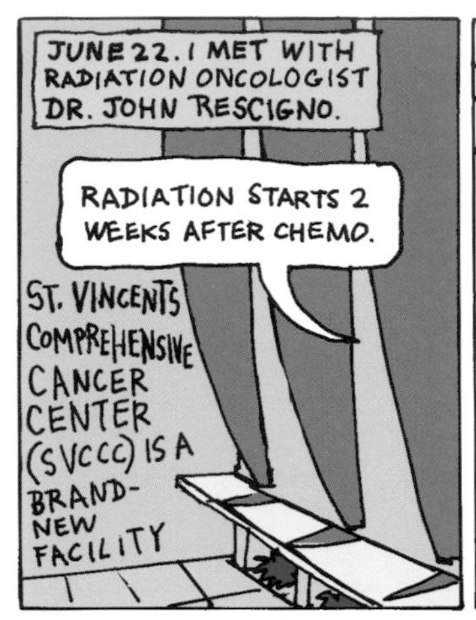
JUNE 22. I MET WITH RADIATION ONCOLOGIST DR. JOHN RESCIGNO.
RADIATION STARTS 2 WEEKS AFTER CHEMO.
ST. VINCENT'S COMPREHENSIVE CANCER CENTER (SVCCC) IS A BRAND-NEW FACILITY

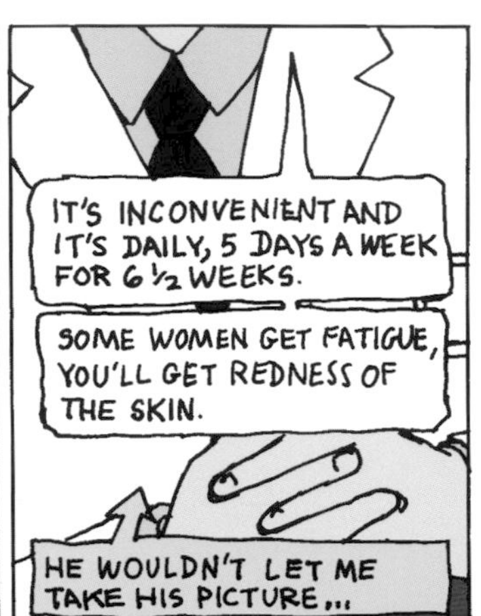
IT'S INCONVENIENT AND IT'S DAILY, 5 DAYS A WEEK FOR 6 ½ WEEKS.
SOME WOMEN GET FATIGUE, YOU'LL GET REDNESS OF THE SKIN.
HE WOULDN'T LET ME TAKE HIS PICTURE...

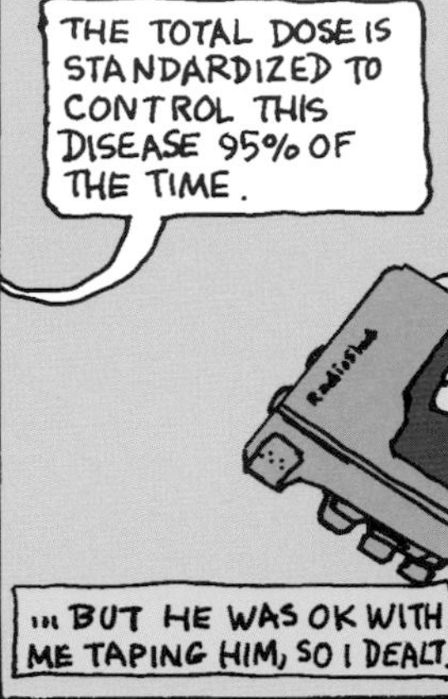
THE TOTAL DOSE IS STANDARDIZED TO CONTROL THIS DISEASE 95% OF THE TIME.
...BUT HE WAS OK WITH ME TAPING HIM, SO I DEALT.

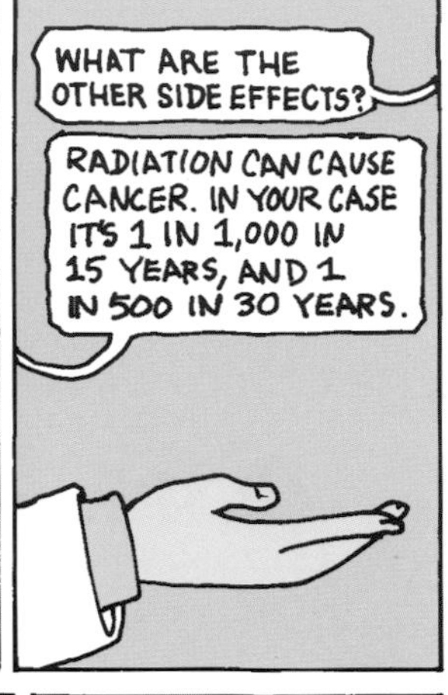
WHAT ARE THE OTHER SIDE EFFECTS?
RADIATION CAN CAUSE CANCER. IN YOUR CASE IT'S 1 IN 1,000 IN 15 YEARS, AND 1 IN 500 IN 30 YEARS.

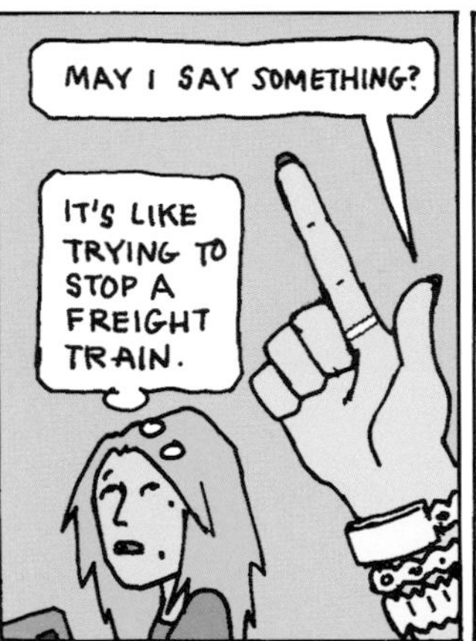
MAY I SAY SOMETHING?
IT'S LIKE TRYING TO STOP A FREIGHT TRAIN.

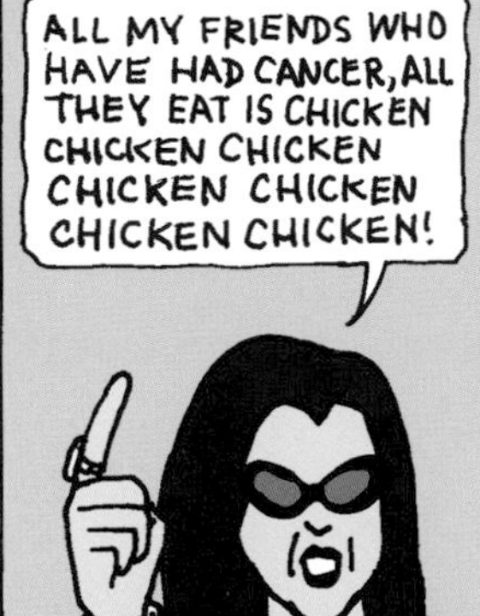
ALL MY FRIENDS WHO HAVE HAD CANCER, ALL THEY EAT IS CHICKEN CHICKEN CHICKEN CHICKEN CHICKEN CHICKEN CHICKEN!

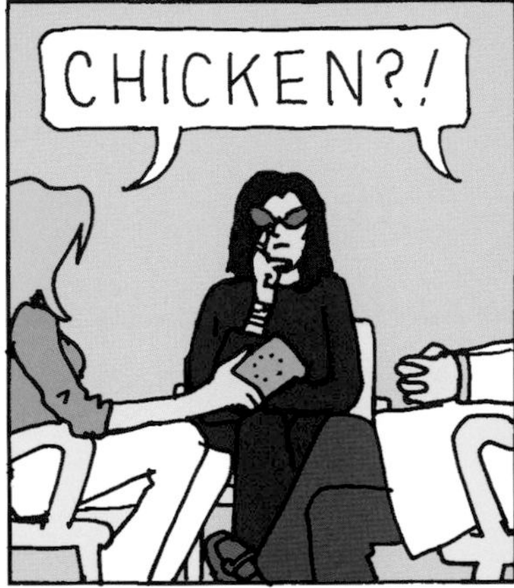
CHICKEN?!

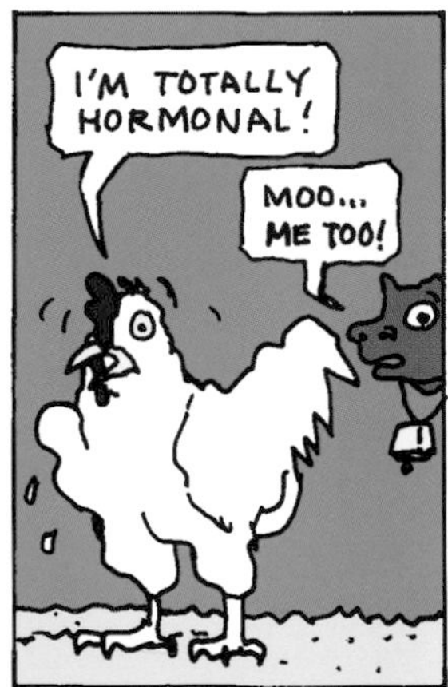
I'M TOTALLY HORMONAL!
MOO... ME TOO!

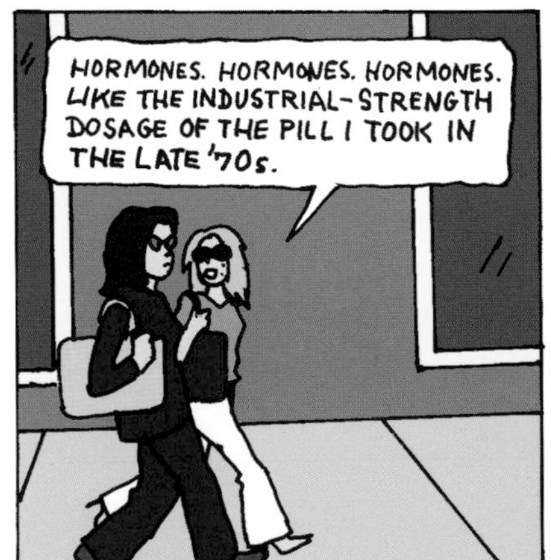
HORMONES. HORMONES. HORMONES. LIKE THE INDUSTRIAL-STRENGTH DOSAGE OF THE PILL I TOOK IN THE LATE '70s.

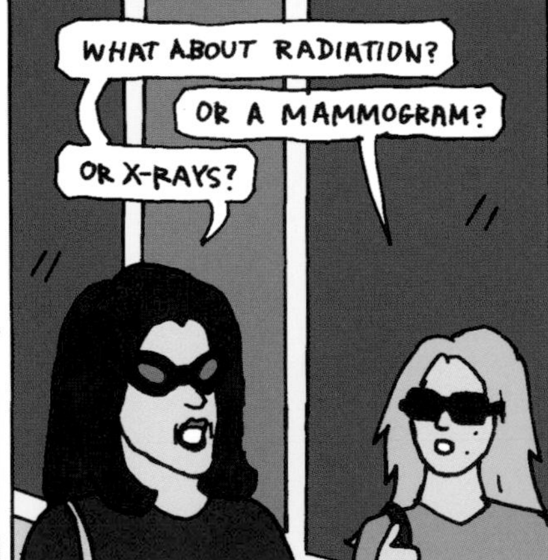
WHAT ABOUT RADIATION?
OR A MAMMOGRAM?
OR X-RAYS?

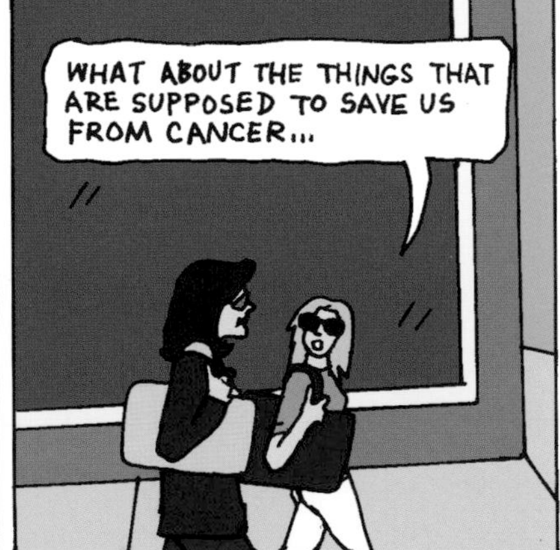
WHAT ABOUT THE THINGS THAT ARE SUPPOSED TO SAVE US FROM CANCER...

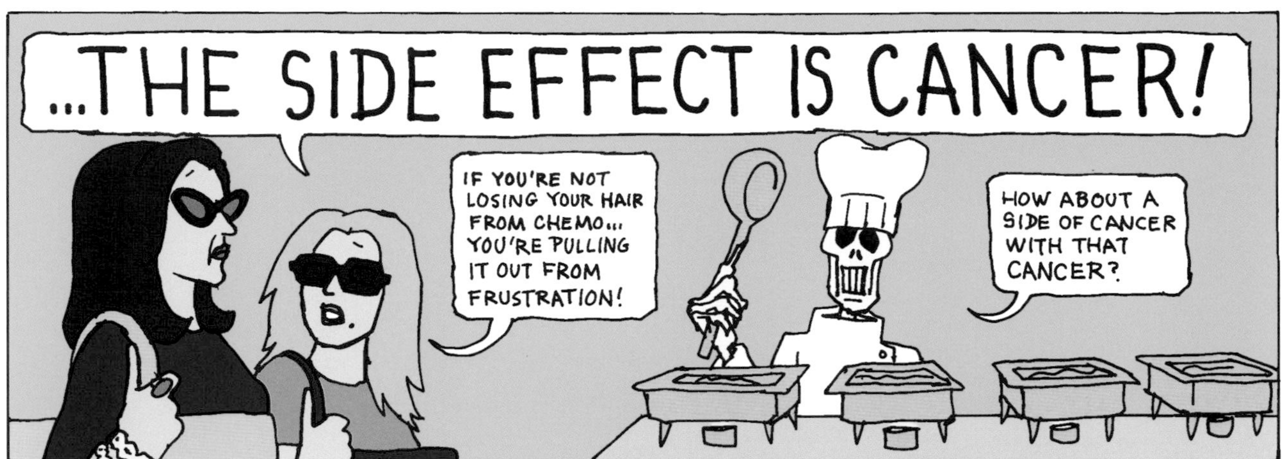
...THE SIDE EFFECT IS CANCER!
IF YOU'RE NOT LOSING YOUR HAIR FROM CHEMO... YOU'RE PULLING IT OUT FROM FRUSTRATION!
HOW ABOUT A SIDE OF CANCER WITH THAT CANCER?

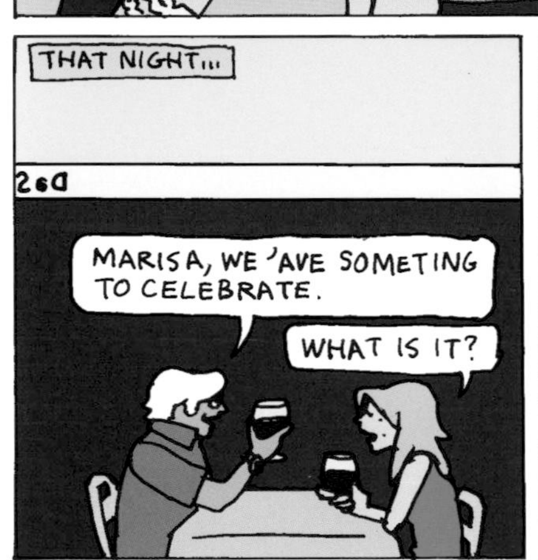
THAT NIGHT...
MARISA, WE 'AVE SOMETING TO CELEBRATE.
WHAT IS IT?

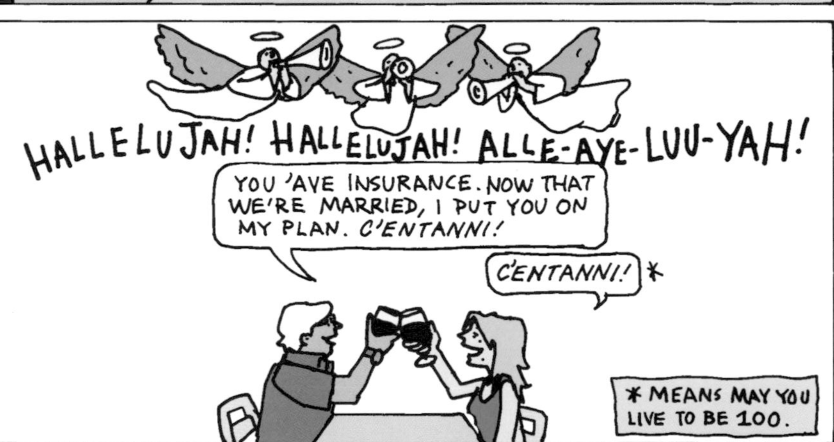
HALLELUJAH! HALLELUJAH! ALLE-AYE-LUU-YAH!
YOU 'AVE INSURANCE. NOW THAT WE'RE MARRIED, I PUT YOU ON MY PLAN. C'ENTANNI!
C'ENTANNI! *
* MEANS MAY YOU LIVE TO BE 100.

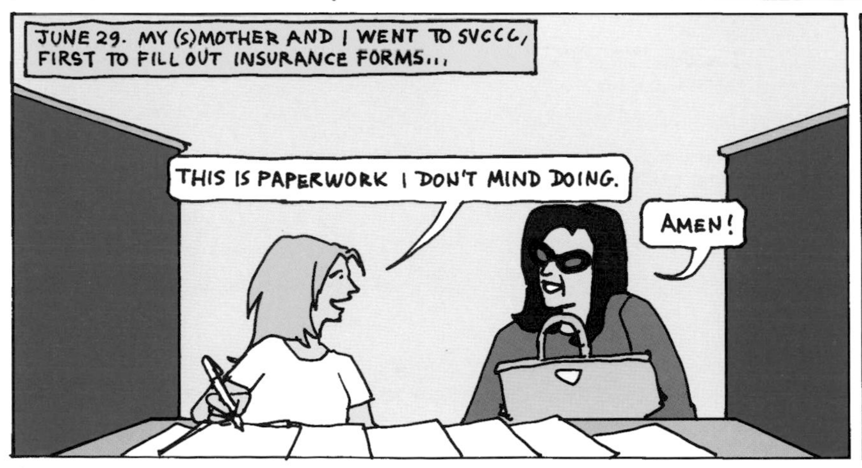
JUNE 29. MY (S)MOTHER AND I WENT TO SVCCC, FIRST TO FILL OUT INSURANCE FORMS...
THIS IS PAPERWORK I DON'T MIND DOING.
AMEN!

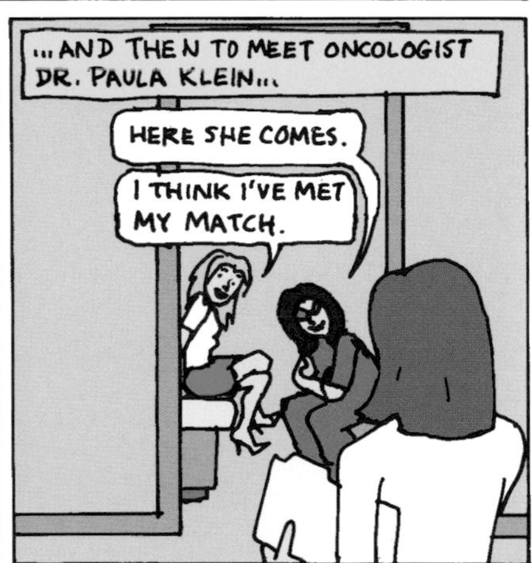
...AND THEN TO MEET ONCOLOGIST DR. PAULA KLEIN...
HERE SHE COMES.
I THINK I'VE MET MY MATCH.

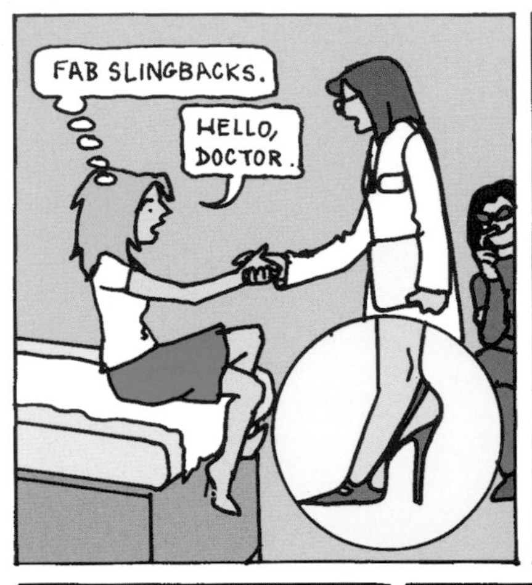
FAB SLINGBACKS.
HELLO, DOCTOR.

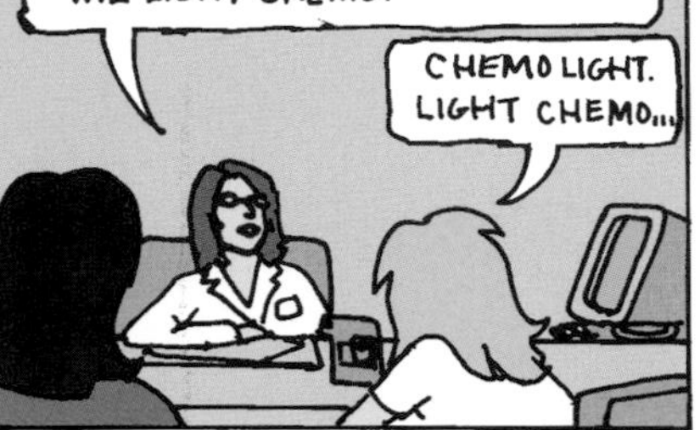
OK, BECAUSE YOU'RE STAGE-1 NODE-NEGATIVE, YOU CAN HAVE EITHER ADRIAMYCIN, "AC," THE HEAVY CHEMO, OR YOU CAN HAVE CYTOXAN, METHOTREXATE AND FLUOROURACIL, "CMF," WHICH IS THE LIGHT CHEMO.
CHEMO LIGHT. LIGHT CHEMO...

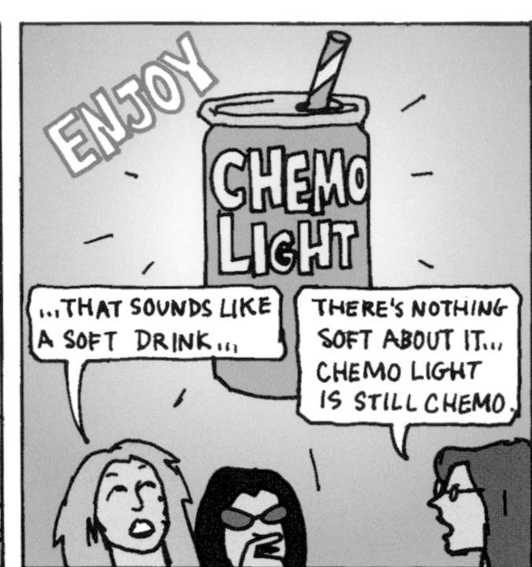
ENJOY
CHEMO LIGHT
...THAT SOUNDS LIKE A SOFT DRINK...
THERE'S NOTHING SOFT ABOUT IT... CHEMO LIGHT IS STILL CHEMO.

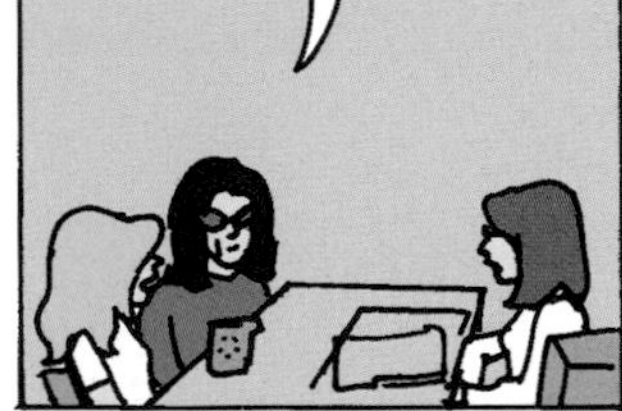
DR. KLEIN, LET ME BE REALLY STRAIGHT. MY HUSBAND OWNS A RESTAURANT WHERE THE MOST BEAUTIFUL WOMEN GO AND I CAN'T LOOK LIKE CRAP!

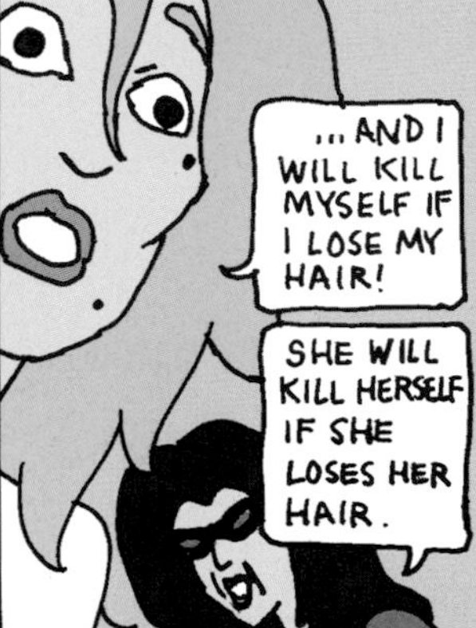
...AND I WILL KILL MYSELF IF I LOSE MY HAIR!
SHE WILL KILL HERSELF IF SHE LOSES HER HAIR.

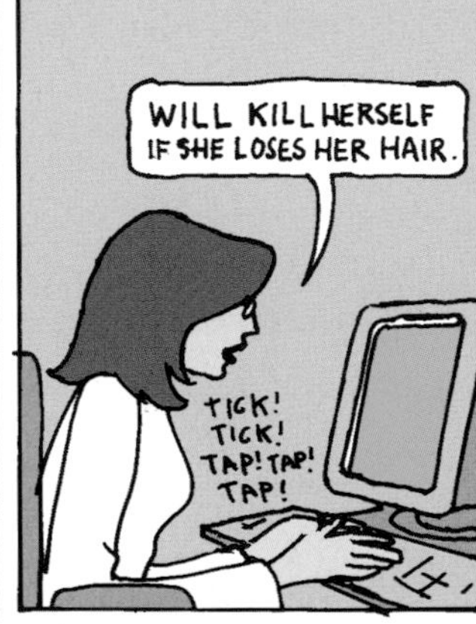
WILL KILL HERSELF IF SHE LOSES HER HAIR.
TICK! TICK! TAP! TAP! TAP!

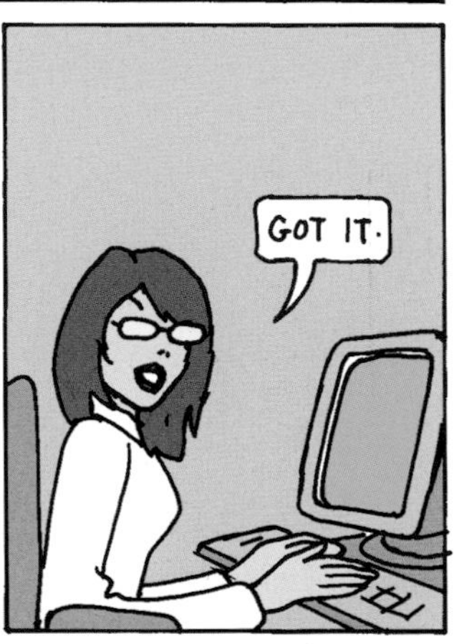
GOT IT.

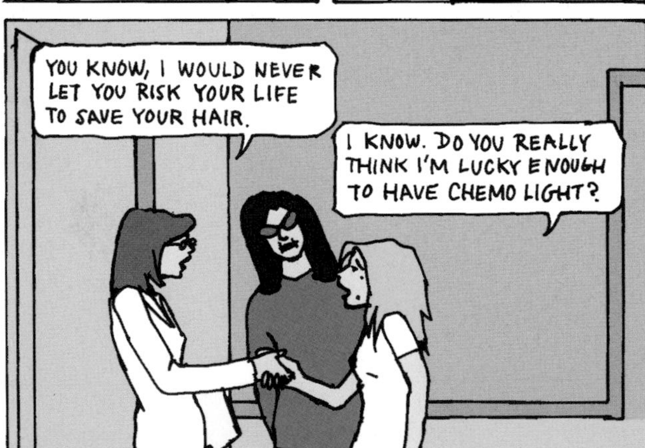
YOU KNOW, I WOULD NEVER LET YOU RISK YOUR LIFE TO SAVE YOUR HAIR.
I KNOW. DO YOU REALLY THINK I'M LUCKY ENOUGH TO HAVE CHEMO LIGHT?

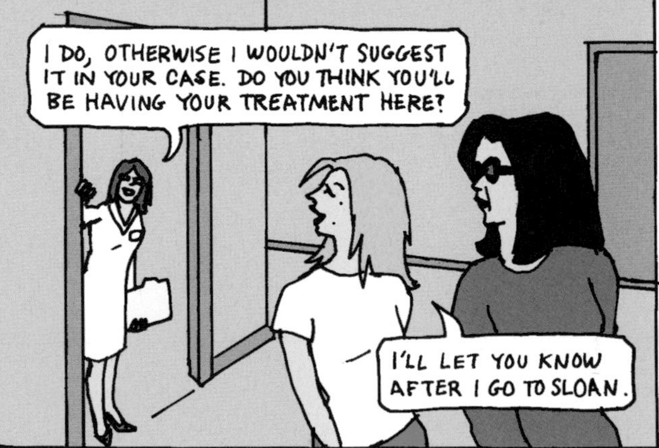
I DO, OTHERWISE I WOULDN'T SUGGEST IT IN YOUR CASE. DO YOU THINK YOU'LL BE HAVING YOUR TREATMENT HERE?
I'LL LET YOU KNOW AFTER I GO TO SLOAN.

JULY 8. MY (S)MOTHER MET ME AT THE EVELYN H. LAUDER BREAST CANCER CENTER AT MEMORIAL SLOAN-KETTERING.*
* COMPLETED IN 1992, THE FIRST-EVER BREAST AND DIAGNOSTIC CENTER WAS EQUIPPED BY A FUND INITIATED BY MRS. LAUDER.
IN OCTOBER 1992, SHE INTRODUCED NATIONAL BREAST CANCER MONTH BY DISTRIBUTING PINK RIBBONS AND BREAST SELF-EXAM CARDS, PLACING BREAST CANCER IN THE FOREFRONT OF PUBLIC AWARENESS.
IN 1993, MRS. LAUDER ESTABLISHED THE BREAST CANCER RESEARCH FOUNDATION, WHICH HAS RAISED OVER $125 MILLION.
SAINT EVELYN
THE PATRON SAINT OF BREAST CANCER**
I AM IN AWE.
HOW MANY LIVES HAS SHE HELPED SAVE?
** NONDENOMINATIONAL.

FIRST, DR. CATHERINE VON POSNIAK, MEDICAL ONCOLOGIST, EXAMINED ME.
I WOULD ALSO SEND YOU TO A DERMATOLOGIST TO LOOK ALL OVER YOUR SKIN, EVEN BETWEEN YOUR TOES, BECAUSE THERE'S A LINK BETWEEN BREAST CANCER AND MELANOMA.

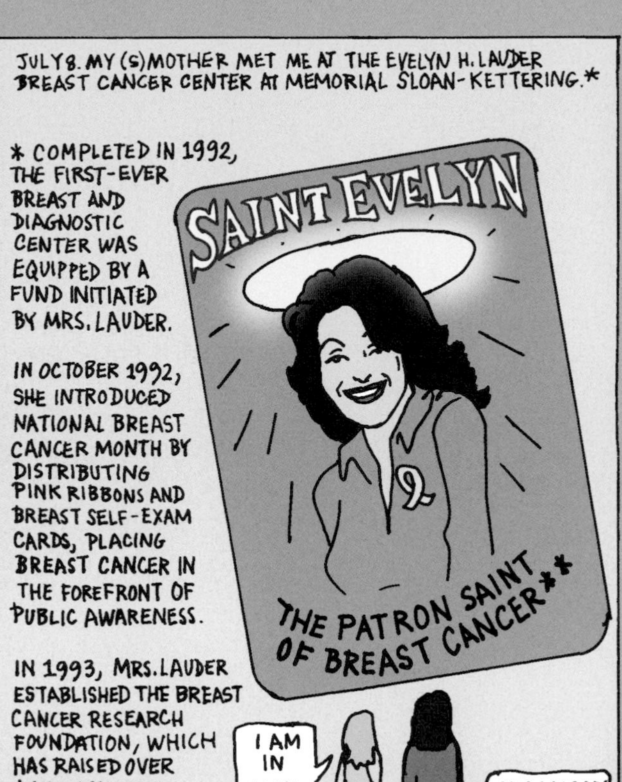

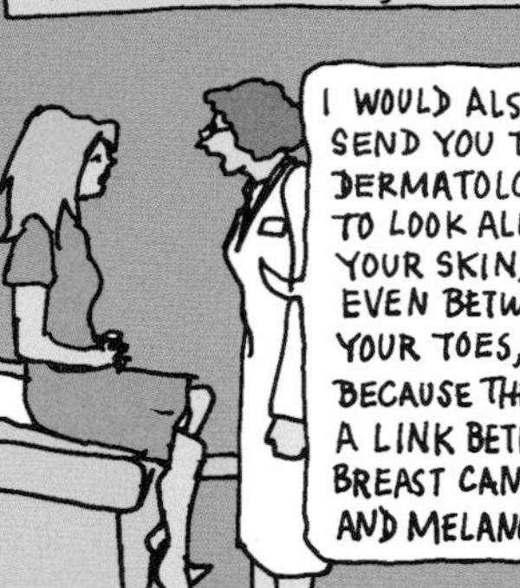

BY THE WAY MSKCC IS THE WINNER! OF THE MOST GLAM GOWN HANDS DOWN!

BACK IN HER OFFICE, DR. VON POSNIAK ADVISED ME ON TREATMENT:
WITH STAGE-1 NODE-NEGATIVE, I WOULD RECOMMEND A CHEMO WHERE YOU WON'T LOSE YOUR HAIR, BUT IT COULD THIN. IT'S CALLED CMF.
THAT'S THE LIGHT CHEMO DR. PAULA KLEIN SUGGESTED.

DR. PAULA KLEIN IS AN EXCELLENT, EXCELLENT DOCTOR. BECAUSE YOU'VE SEEN ME TODAY, YOU'LL ALWAYS BE MY PATIENT, BUT YOU'RE IN GOOD HANDS WITH HER. ANYTHING ELSE?

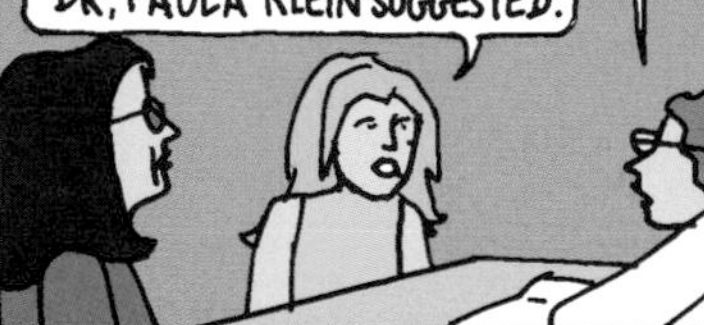

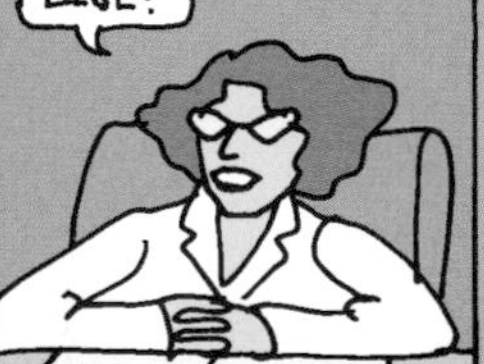

MY HUSBAND AND I HAVEN'T HAD OUR HONEYMOON YET, DO I HAVE TIME NOW?

HMM... IT TAKES 6 TO 8 WEEKS FOR THE TISSUE TO HEAL AFTER SURGERY...

... SO GO TO ITALY NOW, THEN START YOUR TREATMENT IN 2 WEEKS.
NOW?

YOU HAVE TO LIVE YOUR LIFE!
TELL THAT TO YOUR FRIENDS.

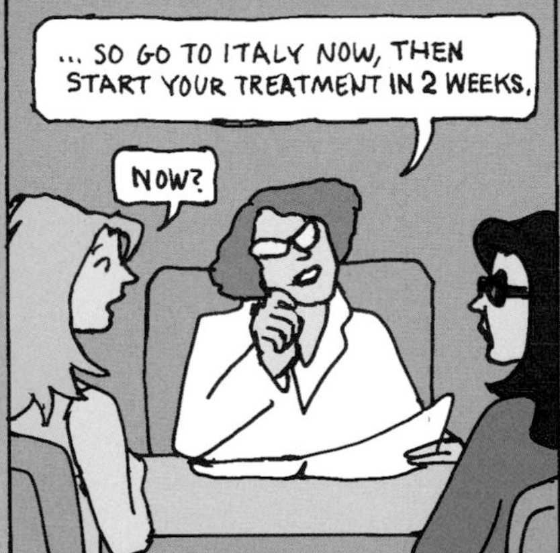

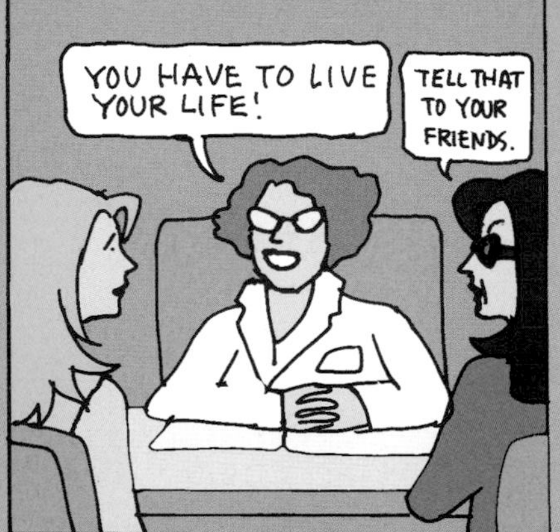

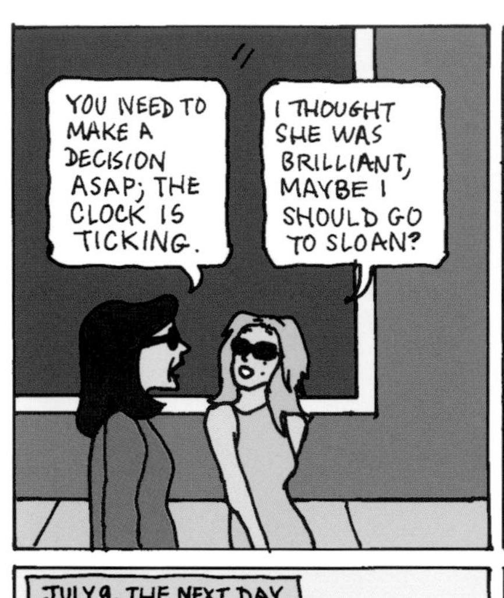
YOU NEED TO MAKE A DECISION ASAP; THE CLOCK IS TICKING.
I THOUGHT SHE WAS BRILLIANT, MAYBE I SHOULD GO TO SLOAN?

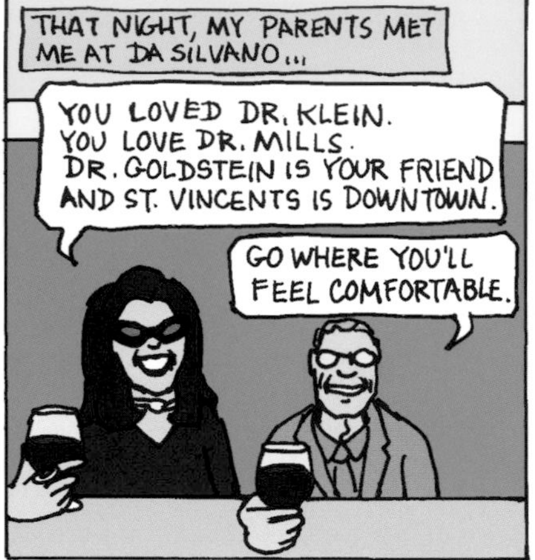
THAT NIGHT, MY PARENTS MET ME AT DA SILVANO...
YOU LOVED DR. KLEIN. YOU LOVE DR. MILLS. DR. GOLDSTEIN IS YOUR FRIEND AND ST. VINCENTS IS DOWNTOWN.
GO WHERE YOU'LL FEEL COMFORTABLE.

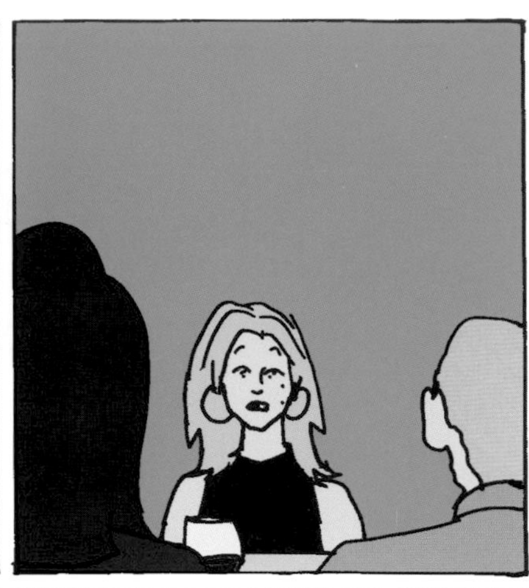

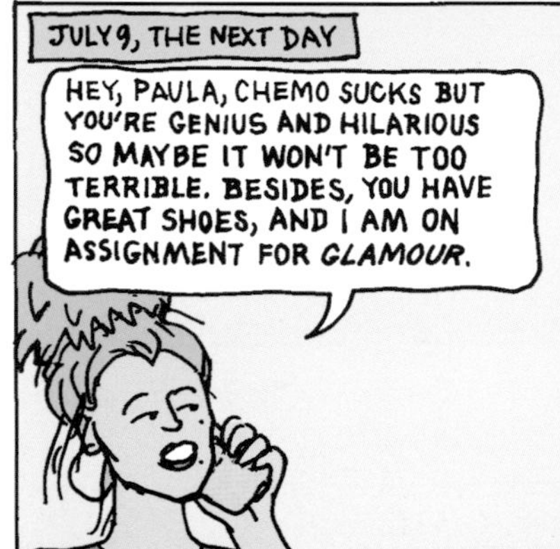
JULY 9, THE NEXT DAY
HEY, PAULA, CHEMO SUCKS BUT YOU'RE GENIUS AND HILARIOUS SO MAYBE IT WON'T BE TOO TERRIBLE. BESIDES, YOU HAVE GREAT SHOES, AND I AM ON ASSIGNMENT FOR *GLAMOUR*.

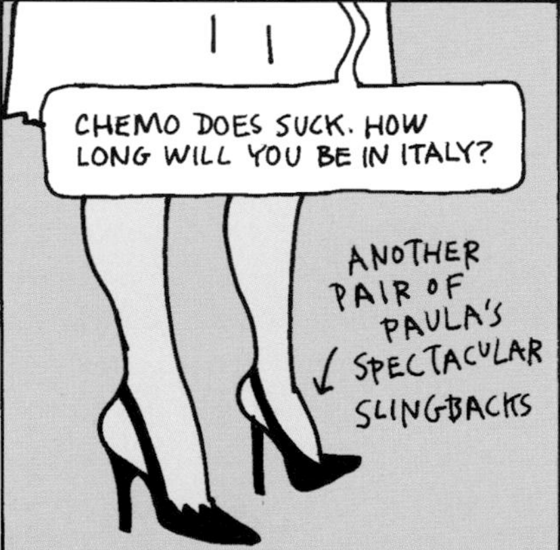
CHEMO DOES SUCK. HOW LONG WILL YOU BE IN ITALY?
ANOTHER PAIR OF PAULA'S SPECTACULAR SLINGBACKS

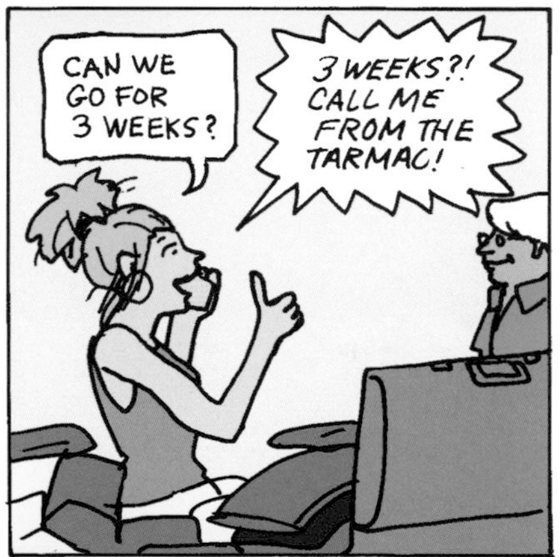
CAN WE GO FOR 3 WEEKS?
3 WEEKS?! CALL ME FROM THE TARMAC!

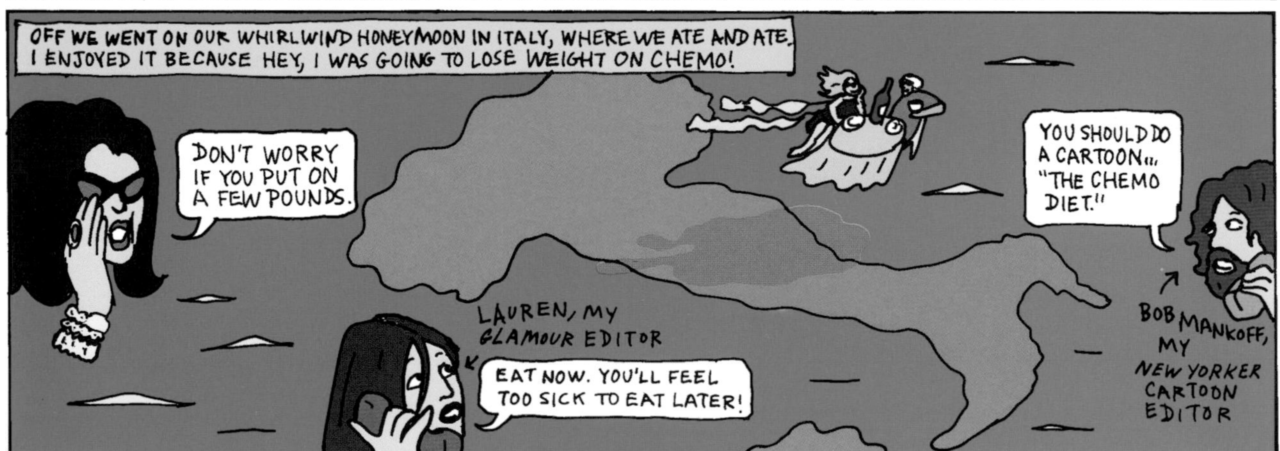
OFF WE WENT ON OUR WHIRLWIND HONEYMOON IN ITALY, WHERE WE ATE AND ATE. I ENJOYED IT BECAUSE HEY, I WAS GOING TO LOSE WEIGHT ON CHEMO!
DON'T WORRY IF YOU PUT ON A FEW POUNDS.
LAUREN, MY *GLAMOUR* EDITOR
EAT NOW. YOU'LL FEEL TOO SICK TO EAT LATER!
YOU SHOULD DO A CARTOON... "THE CHEMO DIET."
BOB MANKOFF, MY *NEW YORKER* CARTOON EDITOR

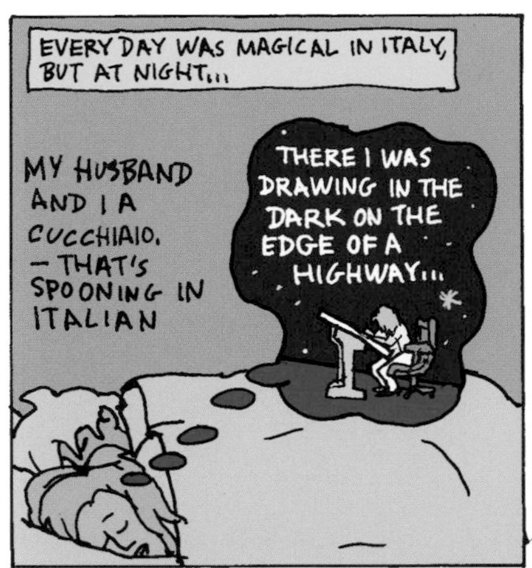
EVERY DAY WAS MAGICAL IN ITALY, BUT AT NIGHT...
MY HUSBAND AND I A CUCCHIAIO. —THAT'S SPOONING IN ITALIAN
THERE I WAS DRAWING IN THE DARK ON THE EDGE OF A HIGHWAY...

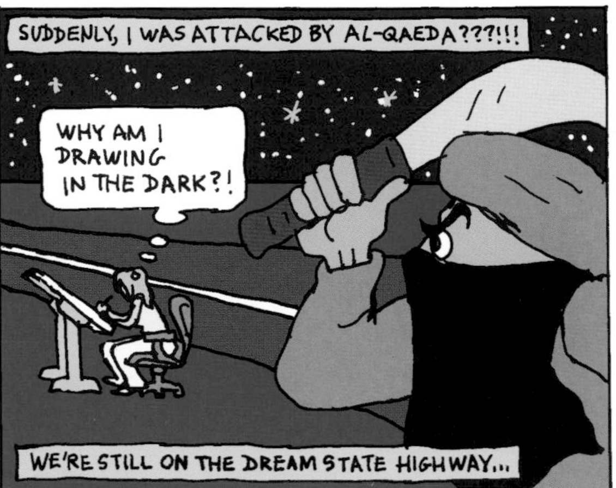
SUDDENLY, I WAS ATTACKED BY AL-QAEDA???!!!
WHY AM I DRAWING IN THE DARK?!
WE'RE STILL ON THE DREAM STATE HIGHWAY...

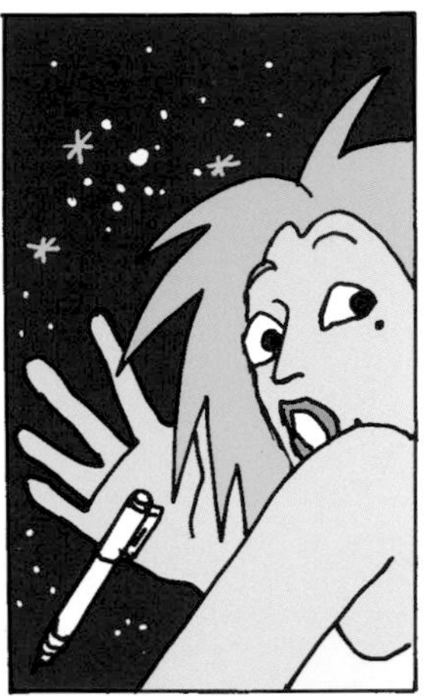

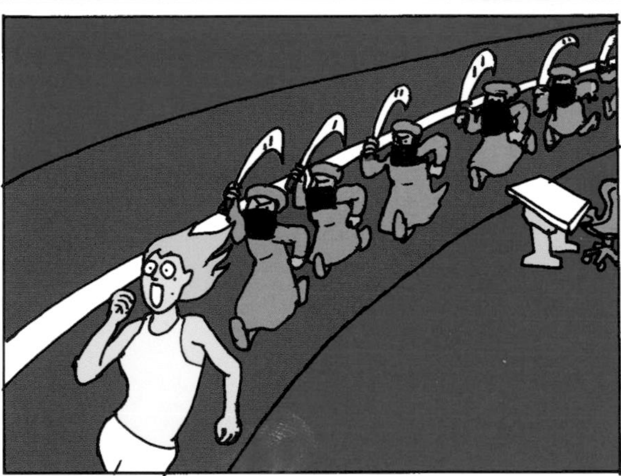

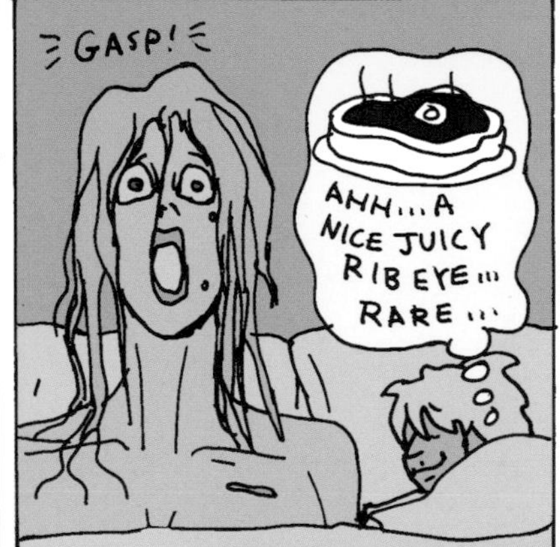
GASP!
AHH...A NICE JUICY RIB EYE... RARE...

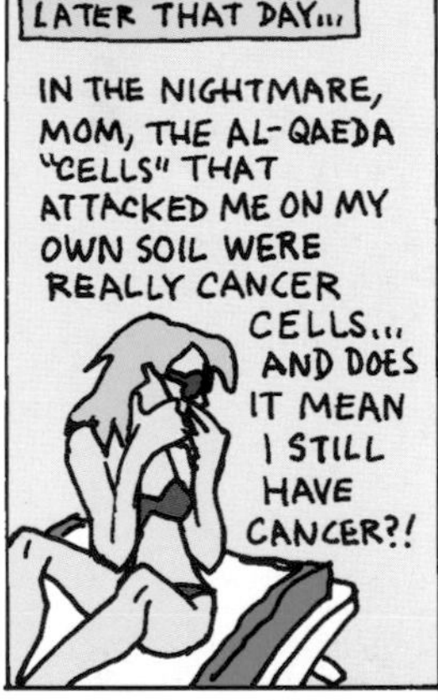
LATER THAT DAY...
IN THE NIGHTMARE, MOM, THE AL-QAEDA "CELLS" THAT ATTACKED ME ON MY OWN SOIL WERE REALLY CANCER CELLS... AND DOES IT MEAN I STILL HAVE CANCER?!

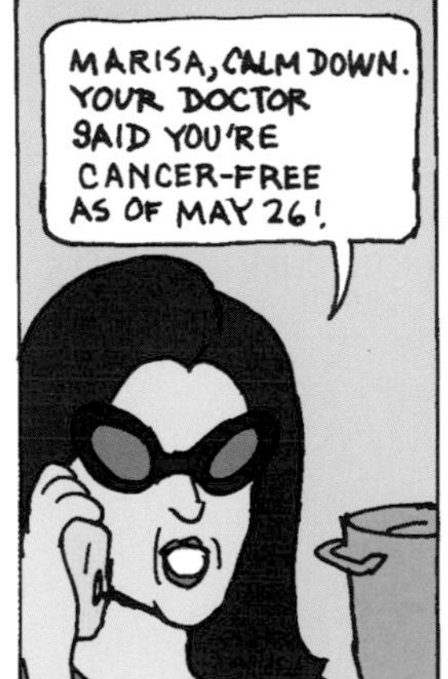
MARISA, CALM DOWN. YOUR DOCTOR SAID YOU'RE CANCER-FREE AS OF MAY 26!

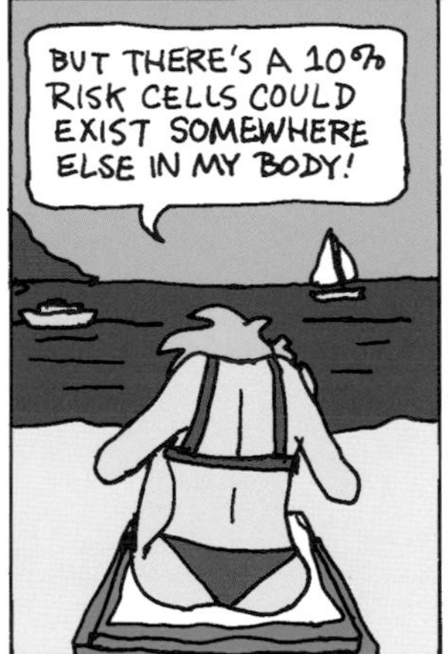
BUT THERE'S A 10% RISK CELLS COULD EXIST SOMEWHERE ELSE IN MY BODY!

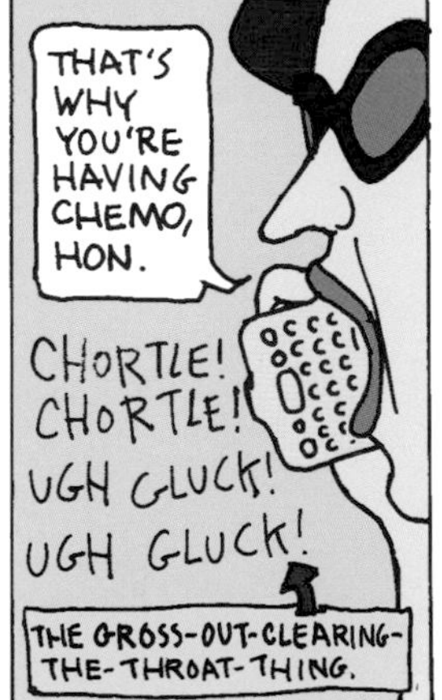
THAT'S WHY YOU'RE HAVING CHEMO, HON.
CHORTLE! CHORTLE! UGH GLUCK! UGH GLUCK!
THE GROSS-OUT-CLEARING-THE-THROAT-THING.

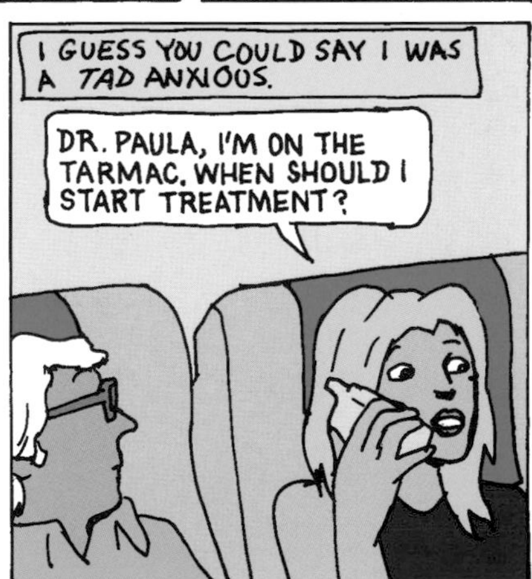
I GUESS YOU COULD SAY I WAS A TAD ANXIOUS.
DR. PAULA, I'M ON THE TARMAC. WHEN SHOULD I START TREATMENT?

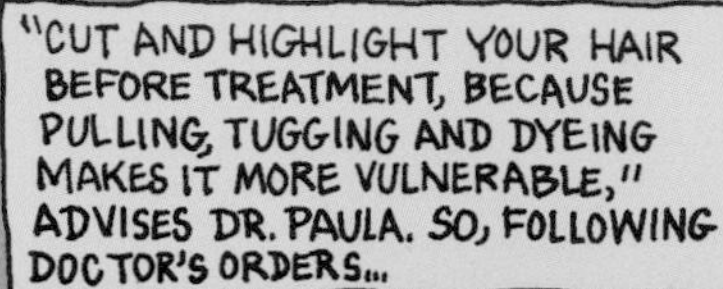

THIS IS MORE IMPORTANT. IF YOU LOOK HEALTHY, YOU'LL FEEL HEALTHY. I LOVE YOU LIKE A SISTER AND I DON'T WANT YOU TO BE SICK.

BUT IF YOU *REALLY* WANT ME TO BE HAPPY, MAKE ME GO BLONDER.

WHILE UNDER THE DRYER...
I HAD BREAST CANCER AND DEVELOPED LYMPHEDEMA. DID ANYONE TELL YOU ABOUT IT?
A LITTLE BIT, HOW DID IT HAPPEN?
IF SHE HAD KNOWN ABOUT LYMPHEDEMA, IT MIGHT HAVE BEEN PREVENTED.

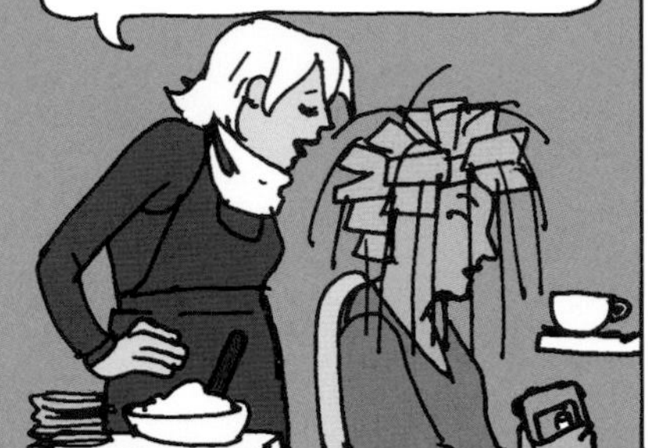

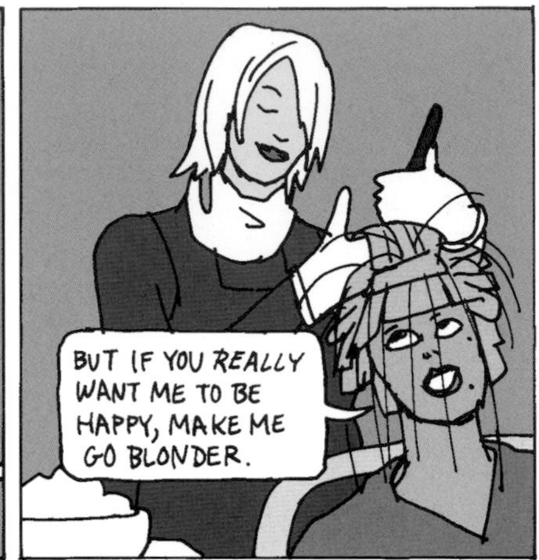

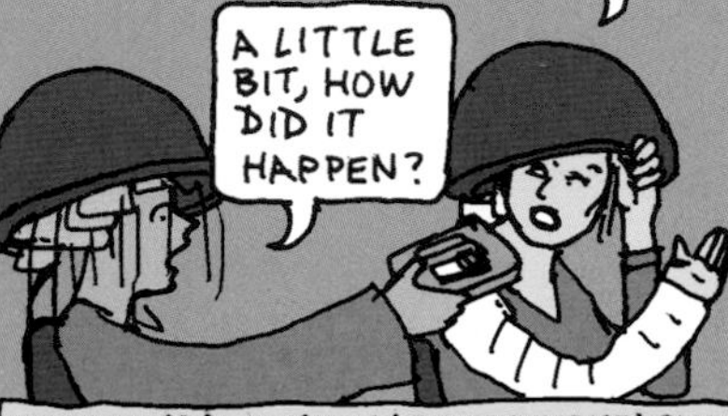

I TOUCHED HOT METAL AND MY ARM PLUMPED UP. NOW I HAVE TO WEAR THIS SLEEVE FOR THE REST OF MY LIFE TO AVOID ELEPHANTIASIS, LOSING MY ARM, OR DEATH...

THIS IS WHAT MADE ME CRY.

SHE HAD A DOUBLE MASTECTOMY AND TOTAL HAIR LOSS 3 YEARS AGO.

SO BE CAREFUL BECAUSE ANY CUT, STRAIN OR EXTREME TEMPERATURE CAN CAUSE IT... AND DON'T LET *ANYONE* CUT YOUR CUTICLES BECAUSE INFECTION CAN TRIGGER LYMPHEDEMA, TOO.

NEXT, BENOIT THE HAIRSTYLIST CUT 6 INCHES. 6 INCHES!
...AND YOU CAN PUT PIECES IN, LIKE PARIS HILTON. ALL HER HAIR IS FAKE.

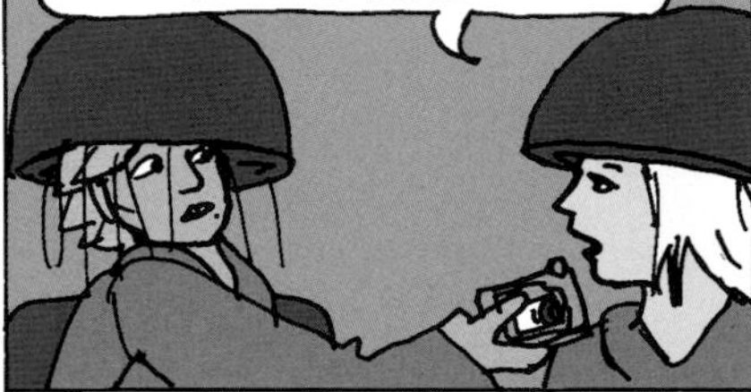

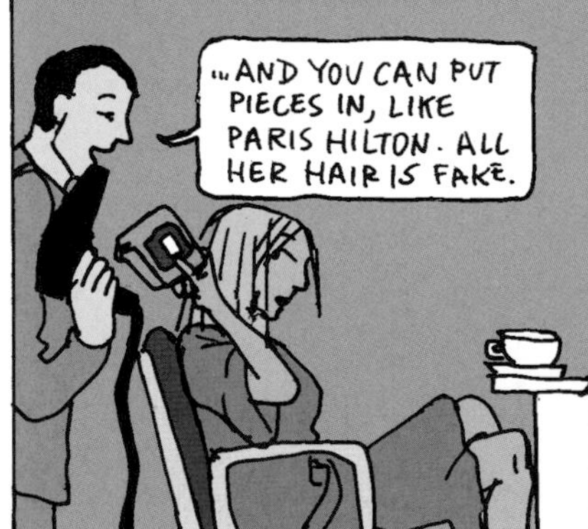

AFTER MY CUT AND COLOR, I MET WITH NEIL, AKA "THE FALL GUY."

IF YOU ARE GOING TO LOSE 20% TO 50% OF YOUR HAIR, YOU CAN CONSIDER

A CLIP-ON, A SEWN-IN, OR A FUSION.

WHAT WOULD *I* NEED? ONLY TIME WOULD TELL...

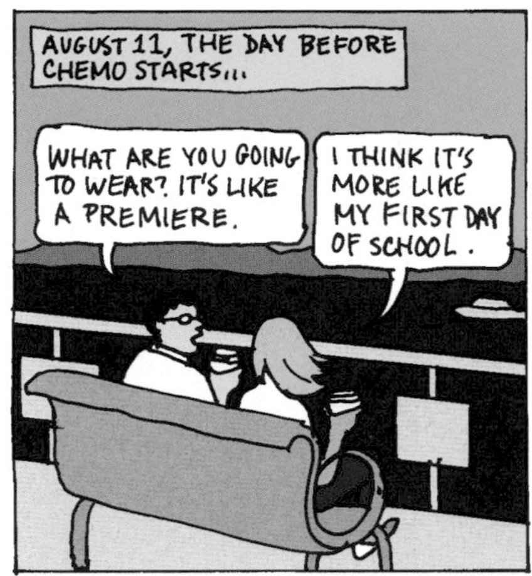

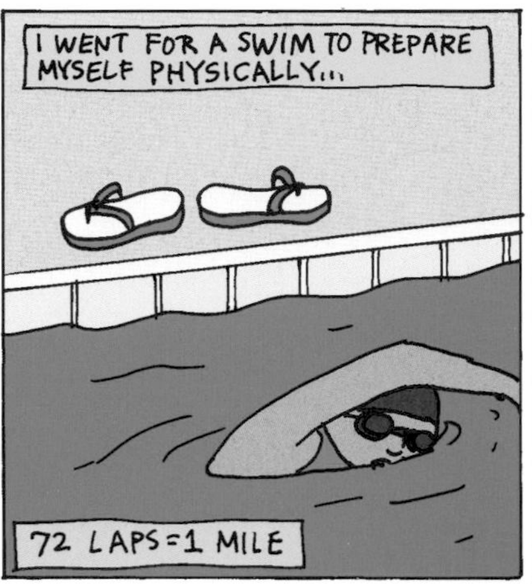

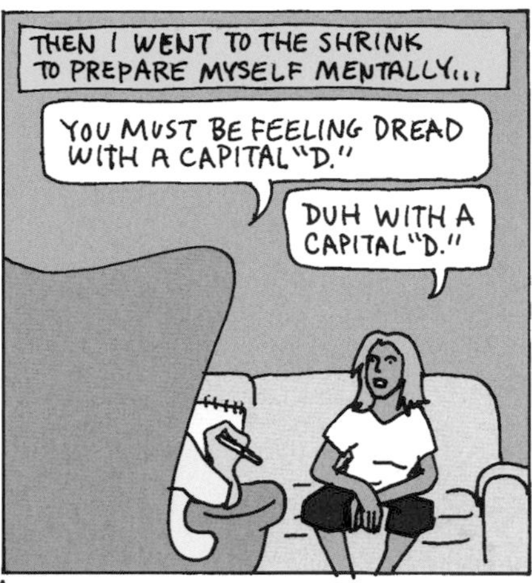

I MADE SURE I HAD ALL MY REPORTER SUPPLIES... THIS TIME I WAS ON ASSIGNMENT FOR *GLAMOUR*.

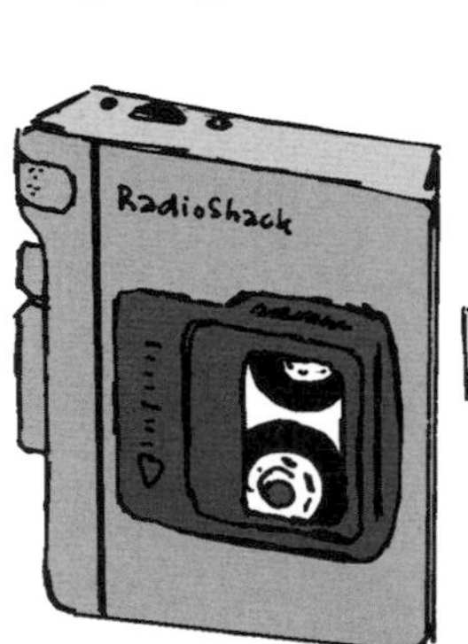

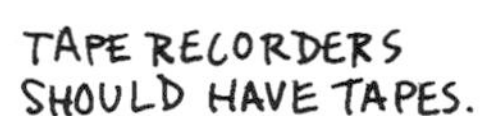

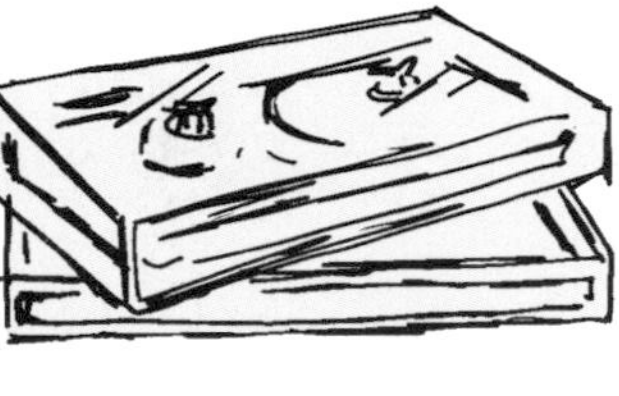

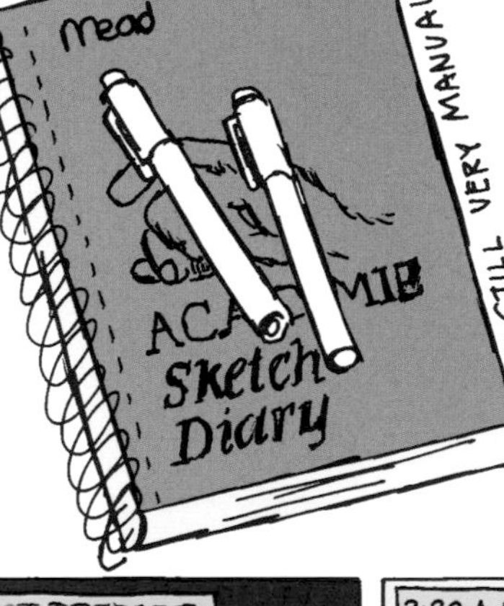

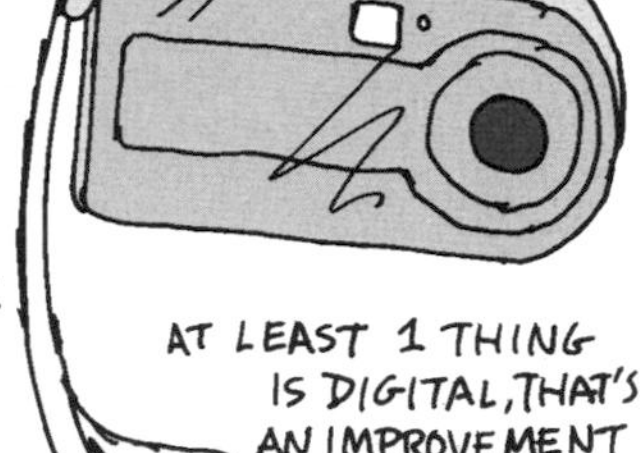

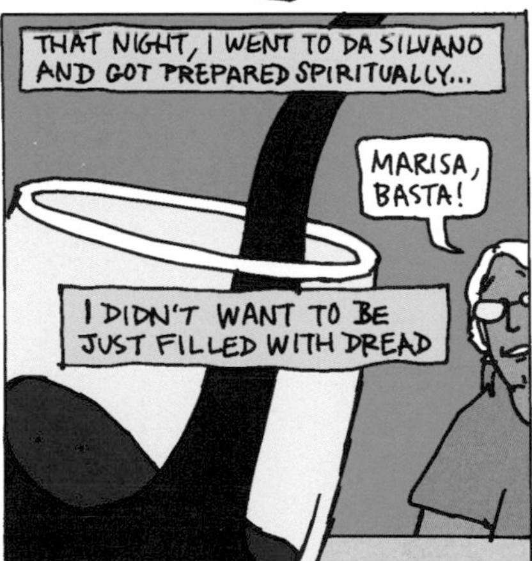

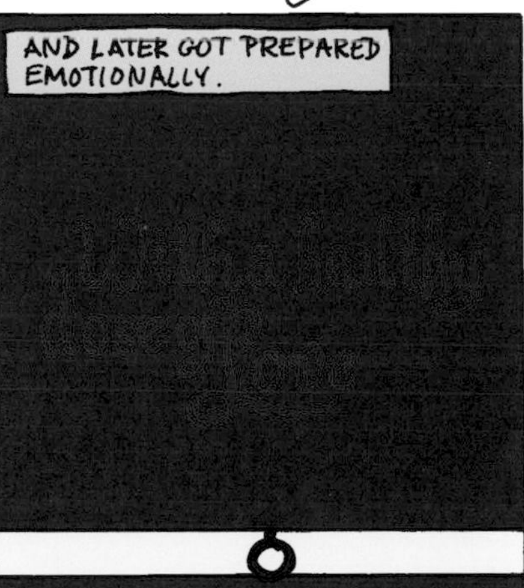

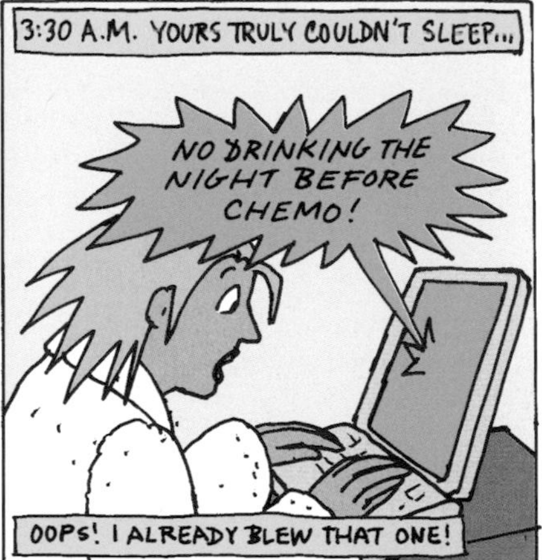

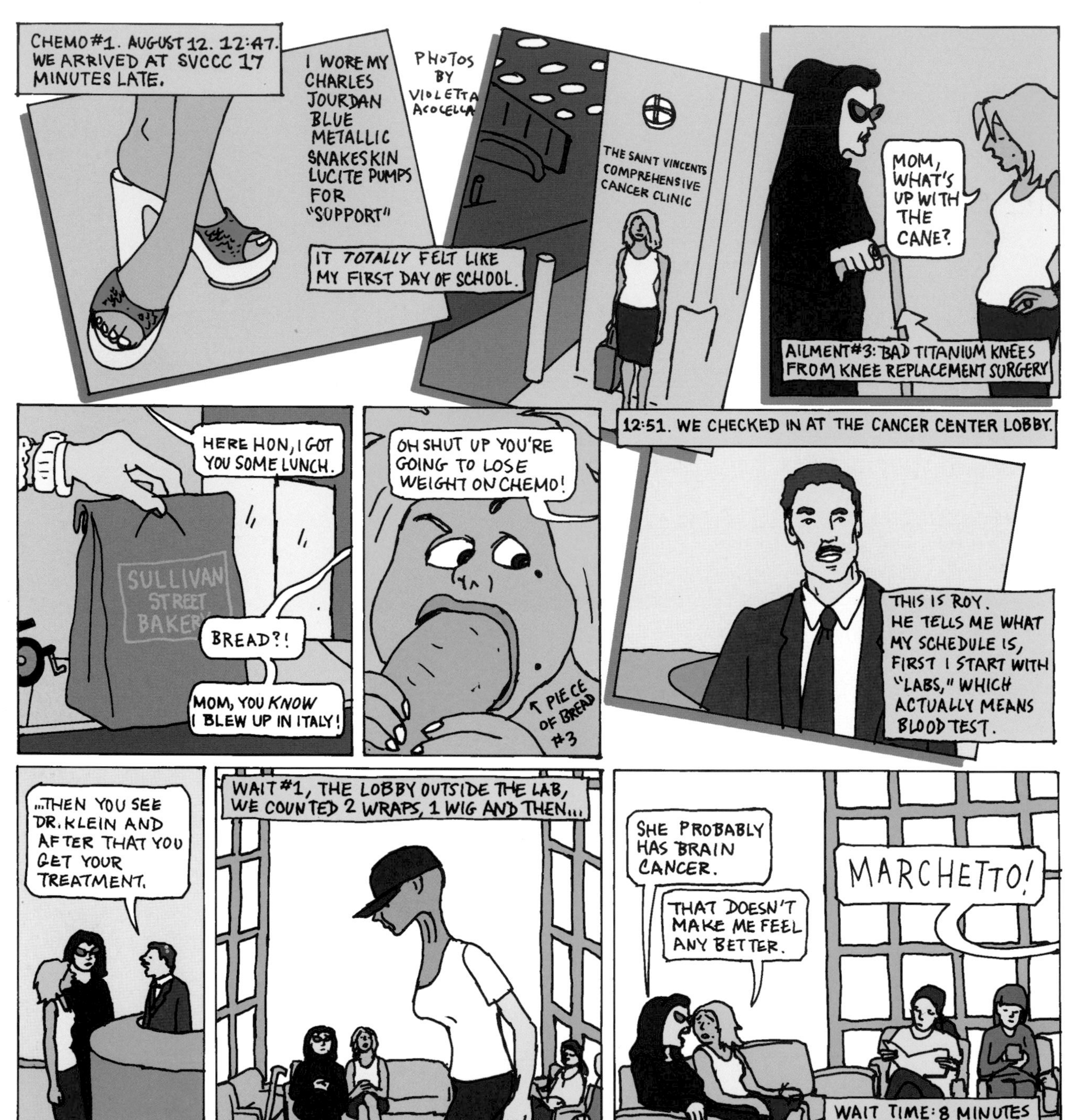
CHEMO #1. AUGUST 12. 12:47. WE ARRIVED AT SVCCC 17 MINUTES LATE.
I WORE MY CHARLES JOURDAN BLUE METALLIC SNAKESKIN LUCITE PUMPS FOR "SUPPORT"
PHOTOS BY VIOLETTA ACOCELLA
IT *TOTALLY* FELT LIKE MY FIRST DAY OF SCHOOL.
THE SAINT VINCENTS COMPREHENSIVE CANCER CLINIC
MOM, WHAT'S UP WITH THE CANE?
AILMENT #3: BAD TITANIUM KNEES FROM KNEE REPLACEMENT SURGERY
HERE HON, I GOT YOU SOME LUNCH.
SULLIVAN STREET BAKERY
BREAD?!
MOM, YOU *KNOW* I BLEW UP IN ITALY!
OH SHUT UP YOU'RE GOING TO LOSE WEIGHT ON CHEMO!
↑ PIECE OF BREAD #3
12:51. WE CHECKED IN AT THE CANCER CENTER LOBBY.
THIS IS ROY. HE TELLS ME WHAT MY SCHEDULE IS, FIRST I START WITH "LABS," WHICH ACTUALLY MEANS BLOOD TEST.
...THEN YOU SEE DR. KLEIN AND AFTER THAT YOU GET YOUR TREATMENT.
WAIT #1, THE LOBBY OUTSIDE THE LAB, WE COUNTED 2 WRAPS, 1 WIG AND THEN...
SHE PROBABLY HAS BRAIN CANCER.
THAT DOESN'T MAKE ME FEEL ANY BETTER.
MARCHETTO!
WAIT TIME: 8 MINUTES

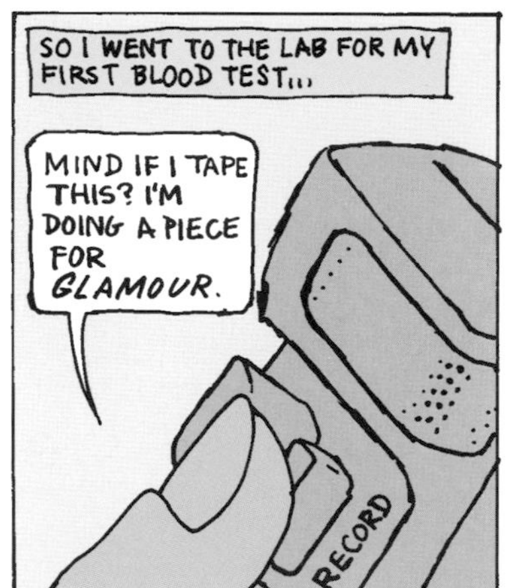

SURE HON, AND YOU CAN TAKE A PICTURE OF ME.

YVONNE "DOESN'T GIVE EVERYONE THAT PRIVILEGE."

WHEN'S YOUR BIRTHDAY?
MY BIRTHDAY? WHY ARE YOU ASKING, ARE YOU INTO ASTROLOGY?

WE ASK YOU THAT TO MAKE SURE YOU'RE YOU, AND YOU'RE GETTING THE RIGHT TREATMENT.
THAT'S OUR WAY OF DOUBLE-CHECKING.

DO YOU HAVE A PORT?
WHAT'S A PORT?
EXCUSE ME...

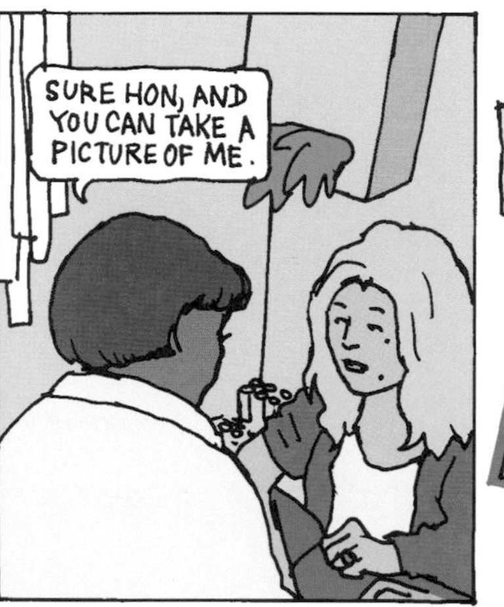

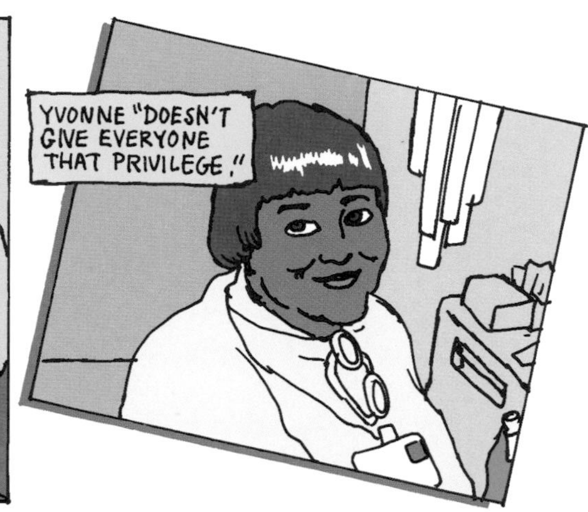

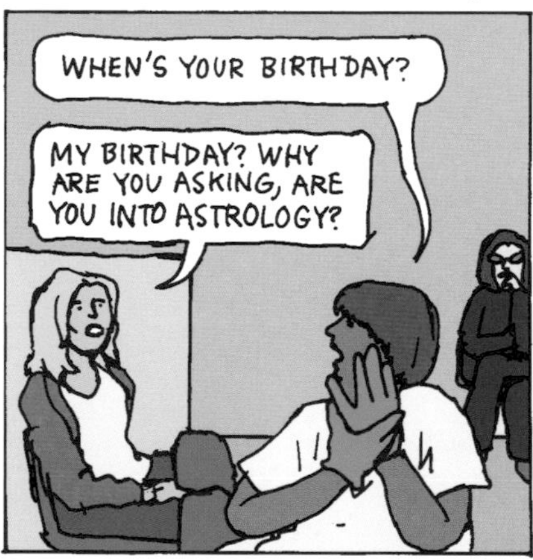

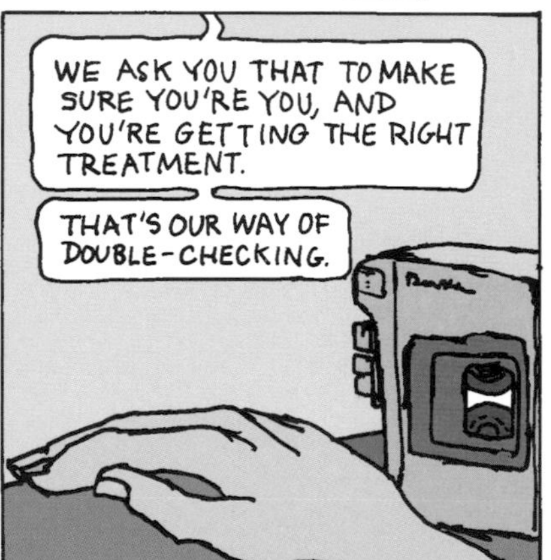

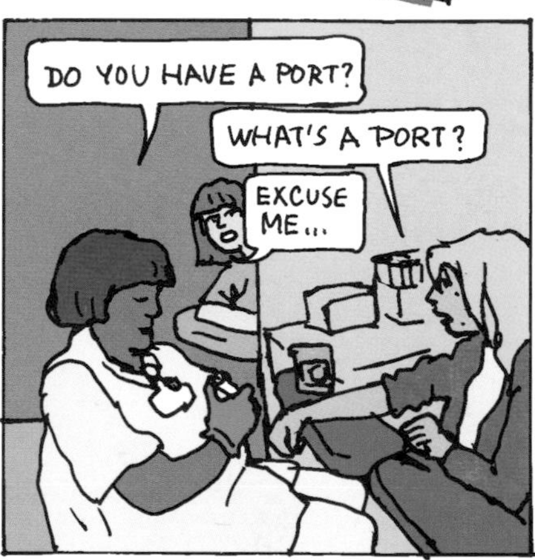

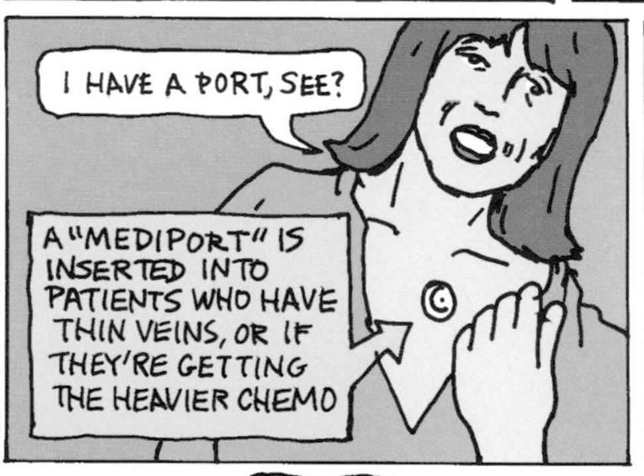

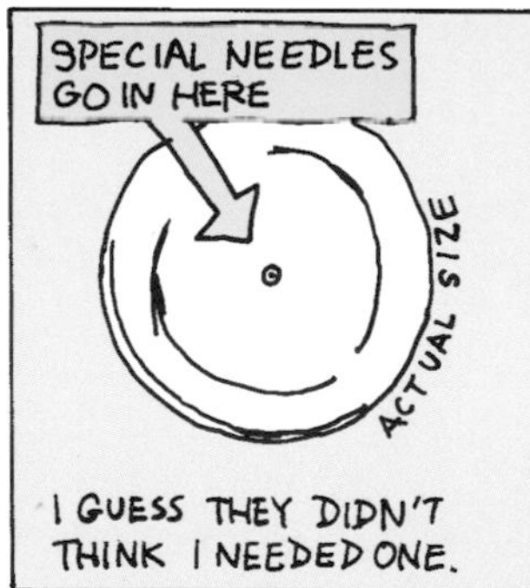

MAKE A FIST FOR ME.

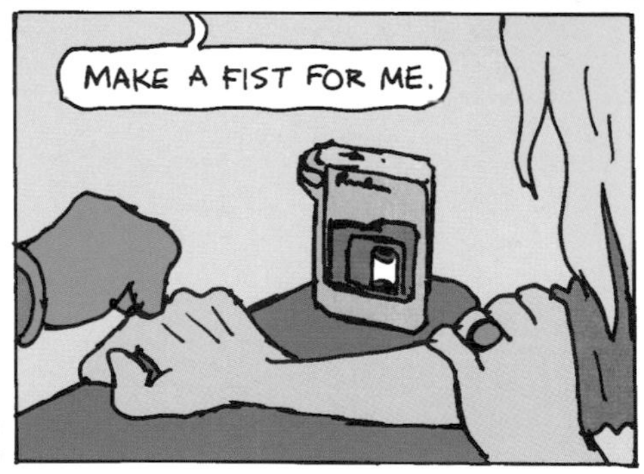

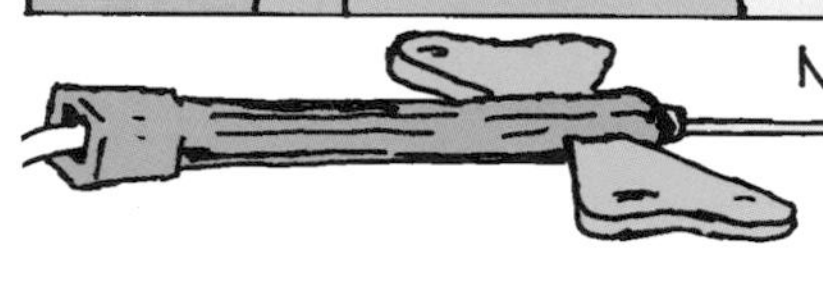

NEEDLE #6

THE "BLOOD-DRAWING NEEDLE"

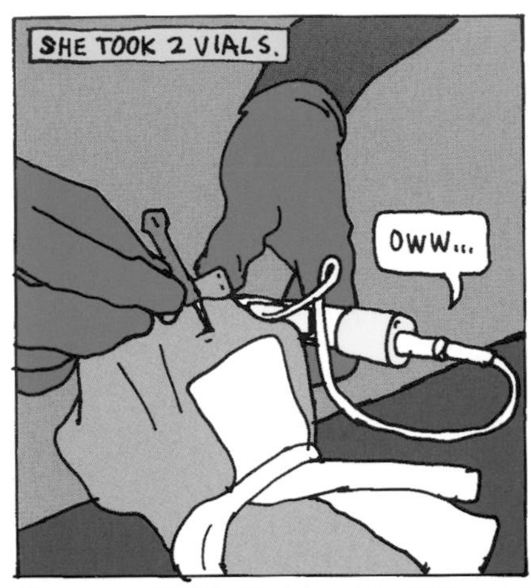
SHE TOOK 2 VIALS.
OWW...

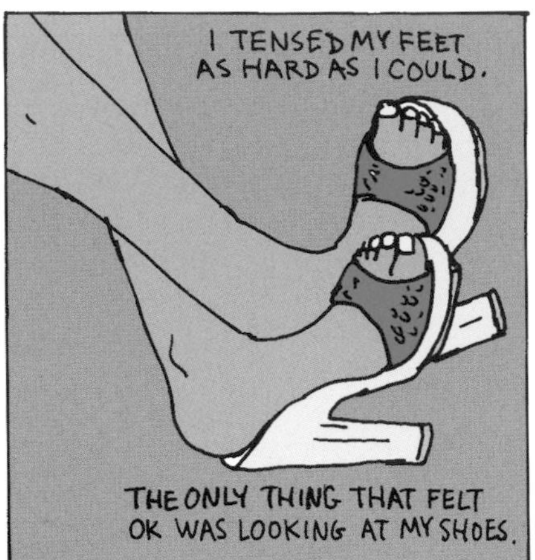
I TENSED MY FEET AS HARD AS I COULD.
THE ONLY THING THAT FELT OK WAS LOOKING AT MY SHOES.

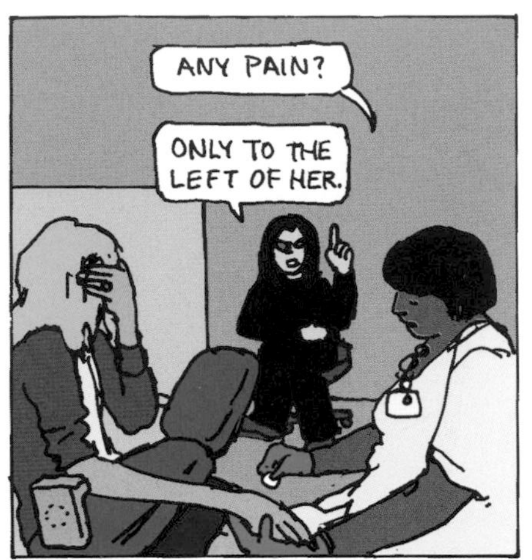
ANY PAIN?
ONLY TO THE LEFT OF HER.

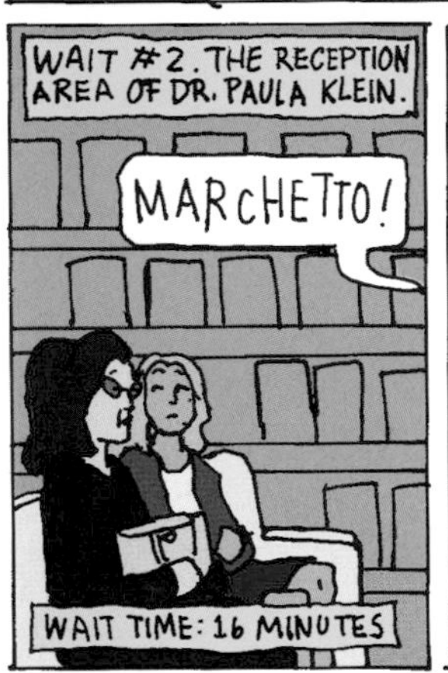
WAIT #2. THE RECEPTION AREA OF DR. PAULA KLEIN.
MARCHETTO!
WAIT TIME: 16 MINUTES

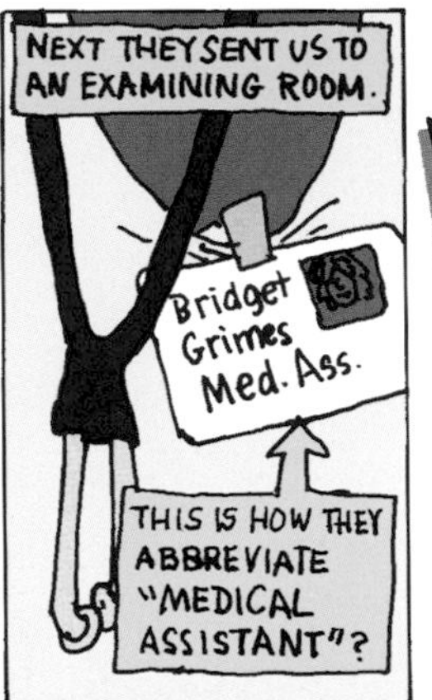
NEXT THEY SENT US TO AN EXAMINING ROOM.
Bridget Grimes Med. Ass.
THIS IS HOW THEY ABBREVIATE "MEDICAL ASSISTANT"?

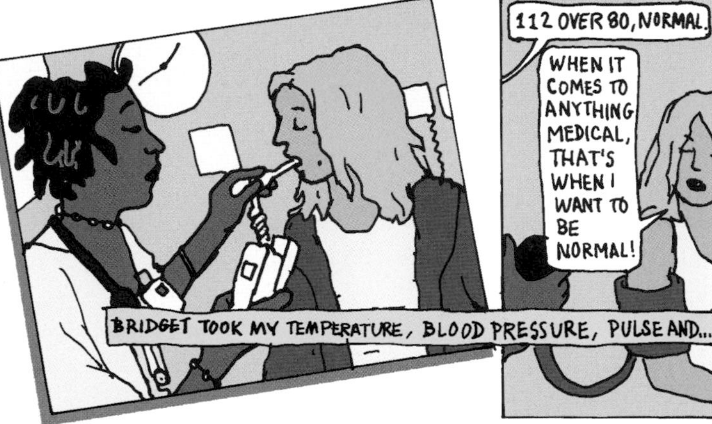
BRIDGET TOOK MY TEMPERATURE, BLOOD PRESSURE, PULSE AND...
112 OVER 80, NORMAL.
WHEN IT COMES TO ANYTHING MEDICAL, THAT'S WHEN I WANT TO BE NORMAL!

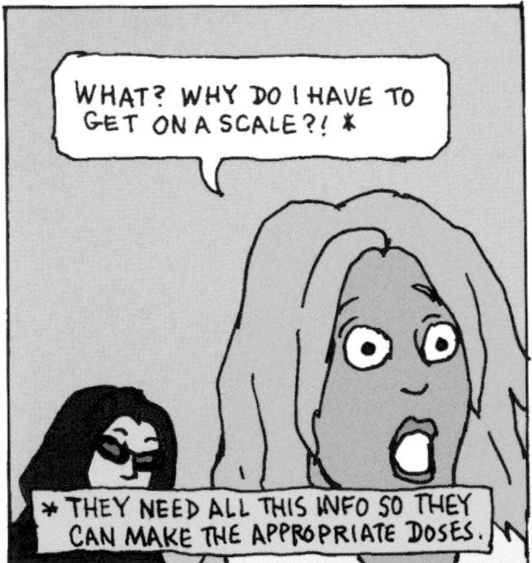
WHAT? WHY DO I HAVE TO GET ON A SCALE?! *
* THEY NEED ALL THIS INFO SO THEY CAN MAKE THE APPROPRIATE DOSES.

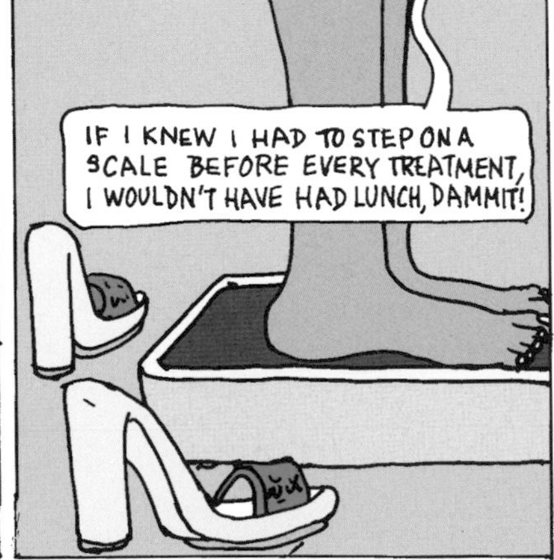
IF I KNEW I HAD TO STEP ON A SCALE BEFORE EVERY TREATMENT, I WOULDN'T HAVE HAD LUNCH, DAMMIT!

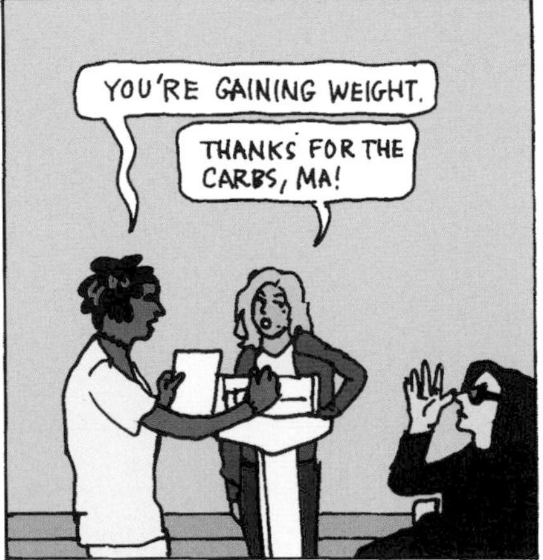
YOU'RE GAINING WEIGHT.
THANKS FOR THE CARBS, MA!

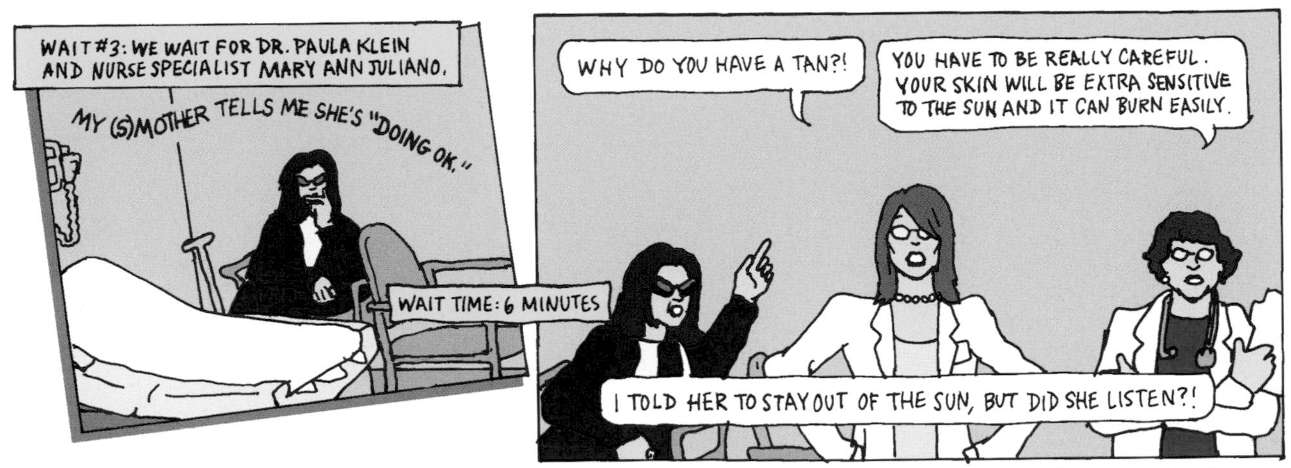

WAIT #3: WE WAIT FOR DR. PAULA KLEIN AND NURSE SPECIALIST MARY ANN JULIANO.
MY (S)MOTHER TELLS ME SHE'S "DOING OK."
WAIT TIME: 6 MINUTES
WHY DO YOU HAVE A TAN?!
YOU HAVE TO BE REALLY CAREFUL. YOUR SKIN WILL BE EXTRA SENSITIVE TO THE SUN AND IT CAN BURN EASILY.
I TOLD HER TO STAY OUT OF THE SUN, BUT DID SHE LISTEN?!

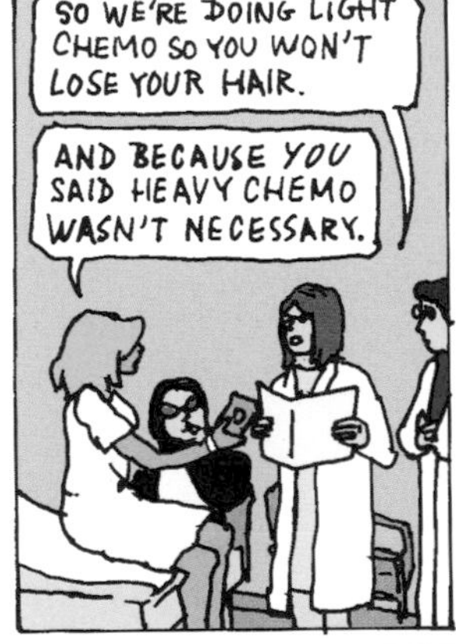

SO WE'RE DOING LIGHT CHEMO SO YOU WON'T LOSE YOUR HAIR.
AND BECAUSE *YOU* SAID HEAVY CHEMO WASN'T NECESSARY.

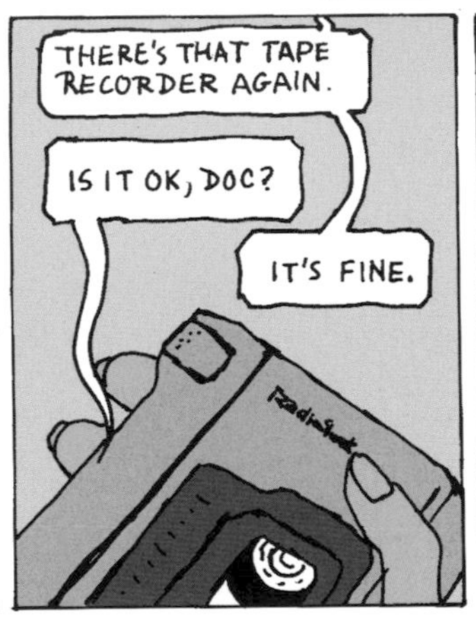

THERE'S THAT TAPE RECORDER AGAIN.
IS IT OK, DOC?
IT'S FINE.
RadioShack

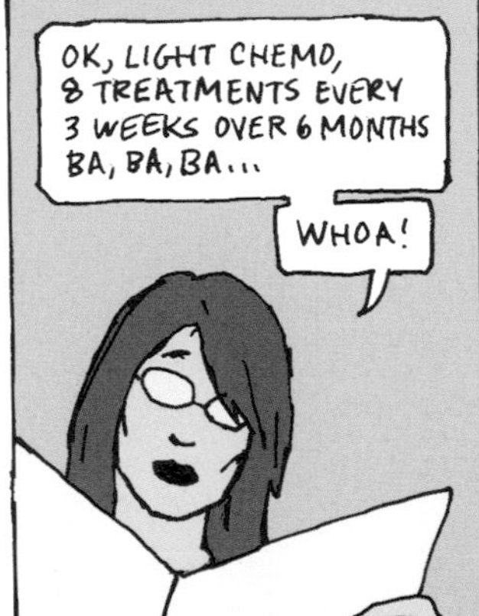

OK, LIGHT CHEMO, 8 TREATMENTS EVERY 3 WEEKS OVER 6 MONTHS BA, BA, BA...
WHOA!

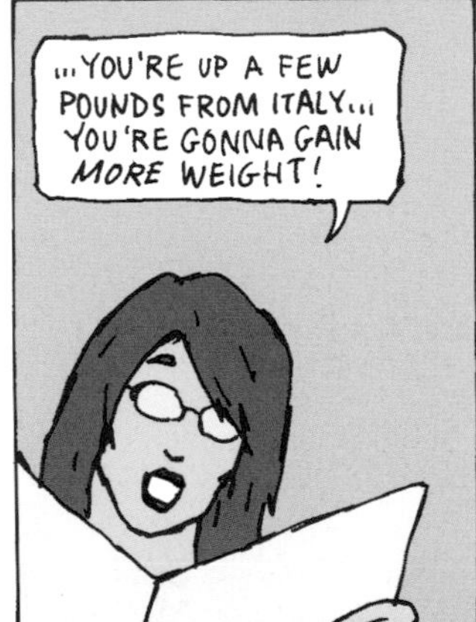

...YOU'RE UP A FEW POUNDS FROM ITALY... YOU'RE GONNA GAIN *MORE* WEIGHT!

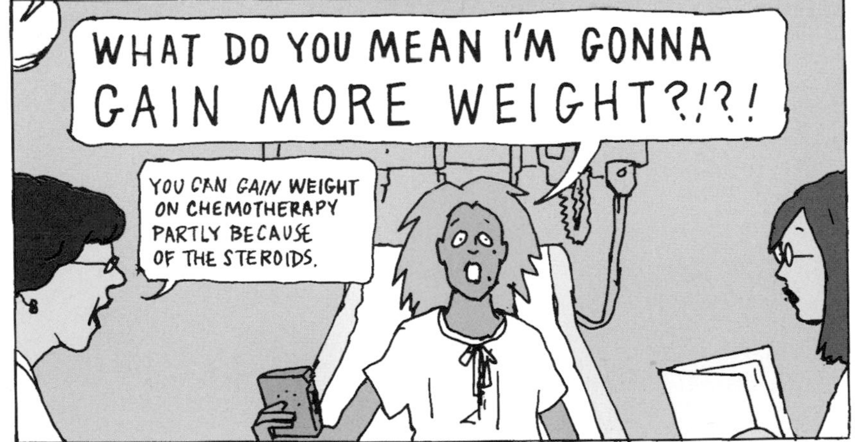

WHAT DO YOU MEAN I'M GONNA GAIN MORE WEIGHT?!?!
YOU CAN *GAIN* WEIGHT ON CHEMOTHERAPY PARTLY BECAUSE OF THE STEROIDS.

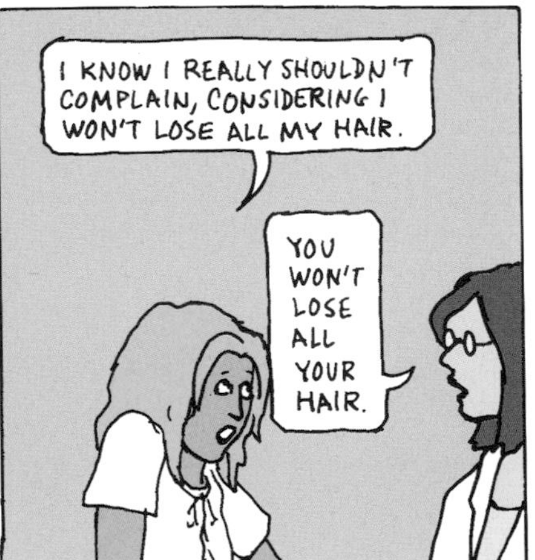

I KNOW I REALLY SHOULDN'T COMPLAIN, CONSIDERING I WON'T LOSE ALL MY HAIR.
YOU WON'T LOSE ALL YOUR HAIR.

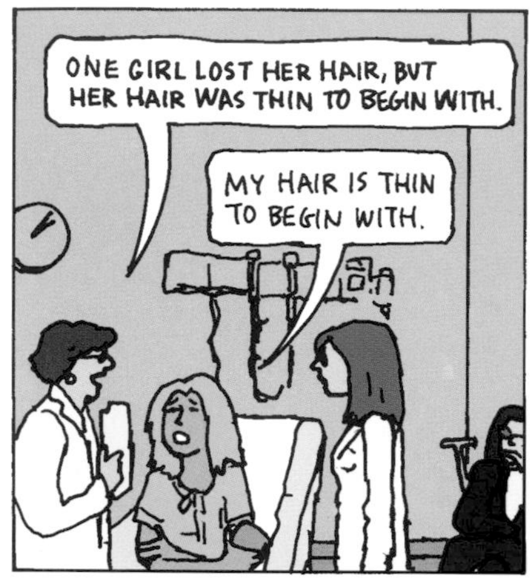
ONE GIRL LOST HER HAIR, BUT HER HAIR WAS THIN TO BEGIN WITH.
MY HAIR IS THIN TO BEGIN WITH.

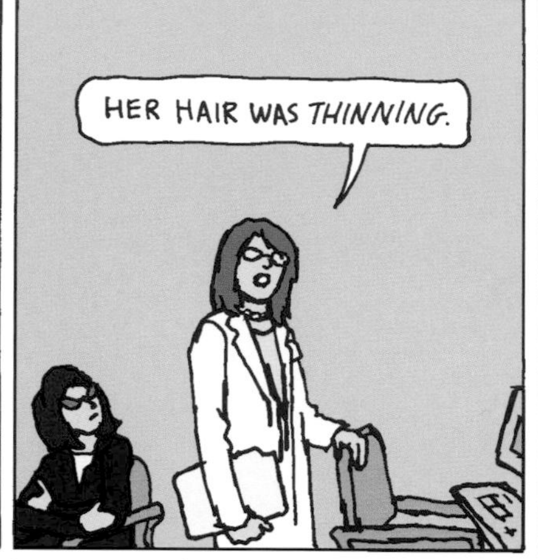
HER HAIR WAS *THINNING*.

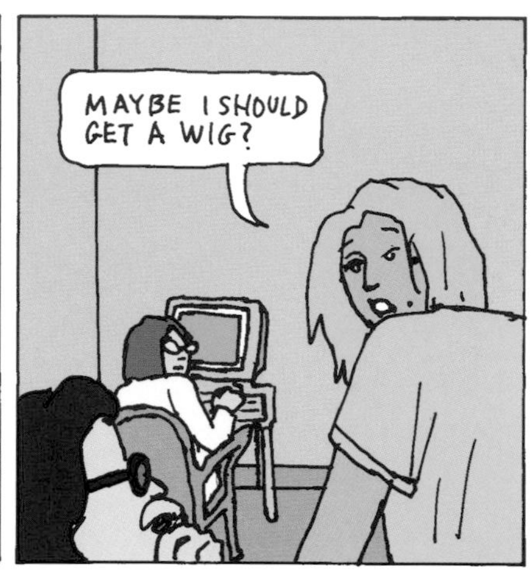
MAYBE I SHOULD GET A WIG?

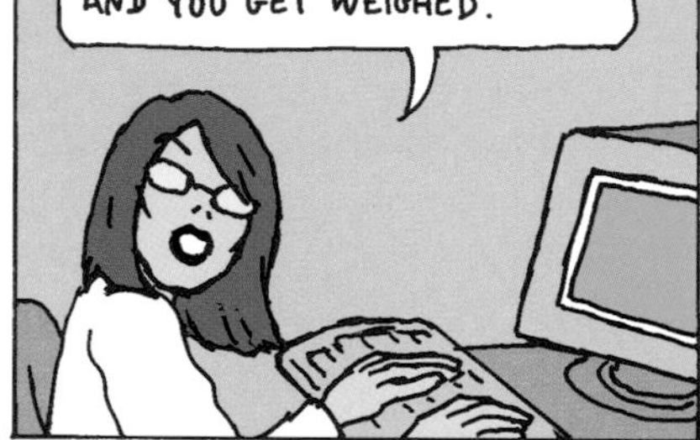
OK, HERE'S THE DRILL. DO YOUR LABS FIRST. WHILE THEY'RE BEING "COOKED" OR TESTED, YOUR BLOOD PRESSURE, PULSE AND TEMPERATURE ARE TAKEN AND YOU GET WEIGHED.

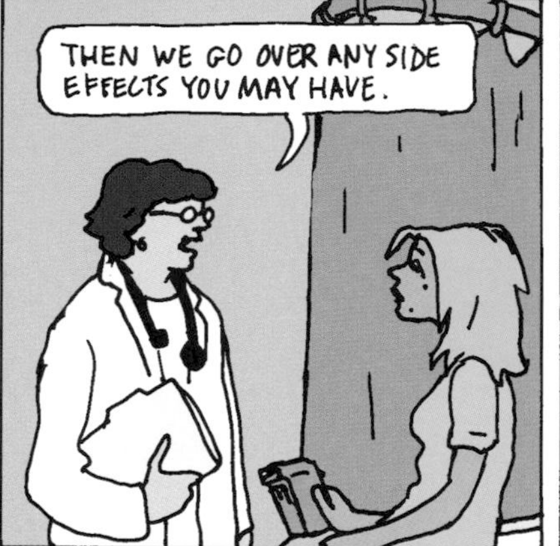
THEN WE GO OVER ANY SIDE EFFECTS YOU MAY HAVE.

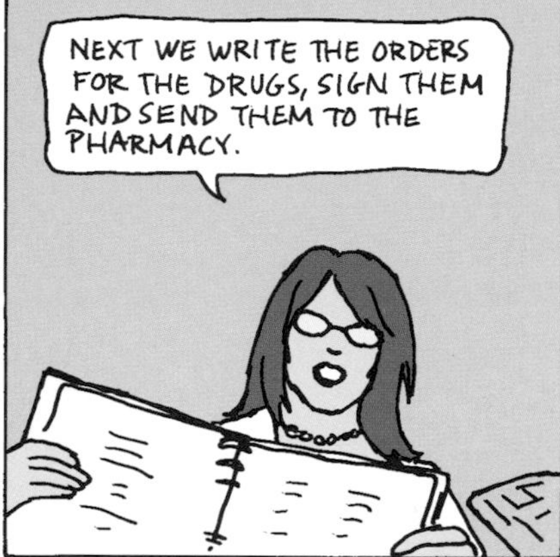
NEXT WE WRITE THE ORDERS FOR THE DRUGS, SIGN THEM AND SEND THEM TO THE PHARMACY.

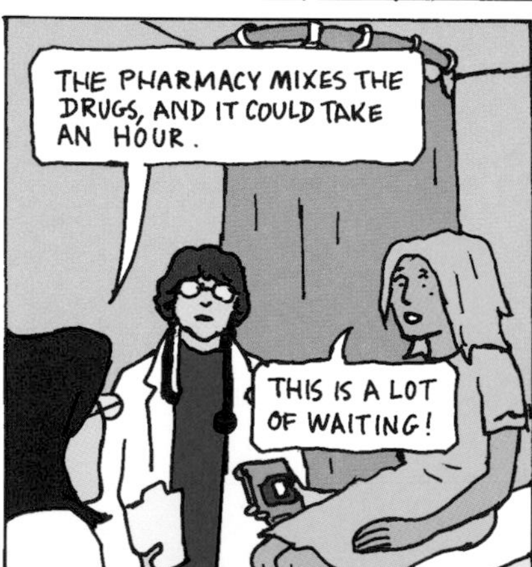
THE PHARMACY MIXES THE DRUGS, AND IT COULD TAKE AN HOUR.
THIS IS A LOT OF WAITING!

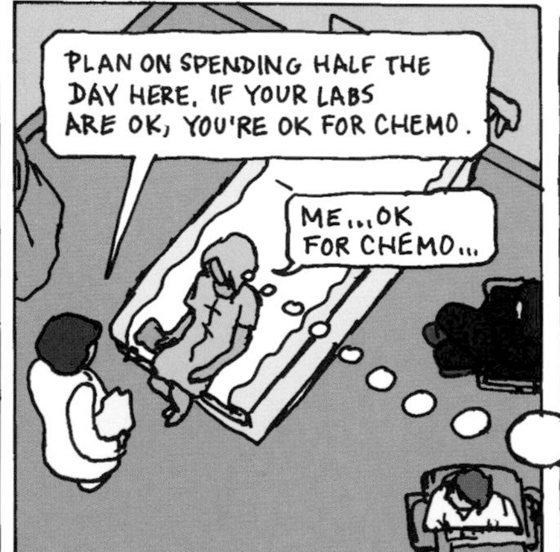
PLAN ON SPENDING HALF THE DAY HERE. IF YOUR LABS ARE OK, YOU'RE OK FOR CHEMO.
ME...OK FOR CHEMO...

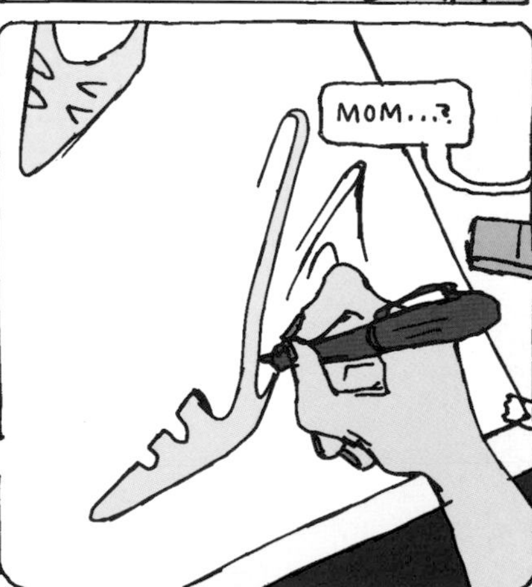
MOM...?

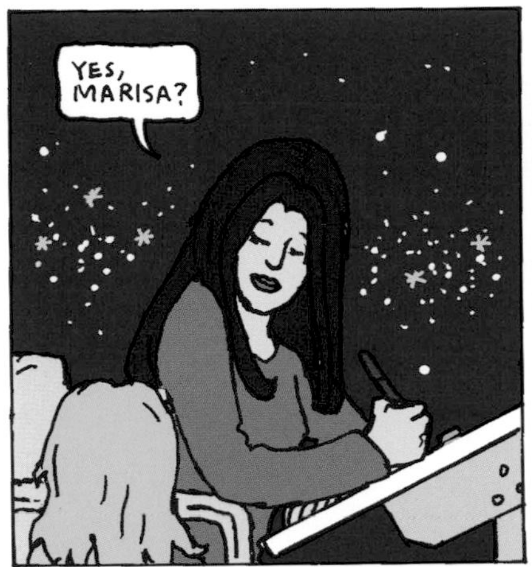
YES, MARISA?

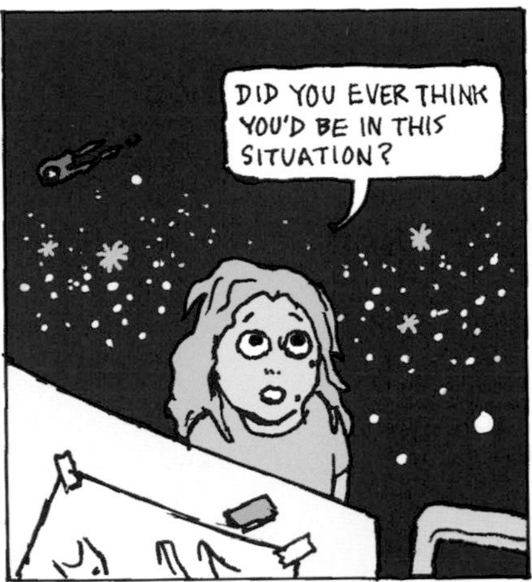
DID YOU EVER THINK YOU'D BE IN THIS SITUATION?

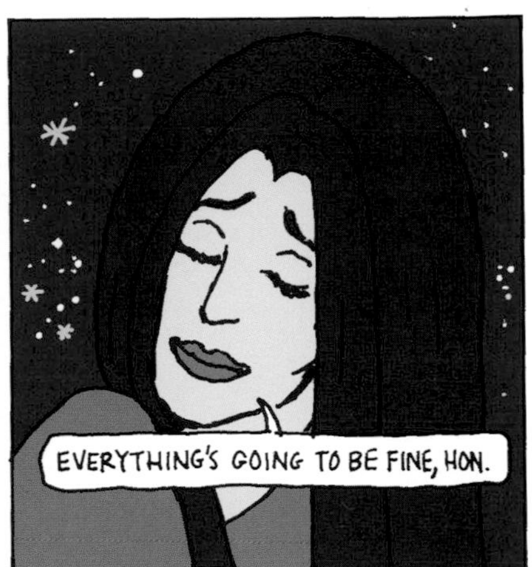
EVERYTHING'S GOING TO BE FINE, HON.

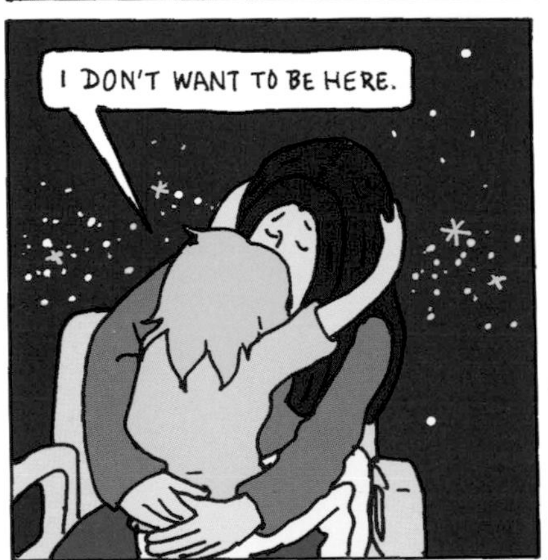
I DON'T WANT TO BE HERE.

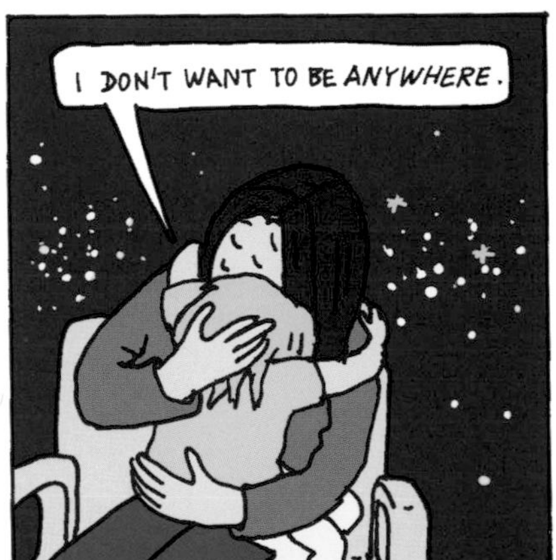
I DON'T WANT TO BE *ANYWHERE*.

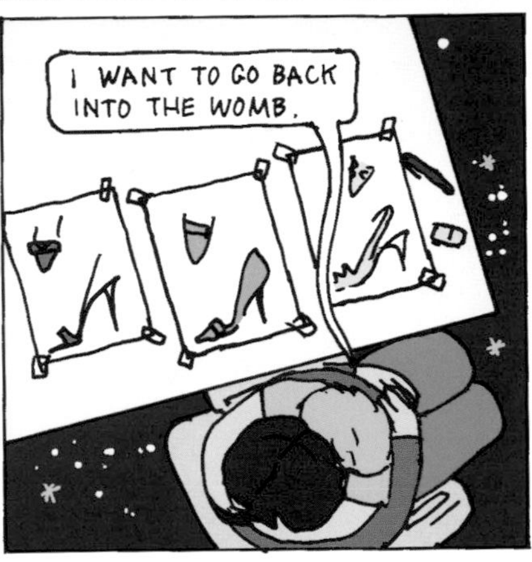
I WANT TO GO BACK INTO THE WOMB.

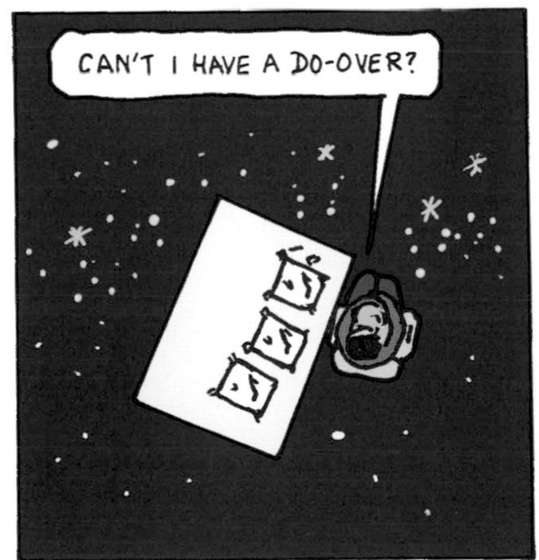
CAN'T I HAVE A DO-OVER?

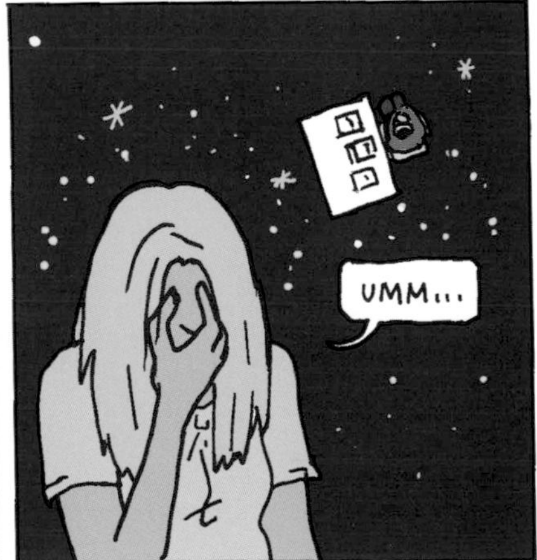
UMM...

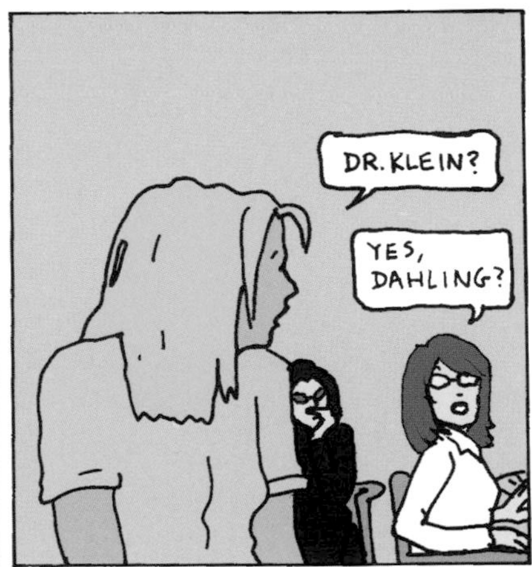
DR. KLEIN?
YES, DAHLING?

How long are treatments?

How often are treatments?

How many treatments will I need?

How will I feel afterward?

Can I exercise? Will I be tired?

What kind of exercise should I do?

Can I keep working?

Does each treatment get progressively worse?

Will I throw up? Can I travel?

How nauseous will I be?

When will this ever end?

DON'T BE SCARED.

OK, SO I'M PUTTING DOWN THAT YOU GAINED 6 POUNDS...

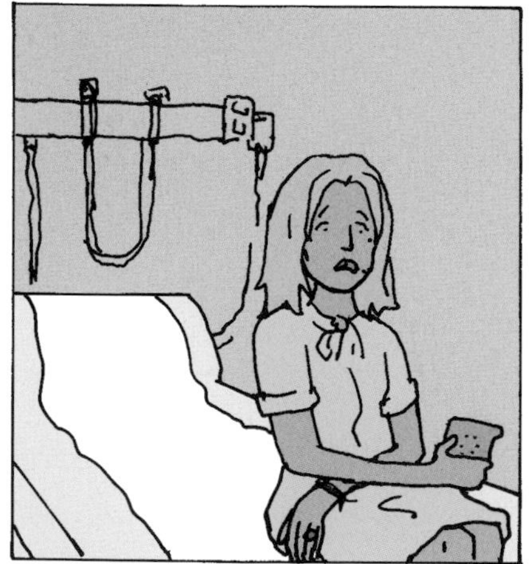

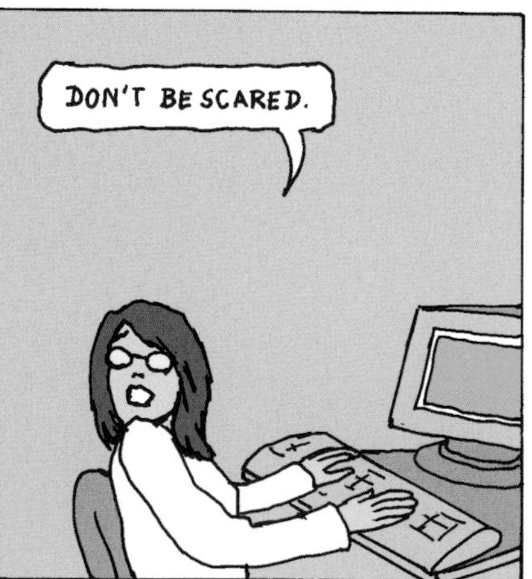

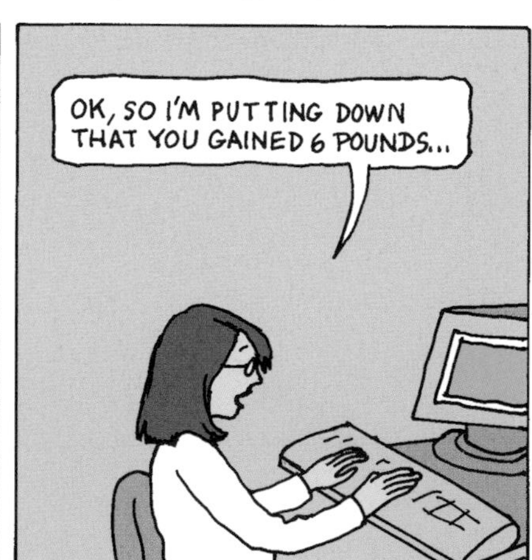

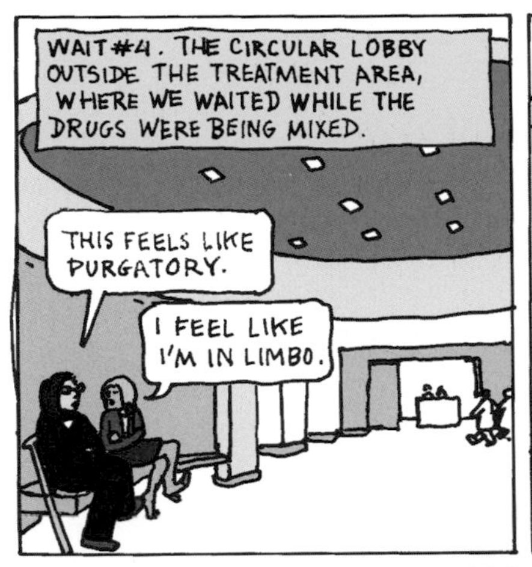
WAIT #4. THE CIRCULAR LOBBY OUTSIDE THE TREATMENT AREA, WHERE WE WAITED WHILE THE DRUGS WERE BEING MIXED.
THIS FEELS LIKE PURGATORY.
I FEEL LIKE I'M IN LIMBO.

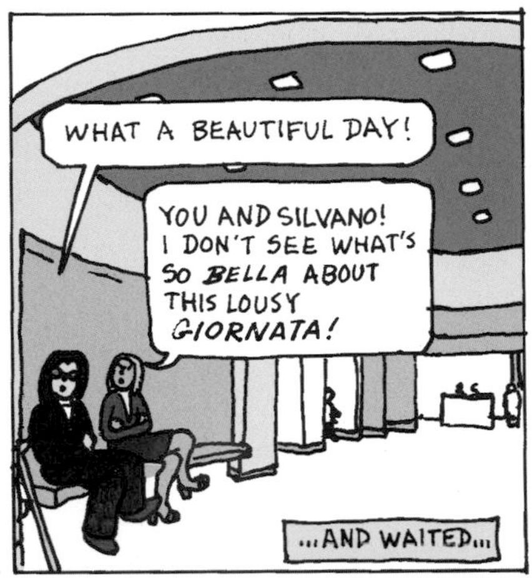
WHAT A BEAUTIFUL DAY!
YOU AND SILVANO! I DON'T SEE WHAT'S SO *BELLA* ABOUT THIS LOUSY *GIORNATA!*
...AND WAITED...

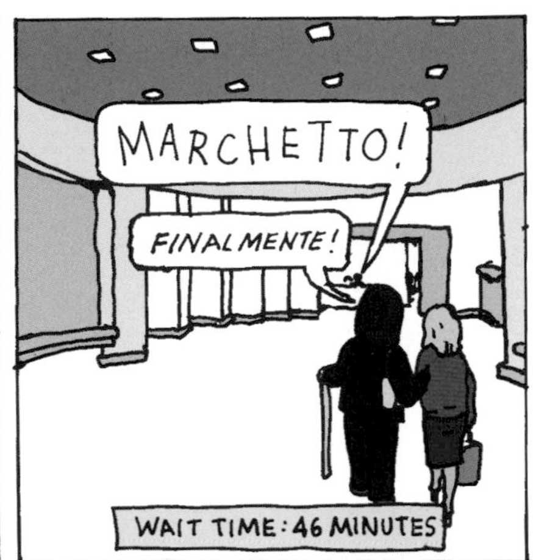
MARCHETTO!
FINALMENTE!
WAIT TIME: 46 MINUTES

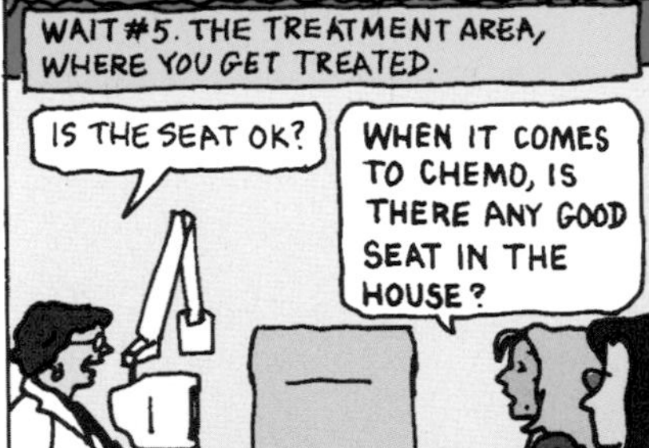
WAIT #5. THE TREATMENT AREA, WHERE YOU GET TREATED.
IS THE SEAT OK?
WHEN IT COMES TO CHEMO, IS THERE ANY GOOD SEAT IN THE HOUSE?

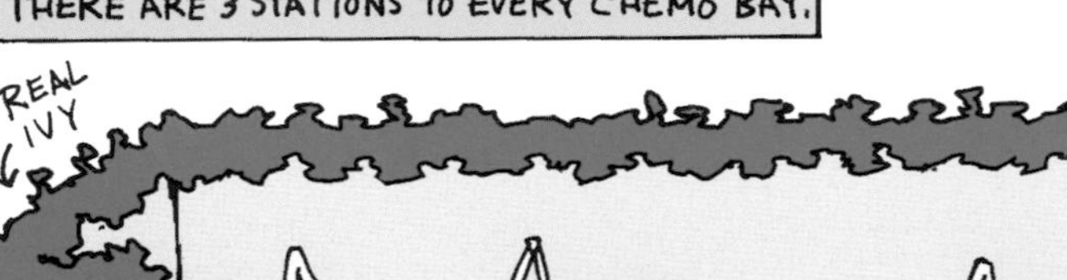
THERE ARE 3 STATIONS TO EVERY CHEMO BAY.
REAL IVY

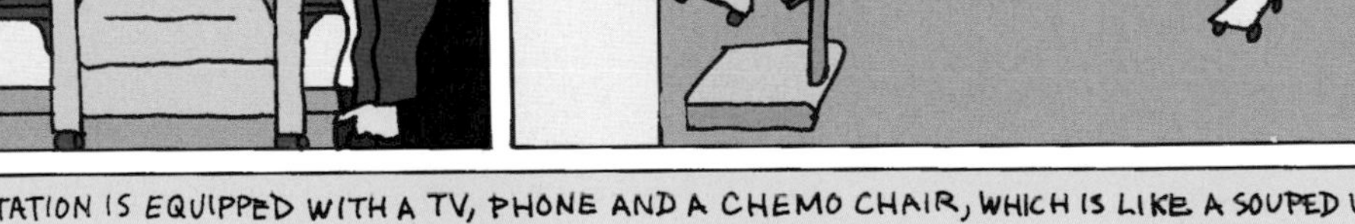
EACH STATION IS EQUIPPED WITH A TV, PHONE AND A CHEMO CHAIR, WHICH IS LIKE A SOUPED UP LA-Z-BOY.

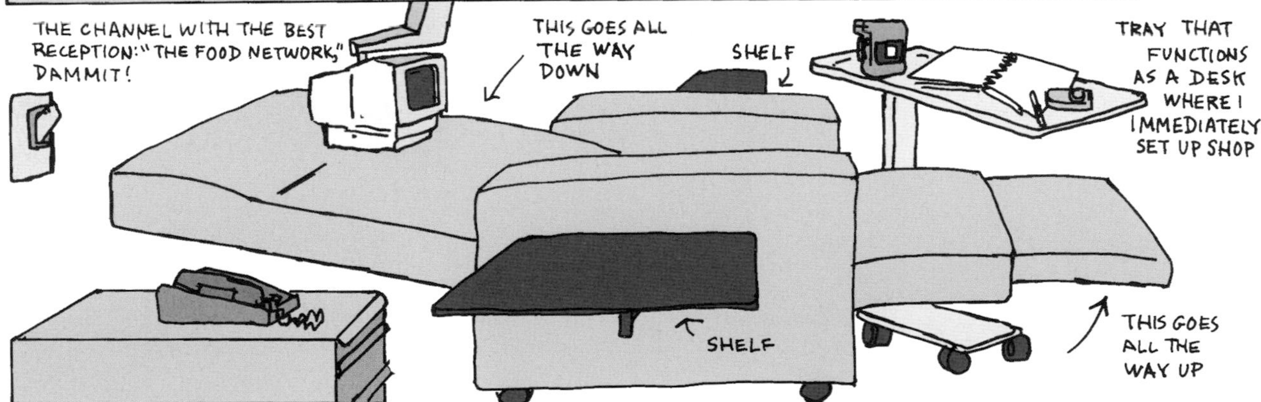
THE CHANNEL WITH THE BEST RECEPTION: "THE FOOD NETWORK," DAMMIT!
THIS GOES ALL THE WAY DOWN
SHELF
TRAY THAT FUNCTIONS AS A DESK WHERE I IMMEDIATELY SET UP SHOP
SHELF
THIS GOES ALL THE WAY UP

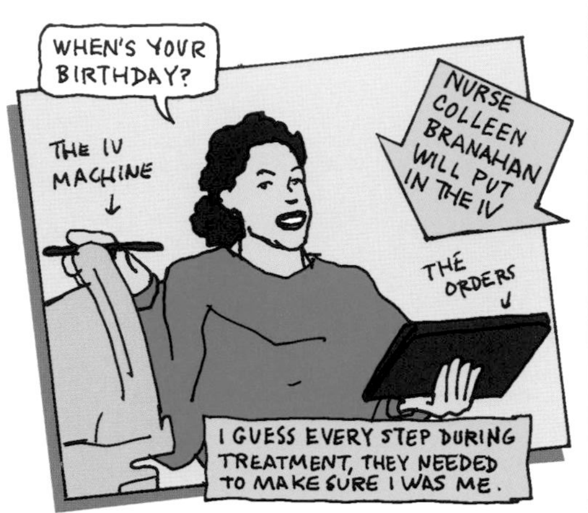

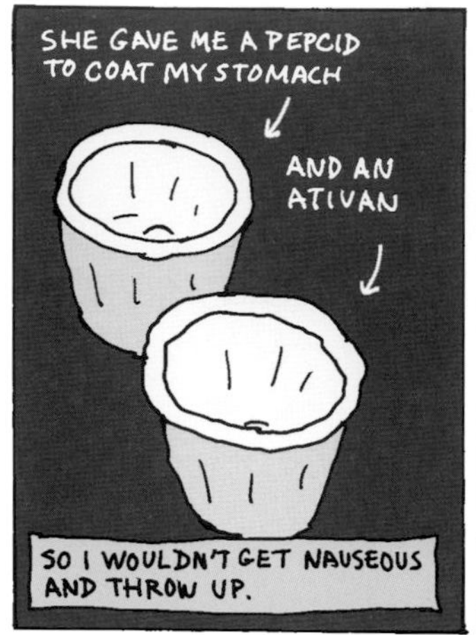

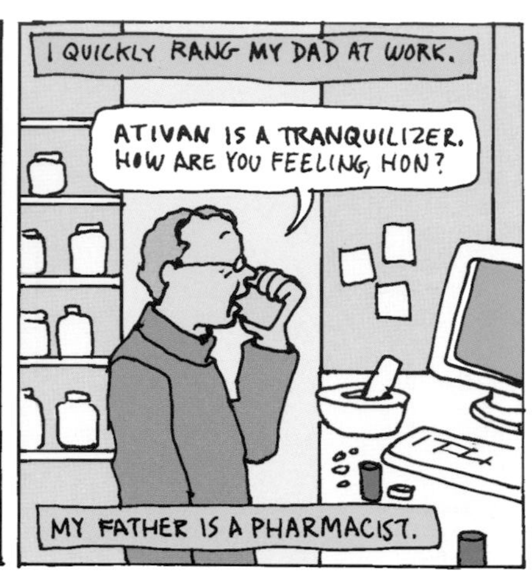

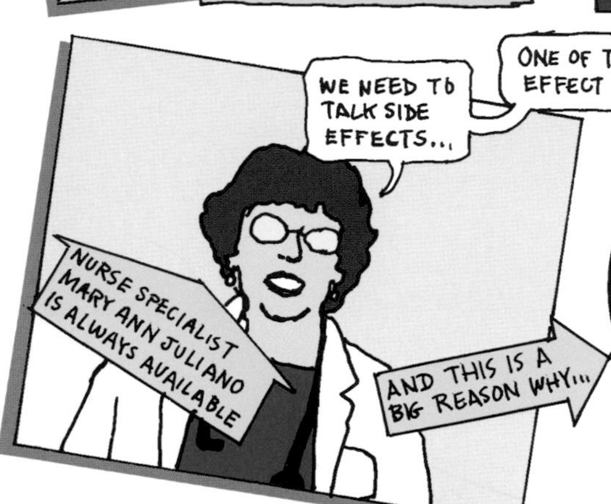

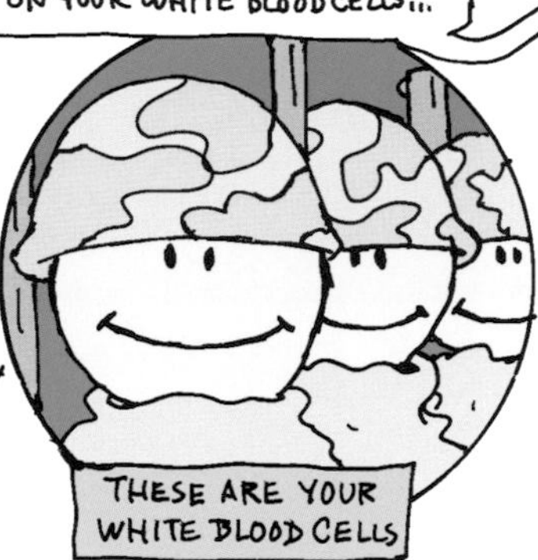

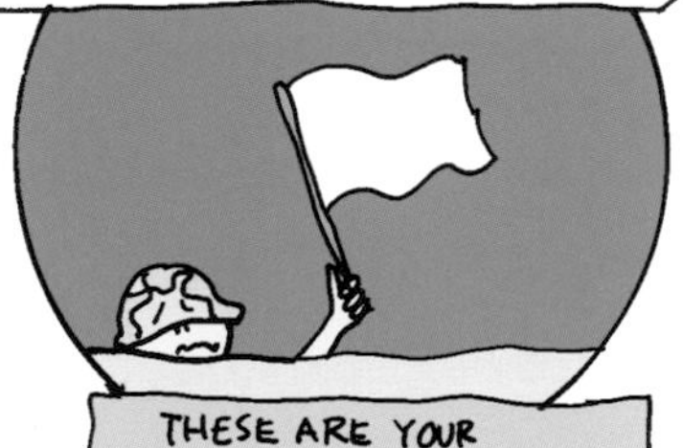

STAY AWAY FROM KIDS, BIG CROWDS, ANYONE WHO'S SICK AND DON'T GO AROUND KISSING EVERYBODY, TELL THEM *YOU* HAVE A SORE THROAT.

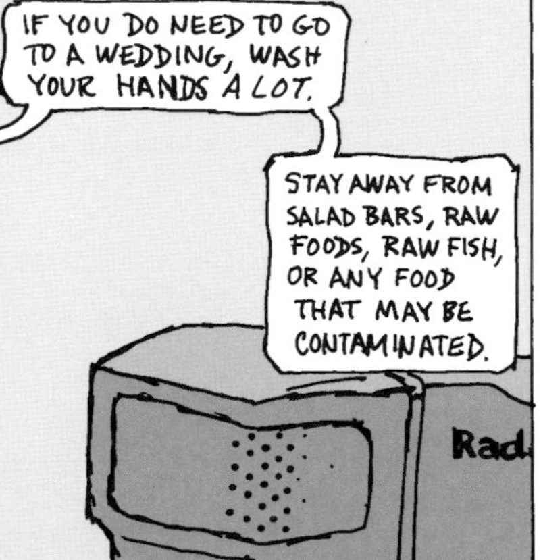

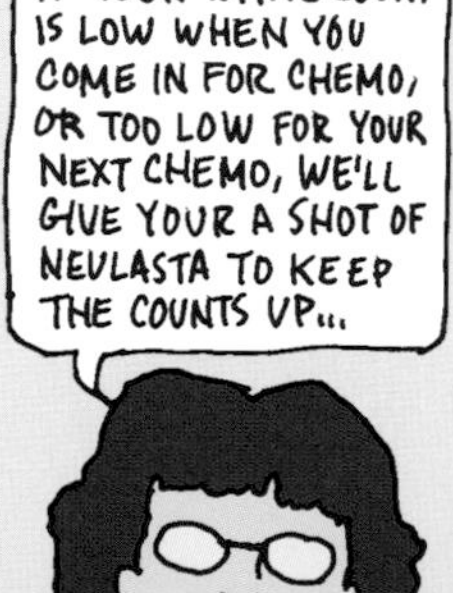

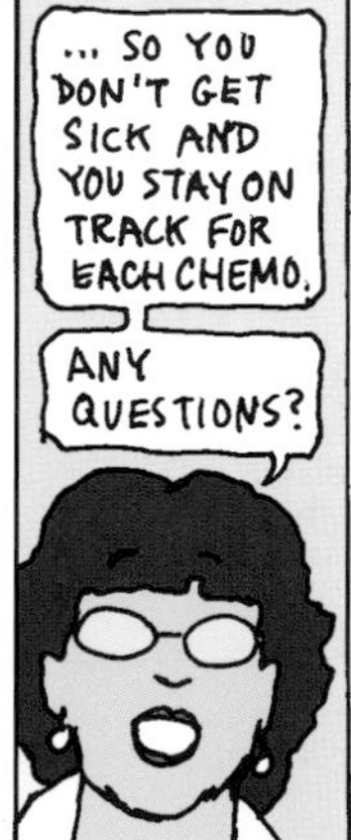

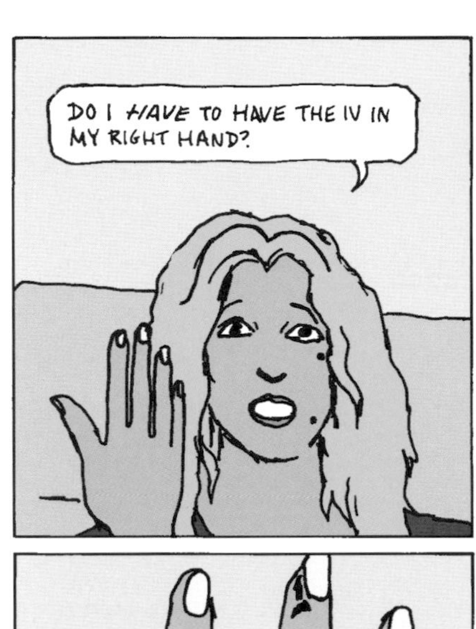

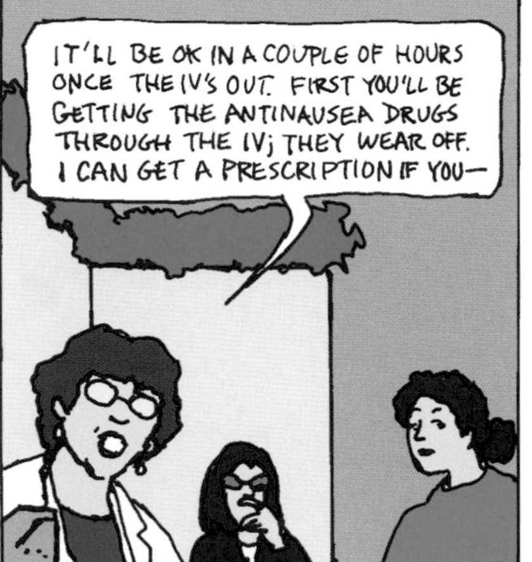

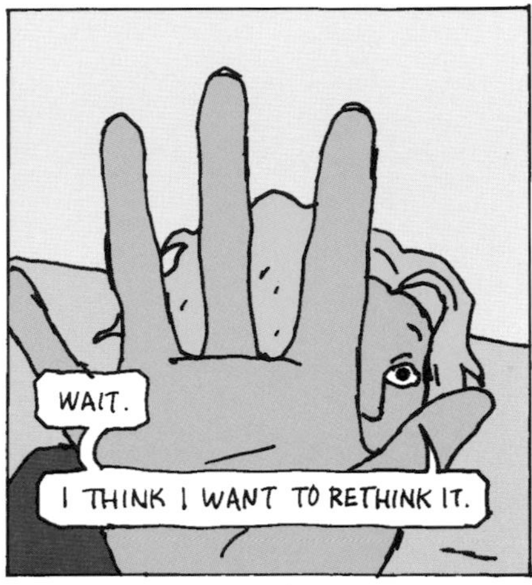

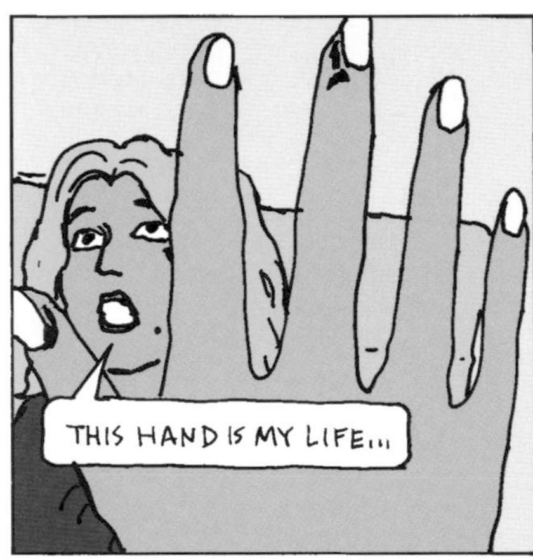

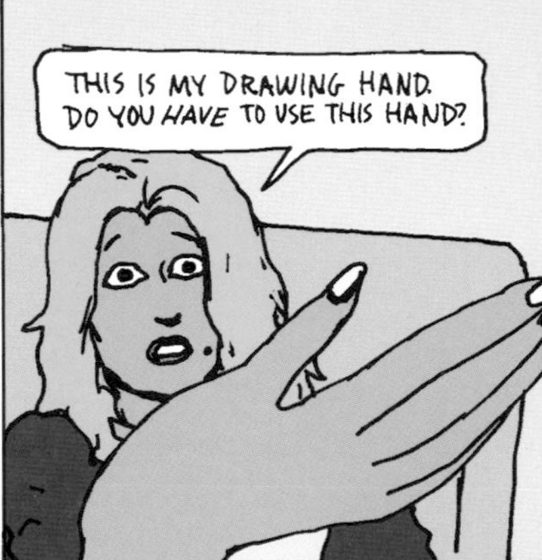

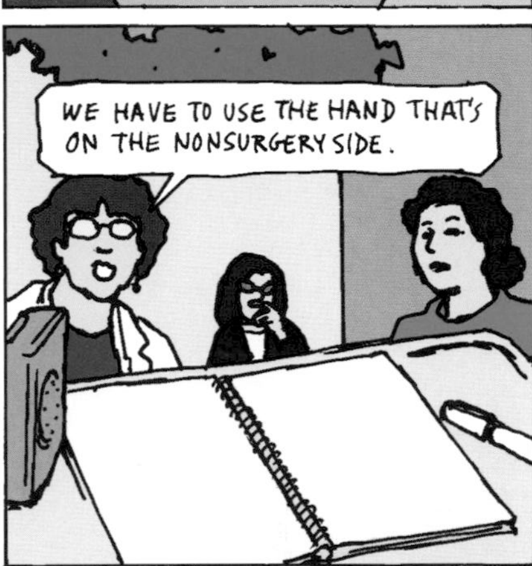

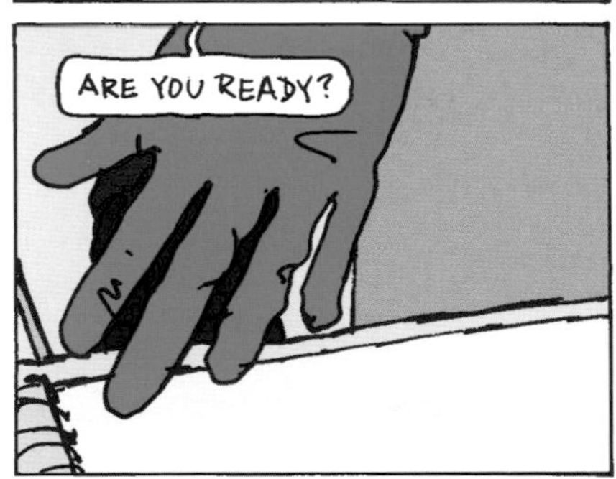

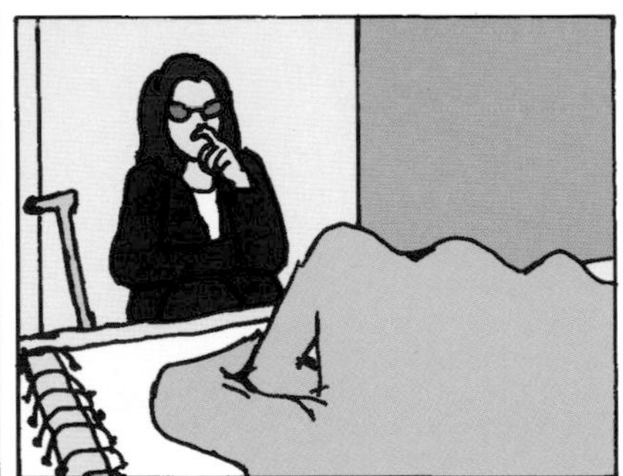

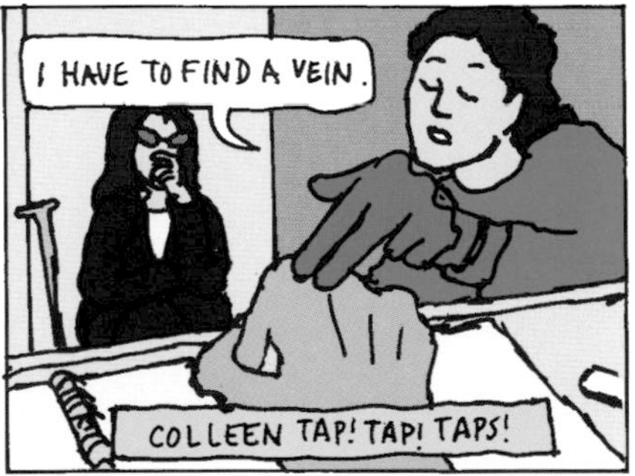

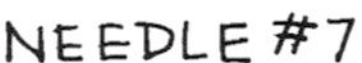

NEEDLE #7

THE CHEMO IV (#1 OF 8 TREATMENTS, EACH 3 WEEKS APART)

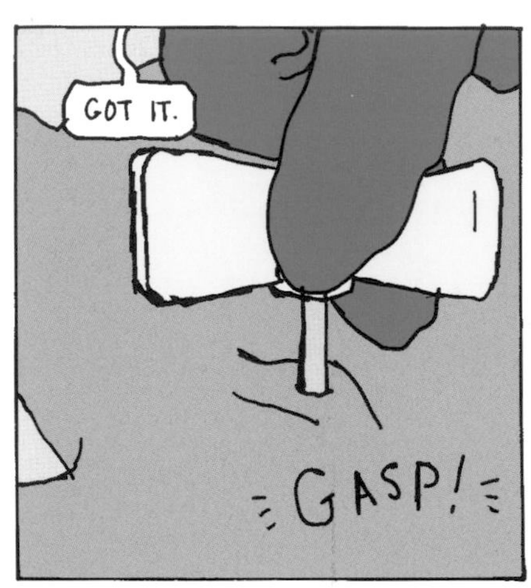
GOT IT.
GASP!

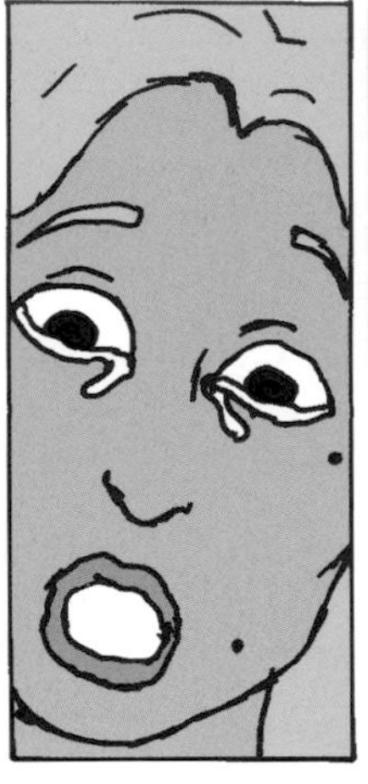

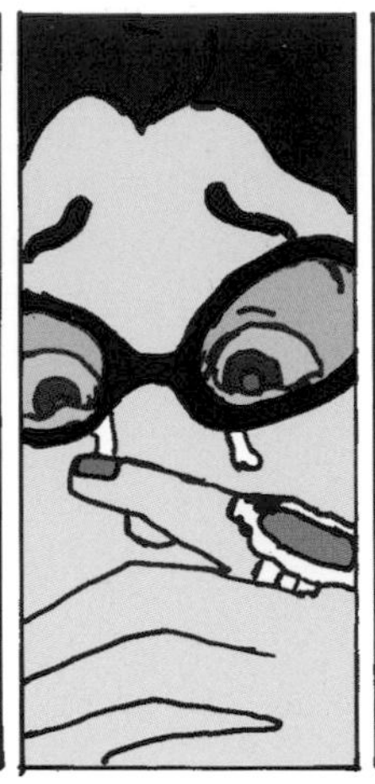

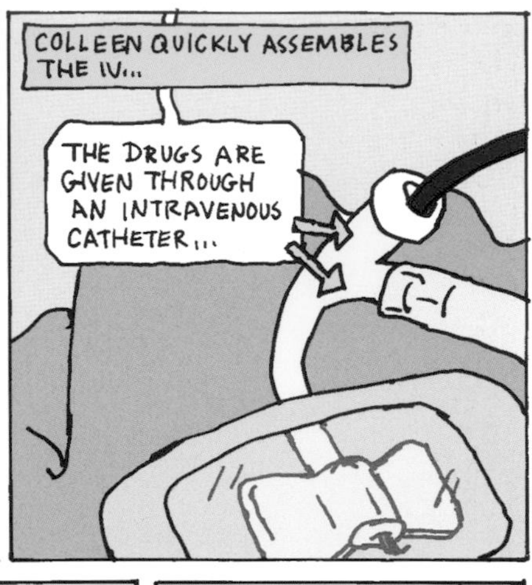
COLLEEN QUICKLY ASSEMBLES THE IV...
THE DRUGS ARE GIVEN THROUGH AN INTRAVENOUS CATHETER...

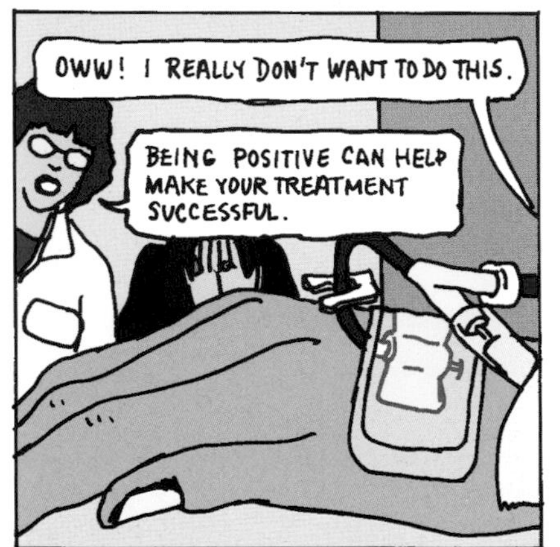
OWW! I REALLY DON'T WANT TO DO THIS.
BEING POSITIVE CAN HELP MAKE YOUR TREATMENT SUCCESSFUL.

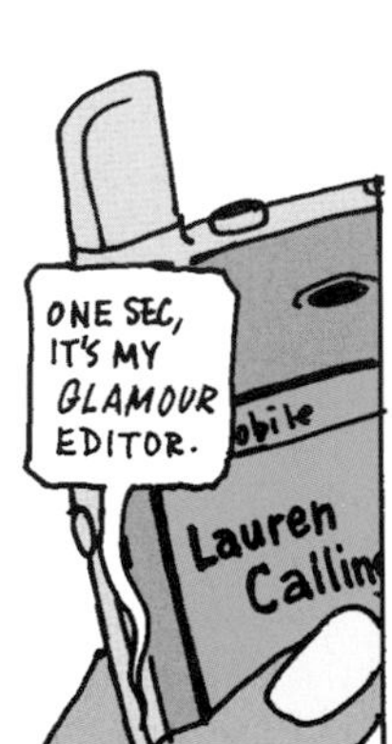
ONE SEC, IT'S MY GLAMOUR EDITOR.
Lauren Callin

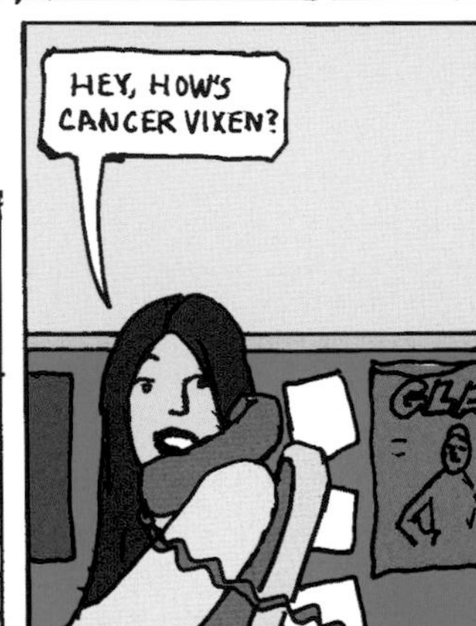
HEY, HOW'S CANCER VIXEN?

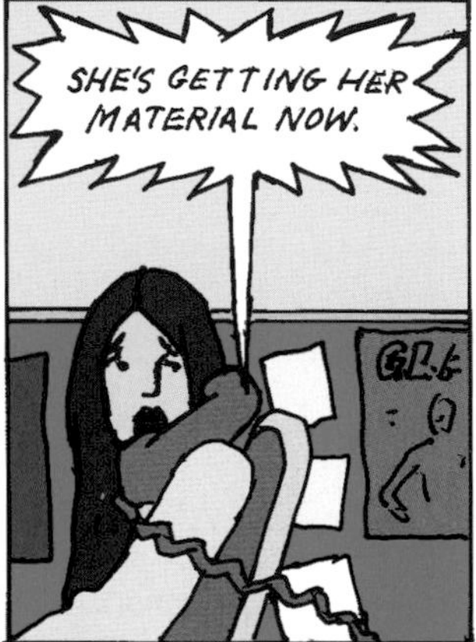
SHE'S GETTING HER MATERIAL NOW.

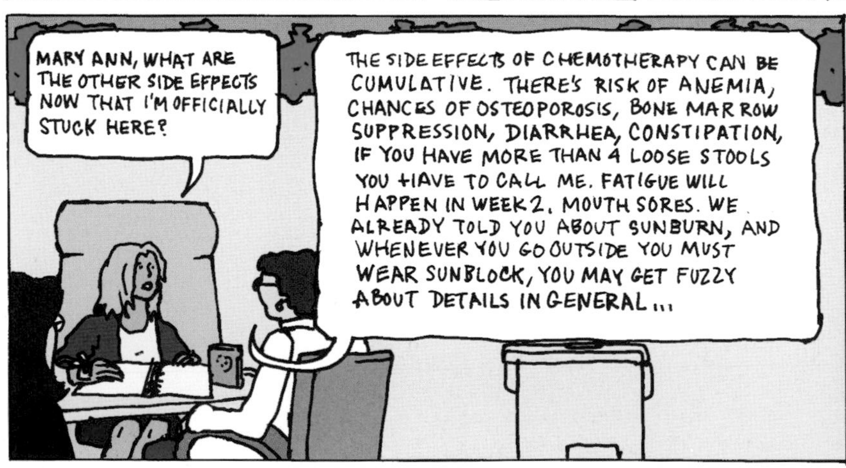
MARY ANN, WHAT ARE THE OTHER SIDE EFFECTS NOW THAT I'M OFFICIALLY STUCK HERE?
THE SIDE EFFECTS OF CHEMOTHERAPY CAN BE CUMULATIVE. THERE'S RISK OF ANEMIA, CHANCES OF OSTEOPOROSIS, BONE MARROW SUPPRESSION, DIARRHEA, CONSTIPATION, IF YOU HAVE MORE THAN 4 LOOSE STOOLS YOU HAVE TO CALL ME. FATIGUE WILL HAPPEN IN WEEK 2. MOUTH SORES. WE ALREADY TOLD YOU ABOUT SUNBURN, AND WHENEVER YOU GO OUTSIDE YOU MUST WEAR SUNBLOCK, YOU MAY GET FUZZY ABOUT DETAILS IN GENERAL...

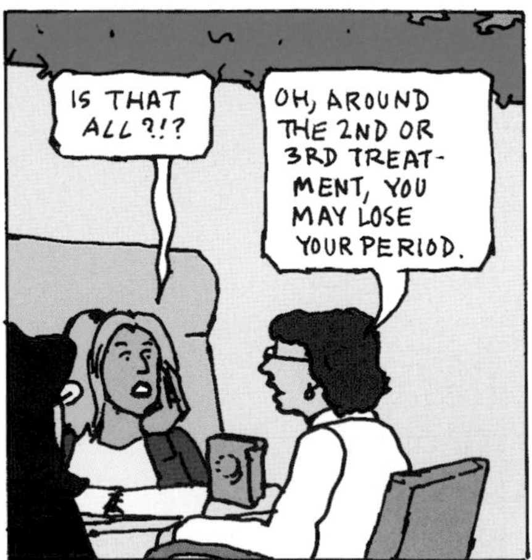
IS THAT ALL?!?
OH, AROUND THE 2ND OR 3RD TREATMENT, YOU MAY LOSE YOUR PERIOD.

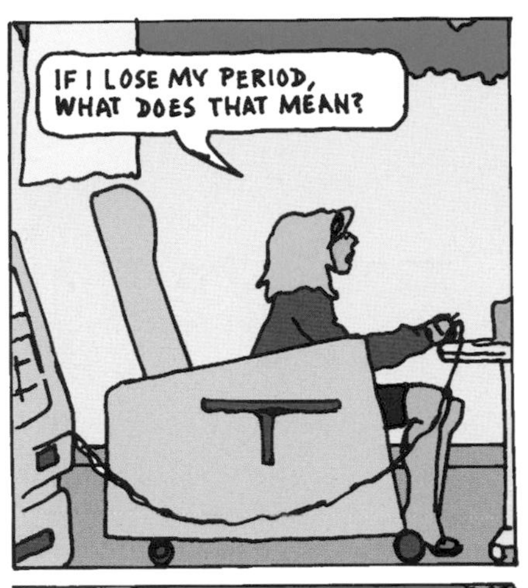
IF I LOSE MY PERIOD, WHAT DOES THAT MEAN?
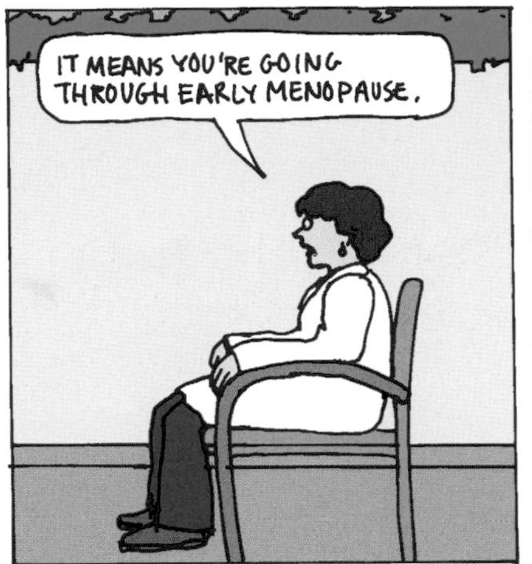
IT MEANS YOU'RE GOING THROUGH EARLY MENOPAUSE.
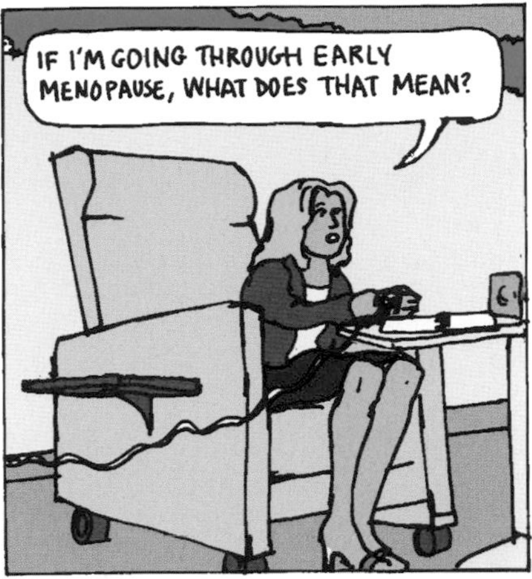
IF I'M GOING THROUGH EARLY MENOPAUSE, WHAT DOES THAT MEAN?
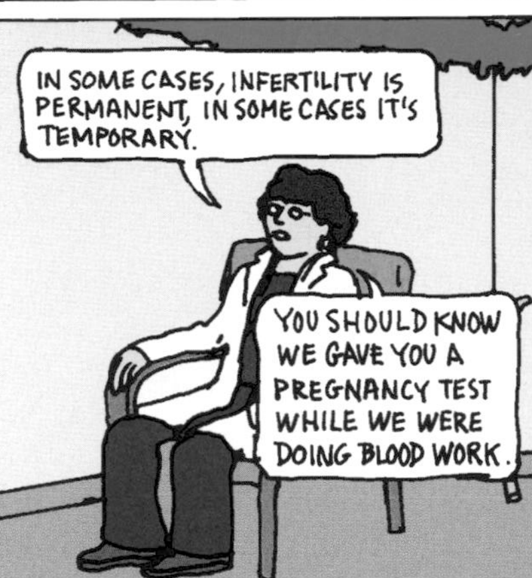
IN SOME CASES, INFERTILITY IS PERMANENT, IN SOME CASES IT'S TEMPORARY.
YOU SHOULD KNOW WE GAVE YOU A PREGNANCY TEST WHILE WE WERE DOING BLOOD WORK.
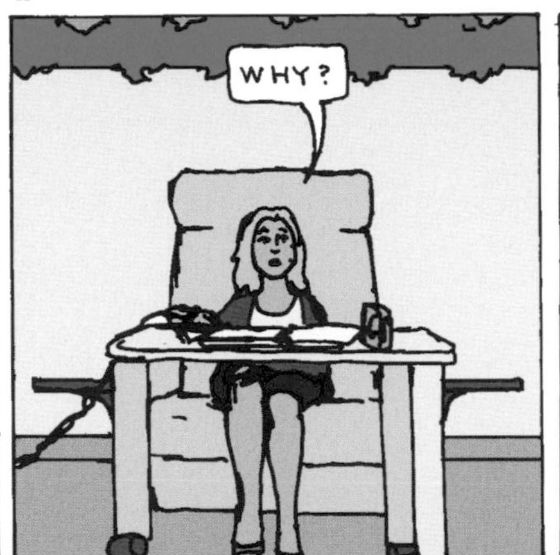
WHY?
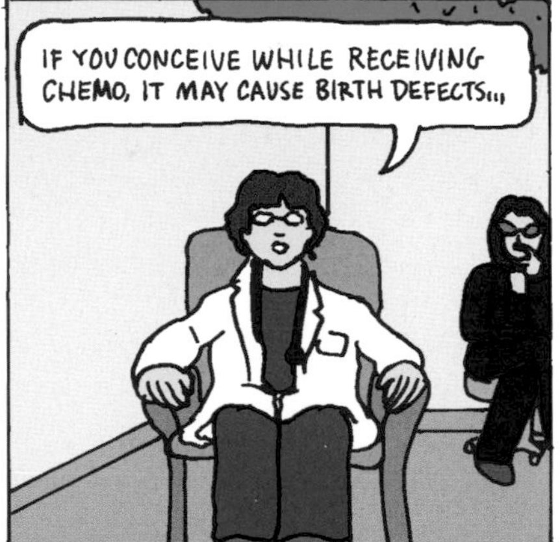
IF YOU CONCEIVE WHILE RECEIVING CHEMO, IT MAY CAUSE BIRTH DEFECTS...
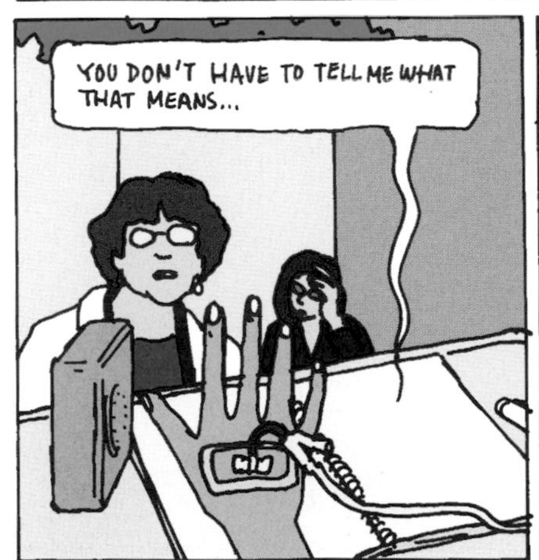
YOU DON'T HAVE TO TELL ME WHAT THAT MEANS...
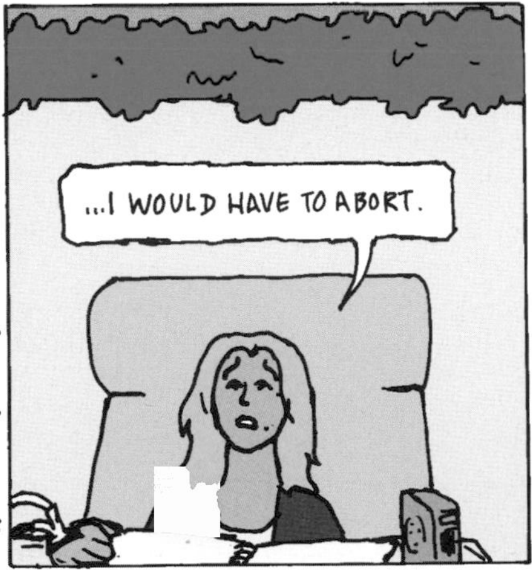
...I WOULD HAVE TO ABORT.
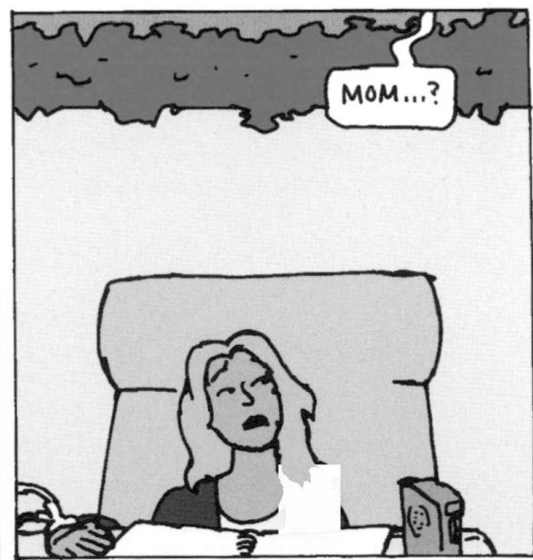
MOM...?

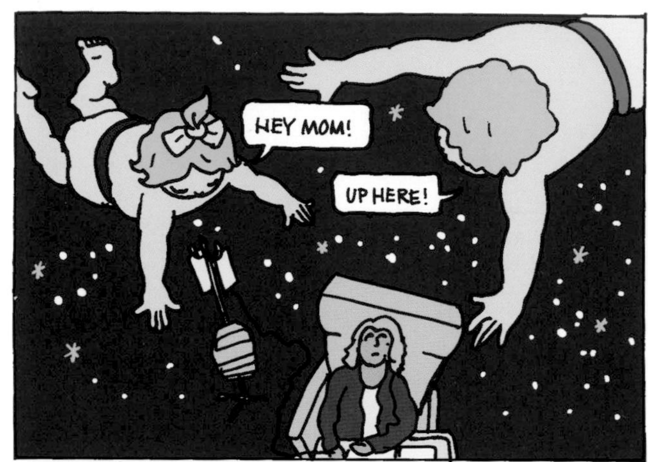
HEY MOM!
UP HERE!

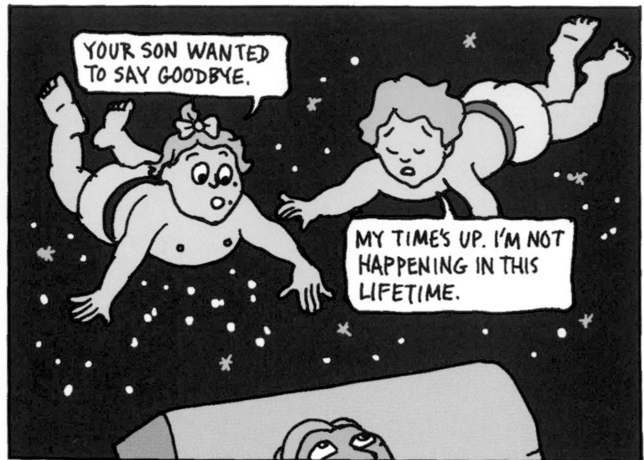
YOUR SON WANTED TO SAY GOODBYE.
MY TIME'S UP. I'M NOT HAPPENING IN THIS LIFETIME.

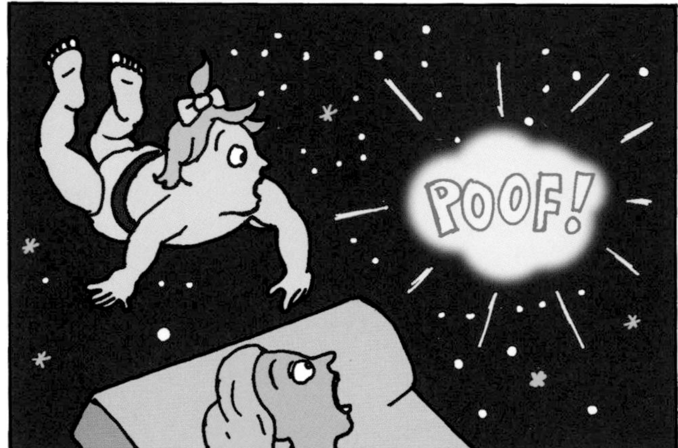
POOF!

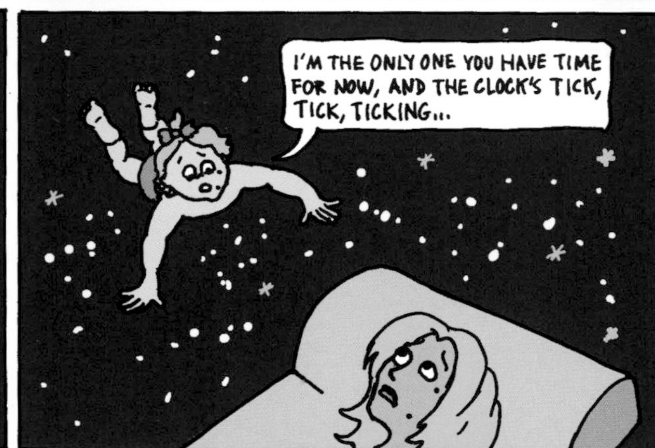
I'M THE ONLY ONE YOU HAVE TIME FOR NOW, AND THE CLOCK'S TICK, TICK, TICKING...

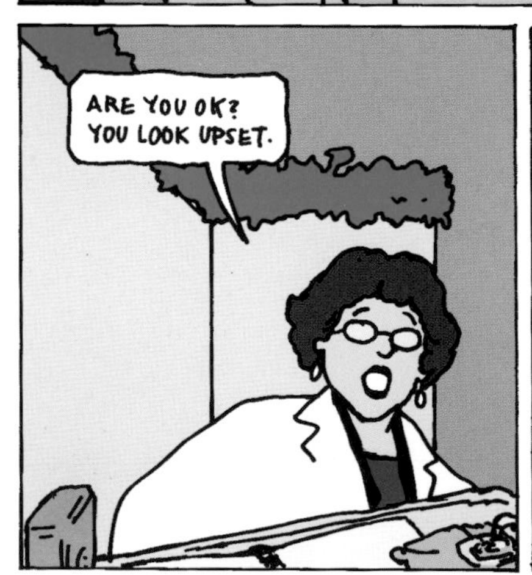
ARE YOU OK? YOU LOOK UPSET.

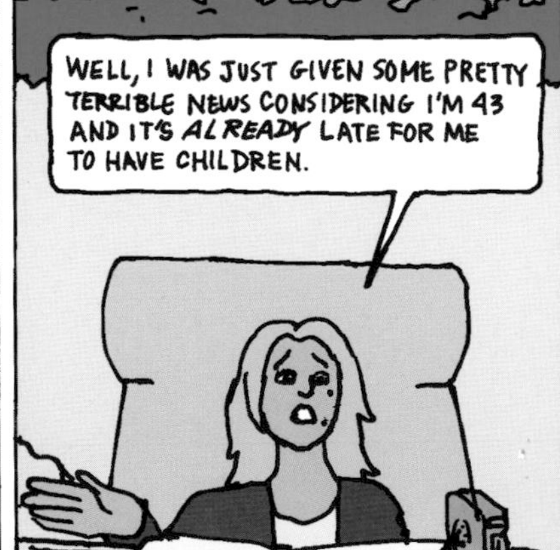
WELL, I WAS JUST GIVEN SOME PRETTY TERRIBLE NEWS CONSIDERING I'M 43 AND IT'S *ALREADY* LATE FOR ME TO HAVE CHILDREN.

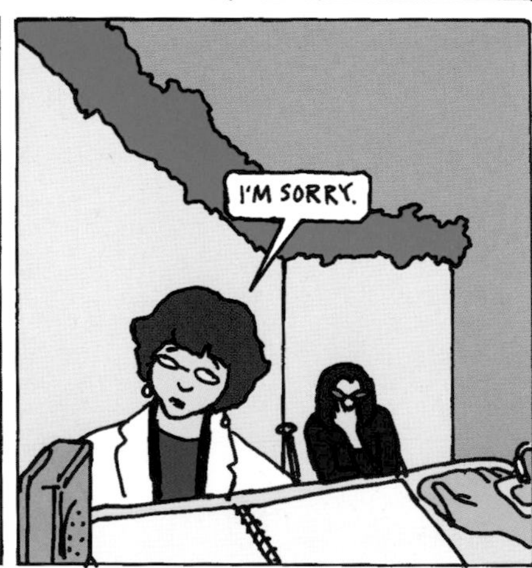
I'M SORRY.

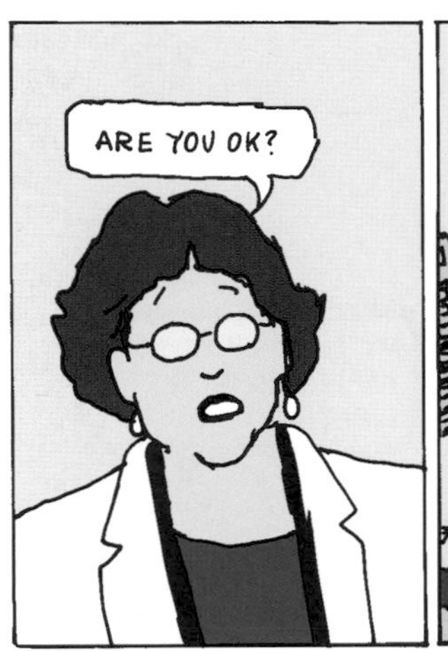
ARE YOU OK?

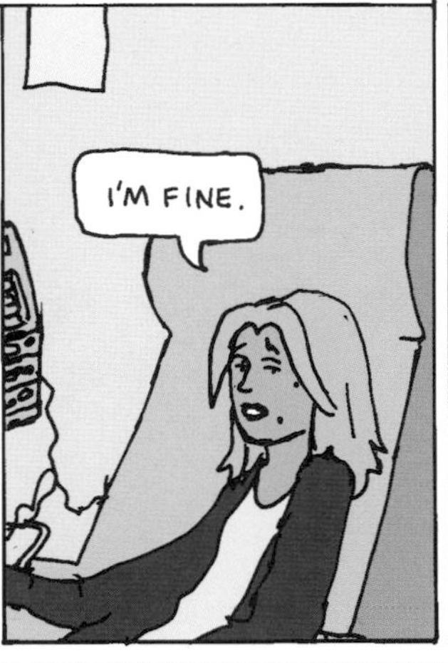
I'M FINE.

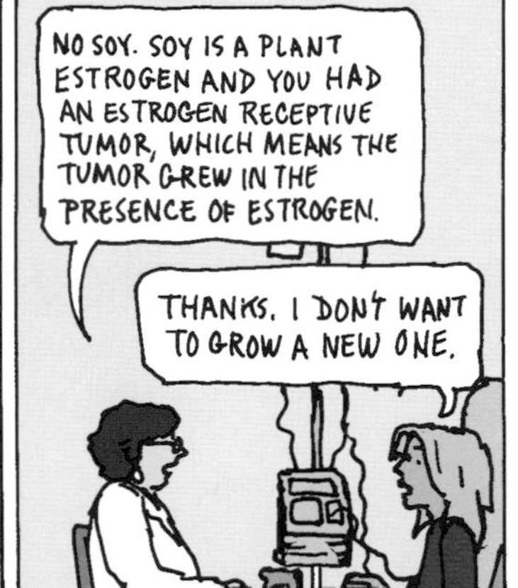
NO SOY. SOY IS A PLANT ESTROGEN AND YOU HAD AN ESTROGEN RECEPTIVE TUMOR, WHICH MEANS THE TUMOR GREW IN THE PRESENCE OF ESTROGEN.
THANKS. I DON'T WANT TO GROW A NEW ONE.

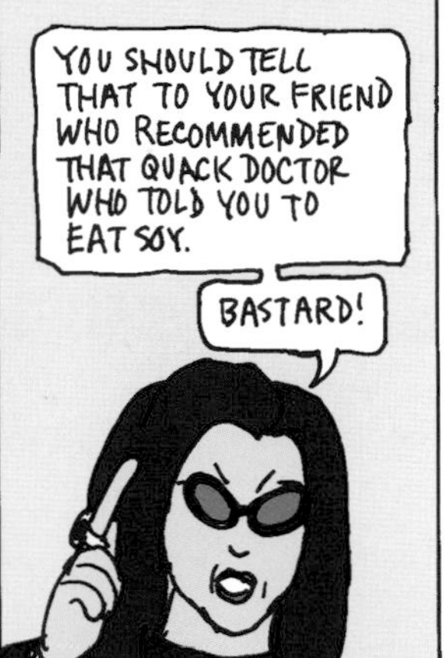
YOU SHOULD TELL THAT TO YOUR FRIEND WHO RECOMMENDED THAT QUACK DOCTOR WHO TOLD YOU TO EAT SOY.
BASTARD!

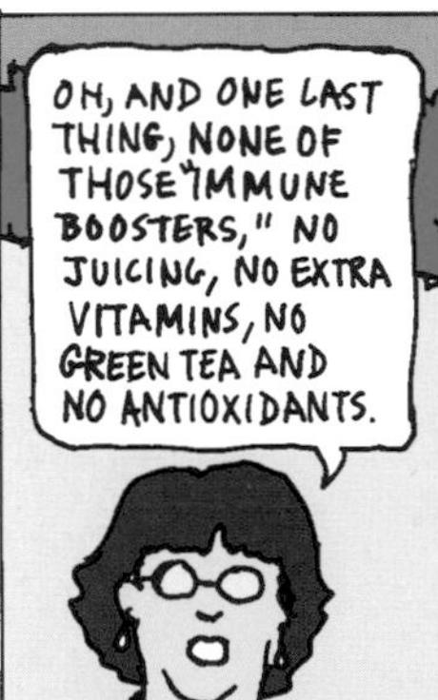
OH, AND ONE LAST THING, NONE OF THOSE "IMMUNE BOOSTERS," NO JUICING, NO EXTRA VITAMINS, NO GREEN TEA AND NO ANTIOXIDANTS.

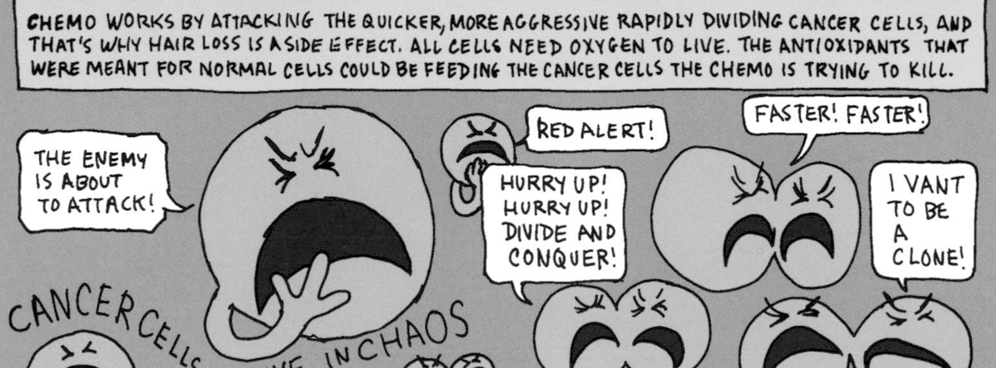
CHEMO WORKS BY ATTACKING THE QUICKER, MORE AGGRESSIVE RAPIDLY DIVIDING CANCER CELLS, AND THAT'S WHY HAIR LOSS IS A SIDE EFFECT. ALL CELLS NEED OXYGEN TO LIVE. THE ANTIOXIDANTS THAT WERE MEANT FOR NORMAL CELLS COULD BE FEEDING THE CANCER CELLS THE CHEMO IS TRYING TO KILL.
THE ENEMY IS ABOUT TO ATTACK!
RED ALERT!
HURRY UP! HURRY UP! DIVIDE AND CONQUER!
FASTER! FASTER!
I VANT TO BE A CLONE!
CANCER CELLS THRIVE IN CHAOS

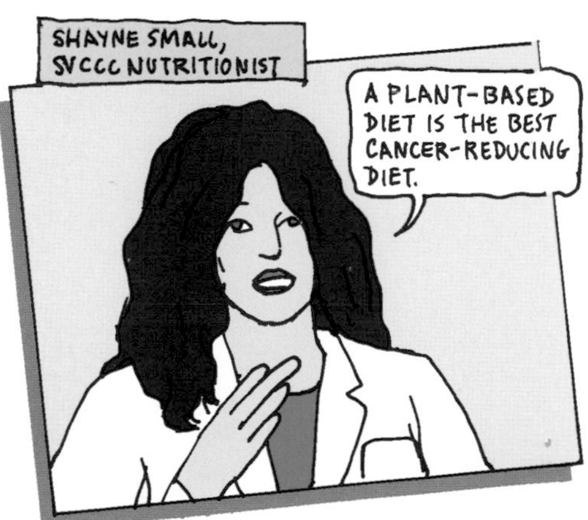
SHAYNE SMALL, SVCCC NUTRITIONIST
A PLANT-BASED DIET IS THE BEST CANCER-REDUCING DIET.

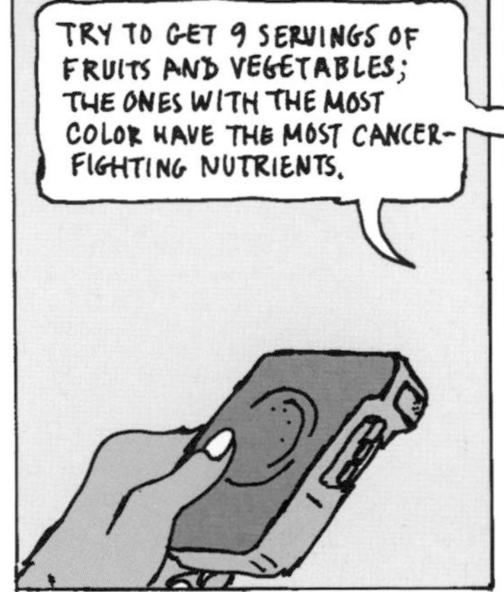
TRY TO GET 9 SERVINGS OF FRUITS AND VEGETABLES; THE ONES WITH THE MOST COLOR HAVE THE MOST CANCER-FIGHTING NUTRIENTS.

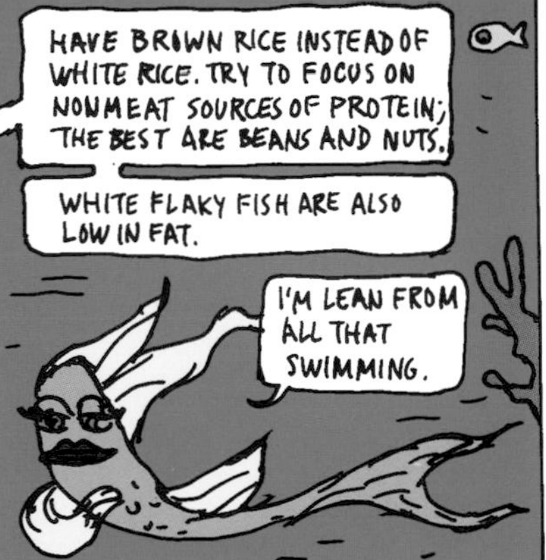
HAVE BROWN RICE INSTEAD OF WHITE RICE. TRY TO FOCUS ON NONMEAT SOURCES OF PROTEIN; THE BEST ARE BEANS AND NUTS.
WHITE FLAKY FISH ARE ALSO LOW IN FAT.
I'M LEAN FROM ALL THAT SWIMMING.

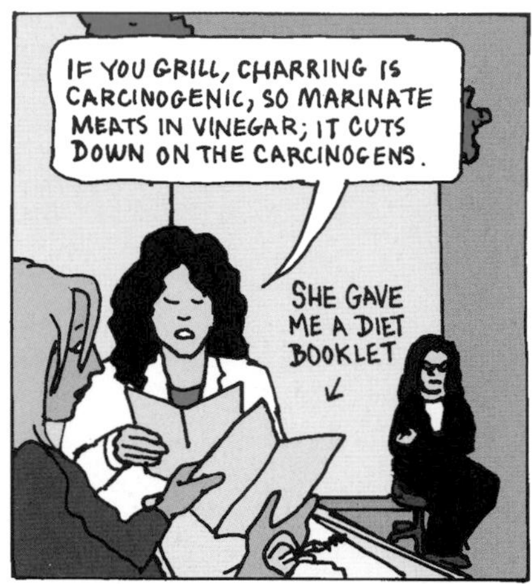
IF YOU GRILL, CHARRING IS CARCINOGENIC, SO MARINATE MEATS IN VINEGAR; IT CUTS DOWN ON THE CARCINOGENS.
SHE GAVE ME A DIET BOOKLET

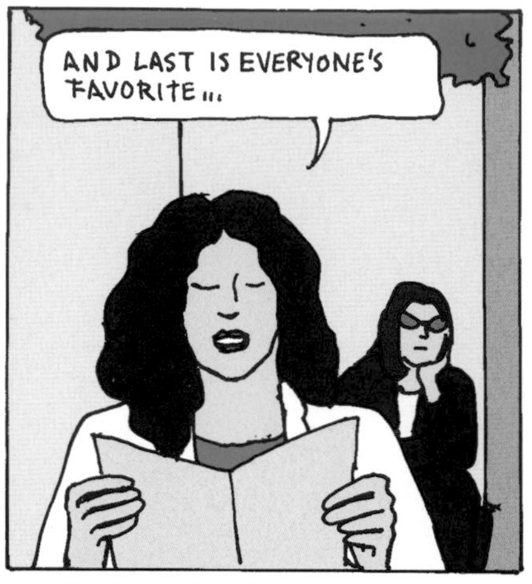
AND LAST IS EVERYONE'S FAVORITE...

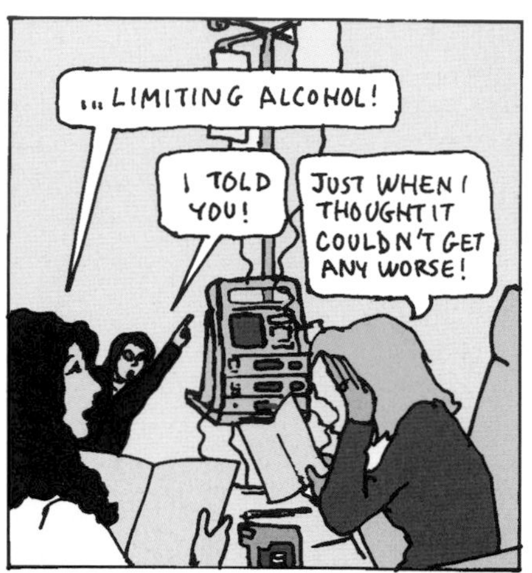
...LIMITING ALCOHOL!
I TOLD YOU!
JUST WHEN I THOUGHT IT COULDN'T GET ANY WORSE!

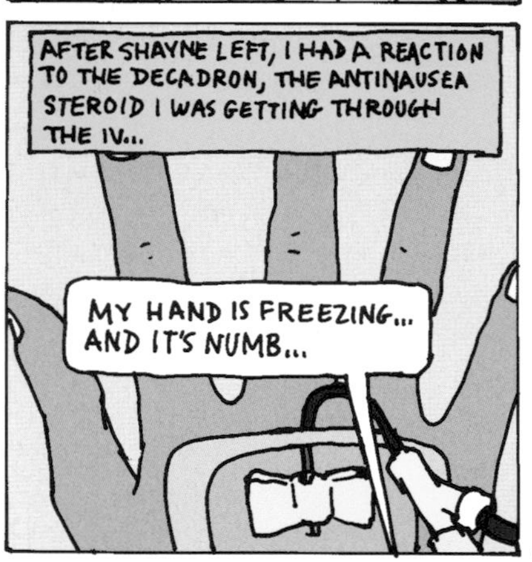
AFTER SHAYNE LEFT, I HAD A REACTION TO THE DECADRON, THE ANTINAUSEA STEROID I WAS GETTING THROUGH THE IV...
MY HAND IS FREEZING... AND IT'S NUMB...

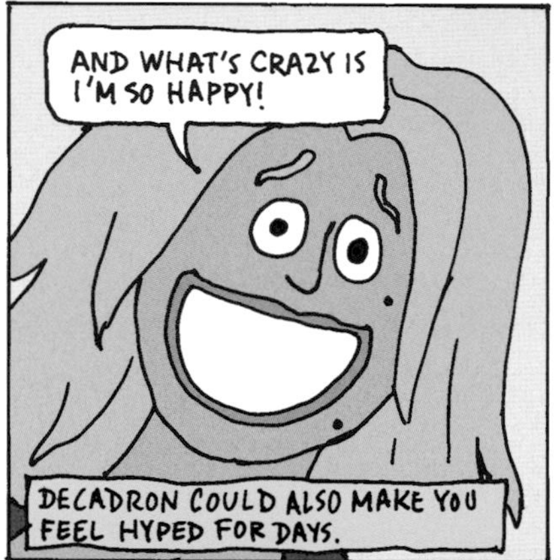
AND WHAT'S CRAZY IS I'M SO HAPPY!
DECADRON COULD ALSO MAKE YOU FEEL HYPED FOR DAYS.

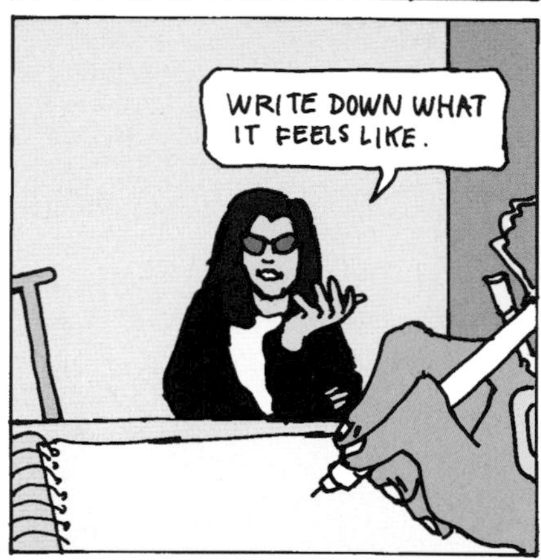
WRITE DOWN WHAT IT FEELS LIKE.

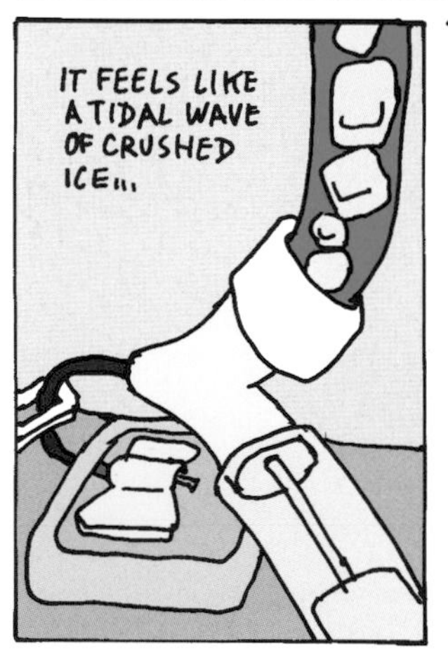
IT FEELS LIKE A TIDAL WAVE OF CRUSHED ICE...

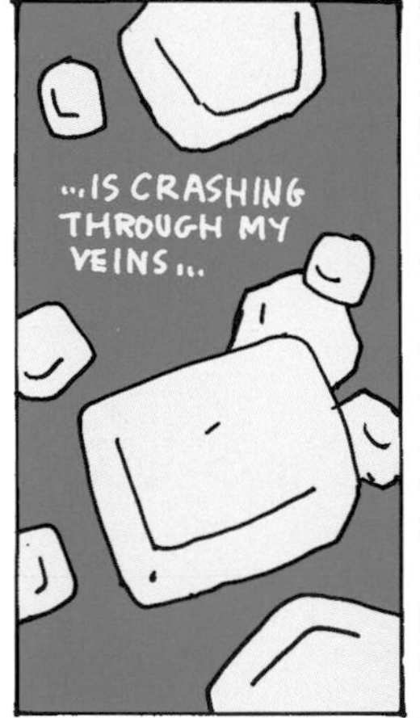
...IS CRASHING THROUGH MY VEINS...

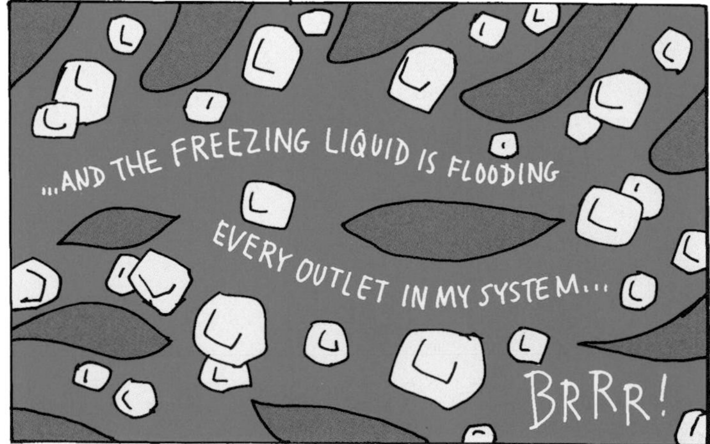
...AND THE FREEZING LIQUID IS FLOODING
EVERY OUTLET IN MY SYSTEM...
BRRR!

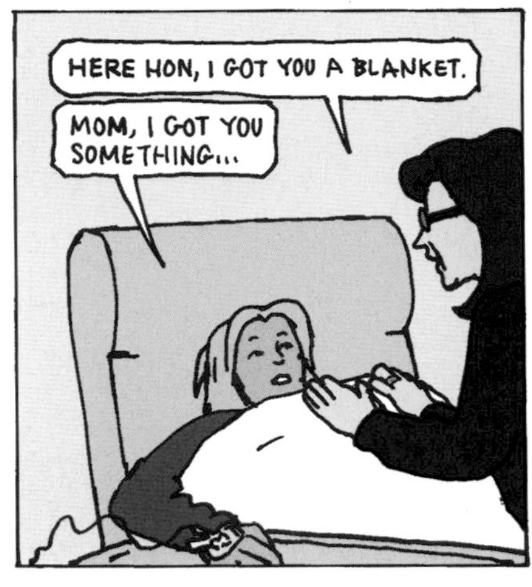
HERE HON, I GOT YOU A BLANKET.
MOM, I GOT YOU SOMETHING...

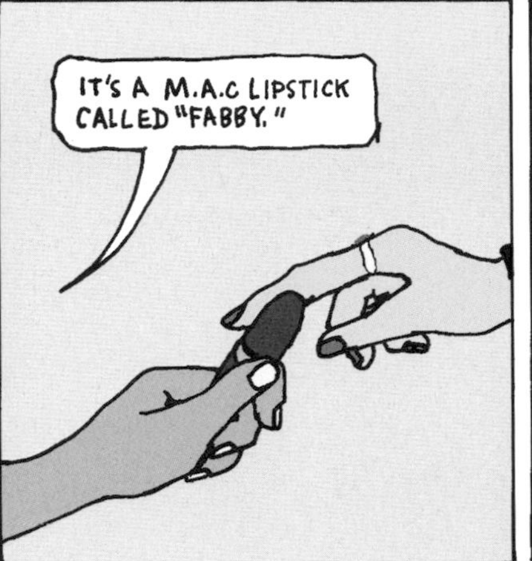
IT'S A M.A.C LIPSTICK CALLED "FABBY."

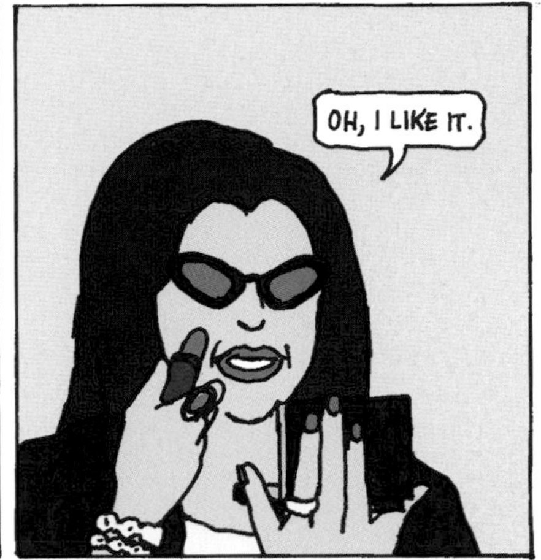
OH, I LIKE IT.

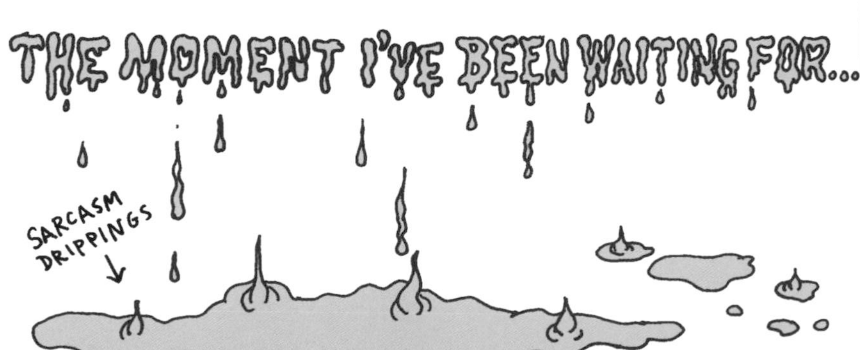
AND NOW,
THE MOMENT I'VE BEEN WAITING FOR...
SARCASM DRIPPINGS

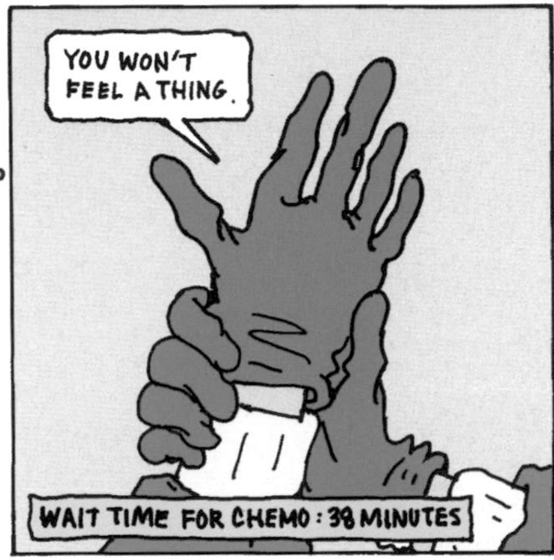
YOU WON'T FEEL A THING.
WAIT TIME FOR CHEMO: 38 MINUTES

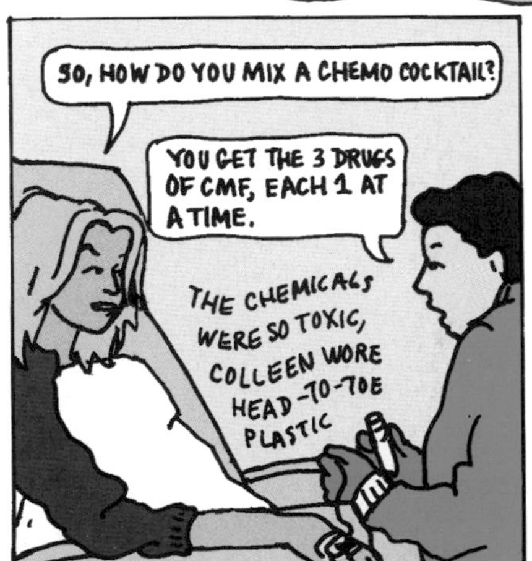
SO, HOW DO YOU MIX A CHEMO COCKTAIL?
YOU GET THE 3 DRUGS OF CMF, EACH 1 AT A TIME.
THE CHEMICALS WERE SO TOXIC, COLLEEN WORE HEAD-TO-TOE PLASTIC

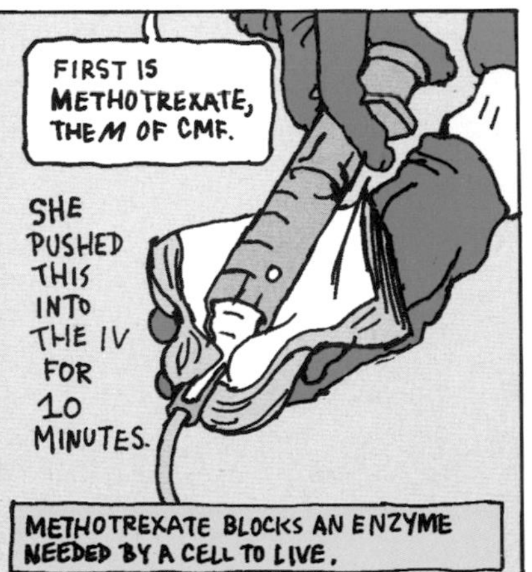
FIRST IS METHOTREXATE, THE M OF CMF.
SHE PUSHED THIS INTO THE IV FOR 10 MINUTES.
METHOTREXATE BLOCKS AN ENZYME NEEDED BY A CELL TO LIVE.

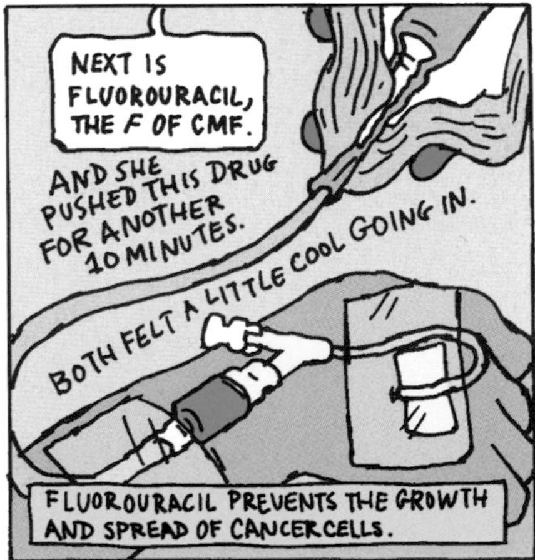
NEXT IS FLUOROURACIL, THE F OF CMF.
AND SHE PUSHED THIS DRUG FOR ANOTHER 10 MINUTES.
BOTH FELT A LITTLE COOL GOING IN.
FLUOROURACIL PREVENTS THE GROWTH AND SPREAD OF CANCER CELLS.

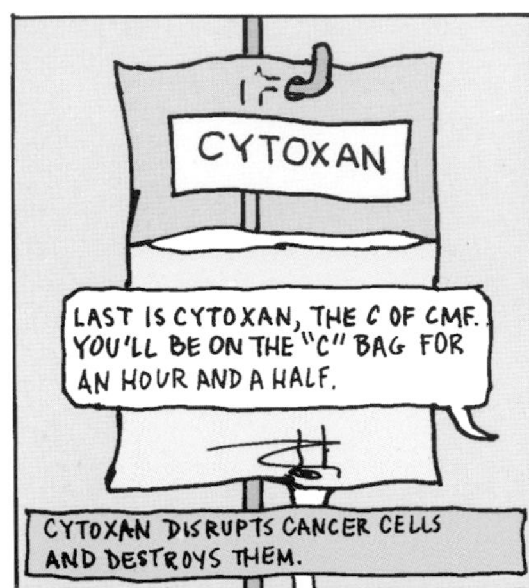

WHILE ON THE "C" BAG...

BEEP!
CHEMO #1 DOWN, 7 MORE TO GO...

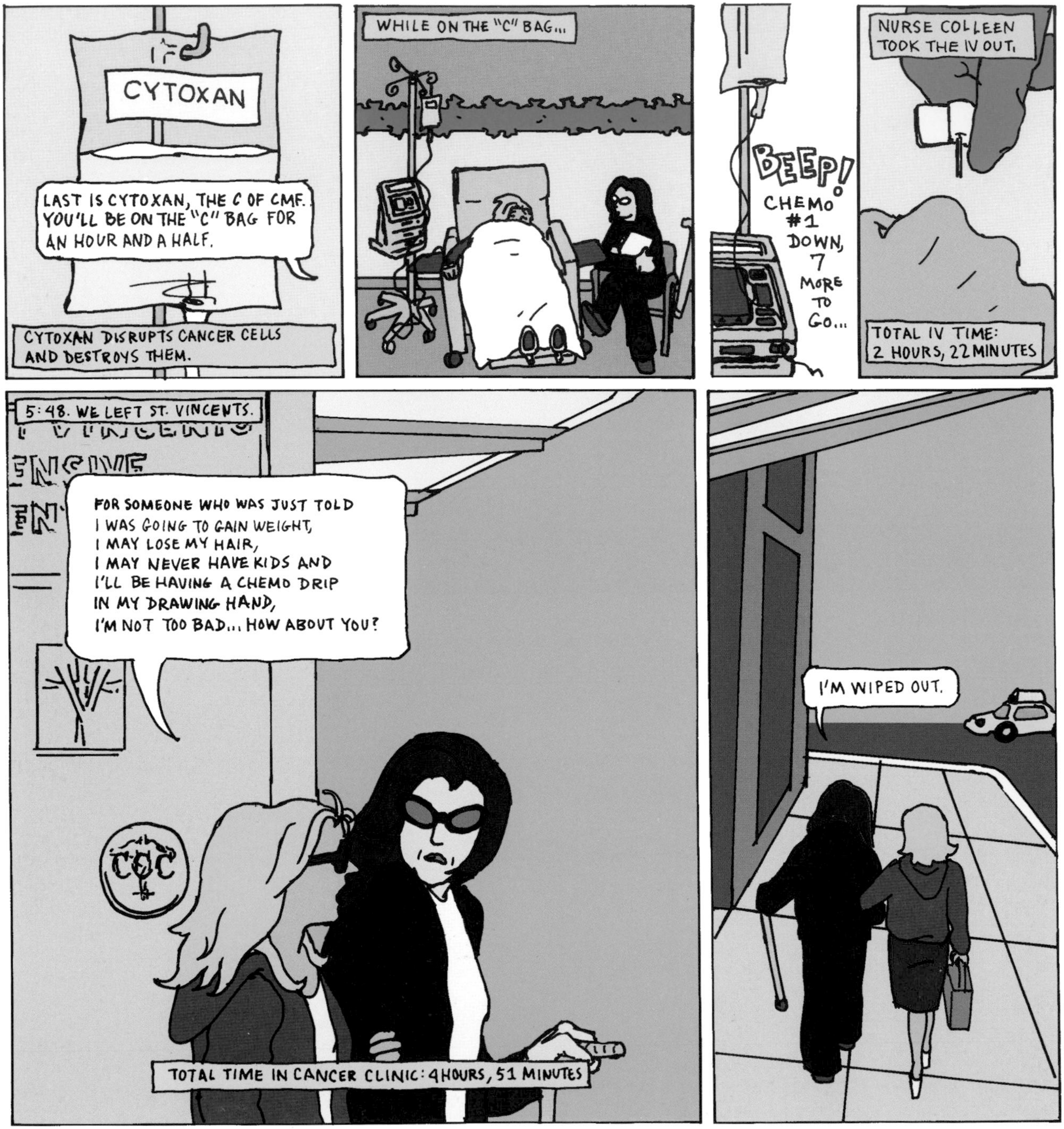

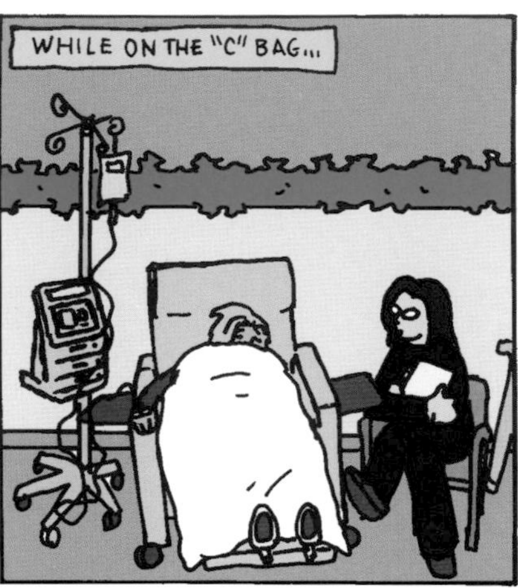

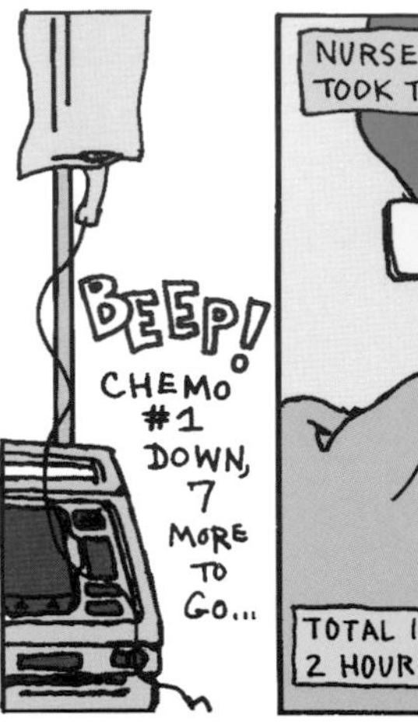

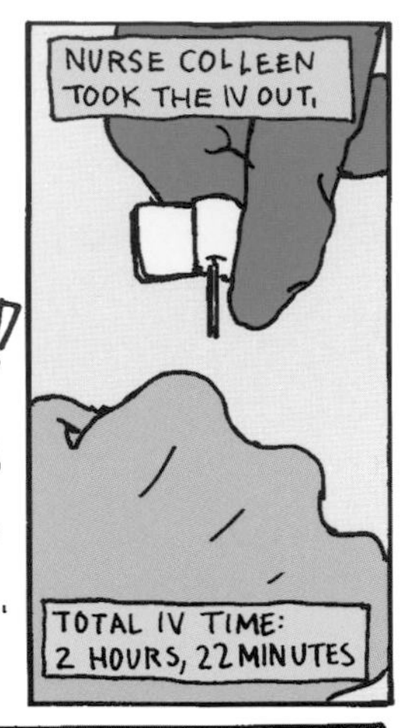

5:48. WE LEFT ST. VINCENTS.

FOR SOMEONE WHO WAS JUST TOLD I WAS GOING TO GAIN WEIGHT, I MAY LOSE MY HAIR, I MAY NEVER HAVE KIDS AND I'LL BE HAVING A CHEMO DRIP IN MY DRAWING HAND, I'M NOT TOO BAD... HOW ABOUT YOU?

TOTAL TIME IN CANCER CLINIC: 4 HOURS, 51 MINUTES

I'M WIPED OUT.

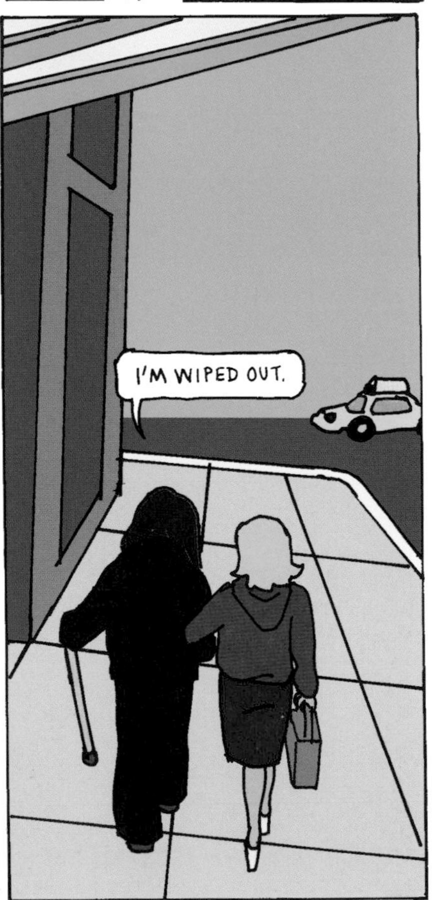

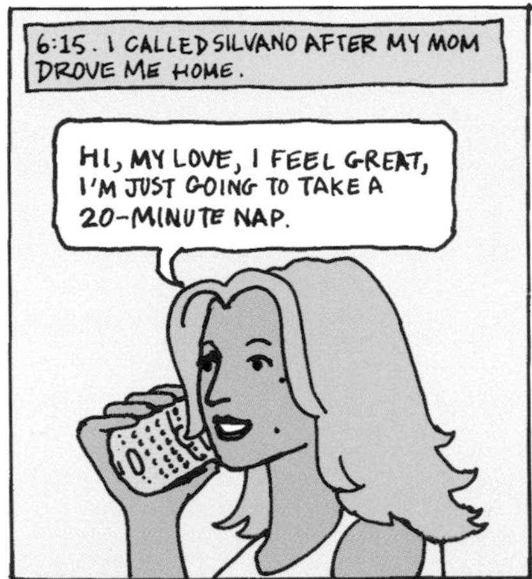
6:15. I CALLED SILVANO AFTER MY MOM DROVE ME HOME.
HI, MY LOVE, I FEEL GREAT, I'M JUST GOING TO TAKE A 20-MINUTE NAP.

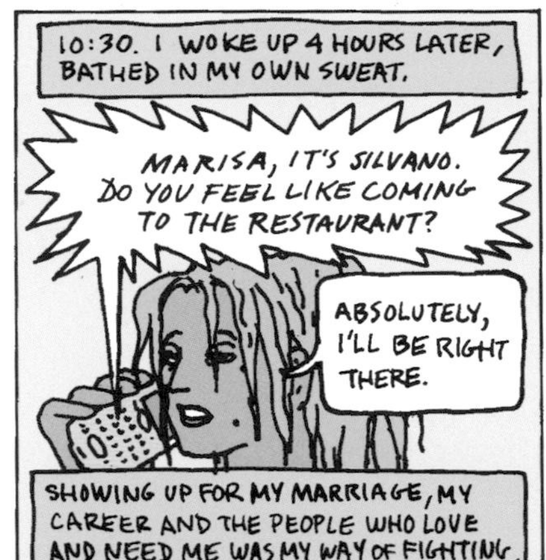
10:30. I WOKE UP 4 HOURS LATER, BATHED IN MY OWN SWEAT.
MARISA, IT'S SILVANO. DO YOU FEEL LIKE COMING TO THE RESTAURANT?
ABSOLUTELY, I'LL BE RIGHT THERE.
SHOWING UP FOR MY MARRIAGE, MY CAREER AND THE PEOPLE WHO LOVE AND NEED ME WAS MY WAY OF FIGHTING.

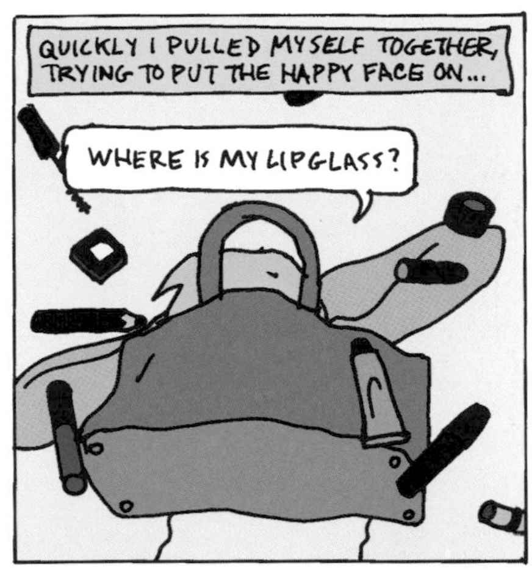
QUICKLY I PULLED MYSELF TOGETHER, TRYING TO PUT THE HAPPY FACE ON...
WHERE IS MY LIPGLASS?

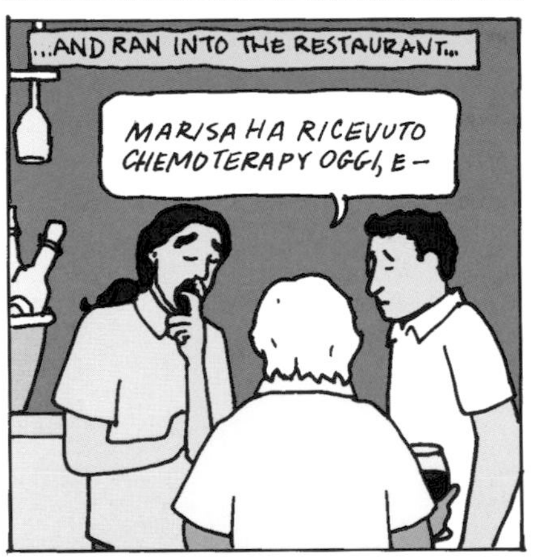
...AND RAN INTO THE RESTAURANT...
MARISA HA RICEVUTO CHEMOTERAPY OGGI, E—

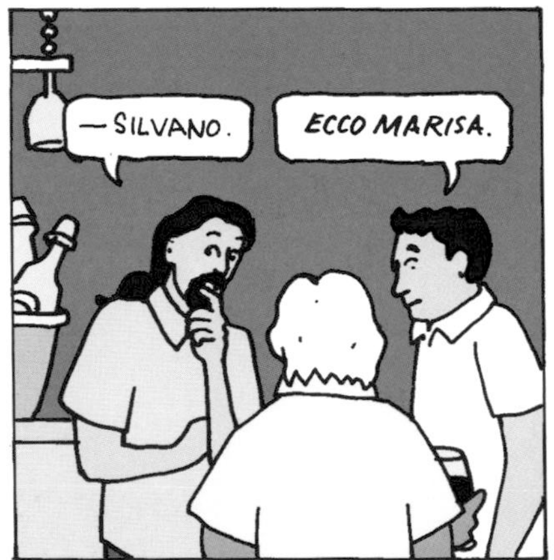
—SILVANO.
ECCO MARISA.

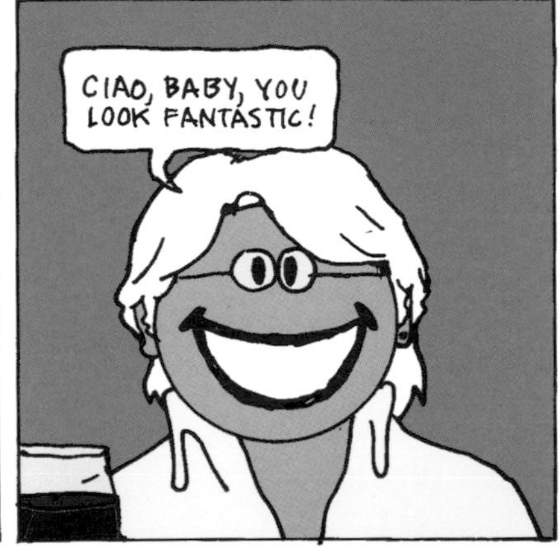
CIAO, BABY, YOU LOOK FANTASTIC!

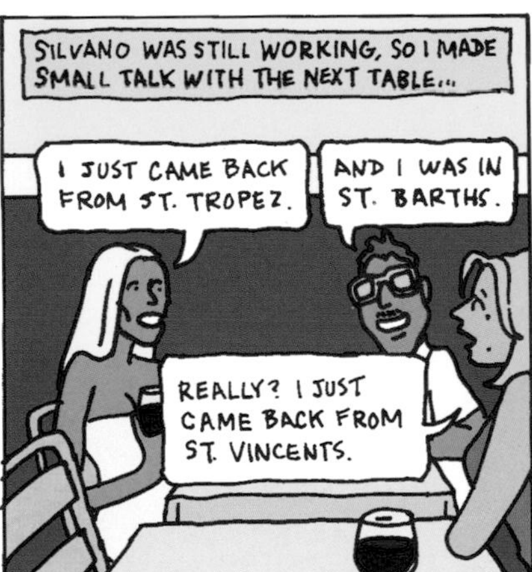
SILVANO WAS STILL WORKING, SO I MADE SMALL TALK WITH THE NEXT TABLE...
I JUST CAME BACK FROM ST. TROPEZ.
AND I WAS IN ST. BARTHS.
REALLY? I JUST CAME BACK FROM ST. VINCENTS.

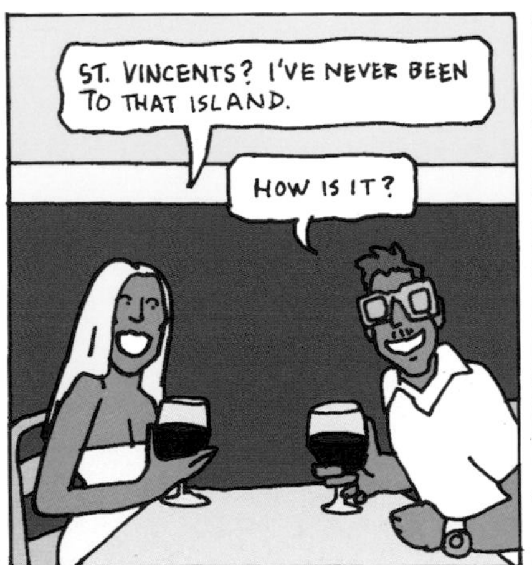
ST. VINCENTS? I'VE NEVER BEEN TO THAT ISLAND.
HOW IS IT?

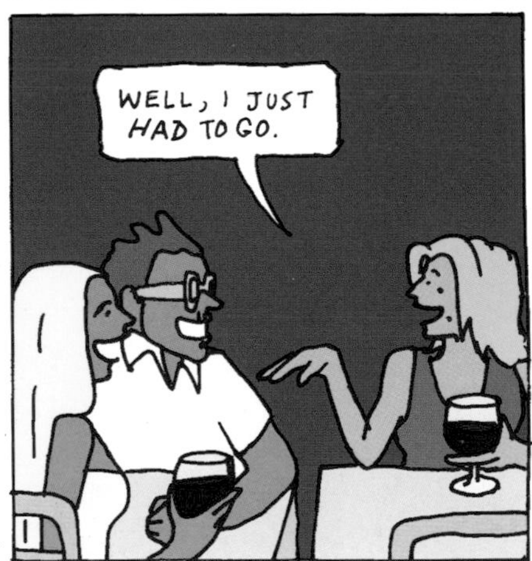
WELL, I JUST HAD TO GO.

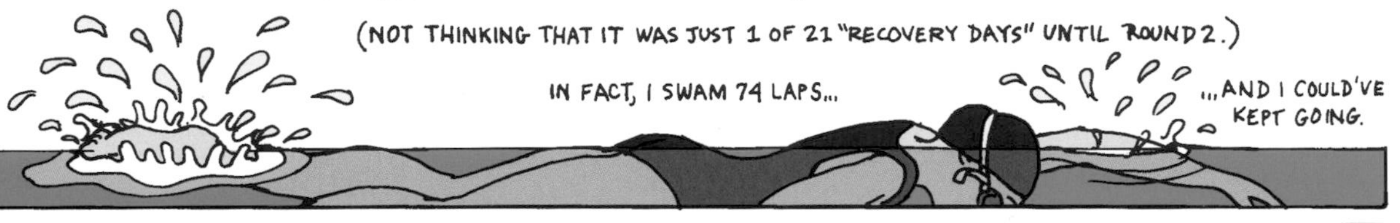
I WAS TO GET TREATED EVERY 3 WEEKS, AND QUICKLY I FOUND OUT THERE WAS A RHYTHM TO IT.
WEEK 1. THE CHEMO HIGH. THE DAY AFTER, I WAS FLYING ON STEROIDS...
(NOT THINKING THAT IT WAS JUST 1 OF 21 "RECOVERY DAYS" UNTIL ROUND 2.)
IN FACT, I SWAM 74 LAPS...
...AND I COULD'VE KEPT GOING.

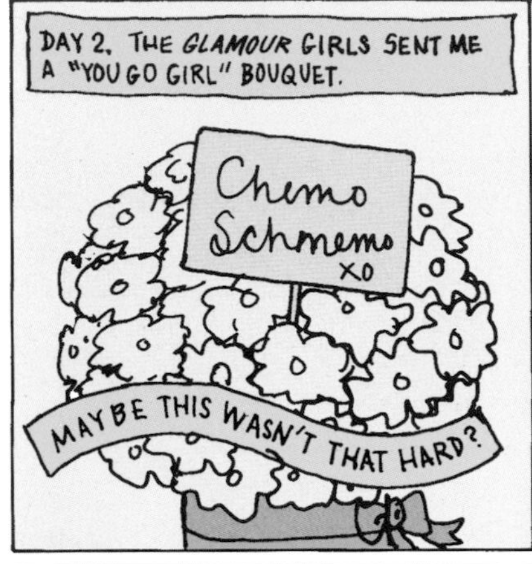
DAY 2. THE GLAMOUR GIRLS SENT ME A "YOU GO GIRL" BOUQUET.
Chemo Schmemo XO
MAYBE THIS WASN'T THAT HARD?

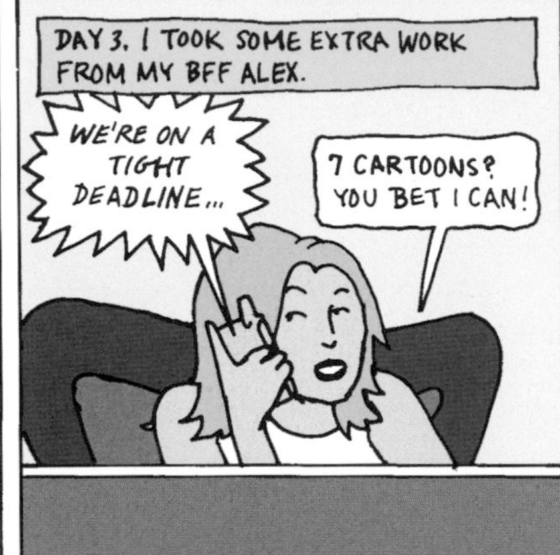
DAY 3. I TOOK SOME EXTRA WORK FROM MY BFF ALEX.
WE'RE ON A TIGHT DEADLINE...
7 CARTOONS? YOU BET I CAN!

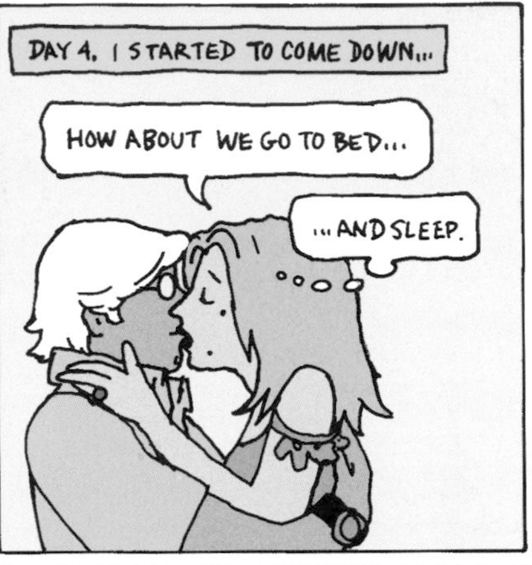
DAY 4. I STARTED TO COME DOWN...
HOW ABOUT WE GO TO BED...
...AND SLEEP.

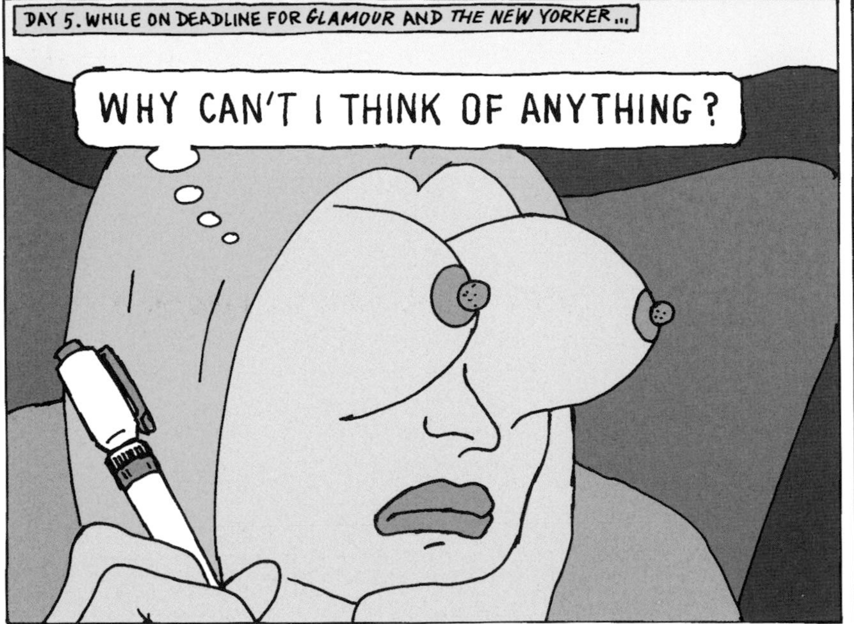
DAY 5. WHILE ON DEADLINE FOR GLAMOUR AND THE NEW YORKER...
WHY CAN'T I THINK OF ANYTHING?

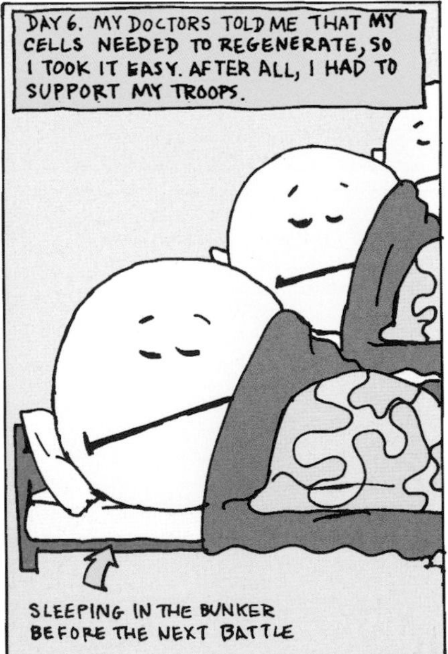
DAY 6. MY DOCTORS TOLD ME THAT MY CELLS NEEDED TO REGENERATE, SO I TOOK IT EASY. AFTER ALL, I HAD TO SUPPORT MY TROOPS.
SLEEPING IN THE BUNKER BEFORE THE NEXT BATTLE

WEEK 2. THE CHEMO LOW. IT SEEMED LIKE I HAD LESS ENERGY WITH EACH DAY.

DAY 7. I SAW MY SHRINK...
I'M SUPPOSED TO GAIN WEIGHT.
AHH... DON'T WORRY ABOUT IT.
BUT I THINK I NEED SOME TOOLS.

DAY 8. I WENT TO THE KABBALAH CENTRE...
WHEN YOU START TO FEEL PITY, FIGHT!
HOW? IT'S SO HARD.

IT'S SO SIMPLE. FAKE IT UNTIL YOU MAKE IT.
AND THEN YOU WON'T HAVE TO FAKE IT ANYMORE.
THIS WAS MY LAST SESSION WITH MEIR. HE WAS RELOCATED TO THE KABBALAH CENTRE IN BOCA RATON.

DAY 9. SHARON AND I WENT FOR A LIGHT SWIM.
I TOLD MY SHRINK ABOUT THE WEIGHT GAIN, SHE TELLS ME NOT TO WORRY ABOUT IT. THAT'S ALL I EVER HEAR... SHE'S THE SLACKER SHRINK.
WHAT WEIGHT GAIN? YOU'RE NOT 7 MONTHS PREGNANT IN MATERNITY CLOTHES.

LOOK AT ME, MAREESE...
I AM HUGE.

YOU'RE HEALTHY! YOU SHOULDN'T BE THINKING OF WEIGHT RIGHT NOW!
LOOK WHO'S TALKING!
BOTH OF US WERE AFFLICTED WITH ACUTE "NEW YORK-ITIS."

I'M HUNGRY.
I'M NAUSEOUS.
I'M HUNGRY AND NAUSEOUS.
SHOULD WE GET SOMETHING TO EAT?
LOVE TO. BUT I CAN'T HAVE SUSHI.
I CAN'T HAVE IT, EITHER.

DAY 10. MY ENERGY WAS AT ITS LOWEST.
DO YOU WANT A CAPPUCCINO?
I NEED A CAPPUCCINO.

DAY 13. I WAS MAKING A COMEBACK— SORT OF.
ALEX, I'LL HAVE FINISHED ART TO YOU BY 6.
JUST IN TIME FOR MY NAP.

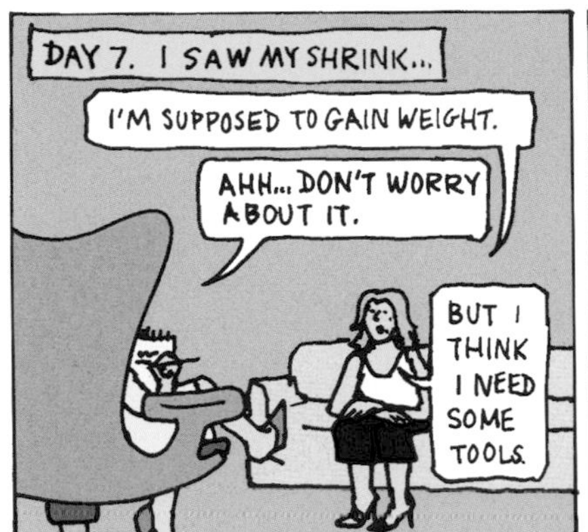

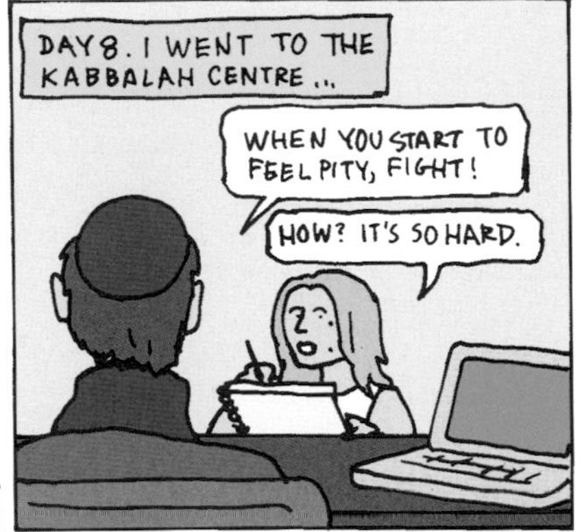

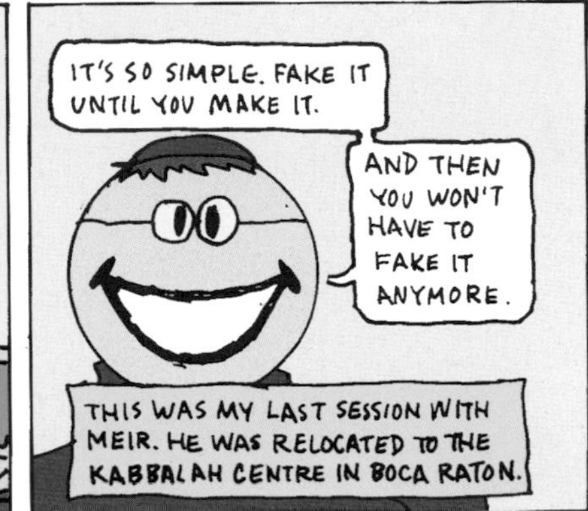

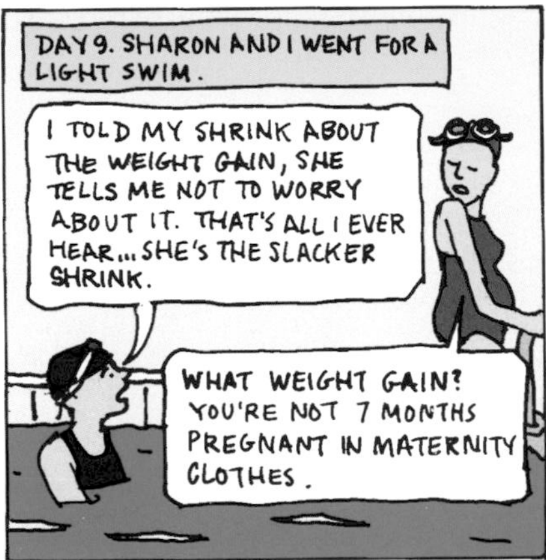

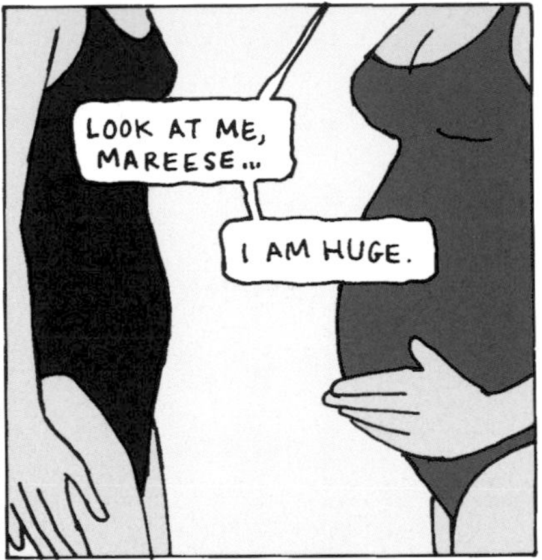

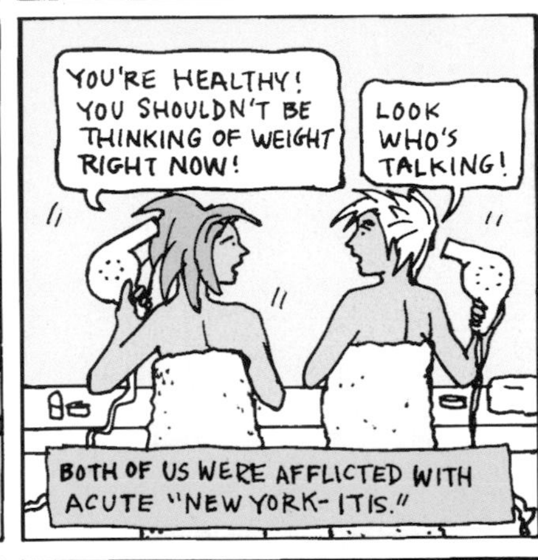

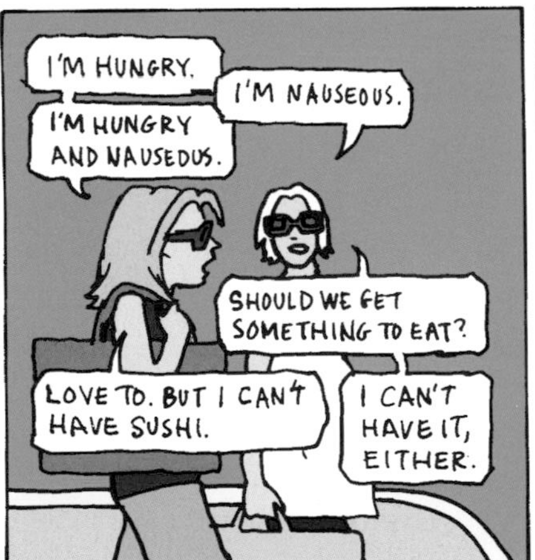

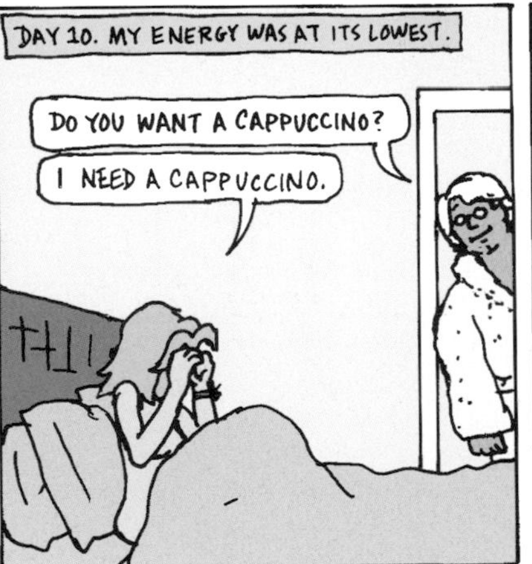

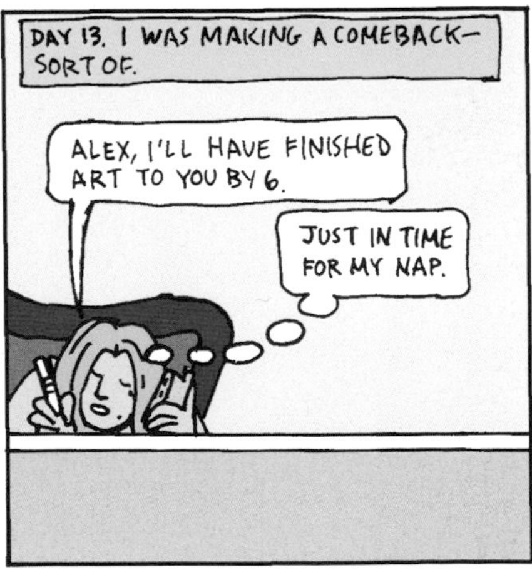

WEEK 3. THE CHEMO LEVELING OFF. JUST WHEN YOU'RE BACK TO YOUR OLD SELF...

BACK TO THOSE CRAZY CARTOONIST LUNCHES...
DIFFEE DOESN'T DRINK; WE'LL SPLIT HIS WINE.
I SHOULDN'T, BUT I WILL.
BACK TO A NAPLESS AFTERNOON...
CARTOONS FOR THE TENTS OF L.A. FASHION WEEK? I'D LOVE TO DO IT.
BACK TO THAT MILE-LONG SWIM 5 TIMES A WEEK...

DAY 17. I THREW A BACHELORETTE PARTY FOR MY FRIEND ANNE.
I'M TIRED. ARE YOU SURE YOU HAD CHEMO?

DAY 20. THE NIGHT BEFORE CHEMO #2, MY (S)MOTHER CALLED...
MARISA, I HAVE A SORE THROAT AND YOU CAN'T BE AROUND ME.
THAT'S OK, MA. I'LL GO BY MYSELF. FEEL BETTER.

CHORTLE! CHORTLE! UGH GLUCK! UGH GLUCK!
THE GROSS-OUT-CLEARING-THE-THROAT-THING.

MUCH LATER...
IT'S 5:30 IN THE MORNING AND YOU NEVER CAME TO BED!
I'VE GOT TO FINISH THIS BEFORE TREATMENT.

1 P.M. THAT DAY...
FERN, I JUST E-MAILED YOU THE ART. WHEN DO THE TENTS GO UP?
TAXI!
DRIVER, CAN YOU TAKE ME TO 15TH BETWEEN 8TH AND 9TH AND STEP ON IT, PLEASE?
OWW... MY EARDRUM!
JUST WHEN YOU'RE BACK TO YOUR OLD SELF, IT'S CHEMO TIME ALL OVER AGAIN...

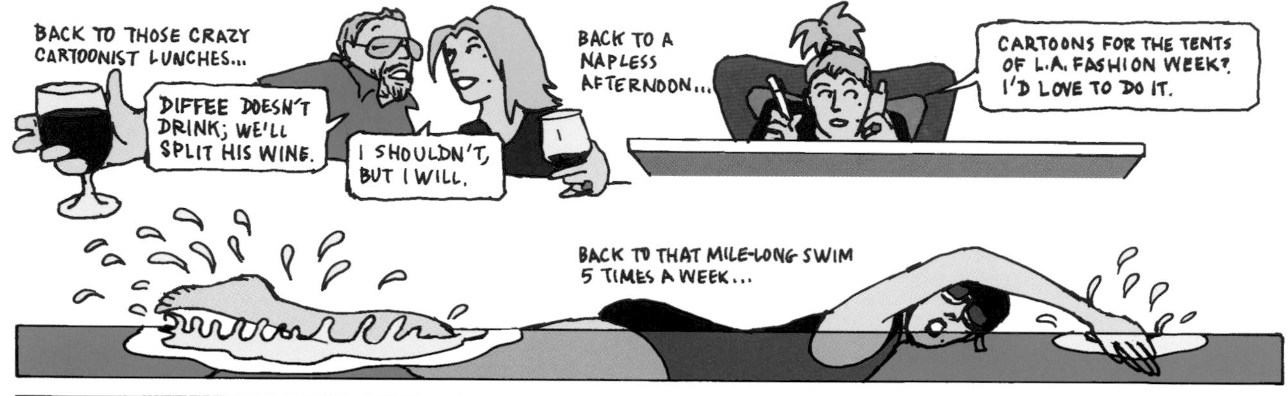

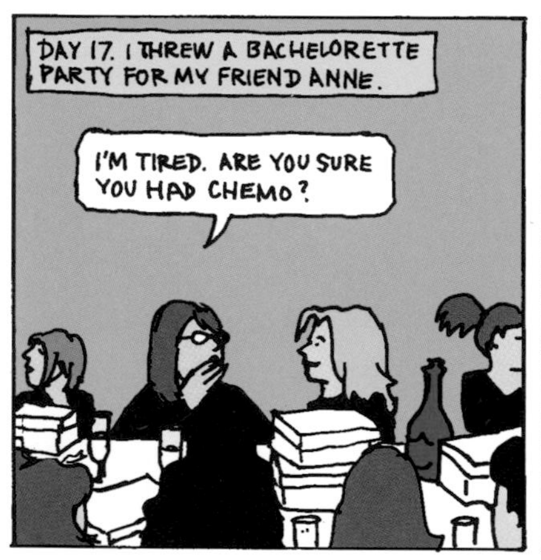

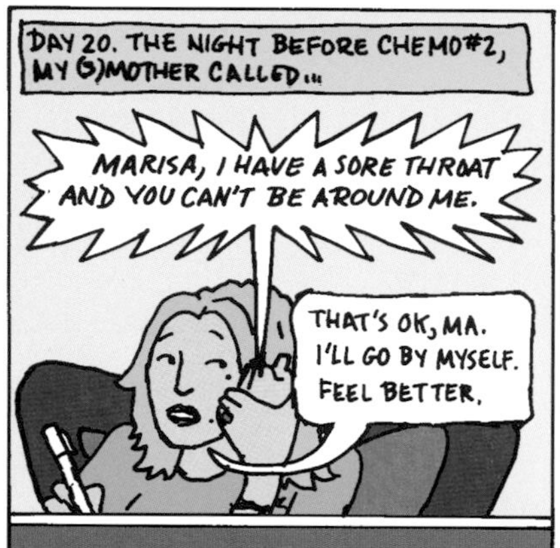

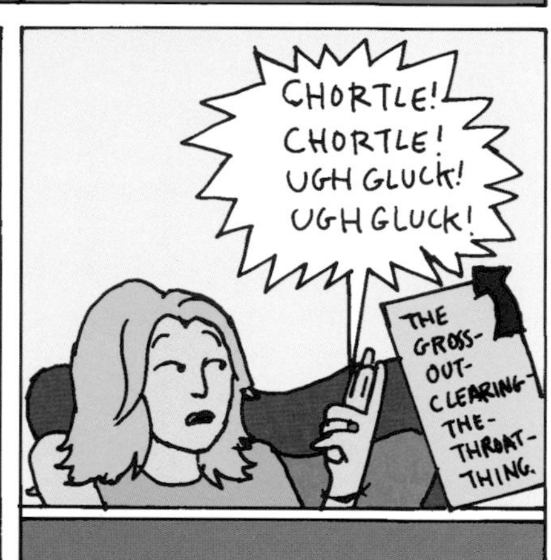

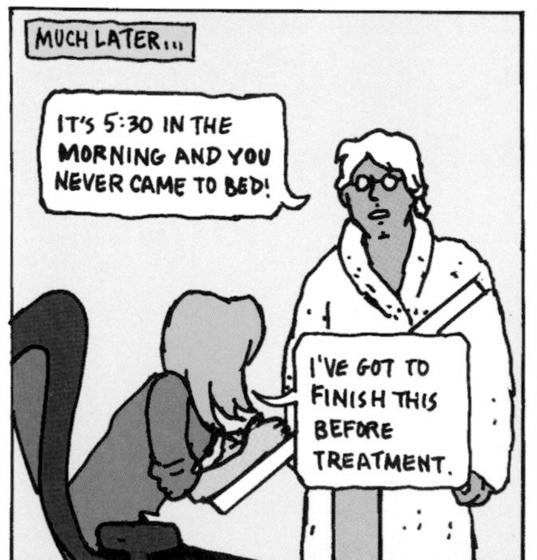

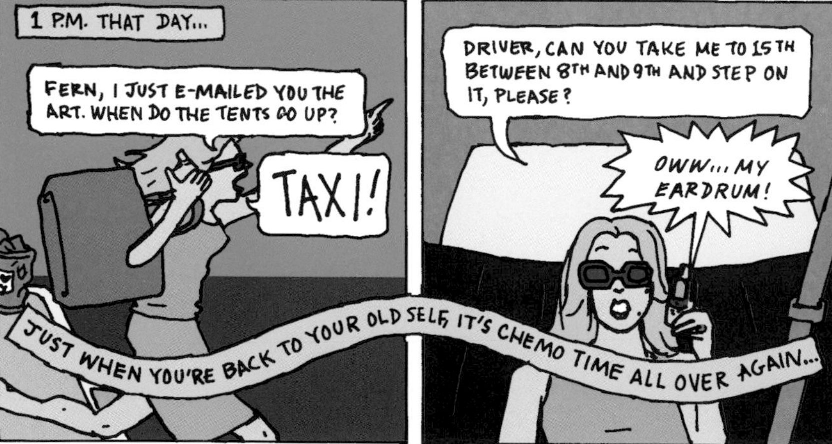

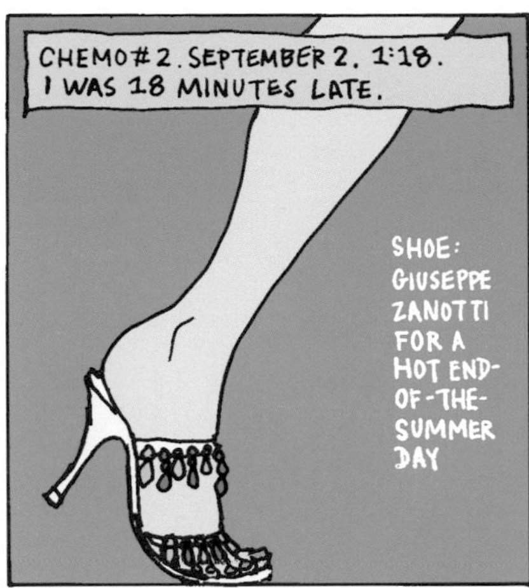
CHEMO #2. SEPTEMBER 2. 1:18.
I WAS 18 MINUTES LATE.
SHOE: GIUSEPPE ZANOTTI FOR A HOT END-OF-THE-SUMMER DAY

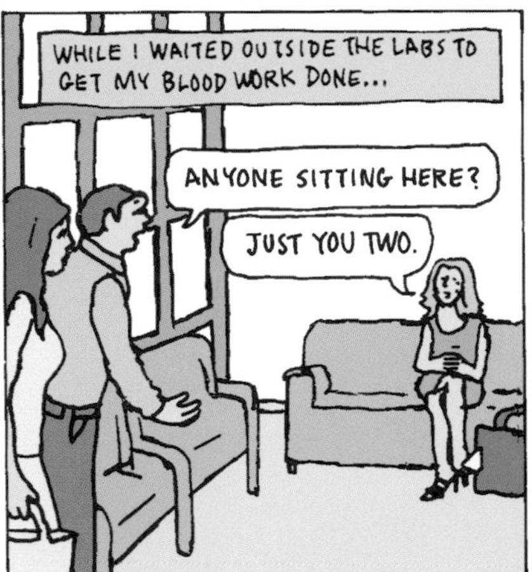
WHILE I WAITED OUTSIDE THE LABS TO GET MY BLOOD WORK DONE...
ANYONE SITTING HERE?
JUST YOU TWO.

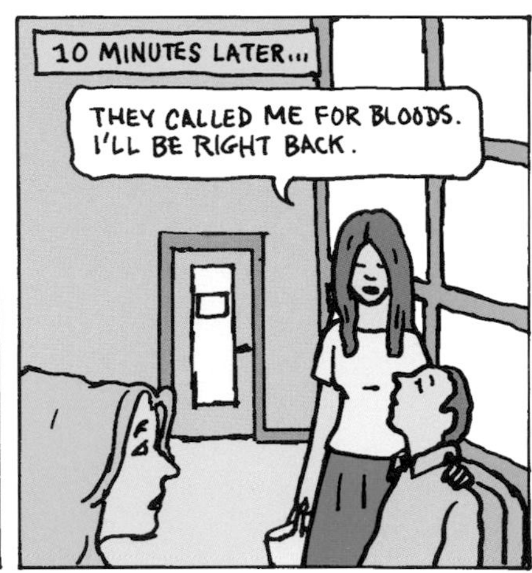
10 MINUTES LATER...
THEY CALLED ME FOR BLOODS. I'LL BE RIGHT BACK.

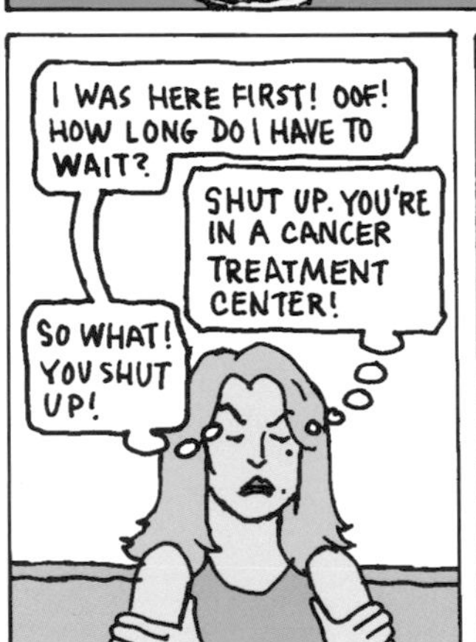
I WAS HERE FIRST! OOF! HOW LONG DO I HAVE TO WAIT?
SHUT UP. YOU'RE IN A CANCER TREATMENT CENTER!
SO WHAT! YOU SHUT UP!

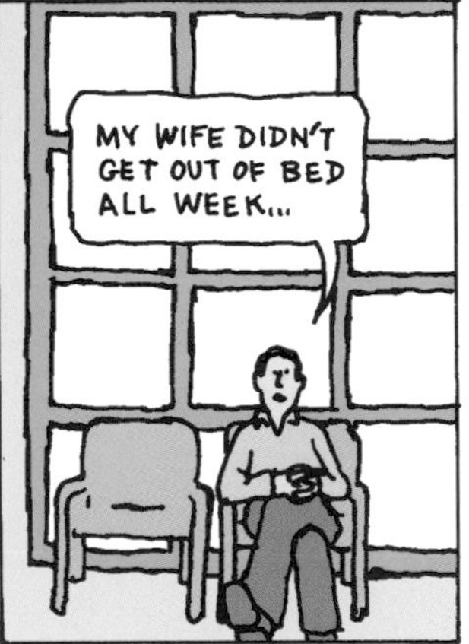
MY WIFE DIDN'T GET OUT OF BED ALL WEEK...

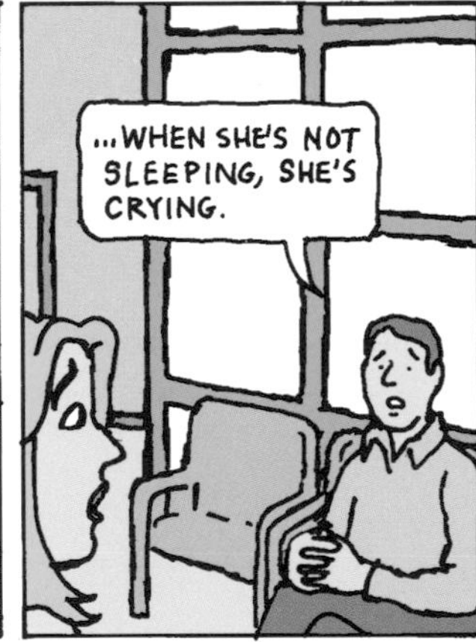
...WHEN SHE'S NOT SLEEPING, SHE'S CRYING.

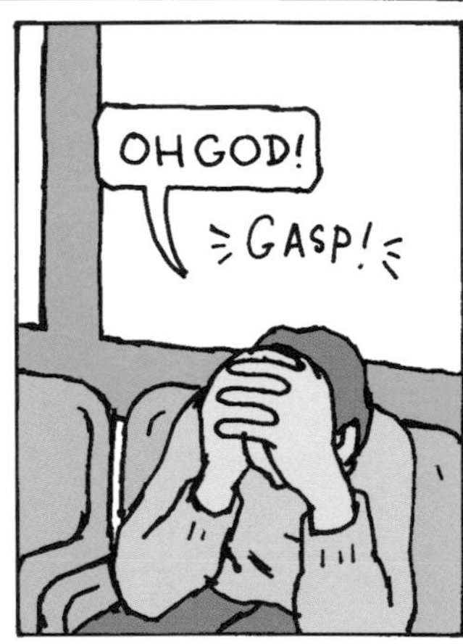
OH GOD!
GASP!

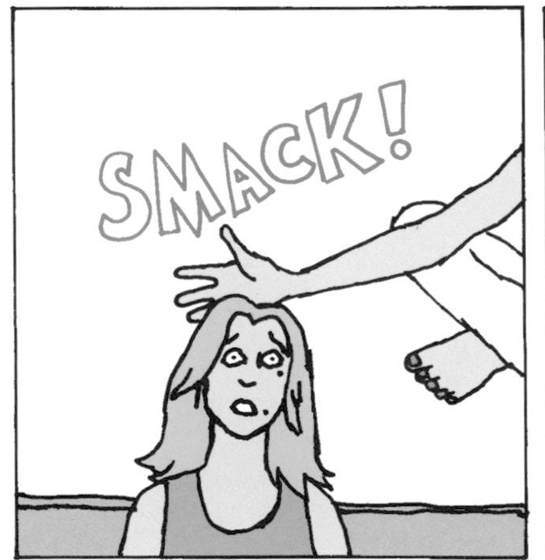
SMACK!

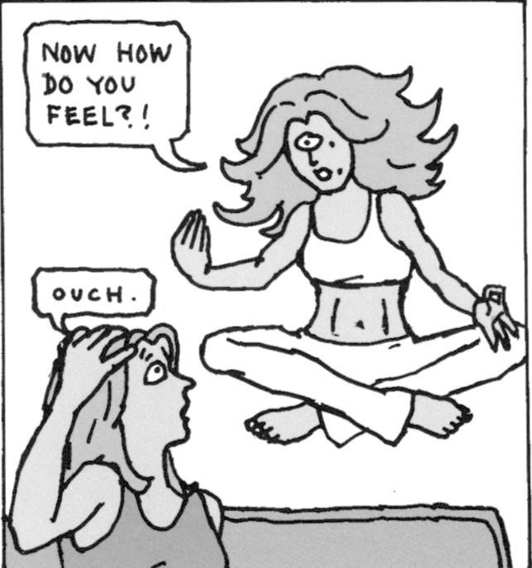
NOW HOW DO YOU FEEL?!
OUCH.

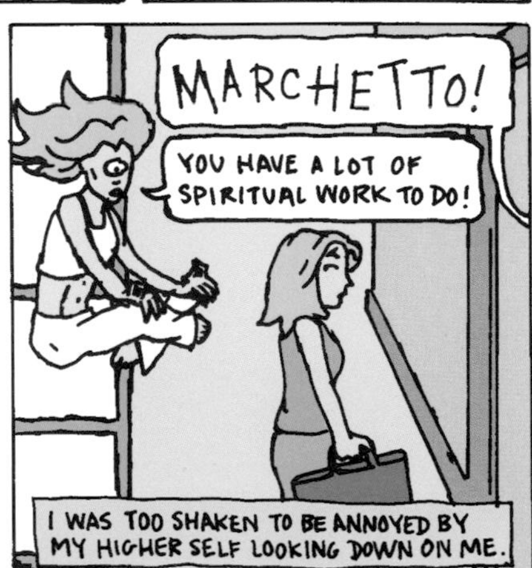
MARCHETTO!
YOU HAVE A LOT OF SPIRITUAL WORK TO DO!
I WAS TOO SHAKEN TO BE ANNOYED BY MY HIGHER SELF LOOKING DOWN ON ME.

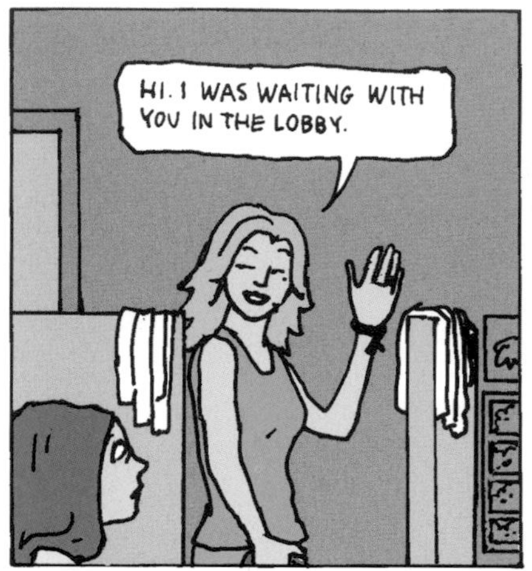
HI. I WAS WAITING WITH YOU IN THE LOBBY.

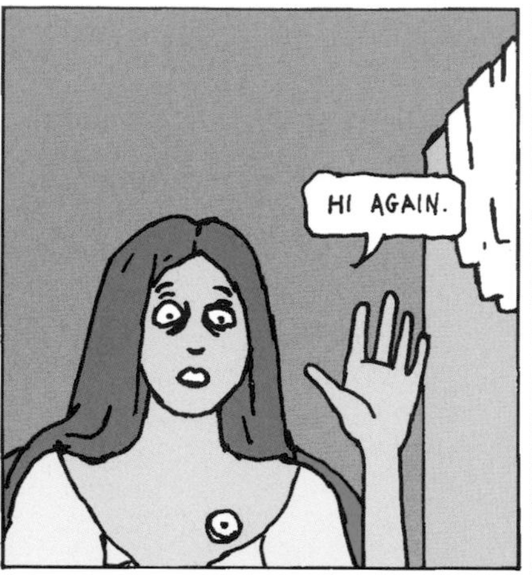
HI AGAIN.

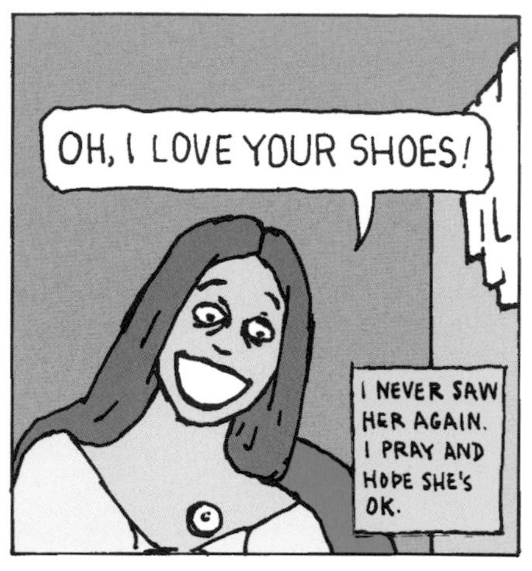
OH, I LOVE YOUR SHOES!
I NEVER SAW HER AGAIN. I PRAY AND HOPE SHE'S OK.

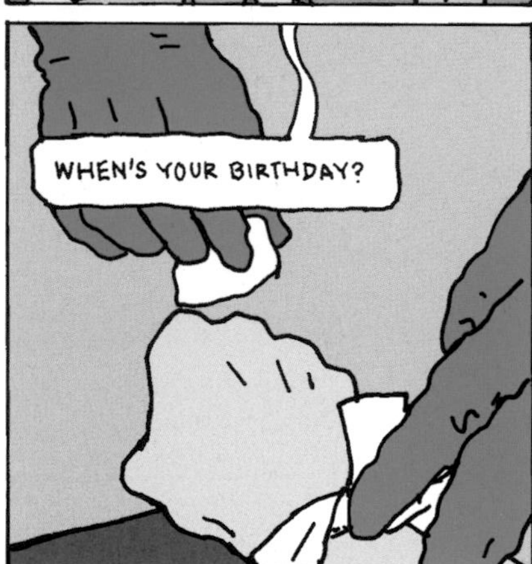
WHEN'S YOUR BIRTHDAY?

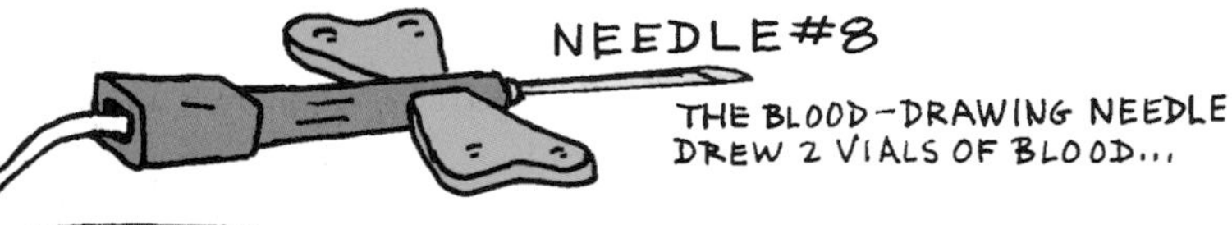
NEEDLE #8
THE BLOOD-DRAWING NEEDLE DREW 2 VIALS OF BLOOD...

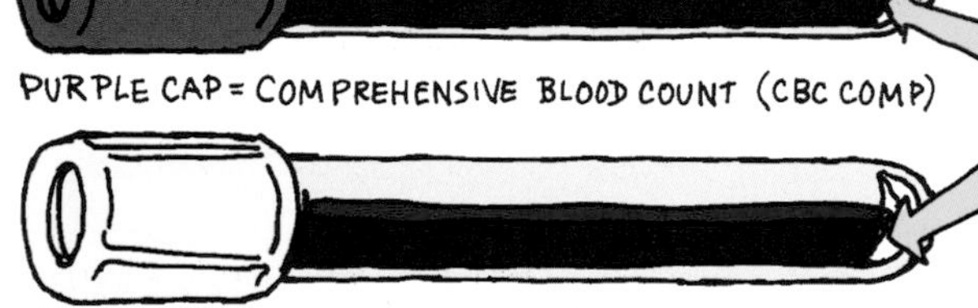
PURPLE CAP = COMPREHENSIVE BLOOD COUNT (CBC COMP)
YELLOW CAP = TUMOR MARGINS
VIALS ARE THEN AGITATED TO DISTRIBUTE A WHITE SUBSTANCE WHICH STOPS THE BLOOD FROM CLOTTING BEFORE IT'S TESTED.

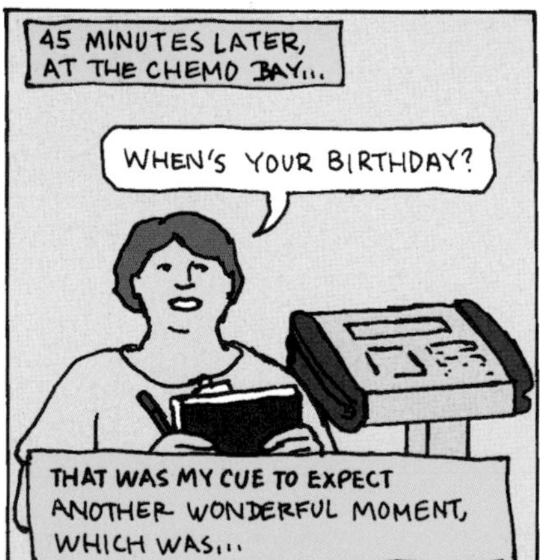
45 MINUTES LATER, AT THE CHEMO BAY...
WHEN'S YOUR BIRTHDAY?
THAT WAS MY CUE TO EXPECT ANOTHER WONDERFUL MOMENT, WHICH WAS...

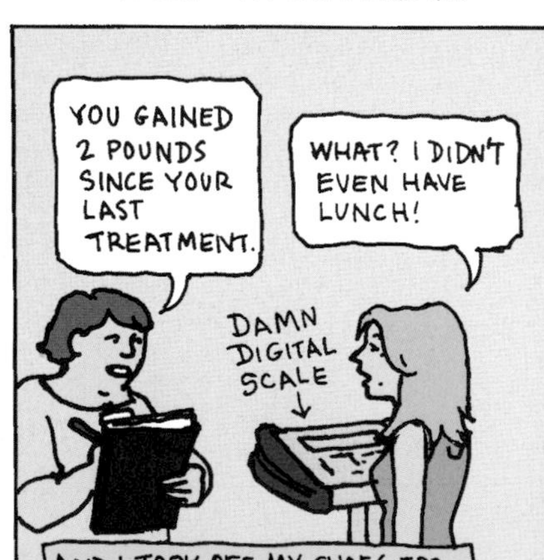
YOU GAINED 2 POUNDS SINCE YOUR LAST TREATMENT.
WHAT? I DIDN'T EVEN HAVE LUNCH!
DAMN DIGITAL SCALE
AND I TOOK OFF MY SHOES, TOO.

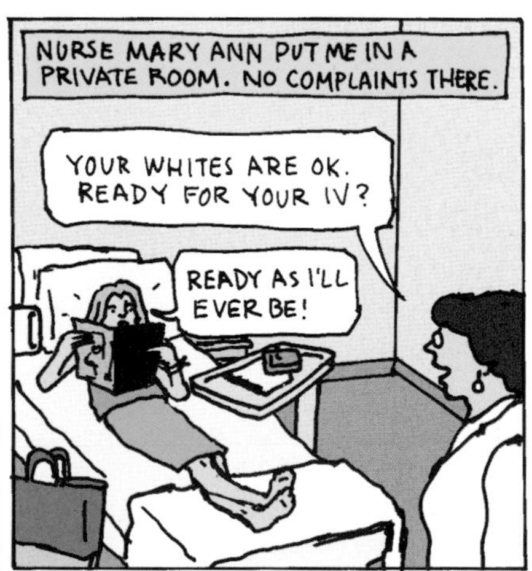
NURSE MARY ANN PUT ME IN A PRIVATE ROOM. NO COMPLAINTS THERE.
YOUR WHITES ARE OK. READY FOR YOUR IV?
READY AS I'LL EVER BE!

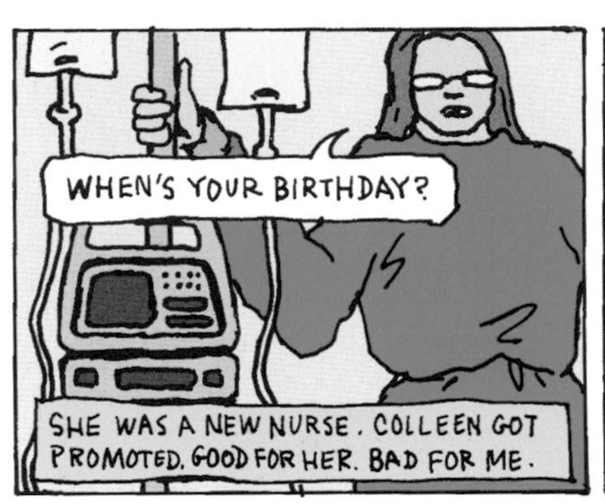

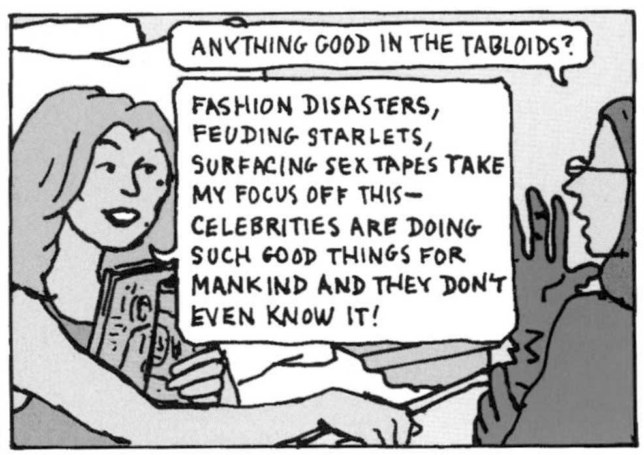

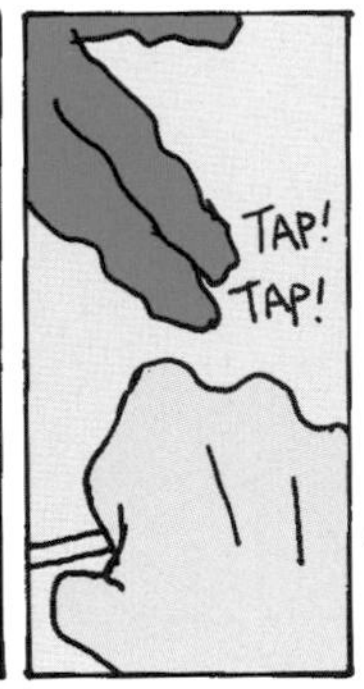

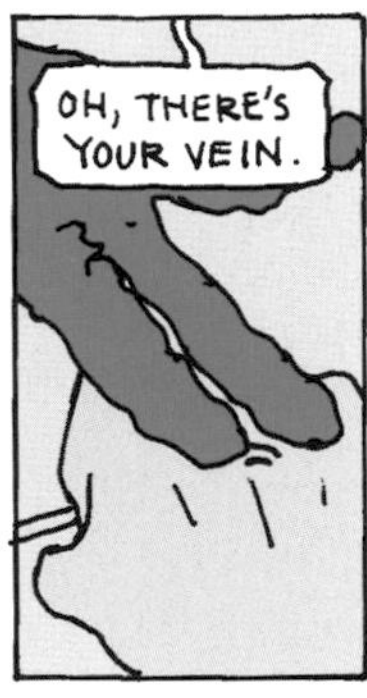

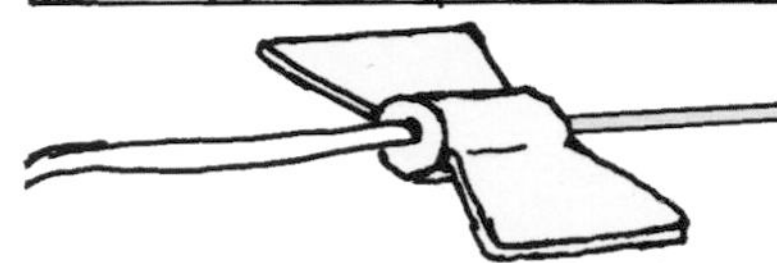

NEEDLE#9

THE CHEMO IV (#2 OF 8)

FOR SOME REASON, THE DRUGS MADE ME HUNGRY. SO I MADE MY WAY TO THE KITCHEN...

TEA BAGS, HOT CHOCOLATE & SOUP MIX

HOT WATER, COLD WATER

COFFEE MACHINE

A VARIETY OF FLAVORED COFFEES

GRAHAM CRACKERS & PEANUT BUTTER CRACKERS

NUTRI-GRAIN BARS

THE IV MACHINE WAS ON WHEELS, SO I WAS MOBILE

I GRABBED A YOGURT

JUICES

SANDWICHES

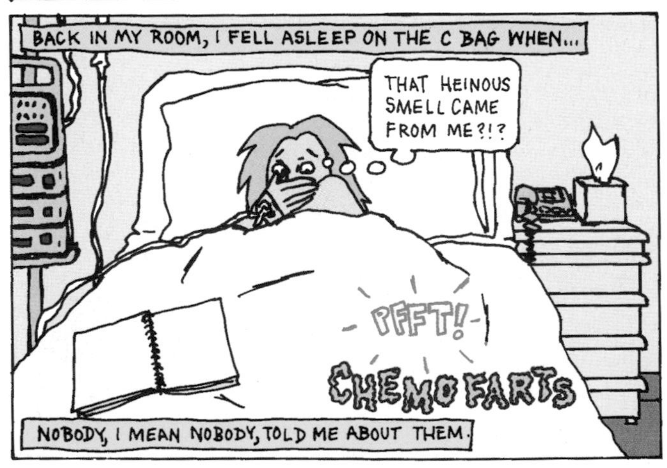

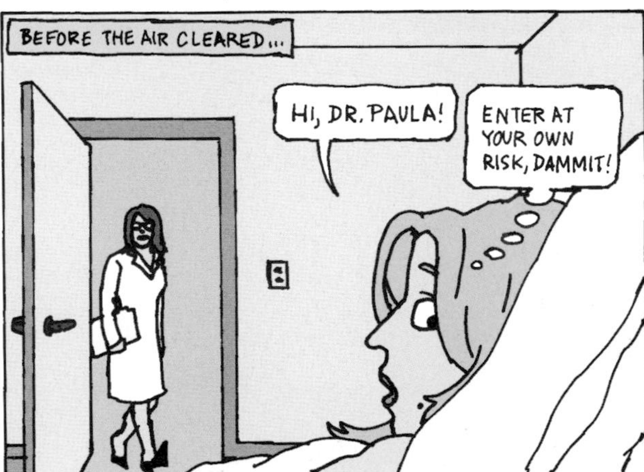

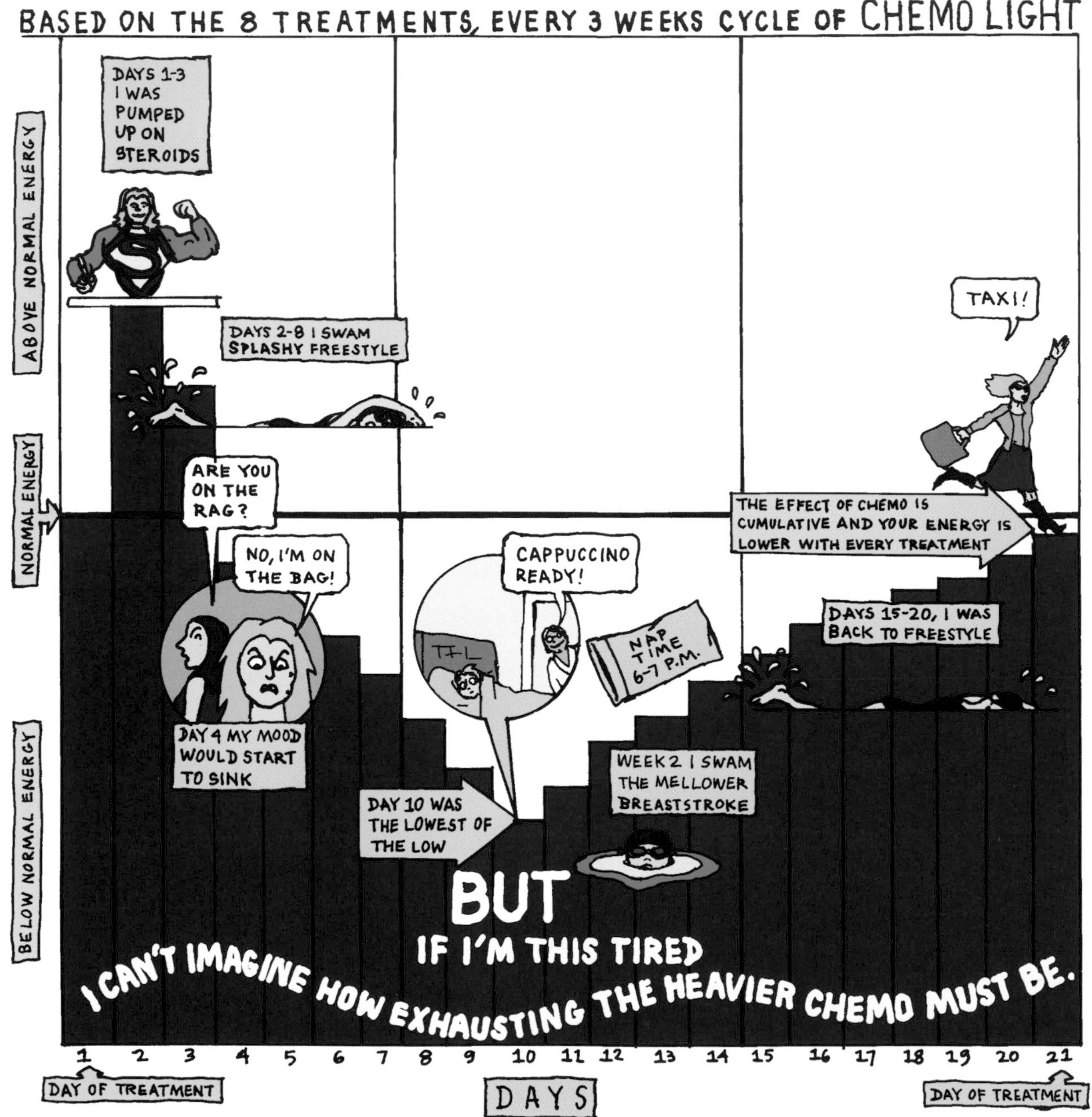
THE CHEMO ENERGY FLOW CHART
BASED ON THE 8 TREATMENTS, EVERY 3 WEEKS CYCLE OF CHEMO LIGHT
ABOVE NORMAL ENERGY
NORMAL ENERGY
BELOW NORMAL ENERGY
DAYS 1-3 I WAS PUMPED UP ON STEROIDS
DAYS 2-8 I SWAM SPLASHY FREESTYLE
ARE YOU ON THE RAG?
NO, I'M ON THE BAG!
DAY 4 MY MOOD WOULD START TO SINK
CAPPUCCINO READY!
NAP TIME 6-7 P.M.
DAY 10 WAS THE LOWEST OF THE LOW
WEEK 2 I SWAM THE MELLOWER BREASTSTROKE
THE EFFECT OF CHEMO IS CUMULATIVE AND YOUR ENERGY IS LOWER WITH EVERY TREATMENT
DAYS 15-20, I WAS BACK TO FREESTYLE
TAXI!
BUT
IF I'M THIS TIRED
I CAN'T IMAGINE HOW EXHAUSTING THE HEAVIER CHEMO MUST BE.
1 2 3 4 5 6 7 8 9 10 11 12 13 14 15 16 17 18 19 20 21
DAY OF TREATMENT
DAYS
DAY OF TREATMENT

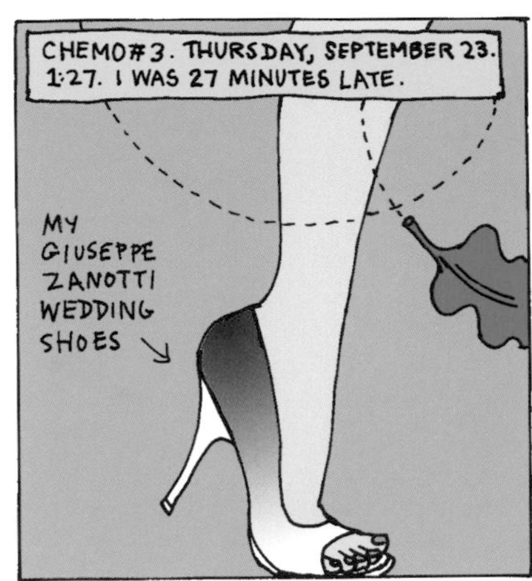

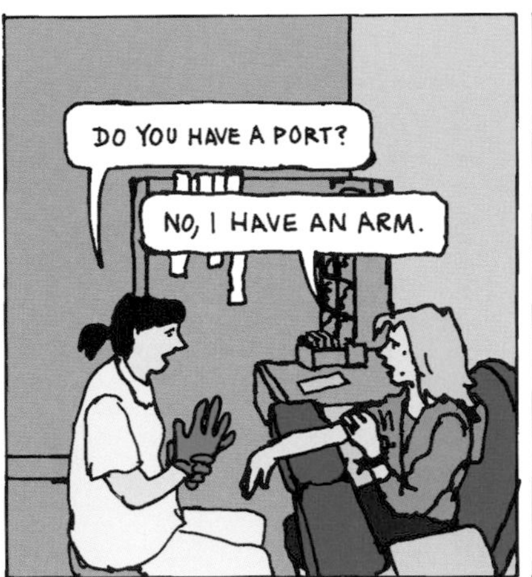

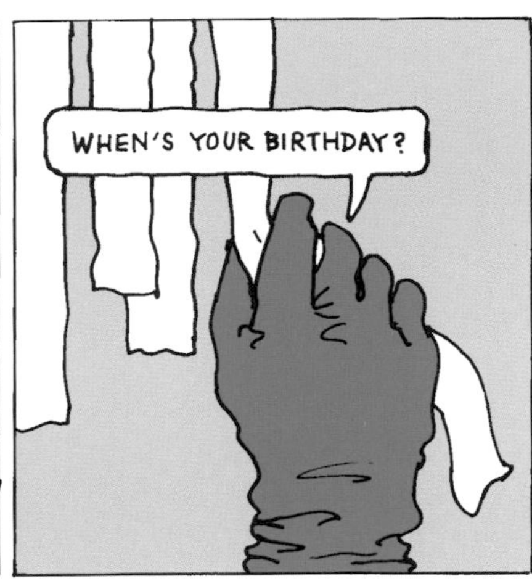

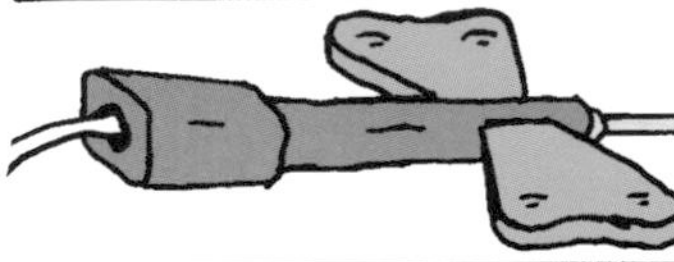

NEEDLE #10

THE BLOOD-DRAWING NEEDLE DREW 2 VIALS OF BLOOD.

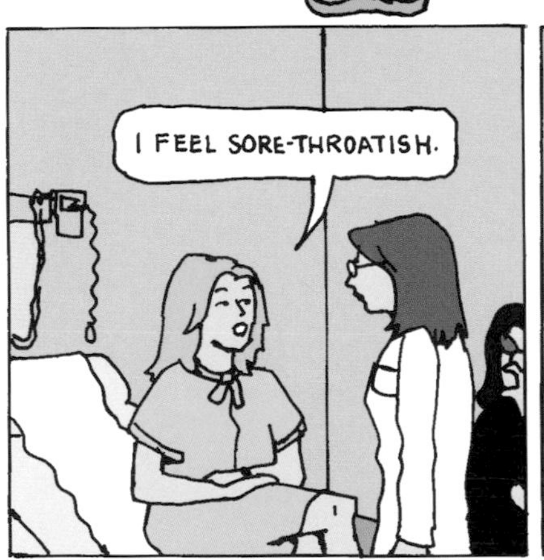

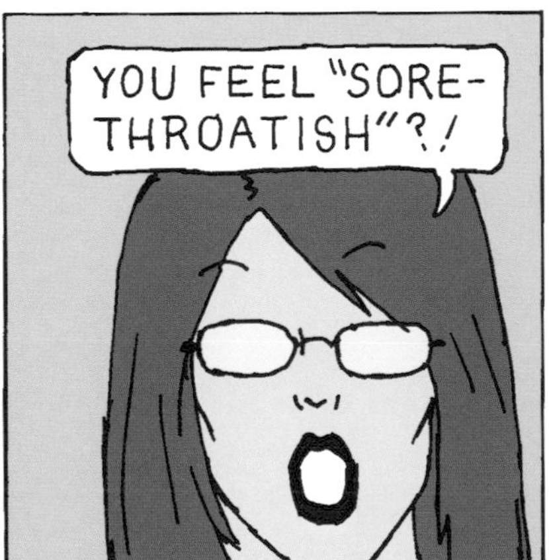

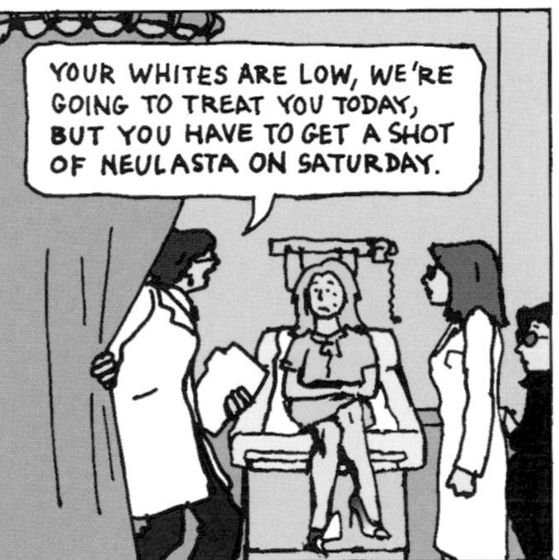

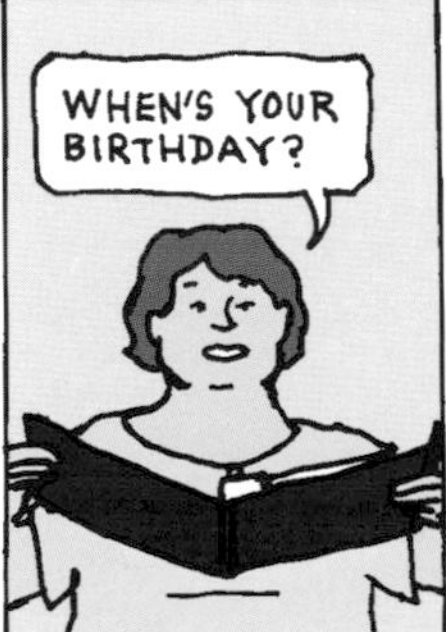

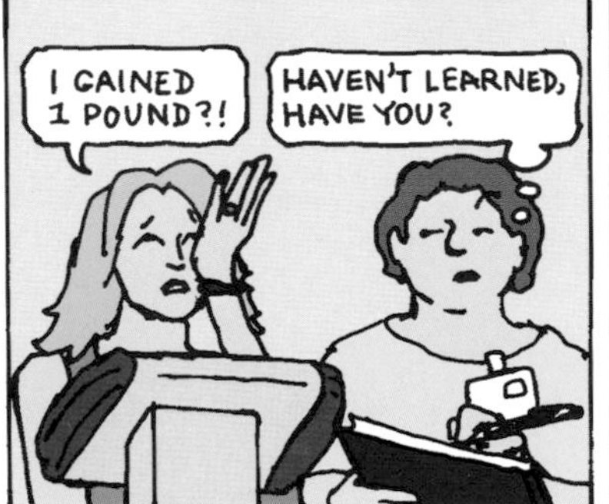

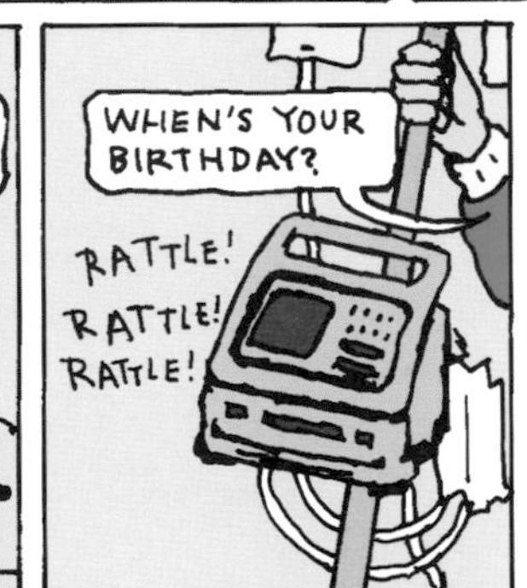

NEEDLE #11

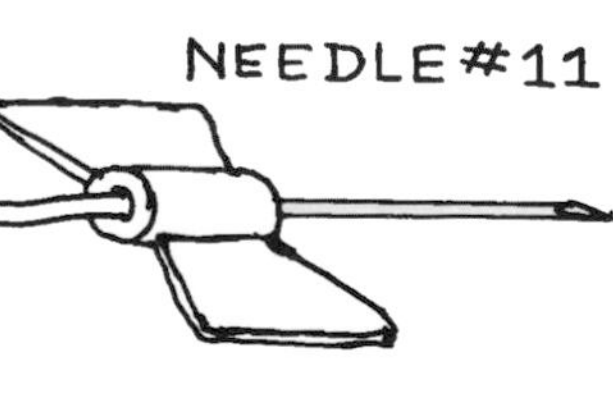

THE CHEMO IV
(#3 OF 8)

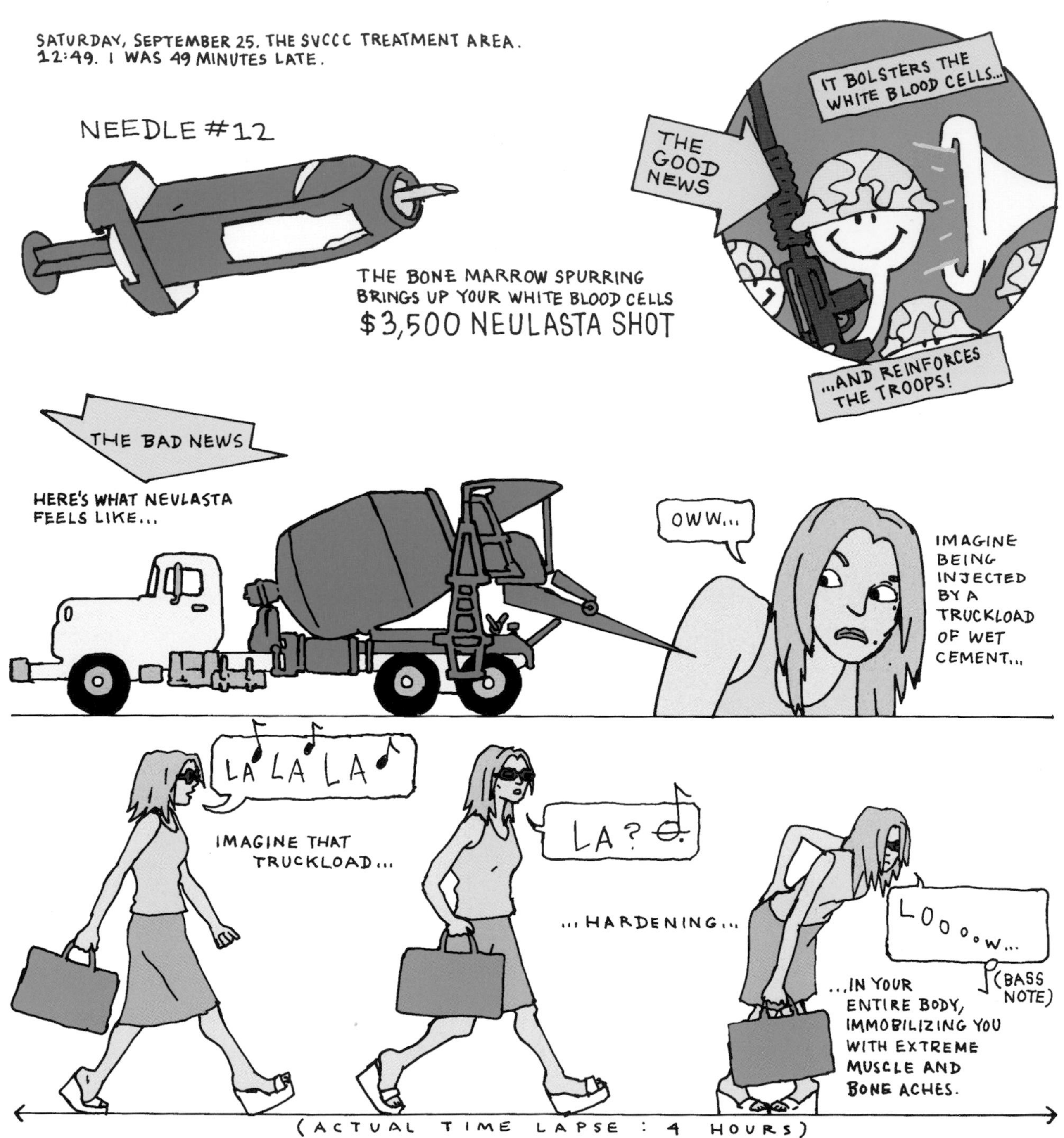
SATURDAY, SEPTEMBER 25. THE SVCCC TREATMENT AREA. 12:49. I WAS 49 MINUTES LATE.
NEEDLE #12
THE BONE MARROW SPURRING BRINGS UP YOUR WHITE BLOOD CELLS
$3,500 NEULASTA SHOT
THE GOOD NEWS
IT BOLSTERS THE WHITE BLOOD CELLS...
...AND REINFORCES THE TROOPS!
THE BAD NEWS
HERE'S WHAT NEULASTA FEELS LIKE...
OWW...
IMAGINE BEING INJECTED BY A TRUCKLOAD OF WET CEMENT...
LA LA LA
IMAGINE THAT TRUCKLOAD...
LA?
...HARDENING...
LOoooW...
(BASS NOTE)
...IN YOUR ENTIRE BODY, IMMOBILIZING YOU WITH EXTREME MUSCLE AND BONE ACHES.
(ACTUAL TIME LAPSE : 4 HOURS)

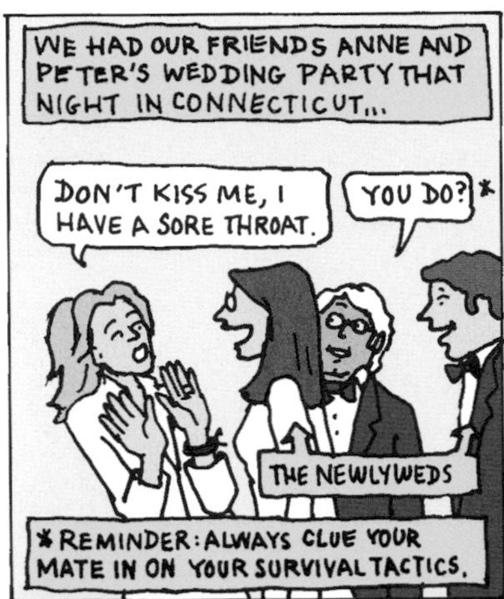
WE HAD OUR FRIENDS ANNE AND PETER'S WEDDING PARTY THAT NIGHT IN CONNECTICUT...
DON'T KISS ME, I HAVE A SORE THROAT.
YOU DO?*
THE NEWLYWEDS
*REMINDER: ALWAYS CLUE YOUR MATE IN ON YOUR SURVIVAL TACTICS.

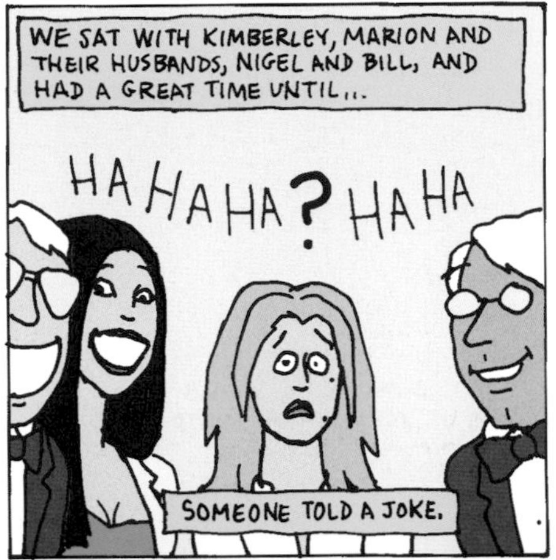
WE SAT WITH KIMBERLEY, MARION AND THEIR HUSBANDS, NIGEL AND BILL, AND HAD A GREAT TIME UNTIL...
HA HA HA HA ? HA HA
SOMEONE TOLD A JOKE.

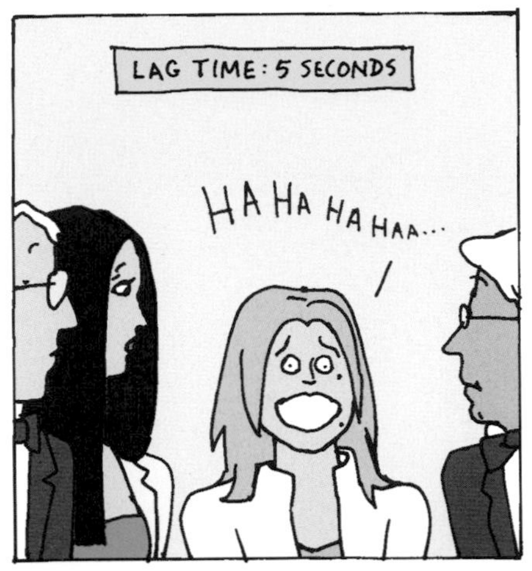
LAG TIME: 5 SECONDS
HA HA HA HAA...

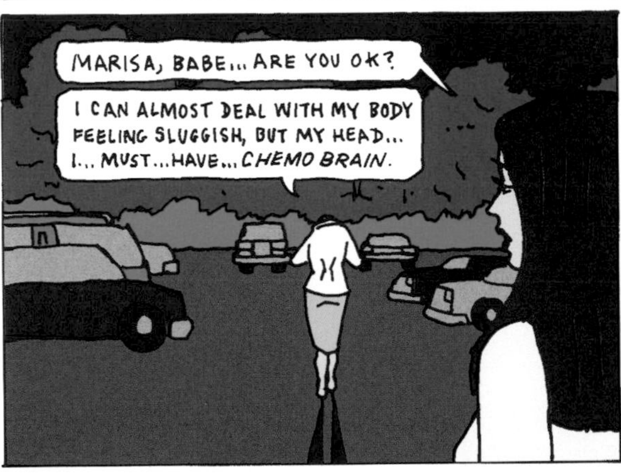
MARISA, BABE... ARE YOU OK?
I CAN ALMOST DEAL WITH MY BODY FEELING SLUGGISH, BUT MY HEAD... I... MUST... HAVE... CHEMO BRAIN.

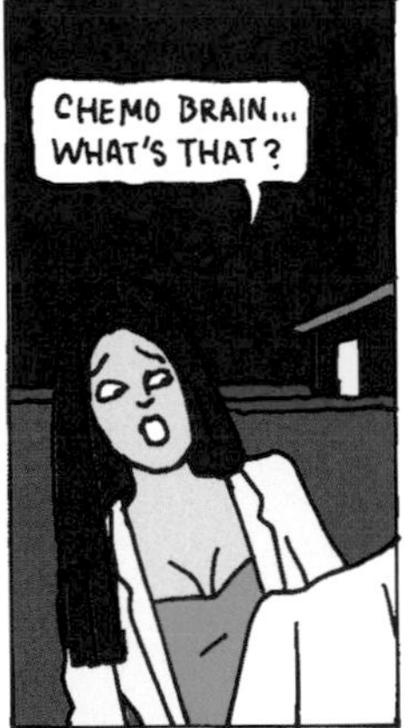
CHEMO BRAIN... WHAT'S THAT?

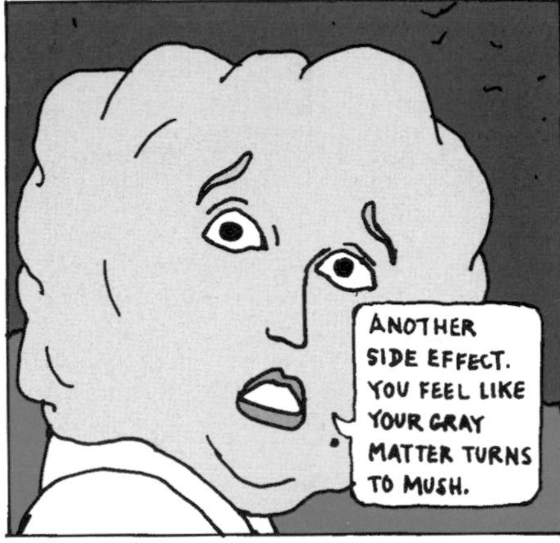
ANOTHER SIDE EFFECT. YOU FEEL LIKE YOUR GRAY MATTER TURNS TO MUSH.

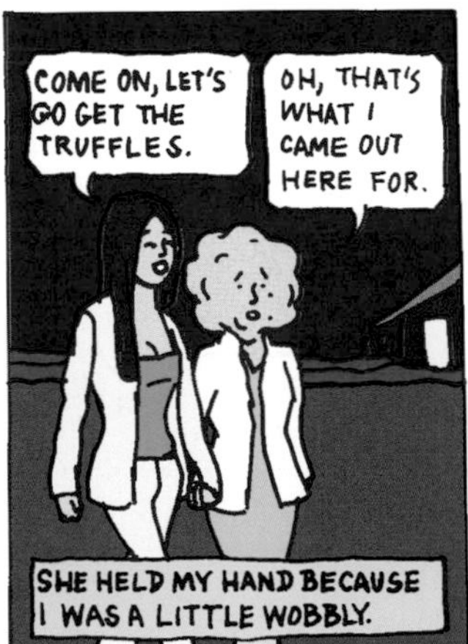
COME ON, LET'S GO GET THE TRUFFLES.
OH, THAT'S WHAT I CAME OUT HERE FOR.
SHE HELD MY HAND BECAUSE I WAS A LITTLE WOBBLY.

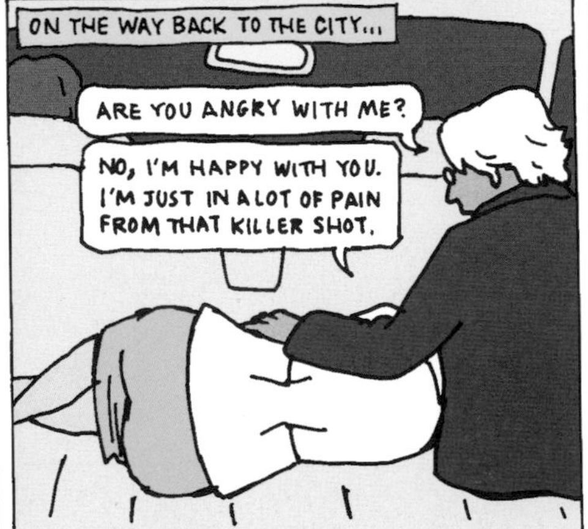
ON THE WAY BACK TO THE CITY...
ARE YOU ANGRY WITH ME?
NO, I'M HAPPY WITH YOU. I'M JUST IN A LOT OF PAIN FROM THAT KILLER SHOT.

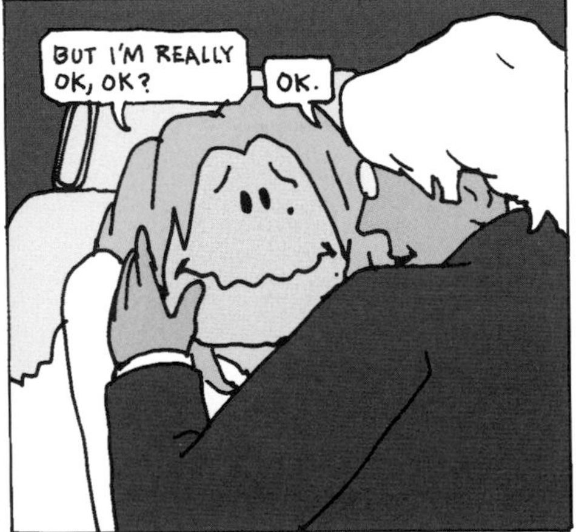
BUT I'M REALLY OK, OK?
OK.

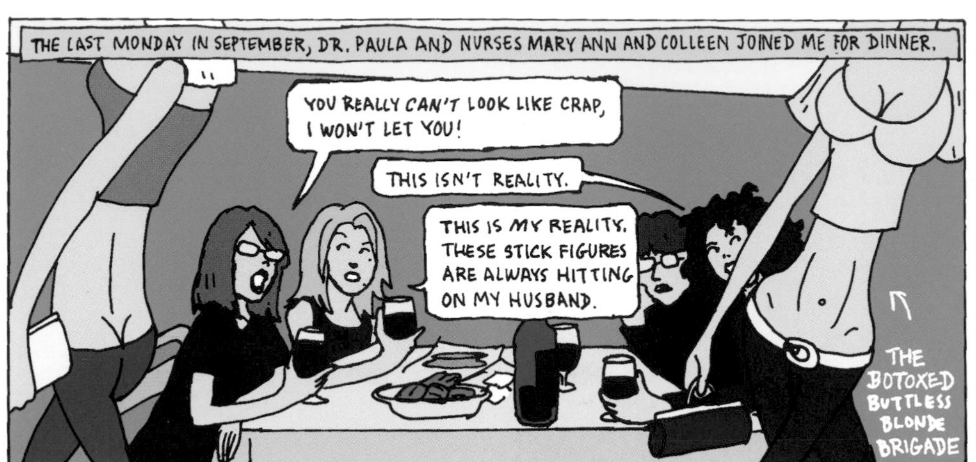
THE LAST MONDAY IN SEPTEMBER, DR. PAULA AND NURSES MARY ANN AND COLLEEN JOINED ME FOR DINNER.
YOU REALLY CAN'T LOOK LIKE CRAP, I WON'T LET YOU!
THIS ISN'T REALITY.
THIS IS MY REALITY. THESE STICK FIGURES ARE ALWAYS HITTING ON MY HUSBAND.
THE BOTOXED BUTTLESS BLONDE BRIGADE

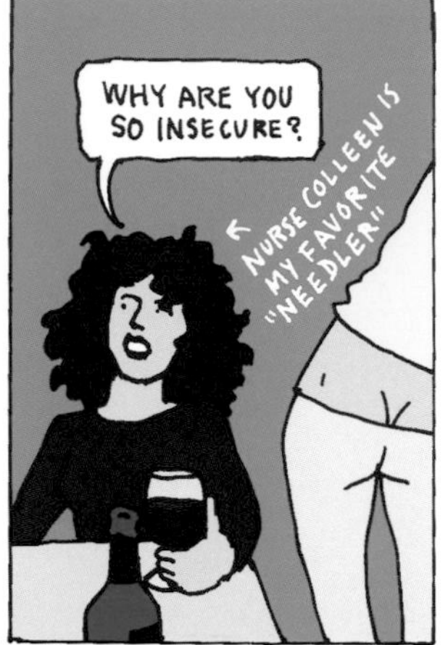
WHY ARE YOU SO INSECURE?
NURSE COLLEEN IS MY FAVORITE "NEEDLER"

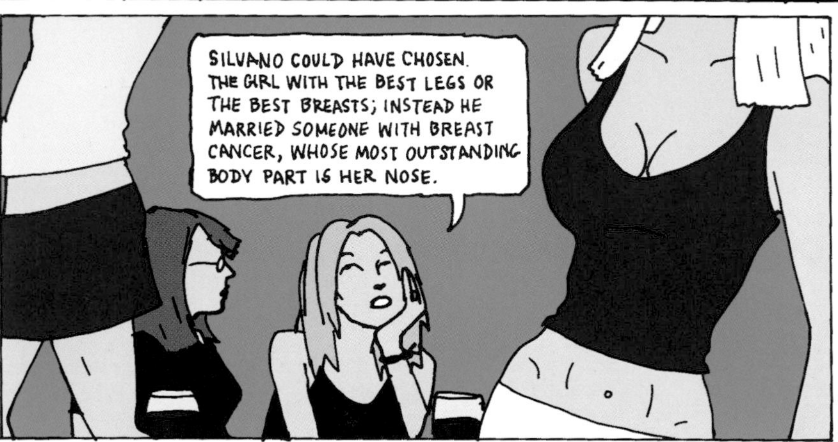
SILVANO COULD HAVE CHOSEN THE GIRL WITH THE BEST LEGS OR THE BEST BREASTS; INSTEAD HE MARRIED SOMEONE WITH BREAST CANCER, WHOSE MOST OUTSTANDING BODY PART IS HER NOSE.

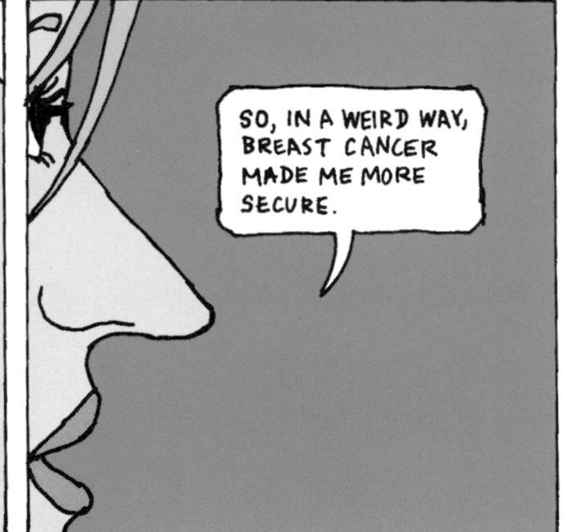
SO, IN A WEIRD WAY, BREAST CANCER MADE ME MORE SECURE.

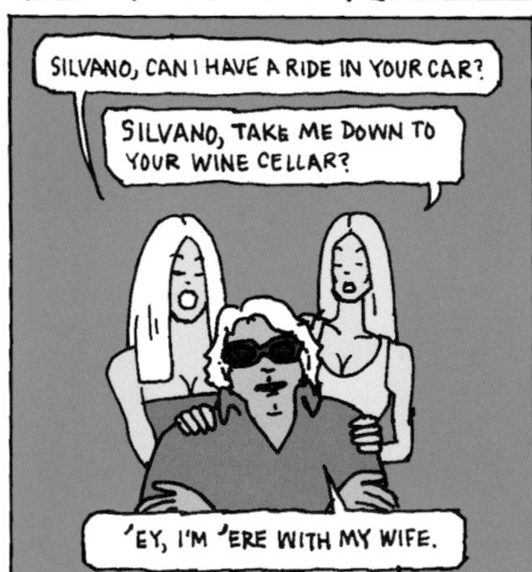
SILVANO, CAN I HAVE A RIDE IN YOUR CAR?
SILVANO, TAKE ME DOWN TO YOUR WINE CELLAR?
'EY, I'M 'ERE WITH MY WIFE.

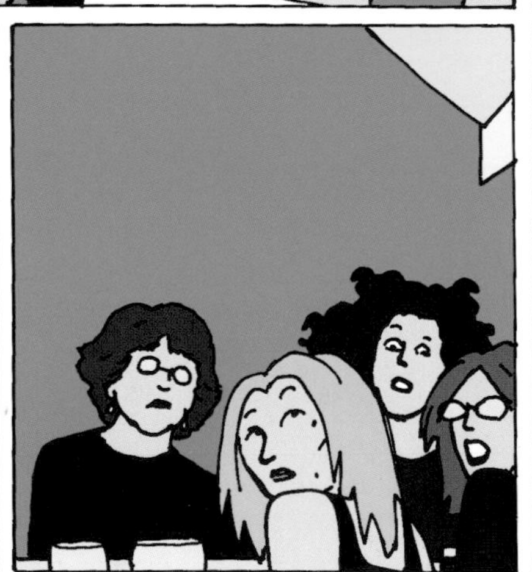

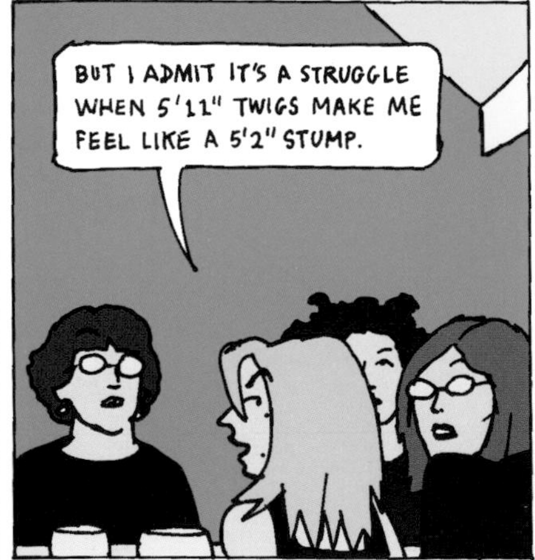
BUT I ADMIT IT'S A STRUGGLE WHEN 5'11" TWIGS MAKE ME FEEL LIKE A 5'2" STUMP.

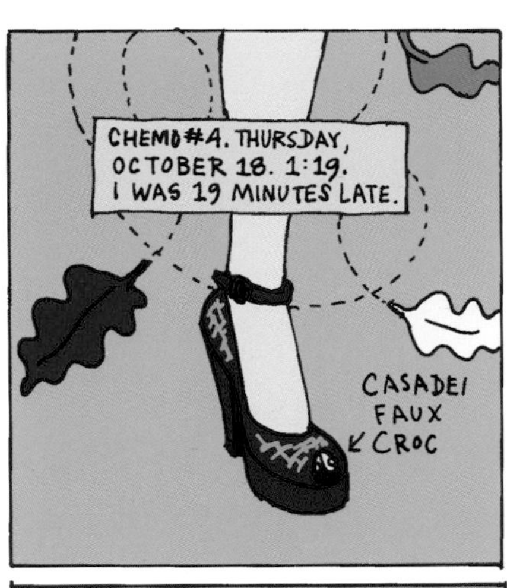
CHEMO #4. THURSDAY, OCTOBER 18. 1:19. I WAS 19 MINUTES LATE.
CASADEI FAUX CROC

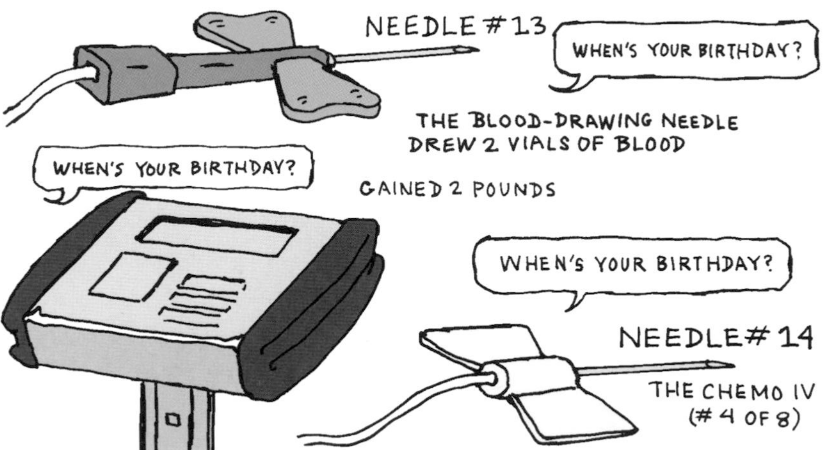
NEEDLE #13
WHEN'S YOUR BIRTHDAY?
THE BLOOD-DRAWING NEEDLE DREW 2 VIALS OF BLOOD
WHEN'S YOUR BIRTHDAY?
GAINED 2 POUNDS
WHEN'S YOUR BIRTHDAY?
NEEDLE # 14
THE CHEMO IV (# 4 OF 8)

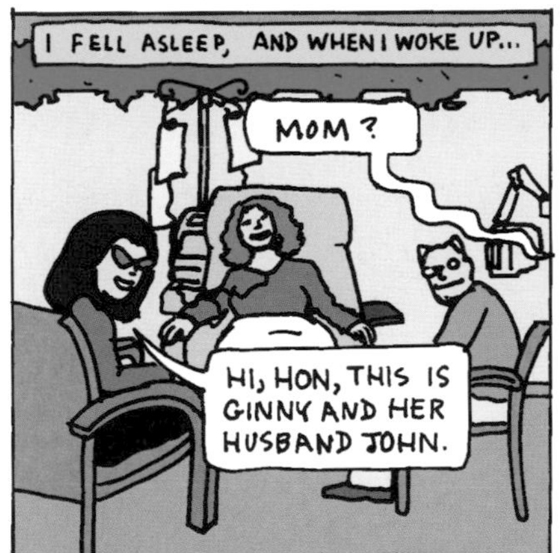
I FELL ASLEEP, AND WHEN I WOKE UP...
MOM?
HI, HON, THIS IS GINNY AND HER HUSBAND JOHN.

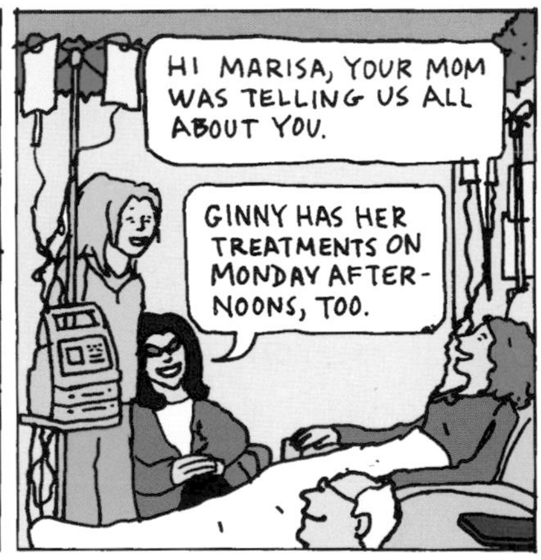
HI MARISA, YOUR MOM WAS TELLING US ALL ABOUT YOU.
GINNY HAS HER TREATMENTS ON MONDAY AFTER-NOONS, TOO.

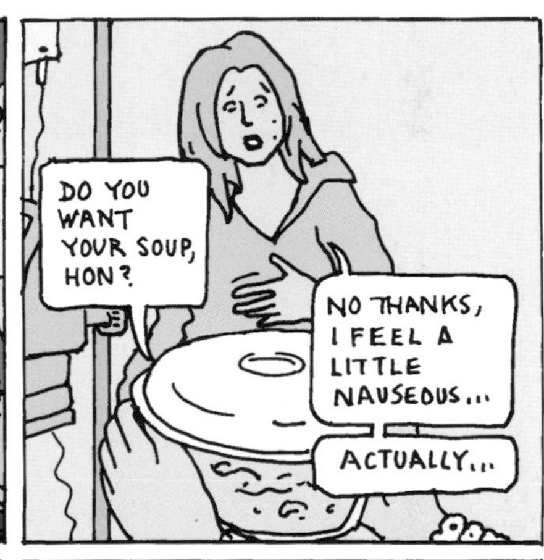
DO YOU WANT YOUR SOUP, HON?
NO THANKS, I FEEL A LITTLE NAUSEOUS...
ACTUALLY...

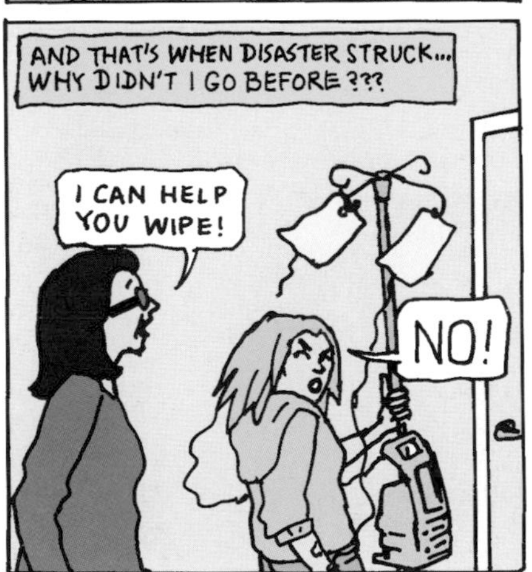
AND THAT'S WHEN DISASTER STRUCK... WHY DIDN'T I GO BEFORE???
I CAN HELP YOU WIPE!
NO!

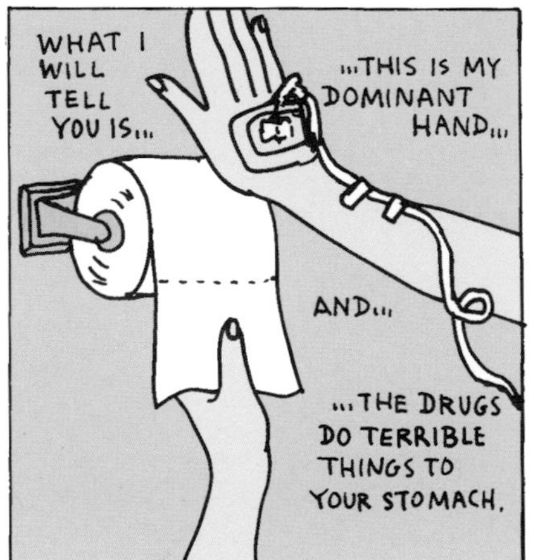
WHAT I WILL TELL YOU IS...
...THIS IS MY DOMINANT HAND...
AND...
...THE DRUGS DO TERRIBLE THINGS TO YOUR STOMACH.

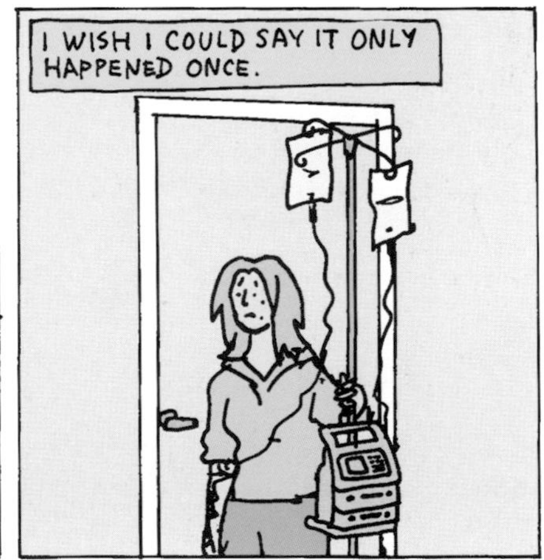
I WISH I COULD SAY IT ONLY HAPPENED ONCE.

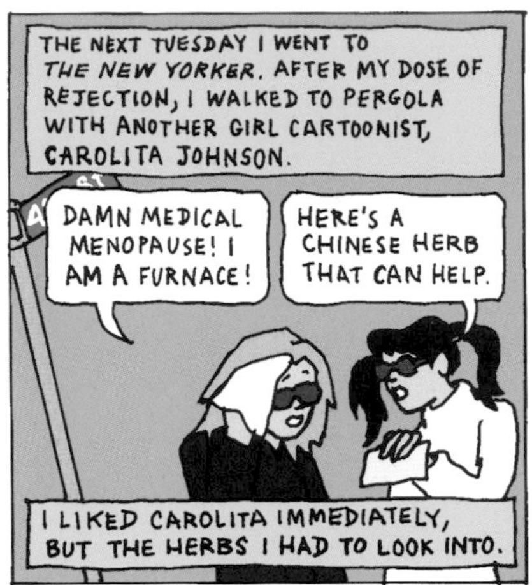

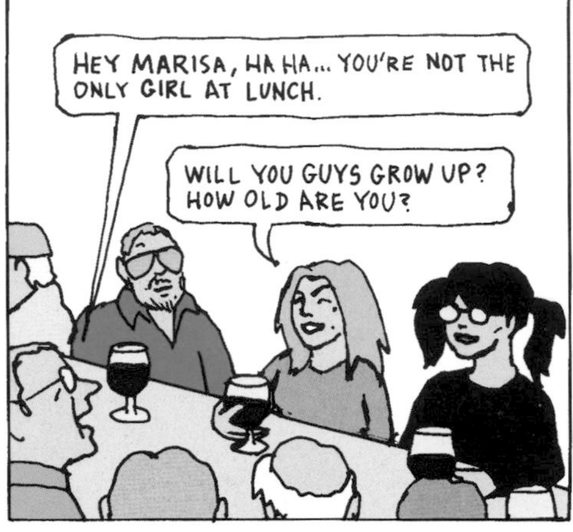

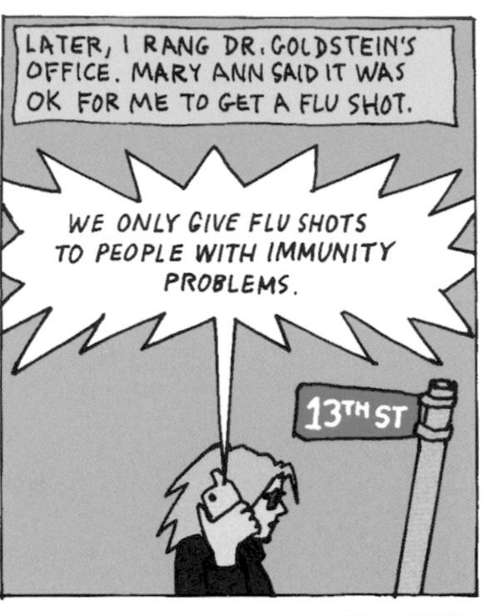

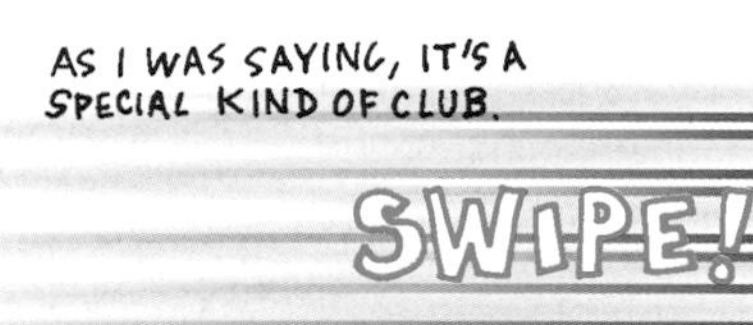

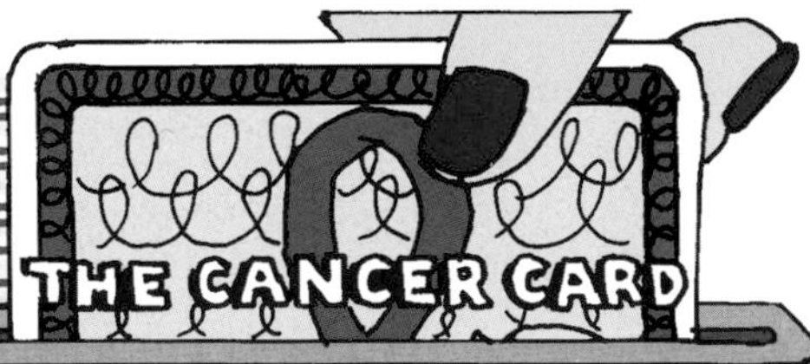

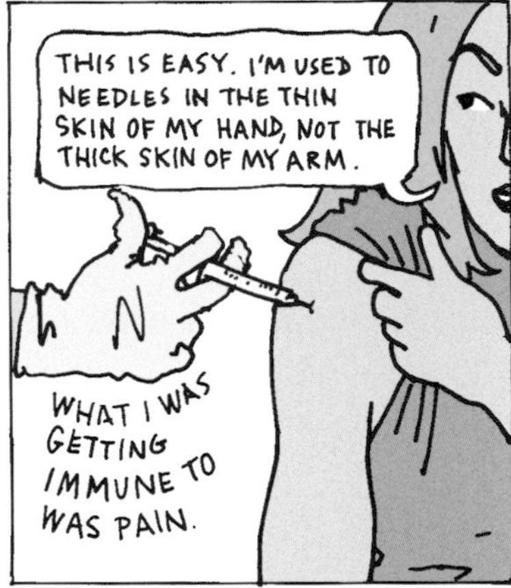

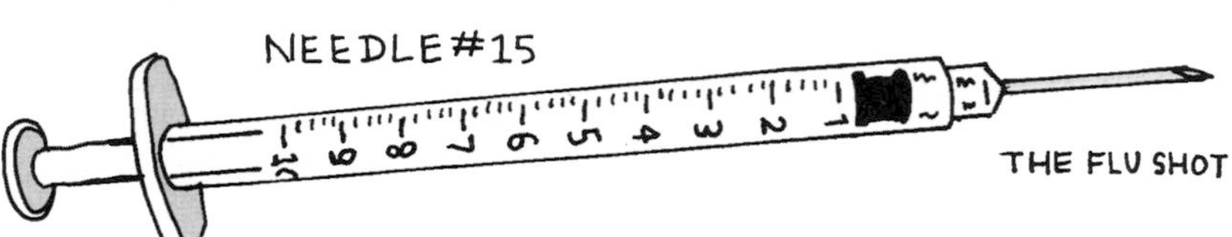

THE NEXT DAY, I WENT TO SVCCC FOR SOME MORE CEMENT-IN-MY-VEINS, WHITE-BLOOD-CELL-SPURRING ACTION.

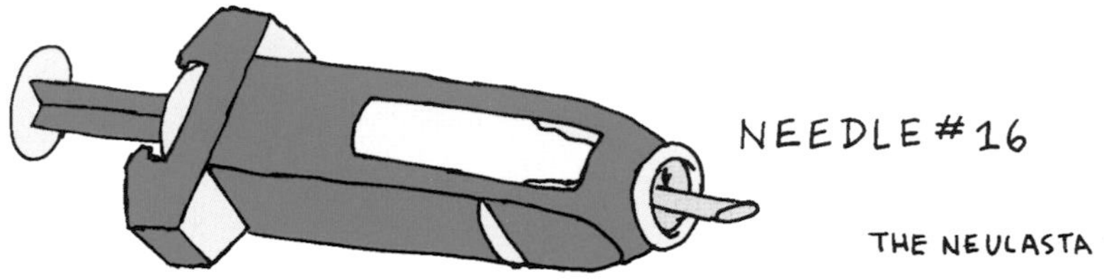

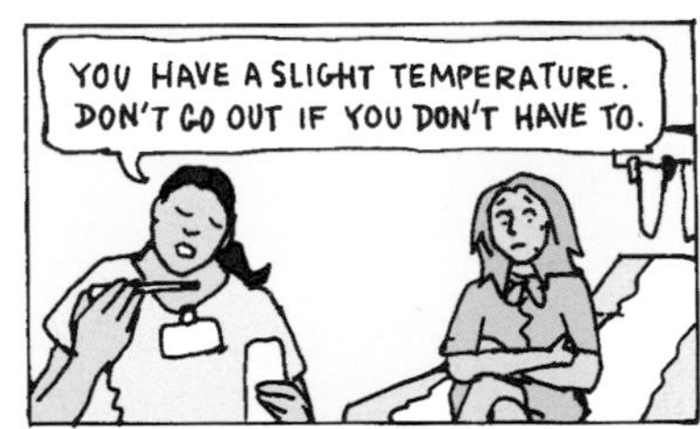

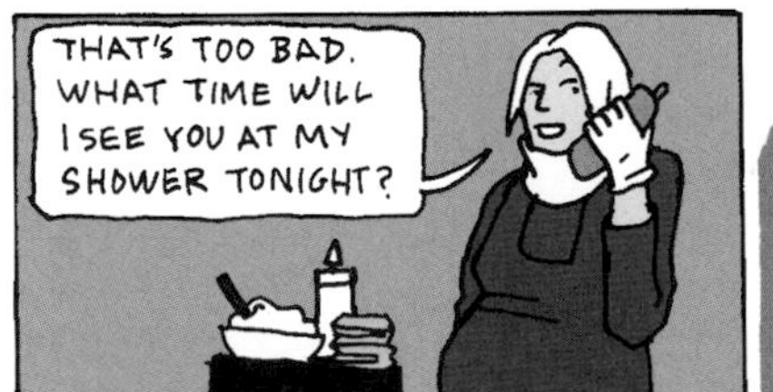

THE CANCER CARD
DECLINED

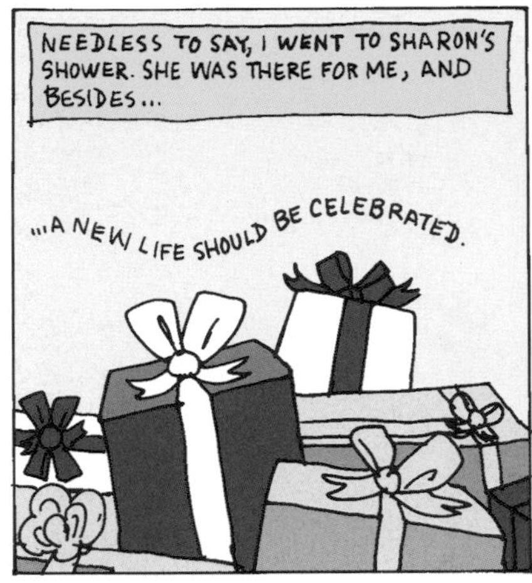

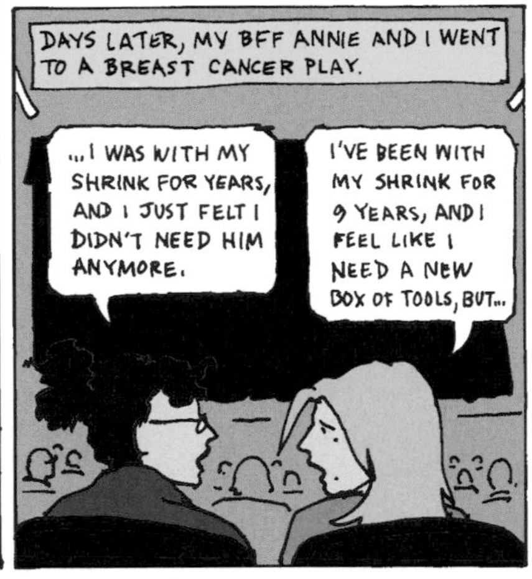

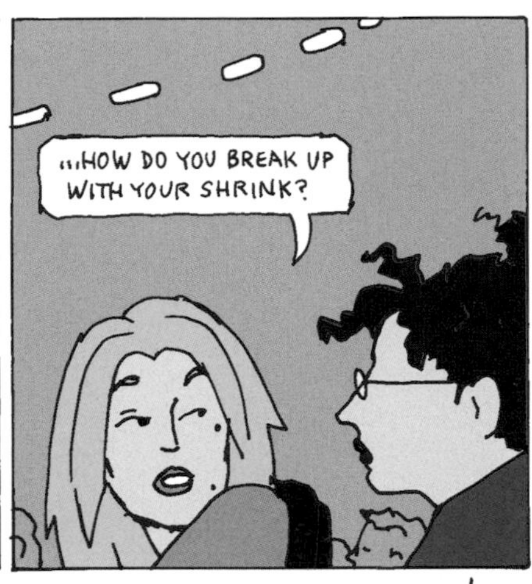

HERE'S HOW. SILVANO AND I WENT TO L.A. FOR FASHION WEEK. MOST PEOPLE GO TO SEE THE SHOWS INSIDE THE TENT, BUT WE WENT TO SEE MY CARTOONS ON THE OUTSIDE OF THE TENT.

WE LEFT FOR LOS ANGELES ON SATURDAY,

HOLLYWOOD

AND TOOK THE RED-EYE BACK ON SUNDAY...

SPEAKING OF RED EYES, YOURS TRULY DIDN'T SLEEP A WINK...

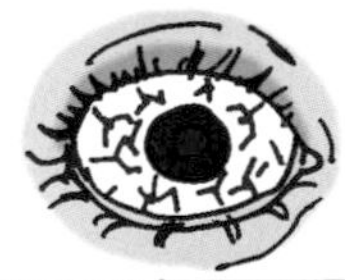
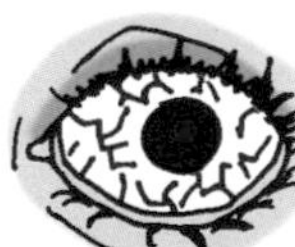

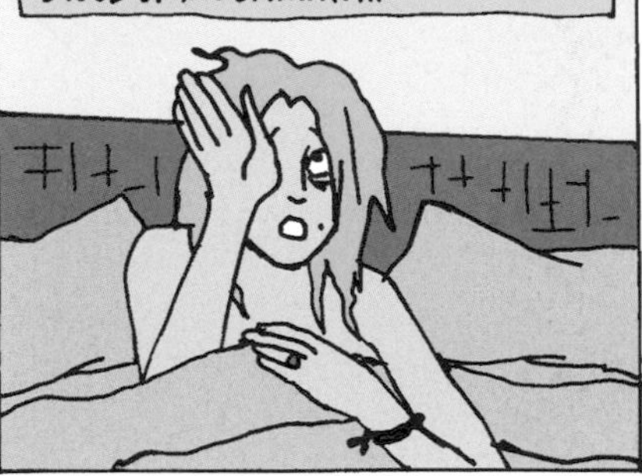

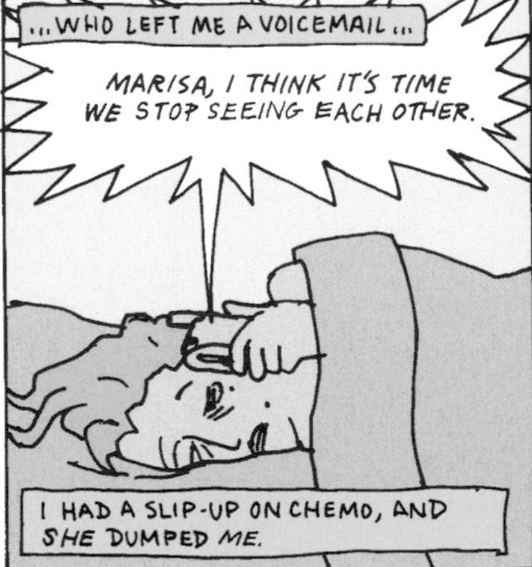

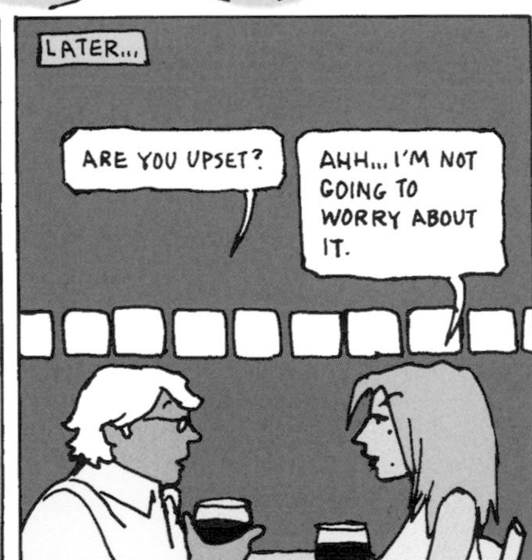

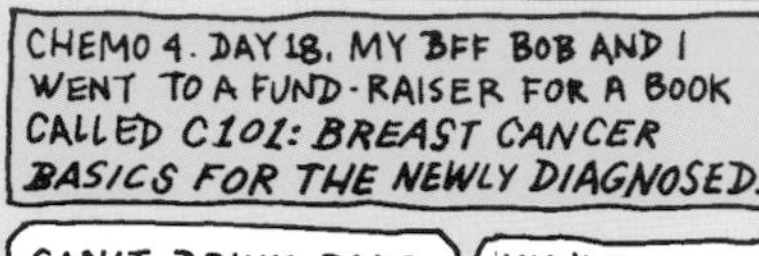
CHEMO 4. DAY 18. MY BFF BOB AND I WENT TO A FUND-RAISER FOR A BOOK CALLED *C101: BREAST CANCER BASICS FOR THE NEWLY DIAGNOSED.*

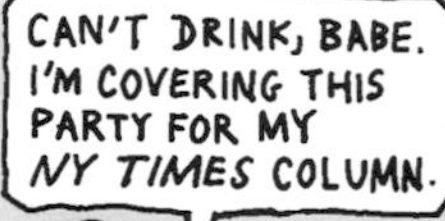
CAN'T DRINK, BABE. I'M COVERING THIS PARTY FOR MY *NY TIMES* COLUMN.

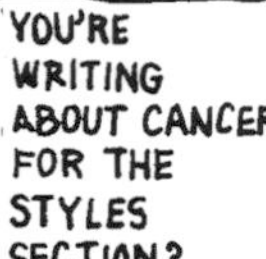
YOU'RE WRITING ABOUT CANCER FOR THE STYLES SECTION?

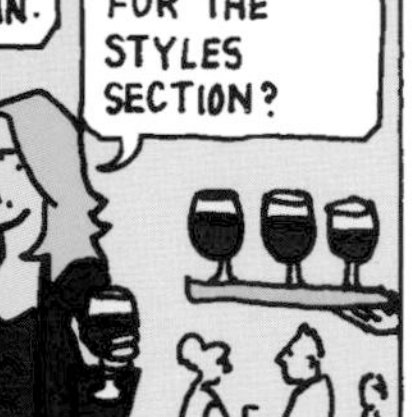

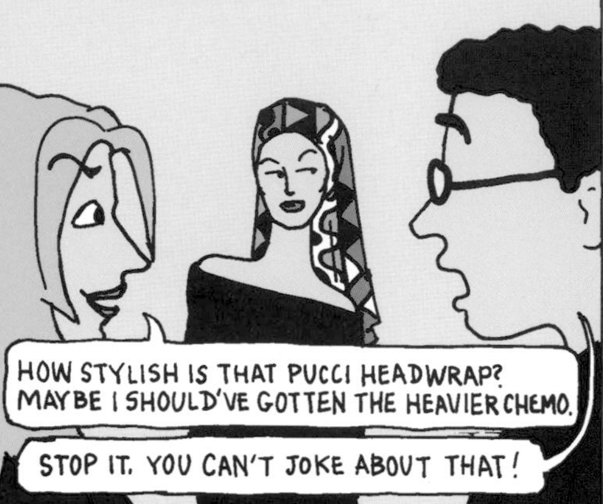
HOW STYLISH IS THAT PUCCI HEADWRAP? MAYBE I SHOULD'VE GOTTEN THE HEAVIER CHEMO.
STOP IT. YOU CAN'T JOKE ABOUT THAT!

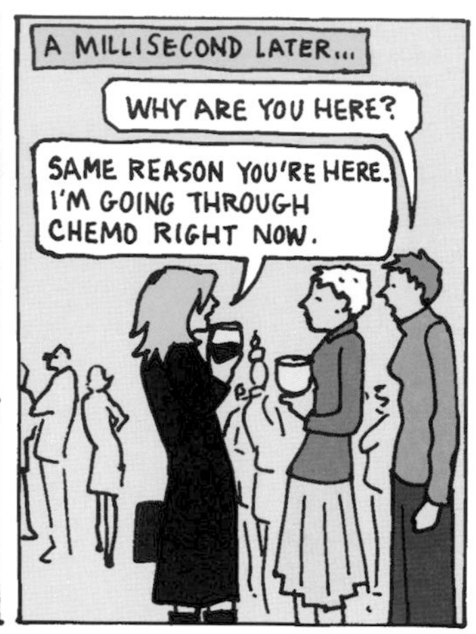
A MILLISECOND LATER...
WHY ARE YOU HERE?
SAME REASON YOU'RE HERE. I'M GOING THROUGH CHEMO RIGHT NOW.

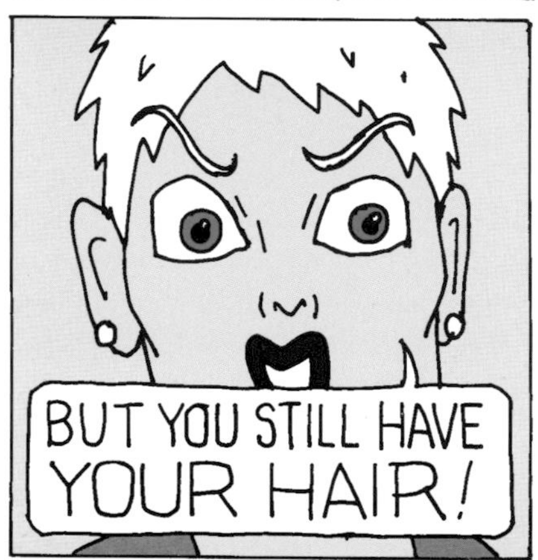
BUT YOU STILL HAVE YOUR HAIR!

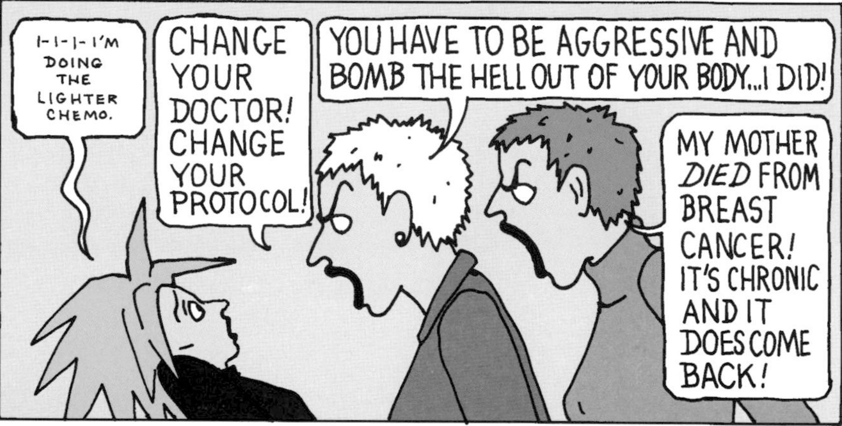
I-I-I-I'M DOING THE LIGHTER CHEMO.
CHANGE YOUR DOCTOR! CHANGE YOUR PROTOCOL!
YOU HAVE TO BE AGGRESSIVE AND BOMB THE HELL OUT OF YOUR BODY...I DID!
MY MOTHER *DIED* FROM BREAST CANCER! IT'S CHRONIC AND IT DOES COME BACK!

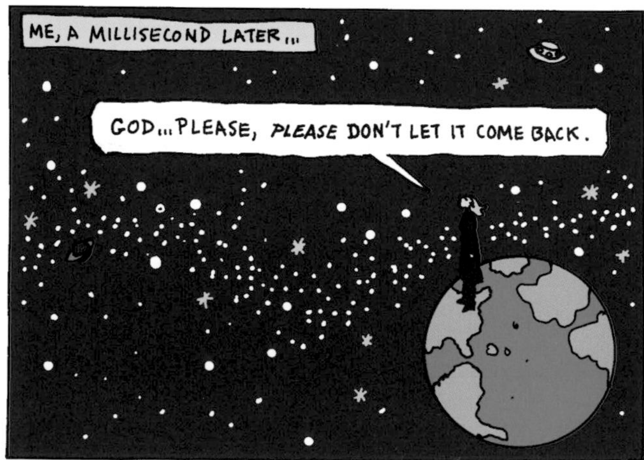
ME, A MILLISECOND LATER...
GOD... PLEASE, *PLEASE* DON'T LET IT COME BACK.

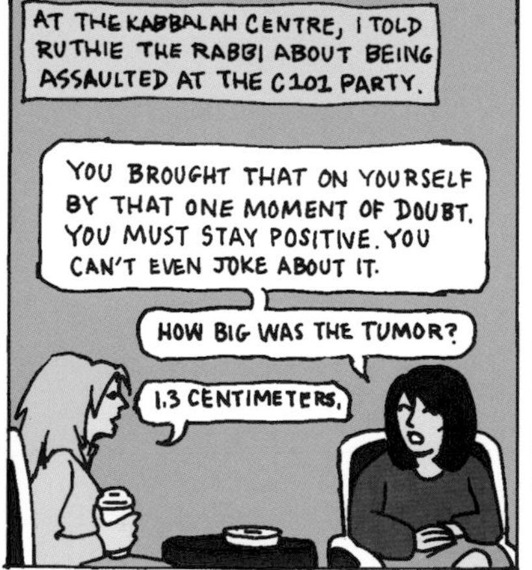
AT THE KABBALAH CENTRE, I TOLD RUTHIE THE RABBI ABOUT BEING ASSAULTED AT THE C101 PARTY.
YOU BROUGHT THAT ON YOURSELF BY THAT ONE MOMENT OF DOUBT. YOU MUST STAY POSITIVE. YOU CAN'T EVEN JOKE ABOUT IT.
HOW BIG WAS THE TUMOR?
1.3 CENTIMETERS.

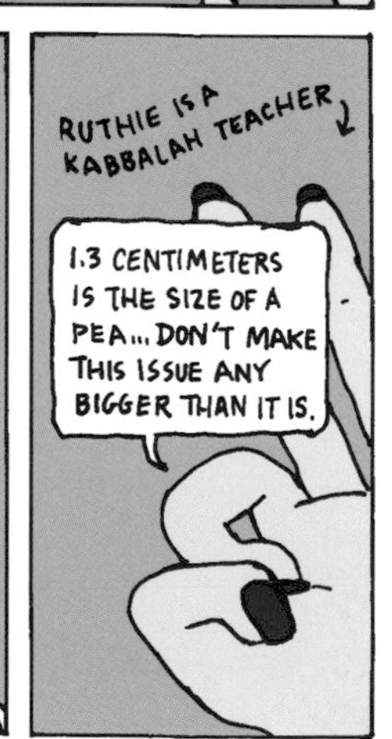
RUTHIE IS A KABBALAH TEACHER
1.3 CENTIMETERS IS THE SIZE OF A PEA... DON'T MAKE THIS ISSUE ANY BIGGER THAN IT IS.

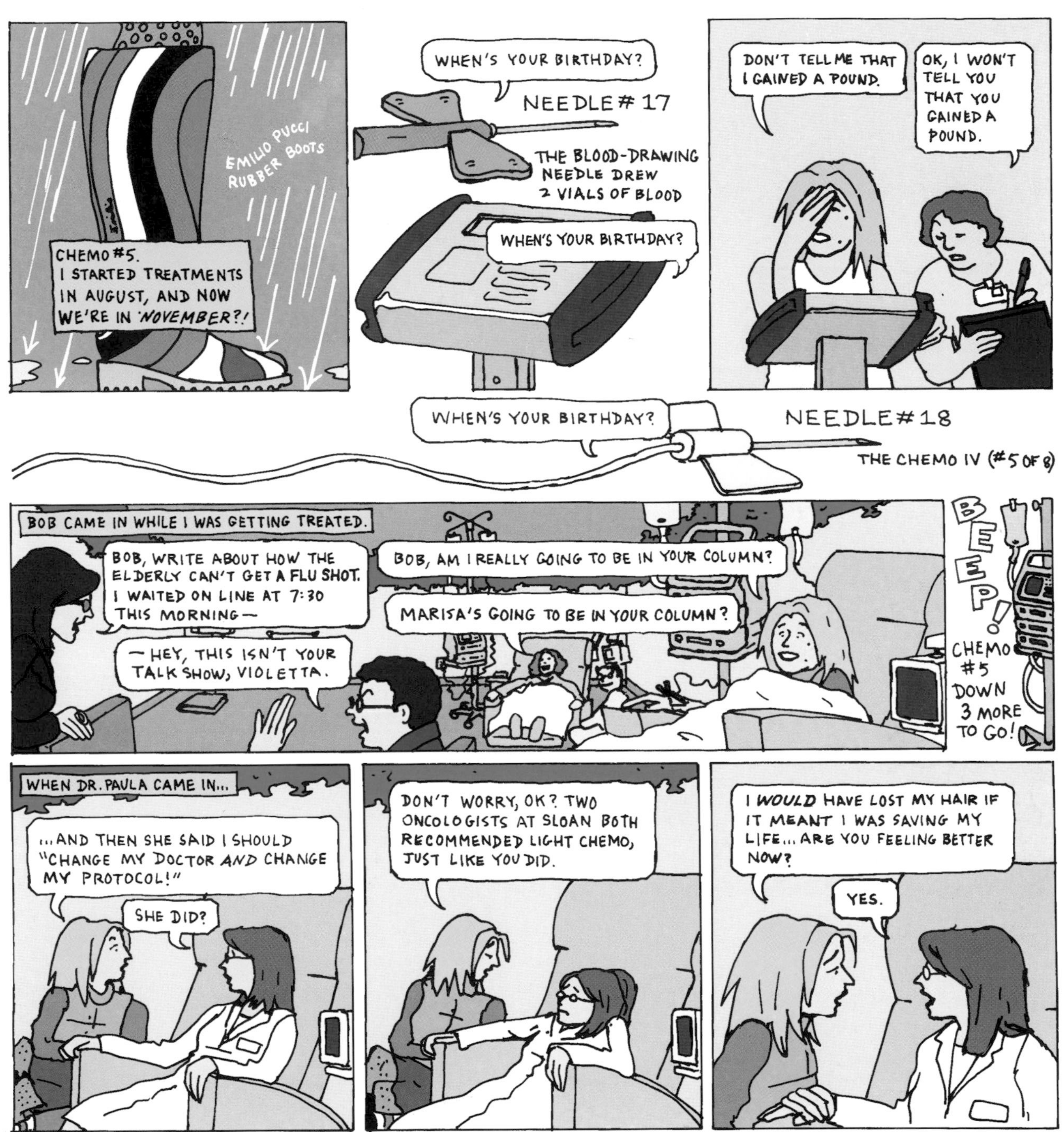
EMILIO PUCCI RUBBER BOOTS
CHEMO #5. I STARTED TREATMENTS IN AUGUST, AND NOW WE'RE IN *NOVEMBER*?!
WHEN'S YOUR BIRTHDAY?
NEEDLE #17
THE BLOOD-DRAWING NEEDLE DREW 2 VIALS OF BLOOD
WHEN'S YOUR BIRTHDAY?
DON'T TELL ME THAT I GAINED A POUND.
OK, I WON'T TELL YOU THAT YOU GAINED A POUND.
WHEN'S YOUR BIRTHDAY?
NEEDLE #18
THE CHEMO IV (#5 OF 8)
BOB CAME IN WHILE I WAS GETTING TREATED.
BOB, WRITE ABOUT HOW THE ELDERLY CAN'T GET A FLU SHOT. I WAITED ON LINE AT 7:30 THIS MORNING—
—HEY, THIS ISN'T YOUR TALK SHOW, VIOLETTA.
BOB, AM I REALLY GOING TO BE IN YOUR COLUMN?
MARISA'S GOING TO BE IN YOUR COLUMN?
BEEP!
CHEMO #5 DOWN 3 MORE TO GO!
WHEN DR. PAULA CAME IN...
...AND THEN SHE SAID I SHOULD "CHANGE MY DOCTOR *AND* CHANGE MY PROTOCOL!"
SHE DID?
DON'T WORRY, OK? TWO ONCOLOGISTS AT SLOAN BOTH RECOMMENDED LIGHT CHEMO, JUST LIKE YOU DID.
I *WOULD* HAVE LOST MY HAIR IF IT MEANT I WAS SAVING MY LIFE... ARE YOU FEELING BETTER NOW?
YES.

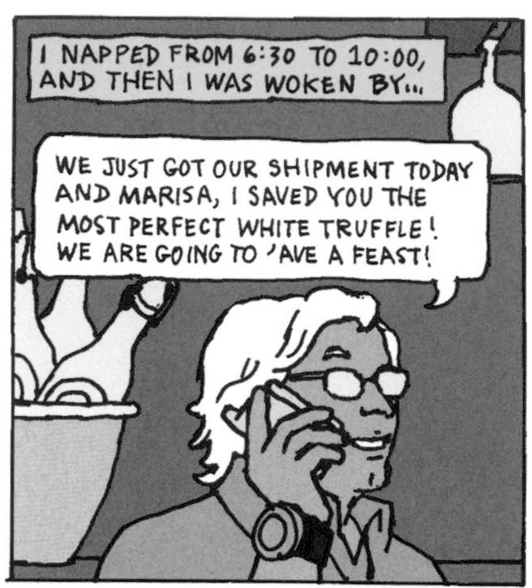
I NAPPED FROM 6:30 TO 10:00, AND THEN I WAS WOKEN BY...
WE JUST GOT OUR SHIPMENT TODAY AND MARISA, I SAVED YOU THE MOST PERFECT WHITE TRUFFLE! WE ARE GOING TO 'AVE A FEAST!

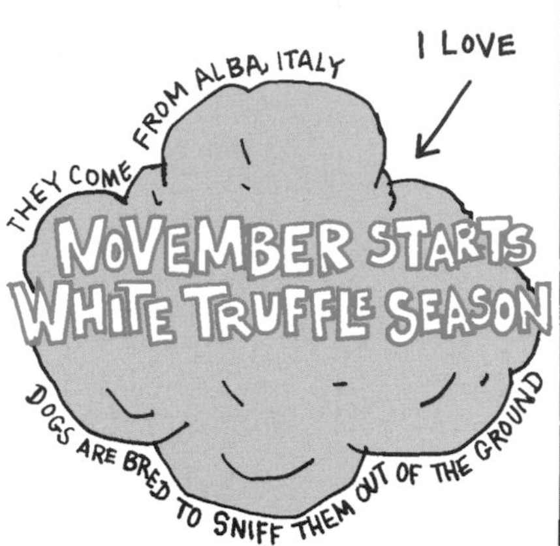
THEY COME FROM ALBA, ITALY
I LOVE
NOVEMBER STARTS WHITE TRUFFLE SEASON
DOGS ARE BRED TO SNIFF THEM OUT OF THE GROUND

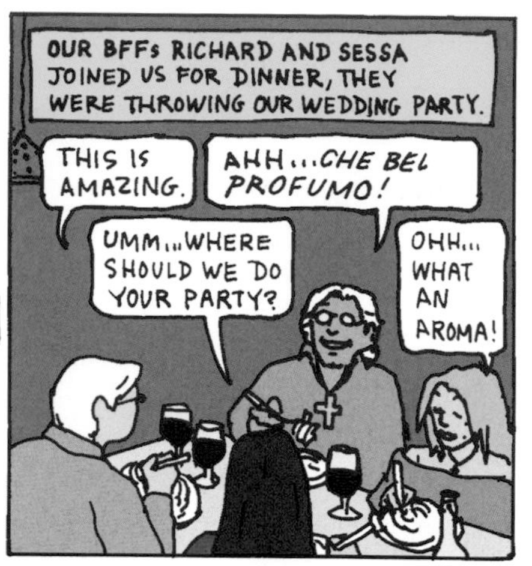
OUR BFFs RICHARD AND SESSA JOINED US FOR DINNER, THEY WERE THROWING OUR WEDDING PARTY.
THIS IS AMAZING.
AHH... *CHE BEL PROFUMO!*
UMM... WHERE SHOULD WE DO YOUR PARTY?
OHH... WHAT AN AROMA!

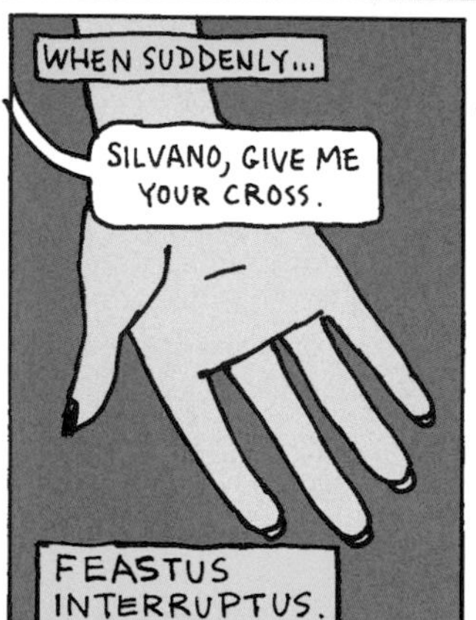
WHEN SUDDENLY...
SILVANO, GIVE ME YOUR CROSS.
FEASTUS INTERRUPTUS.

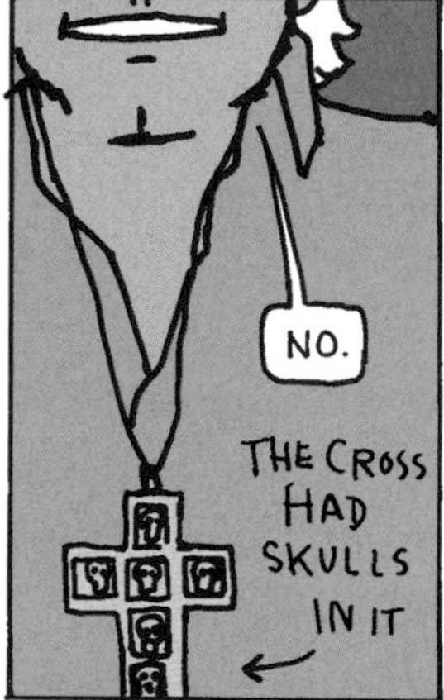
NO.
THE CROSS HAD SKULLS IN IT

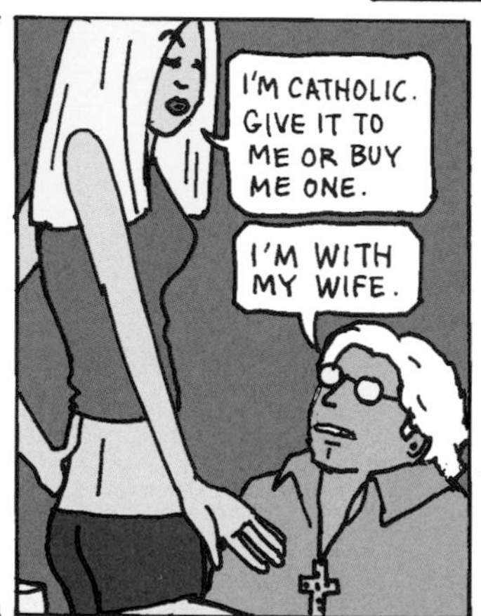
I'M CATHOLIC. GIVE IT TO ME OR BUY ME ONE.
I'M WITH MY WIFE.

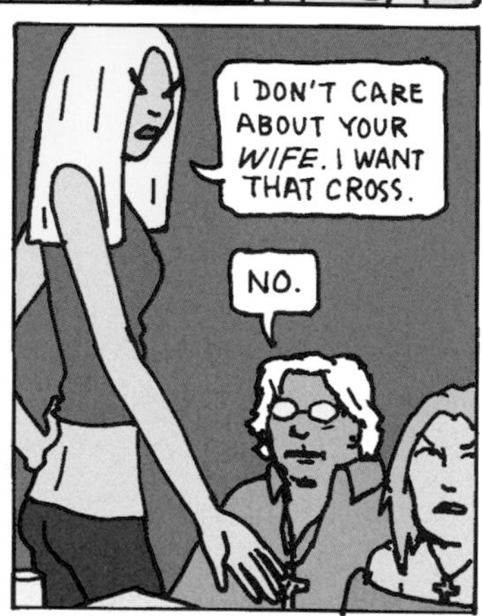
I DON'T CARE ABOUT YOUR *WIFE*. I WANT THAT CROSS.
NO.

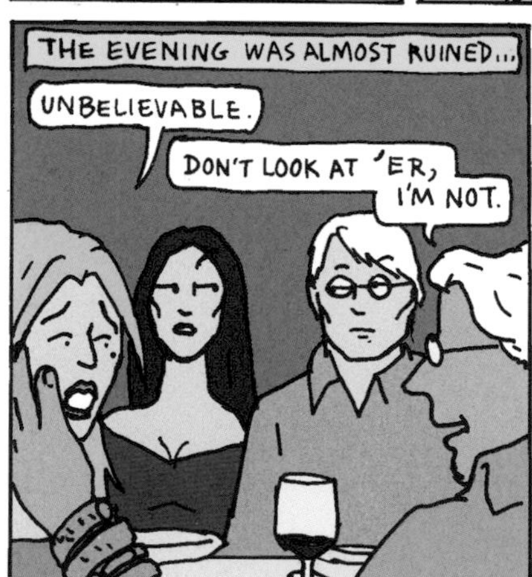
THE EVENING WAS ALMOST RUINED...
UNBELIEVABLE.
DON'T LOOK AT 'ER, I'M NOT.

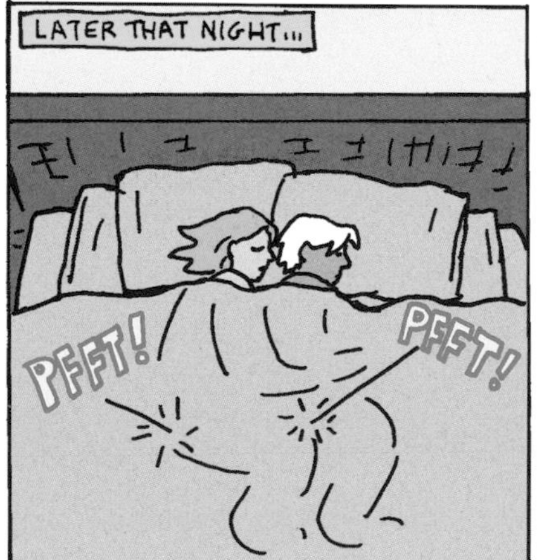
LATER THAT NIGHT...
PFFT!
PFFT!

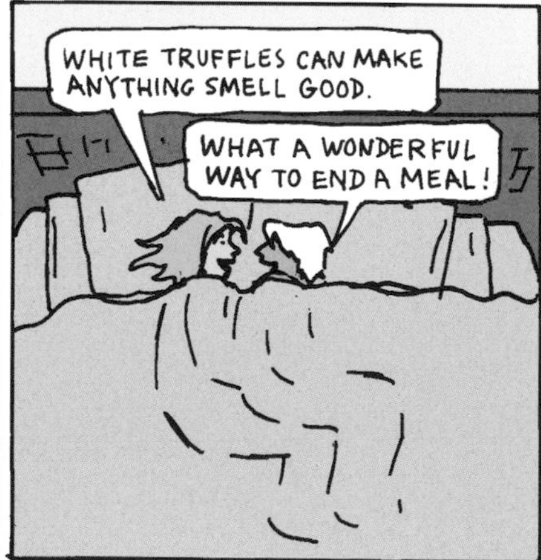
WHITE TRUFFLES CAN MAKE ANYTHING SMELL GOOD.
WHAT A WONDERFUL WAY TO END A MEAL!

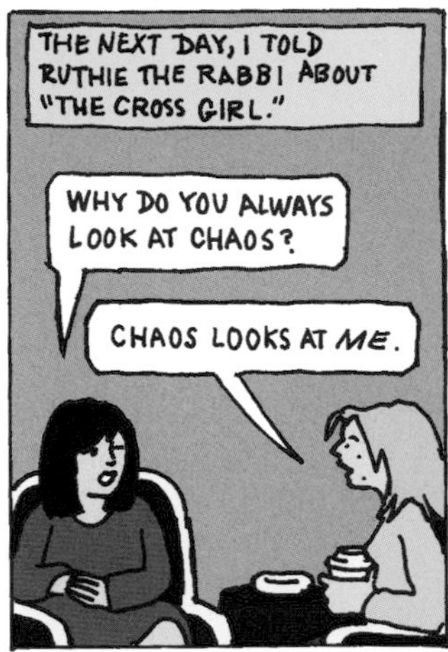
THE NEXT DAY, I TOLD RUTHIE THE RABBI ABOUT "THE CROSS GIRL."
WHY DO YOU ALWAYS LOOK AT CHAOS?
CHAOS LOOKS AT ME.
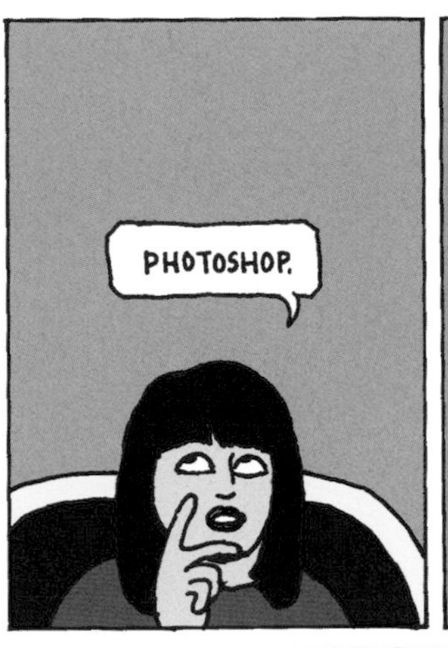
PHOTOSHOP.
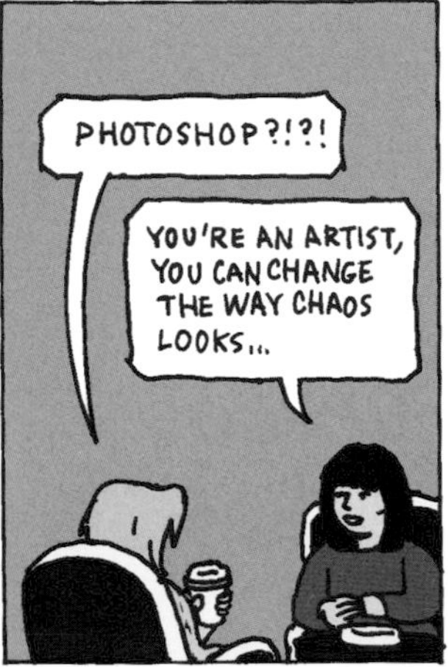
PHOTOSHOP?!?!
YOU'RE AN ARTIST, YOU CAN CHANGE THE WAY CHAOS LOOKS...
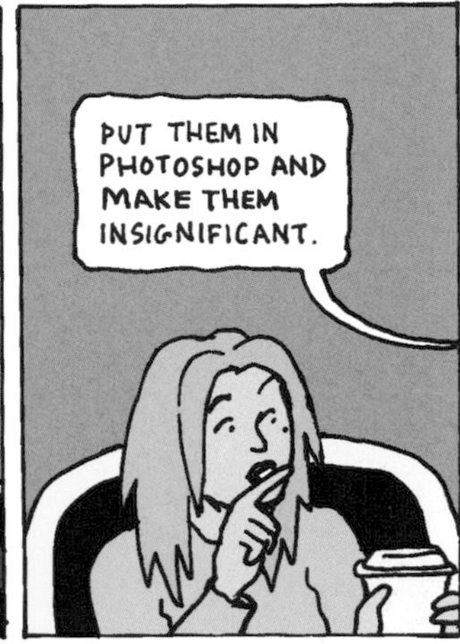
PUT THEM IN PHOTOSHOP AND MAKE THEM INSIGNIFICANT.
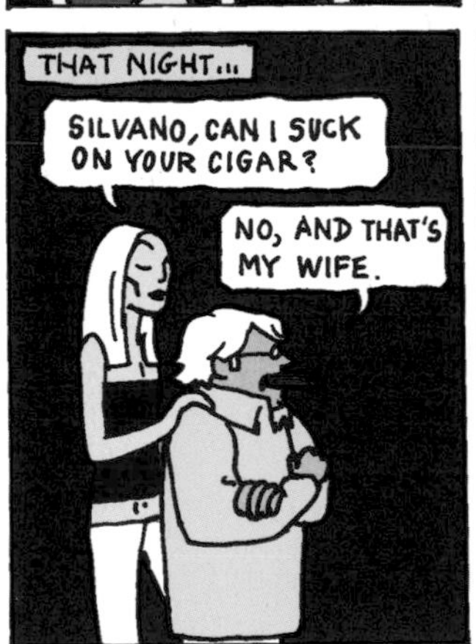
THAT NIGHT...
SILVANO, CAN I SUCK ON YOUR CIGAR?
NO, AND THAT'S MY WIFE.
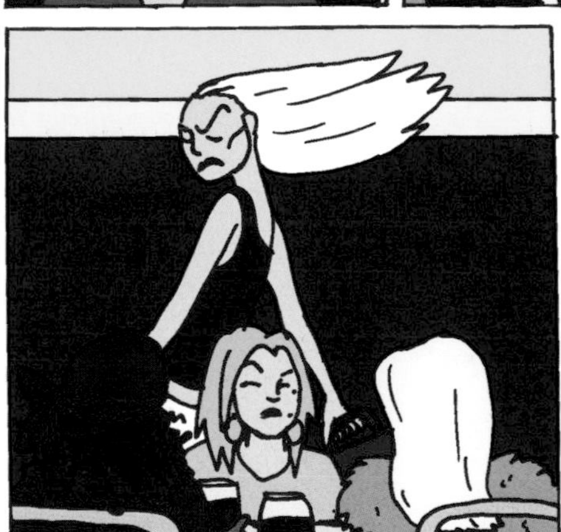
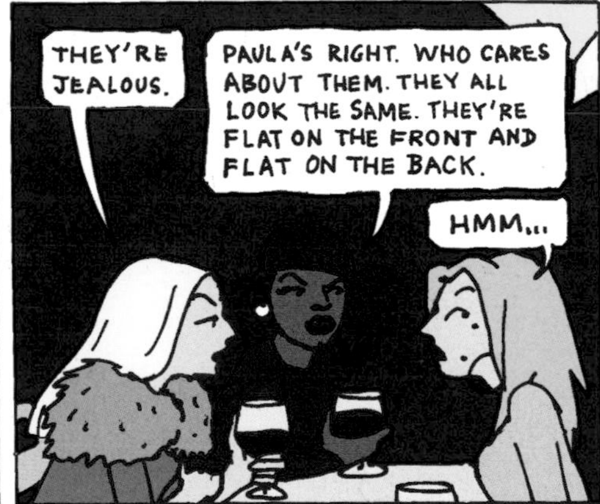
THEY'RE JEALOUS.
PAULA'S RIGHT. WHO CARES ABOUT THEM. THEY ALL LOOK THE SAME. THEY'RE FLAT ON THE FRONT AND FLAT ON THE BACK.
HMM...
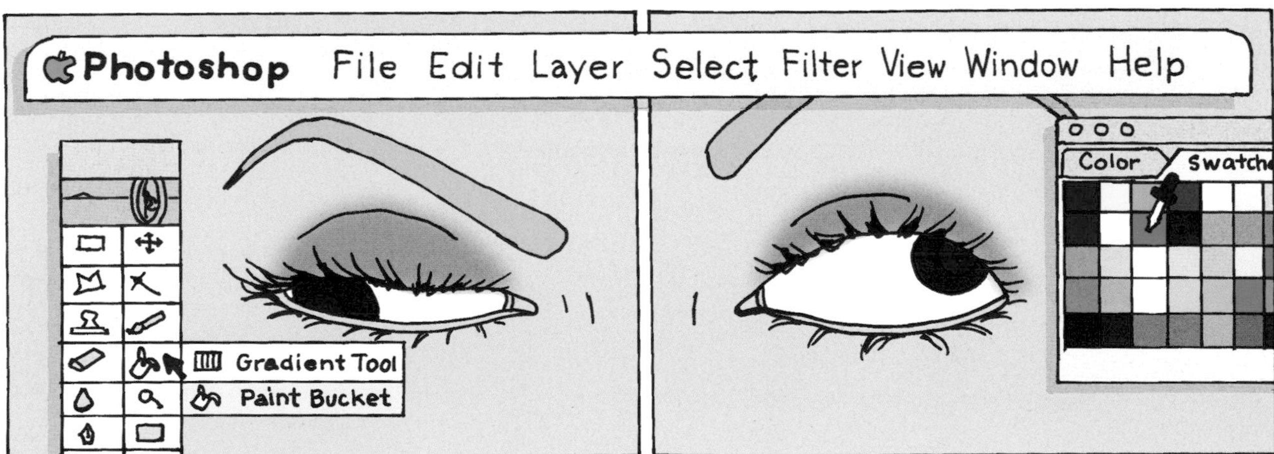
Photoshop File Edit Layer Select Filter View Window Help
Gradient Tool
Paint Bucket
Color

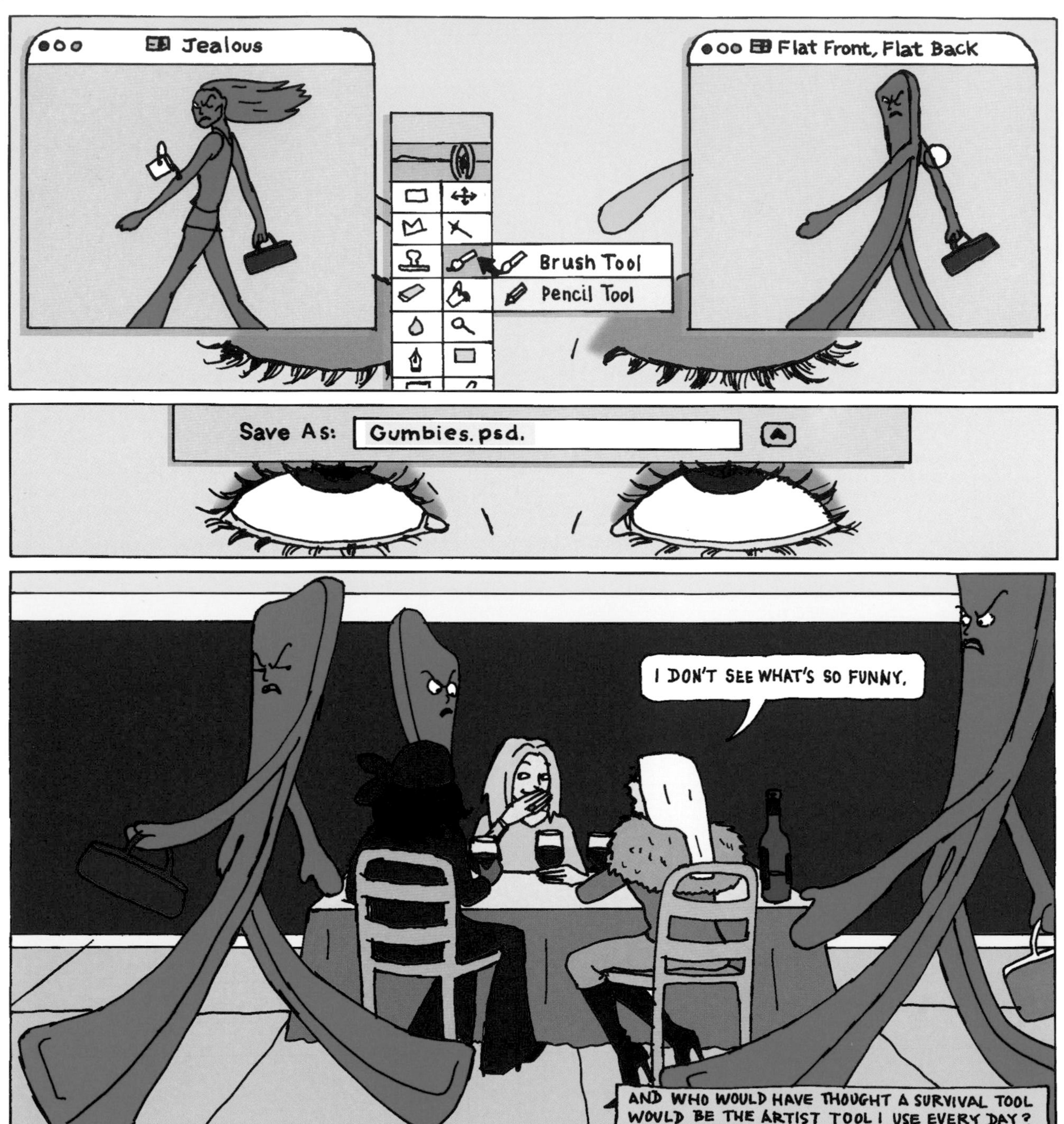
Jealous
Flat Front, Flat Back
Brush Tool
Pencil Tool
Save As: Gumbies.psd.
I DON'T SEE WHAT'S SO FUNNY.
AND WHO WOULD HAVE THOUGHT A SURVIVAL TOOL WOULD BE THE ARTIST TOOL I USE EVERY DAY?

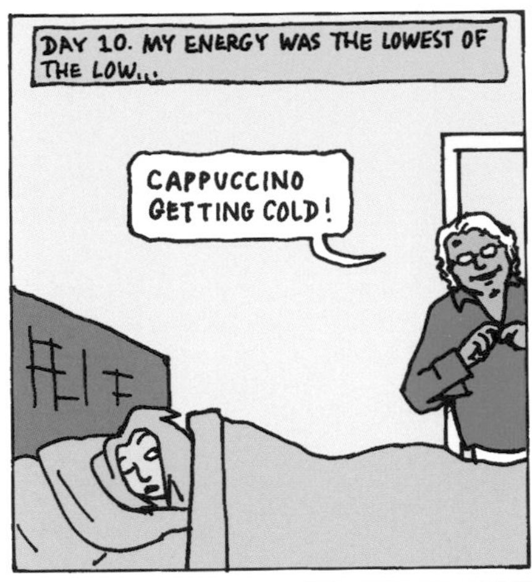
DAY 10. MY ENERGY WAS THE LOWEST OF THE LOW...
CAPPUCCINO GETTING COLD!

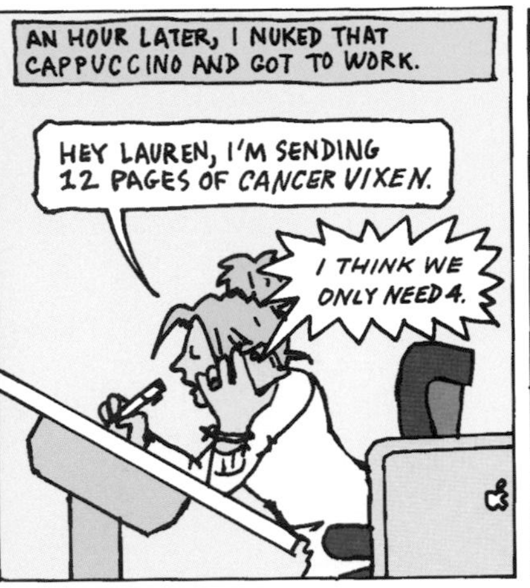
AN HOUR LATER, I NUKED THAT CAPPUCCINO AND GOT TO WORK.
HEY LAUREN, I'M SENDING 12 PAGES OF CANCER VIXEN.
I THINK WE ONLY NEED 4.

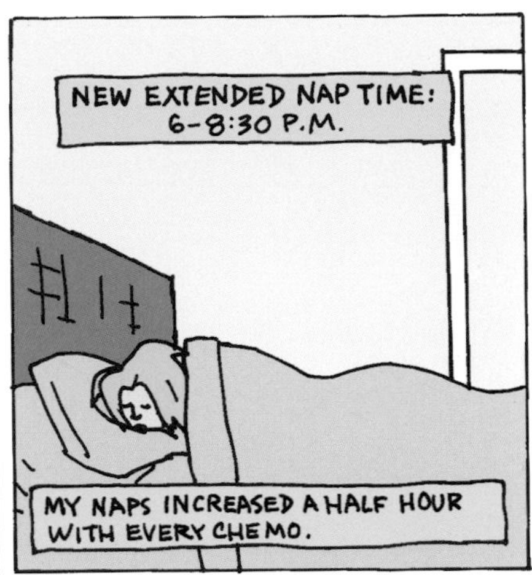
NEW EXTENDED NAP TIME: 6-8:30 P.M.
MY NAPS INCREASED A HALF HOUR WITH EVERY CHEMO.

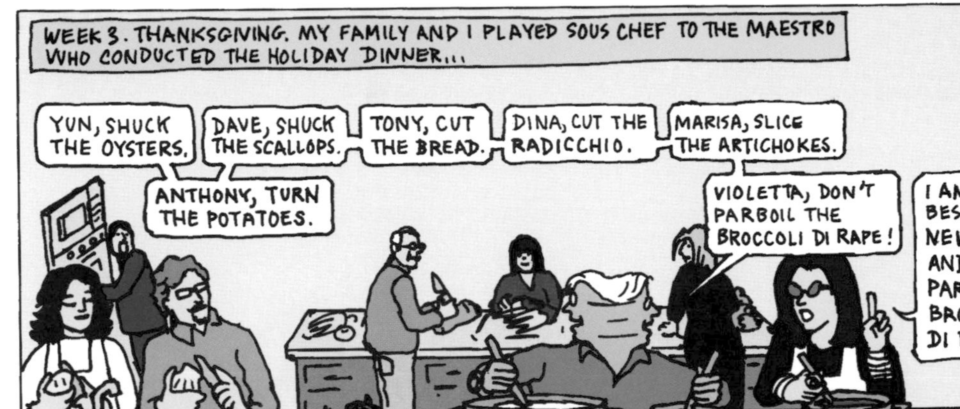
WEEK 3. THANKSGIVING. MY FAMILY AND I PLAYED SOUS CHEF TO THE MAESTRO WHO CONDUCTED THE HOLIDAY DINNER...
YUN, SHUCK THE OYSTERS.
ANTHONY, TURN THE POTATOES.
DAVE, SHUCK THE SCALLOPS.
TONY, CUT THE BREAD.
DINA, CUT THE RADICCHIO.
MARISA, SLICE THE ARTICHOKES.
VIOLETTA, DON'T PARBOIL THE BROCCOLI DI RAPE!
I AM THE BEST COOK IN NEW JERSEY, AND I ALWAYS PARBOIL BROCCOLI DI RAPE!

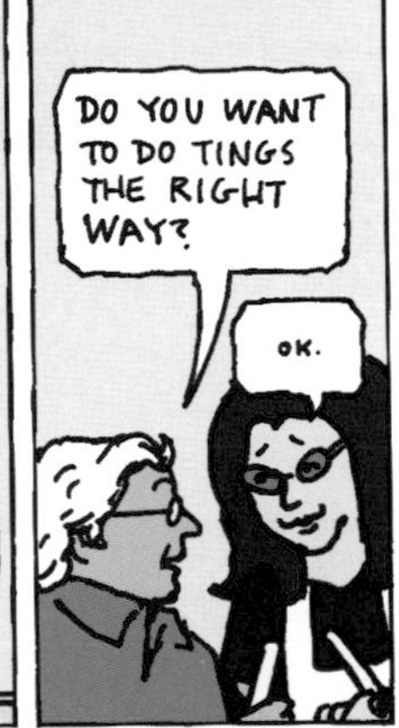
DO YOU WANT TO DO TINGS THE RIGHT WAY?
OK.

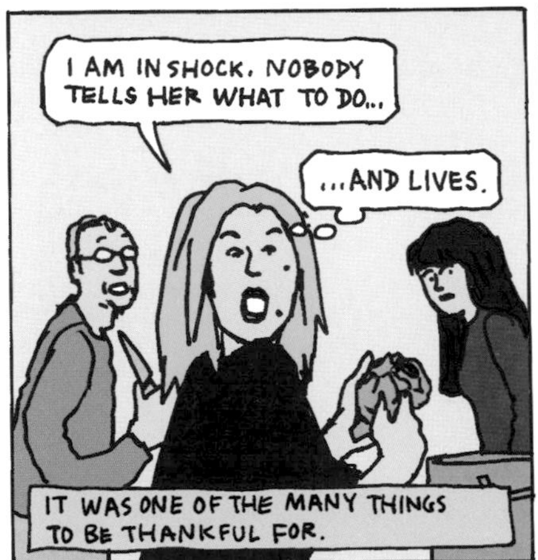
I AM IN SHOCK. NOBODY TELLS HER WHAT TO DO...
...AND LIVES.
IT WAS ONE OF THE MANY THINGS TO BE THANKFUL FOR.

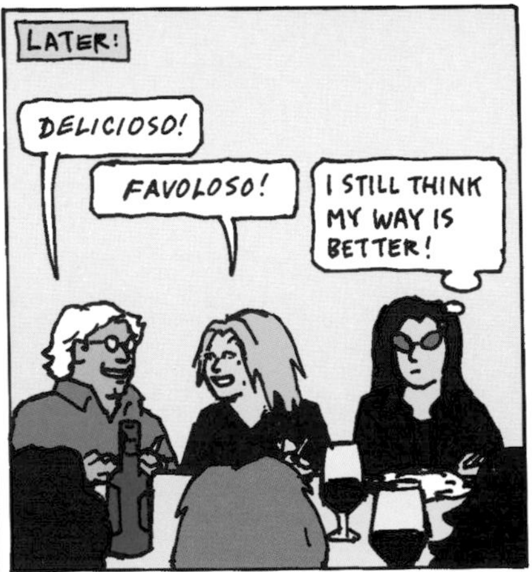
LATER!
DELICIOSO!
FAVOLOSO!
I STILL THINK MY WAY IS BETTER!

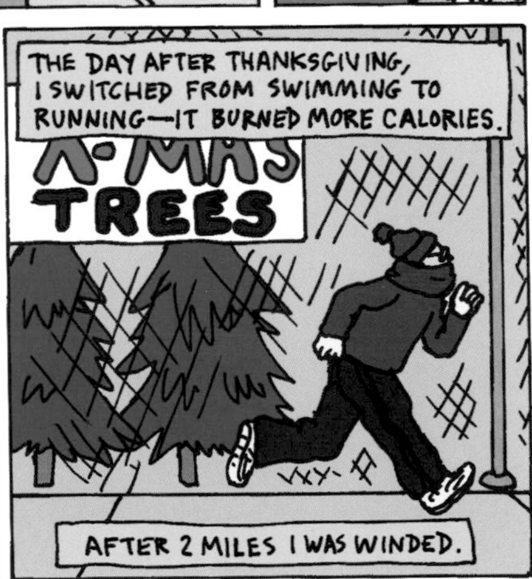
THE DAY AFTER THANKSGIVING, I SWITCHED FROM SWIMMING TO RUNNING—IT BURNED MORE CALORIES.
X-MAS TREES
AFTER 2 MILES I WAS WINDED.

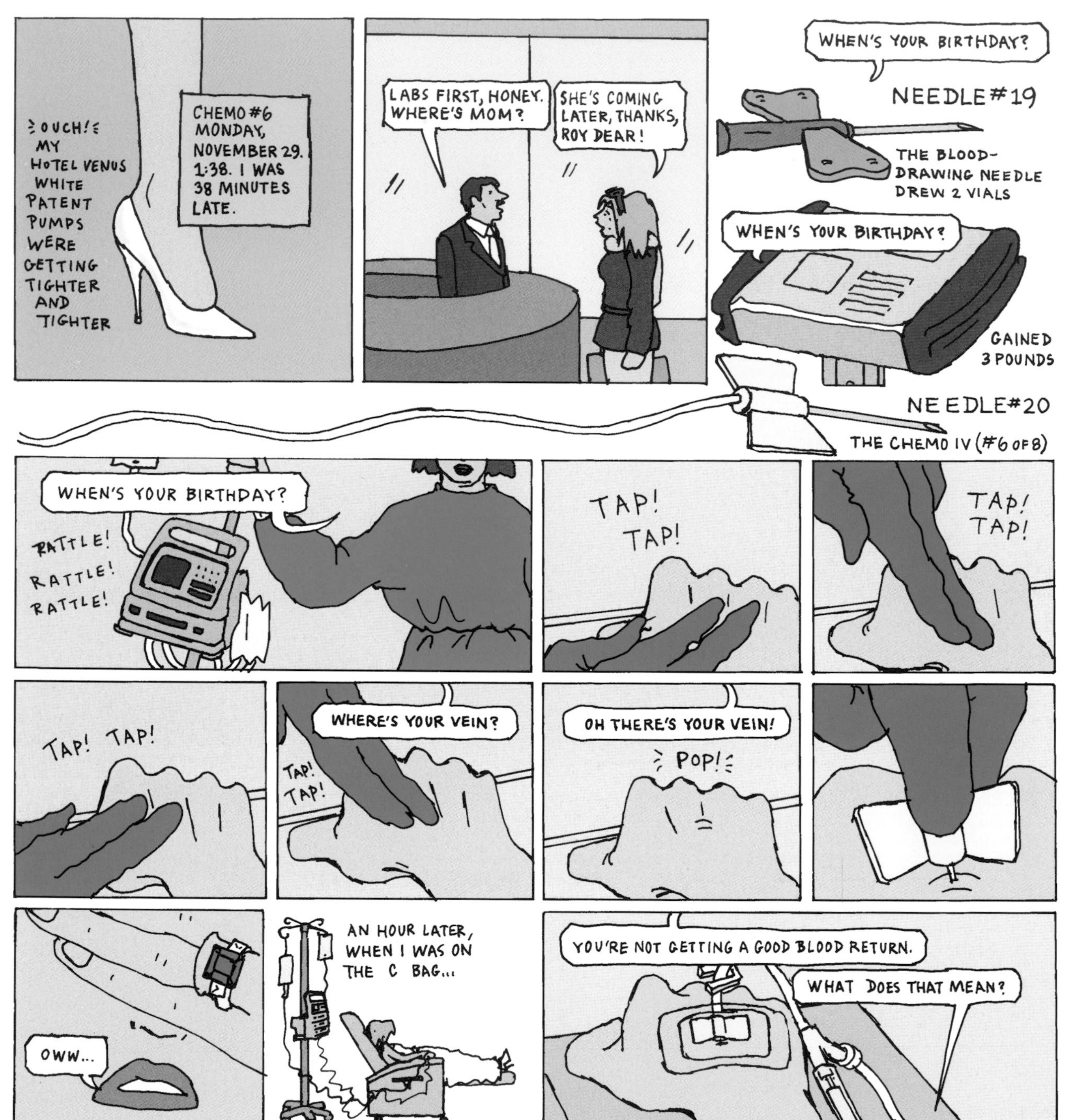
OUCH! MY HOTEL VENUS WHITE PATENT PUMPS WERE GETTING TIGHTER AND TIGHTER
CHEMO #6 MONDAY, NOVEMBER 29. 1:38. I WAS 38 MINUTES LATE.
LABS FIRST, HONEY. WHERE'S MOM?
SHE'S COMING LATER, THANKS, ROY DEAR!
WHEN'S YOUR BIRTHDAY?
NEEDLE #19
THE BLOOD-DRAWING NEEDLE DREW 2 VIALS
WHEN'S YOUR BIRTHDAY?
GAINED 3 POUNDS
NEEDLE #20
THE CHEMO IV (#6 OF 8)
WHEN'S YOUR BIRTHDAY?
RATTLE! RATTLE! RATTLE!
TAP! TAP!
TAP! TAP!
TAP! TAP!
WHERE'S YOUR VEIN?
TAP! TAP!
OH THERE'S YOUR VEIN!
POP!
OWW...
AN HOUR LATER, WHEN I WAS ON THE C BAG...
YOU'RE NOT GETTING A GOOD BLOOD RETURN.
WHAT DOES THAT MEAN?

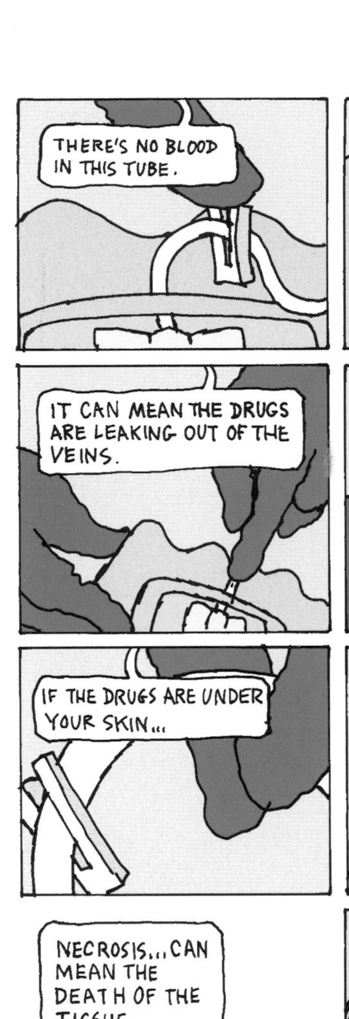
THERE'S NO BLOOD IN THIS TUBE.
IT CAN MEAN THE DRUGS ARE LEAKING OUT OF THE VEINS.
IF THE DRUGS ARE UNDER YOUR SKIN...

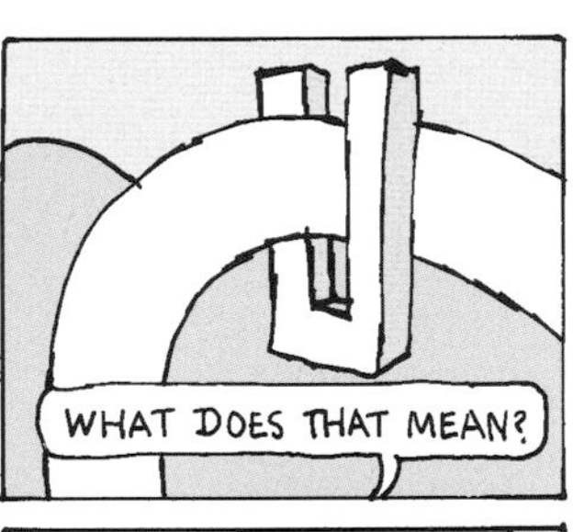
WHAT DOES THAT MEAN?

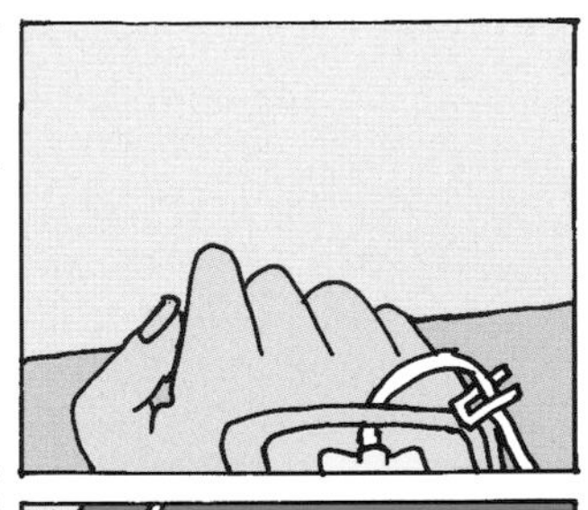

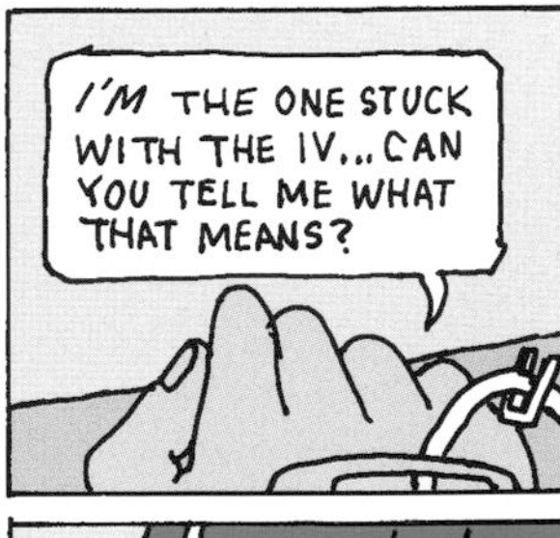
I'M THE ONE STUCK WITH THE IV... CAN YOU TELL ME WHAT THAT MEANS?

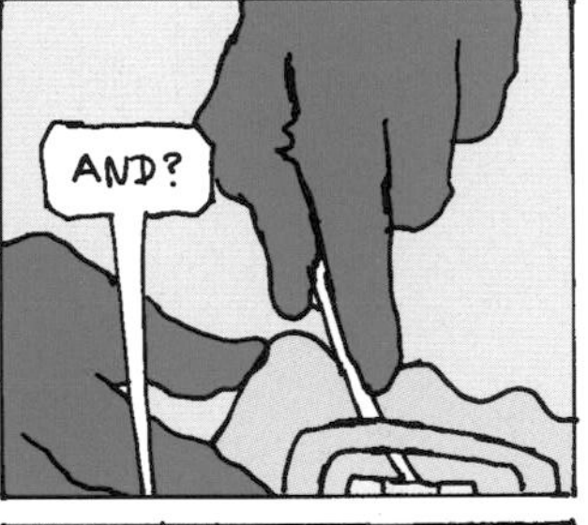
AND?

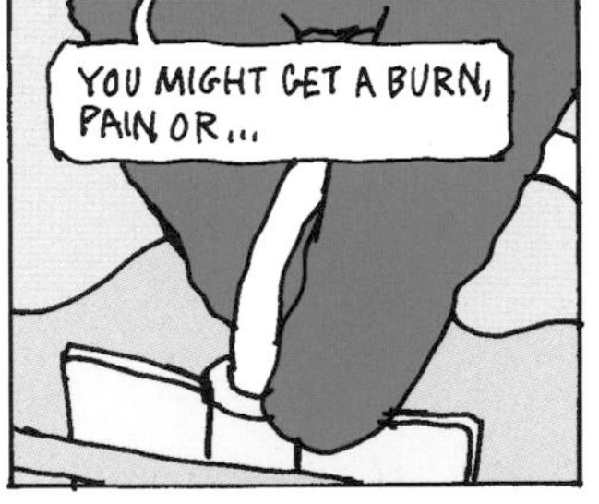
YOU MIGHT GET A BURN, PAIN OR...

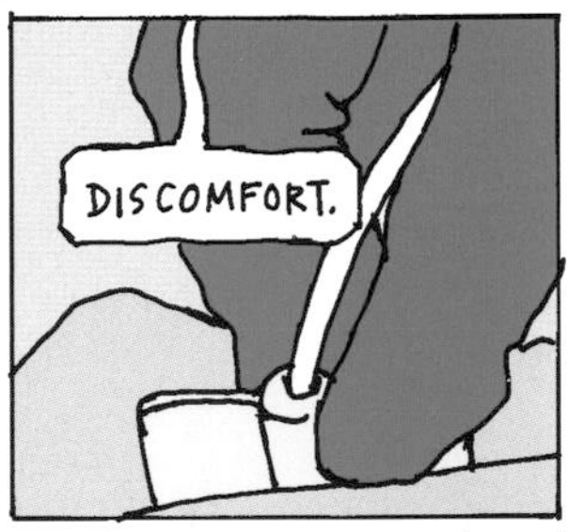
DISCOMFORT.

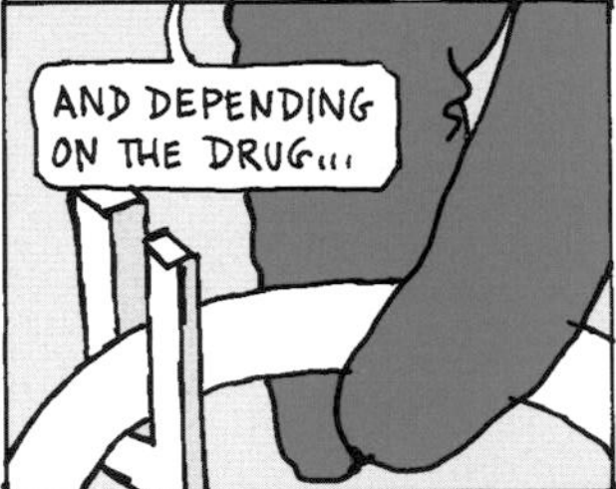
AND DEPENDING ON THE DRUG...

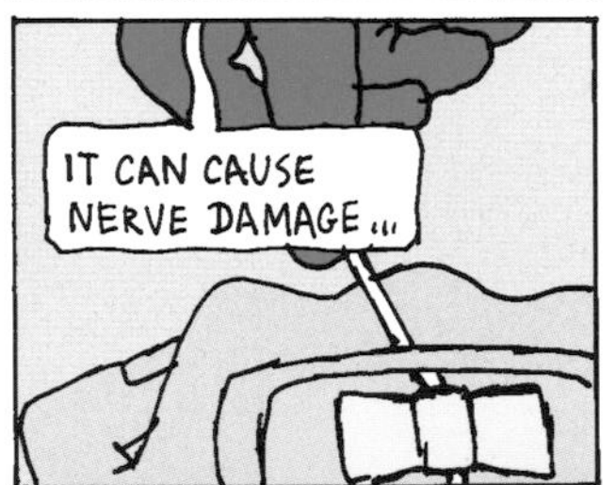
IT CAN CAUSE NERVE DAMAGE...

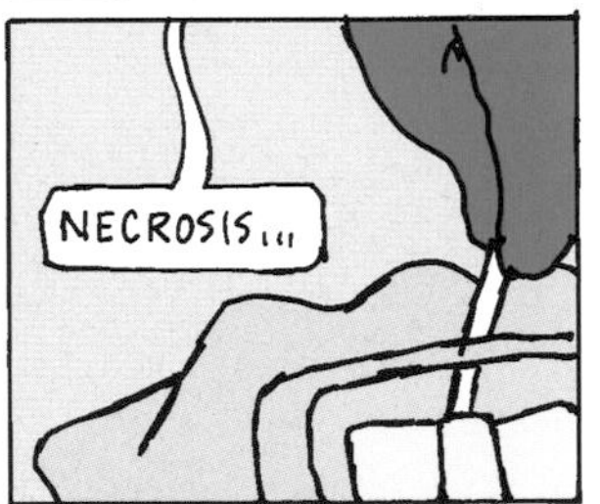
NECROSIS...

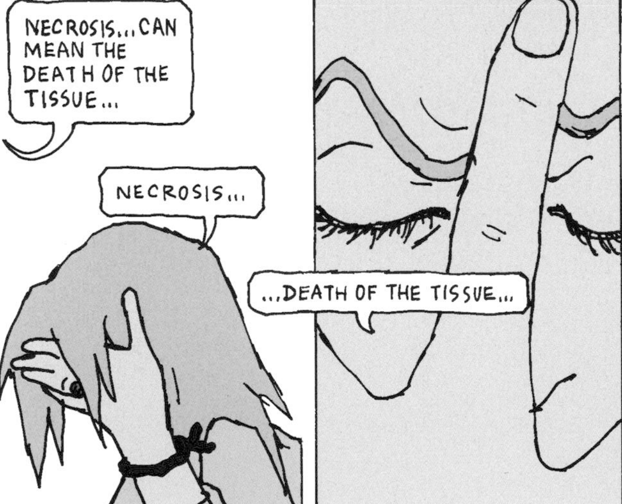
NECROSIS... CAN MEAN THE DEATH OF THE TISSUE...
NECROSIS...
...DEATH OF THE TISSUE...

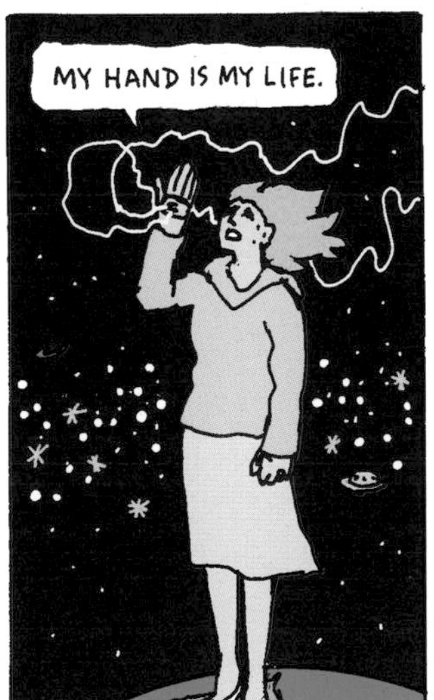
MY HAND IS MY LIFE.

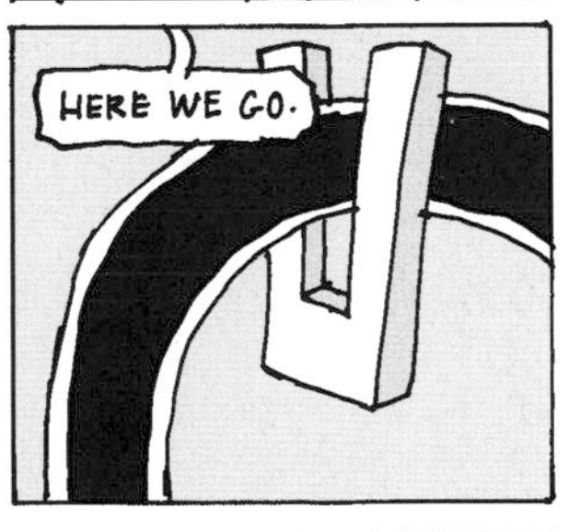
HERE WE GO.

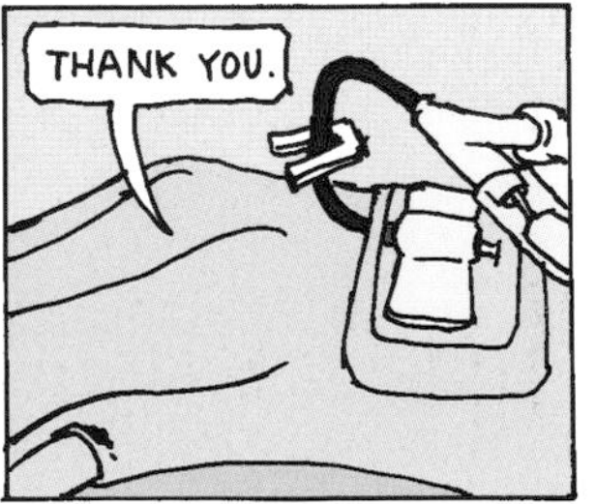
THANK YOU.

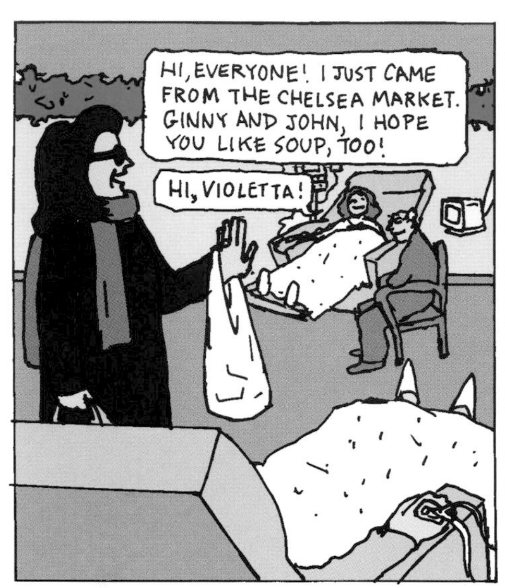
HI, EVERYONE! I JUST CAME FROM THE CHELSEA MARKET. GINNY AND JOHN, I HOPE YOU LIKE SOUP, TOO!
HI, VIOLETTA!

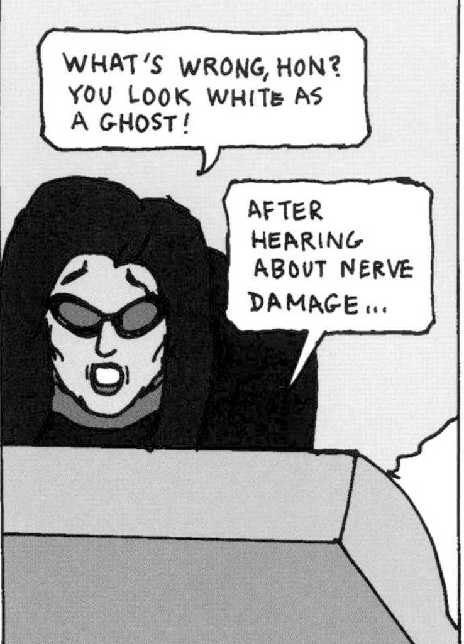
WHAT'S WRONG, HON? YOU LOOK WHITE AS A GHOST!
AFTER HEARING ABOUT NERVE DAMAGE...

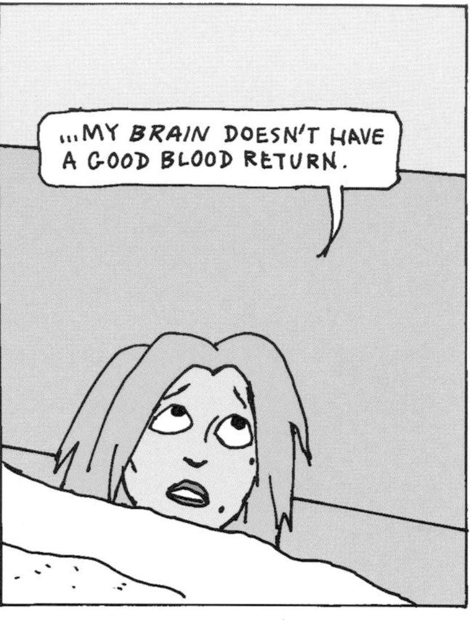
...MY *BRAIN* DOESN'T HAVE A GOOD BLOOD RETURN.

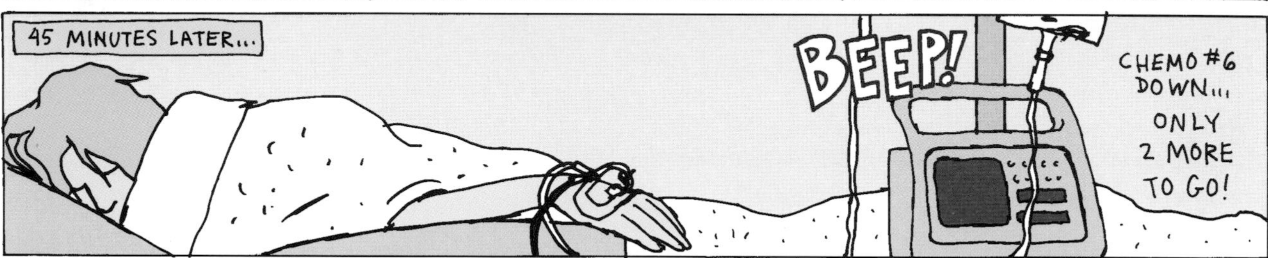
45 MINUTES LATER...
BEEP!
CHEMO #6 DOWN... ONLY 2 MORE TO GO!

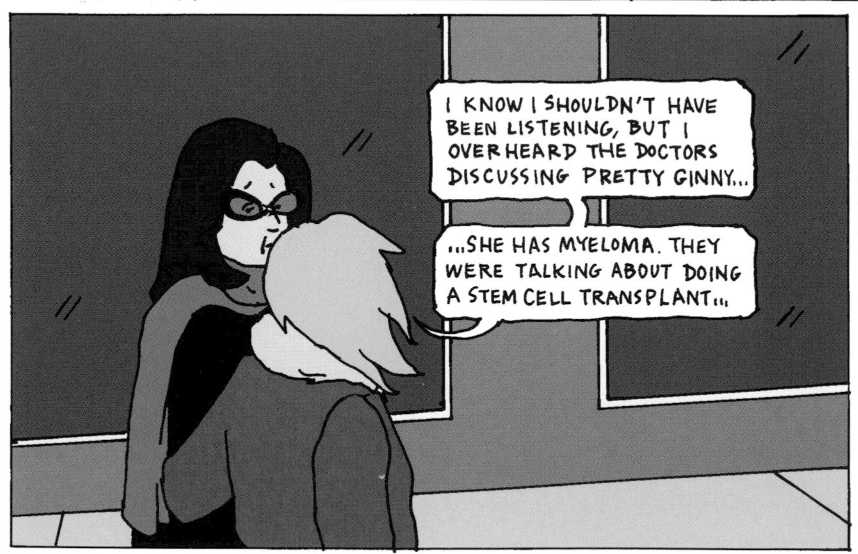
I KNOW I SHOULDN'T HAVE BEEN LISTENING, BUT I OVERHEARD THE DOCTORS DISCUSSING PRETTY GINNY...
...SHE HAS MYELOMA. THEY WERE TALKING ABOUT DOING A STEM CELL TRANSPLANT...

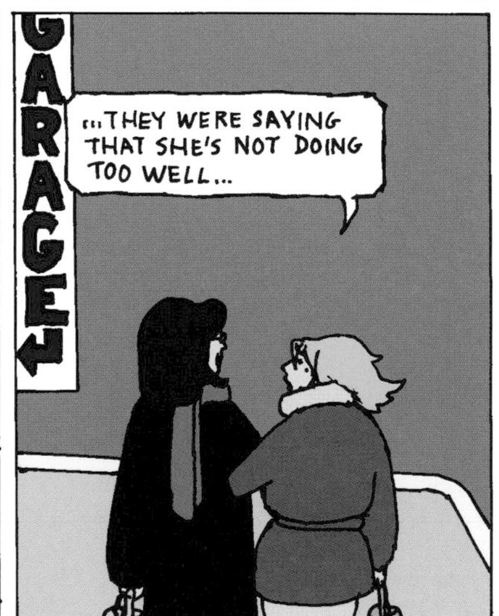
GARAGE
...THEY WERE SAYING THAT SHE'S NOT DOING TOO WELL...

I COLLAPSED AFTER THAT CHEMO. AT 10:30 SILVANO CALLED...
MARISA, YOU DON'T 'AVE TO COME DOWN, I CAN SEND SOMETING UP... I MADE A NICE CAULIFLOWER AND BRUSSEL SPROUT SOUP, I KNOW 'OW YOU LOVE THEM! *
NO, I'LL COME OVER.
*CRUCIFEROUS VEGETABLES COMBAT CANCER.

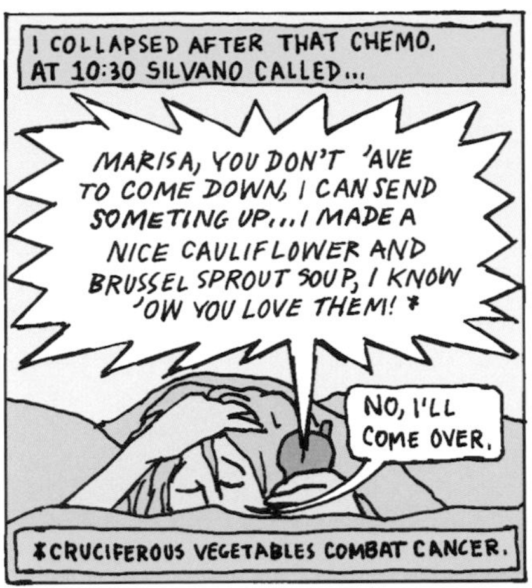

WEDNESDAY, DECEMBER 1.

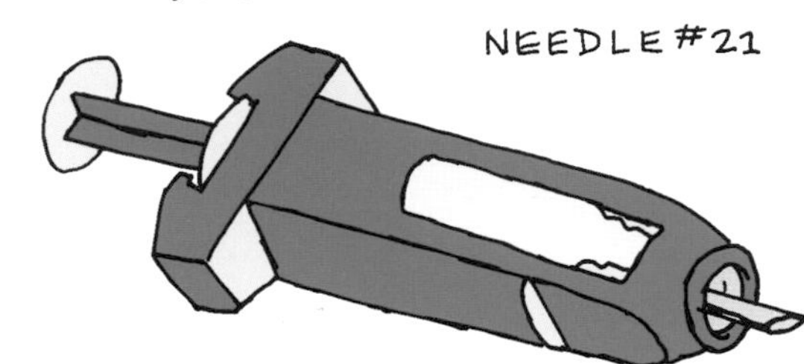

THAT CREAKY-CEMENT-HARDENING-IN-MY-BONE-MARROW-NOT-SO-EASY-TO-MOVE-$3,500 SHOT OF NEULASTA ALMOST RUINED MY CHEMO HIGH...

NOTICE I SAID "ALMOST." THE NEXT DAY...
CONGRATULATIONS, BABY!
THANK YOU!
...I GOT AN OK FROM *THE NEW YORKER*.

I GOT MY ASS OUT 2 DAYS AFTER NEULASTA. NURSE MARY ANN SUGGESTED I WALK BECAUSE RUNNING MADE ME WINDED.
TOTAL MILES: 6
AND JUST WHEN YOU'RE (SORTA) BACK TO YOUR OLD SELF... IT'S CHEMO TIME ALL OVER AGAIN...

DAY 10. MY ENERGY HIT A NEW LOW ON THE DAY IT WAS USUALLY ITS LOWEST.
CAPPUCCINO IS COLD NOW!

AN HOUR AND A HALF LATER, I ADDED A SHOT OF ESPRESSO TO THAT CAPPUCCINO, NUKED IT AND WENT TO WORK.
I HAD TO FINISH THAT OK I GOT FROM *THE NEW YORKER*.

NEW EXTENDED NAP TIME: 6-9:30 P.M.

AND THEN,
AFTER I PASSED THE HALFWAY POINT,
JUST WHEN I COULD SEE THE LIGHT AT THE END OF THE TUNNEL,
THE FINISH LINE,
JUST WHEN I WAS ALMOST DONE WITH CHEMOTHERAPY, WHICH I'LL *NEVER REALLY KNOW* IF I NEEDED TO PREVENT A RECURRENCE OR NOT...
...A STORY APPEARED IN *THE NEW YORK TIMES*...
I READ A PAPER-LESS PAPER →

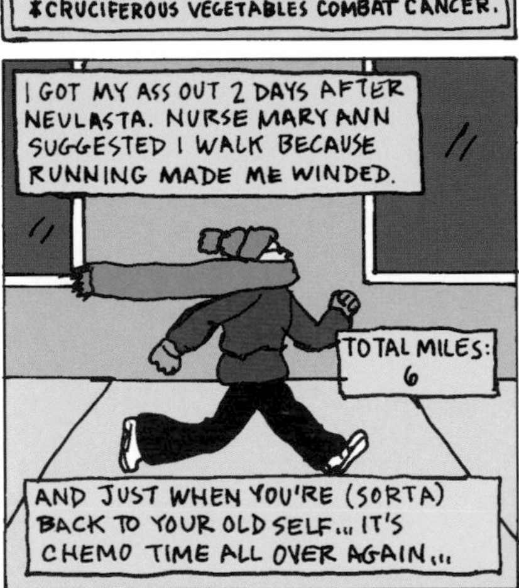

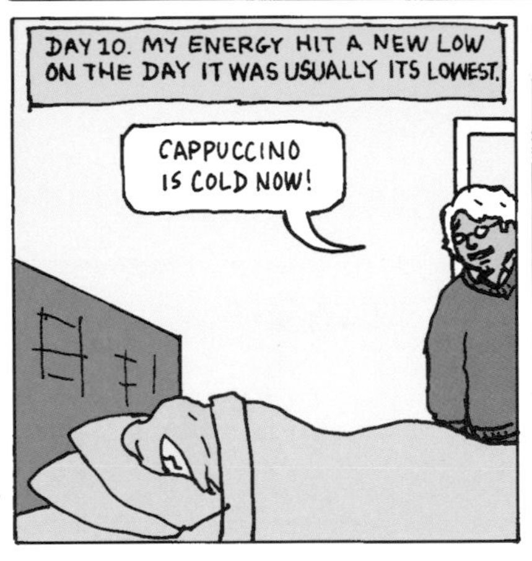

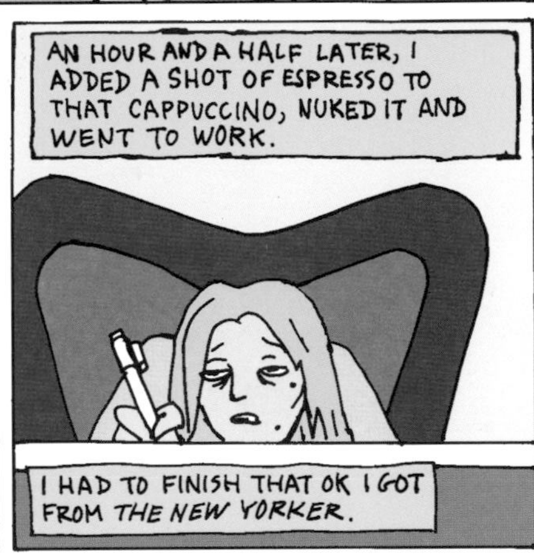

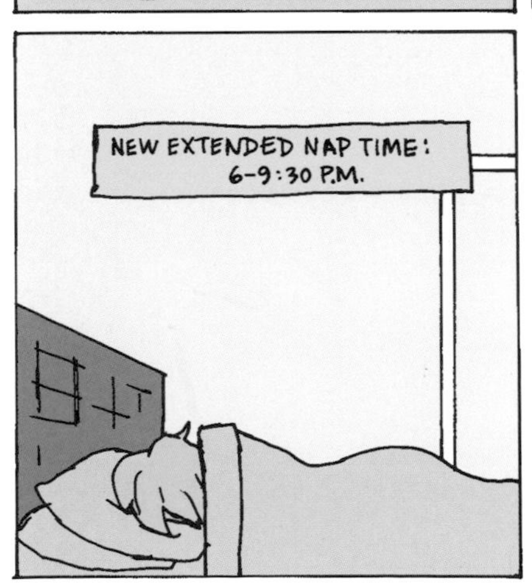

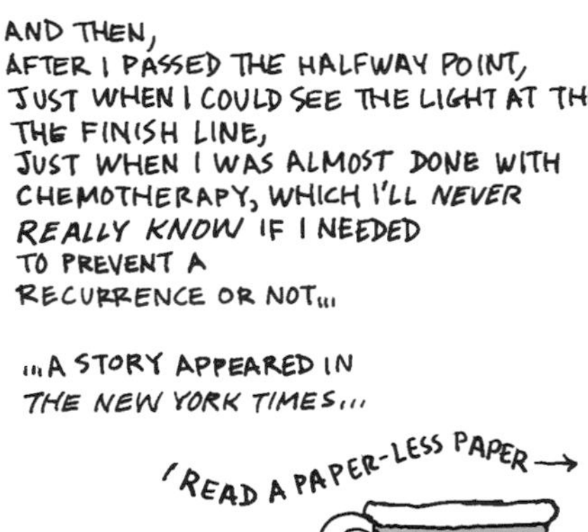

The New York Times

nytimes.com

December 11, 2004

Data Mounts on Avoiding Chemotherapy

By ANDREW POLLACK

New findings add to the evidence that genetic tests can help predict whether breast cancer will recur, giving valuable guidance to doctors and patients about whether potentially toxic chemotherapy will be useful or can safely be avoided, researchers said yesterday.

SO I ASKED DR. PAULA...
IT'S TOO LATE FOR YOU TO BE TESTED, YOU'RE ALMOST DONE WITH CHEMO.
OH WELL, I HOPE IT HELPS SOMEONE ELSE.

WEEK 3.
IT'S MY FAVORITE TIME OF THE YEAR...
I LOVE THE TREE...
I LOVE THE BIG SNOWFLAKES ON 57TH AND 5TH...
I LOVE THE DEPARTMENT STORE WINDOWS...
BUT THE DEPARTMENT STORES...
DAMN MEDICAL MENOPAUSE!

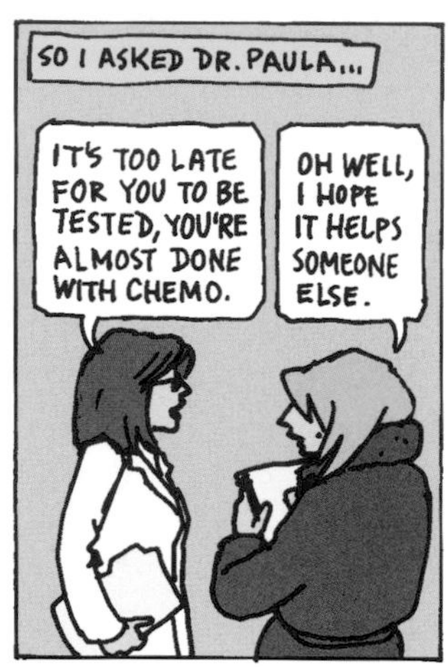

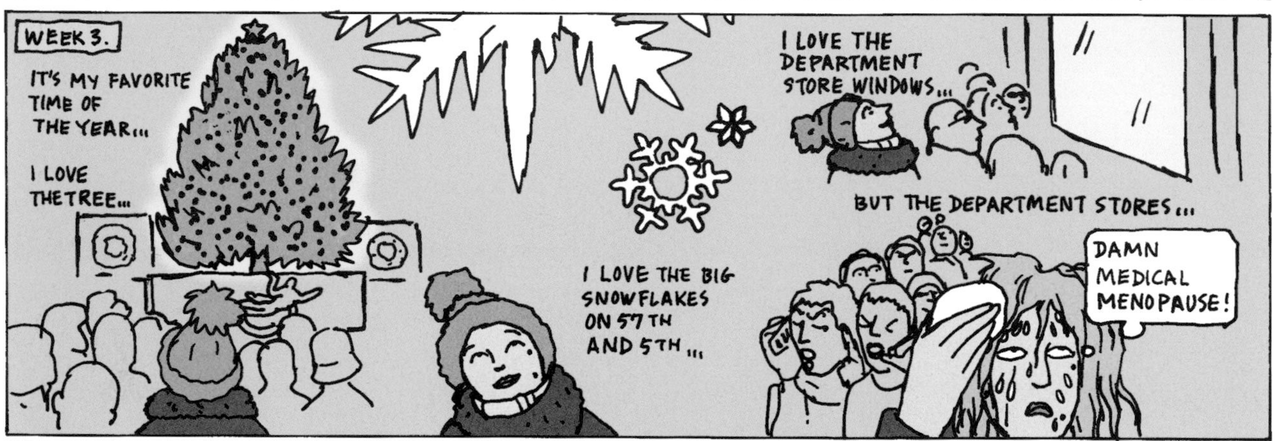

...CHRISTMAS SHOPPING AT BLOOMINGDALE'S. EXHAUSTING EVEN IF YOU'RE NOT ON CHEMO...

LYMPHEDEMA ALERT: I ONLY CARRY THINGS ON MY NON SURGERY SIDE.

YOU NEED THIS MORE THAN I DO. HAPPY HOLIDAYS!
WHO WAS MORE EMBARRASSED, THAT MAN FOR THINKING I WAS A BAG LADY, OR ME FOR LOOKING LIKE ONE?

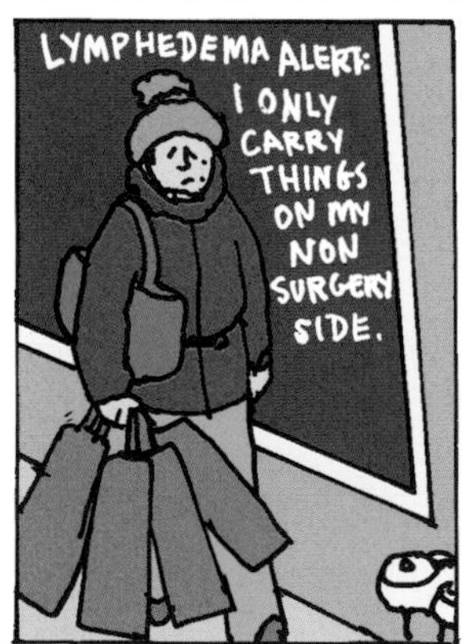

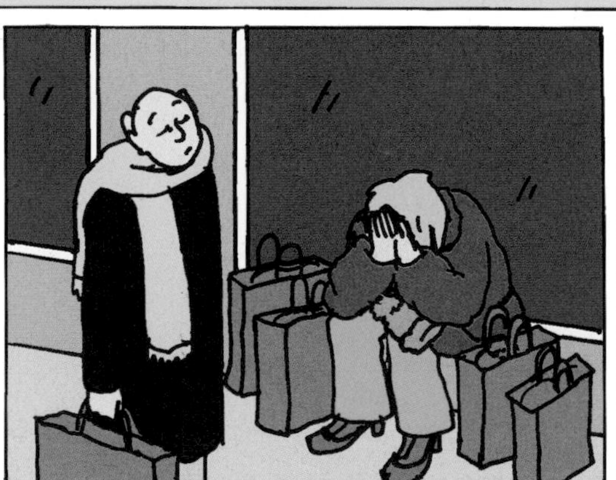

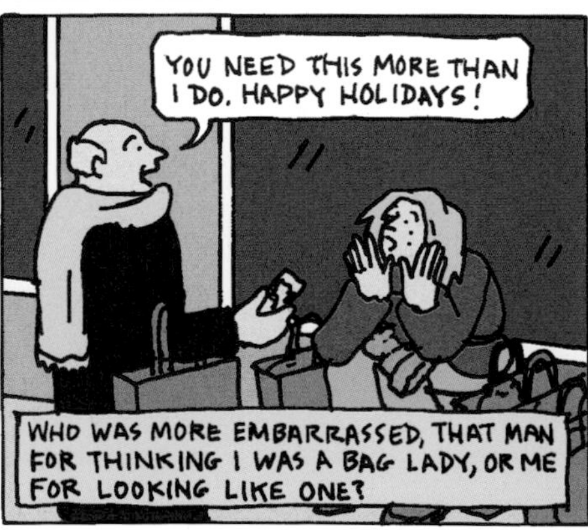

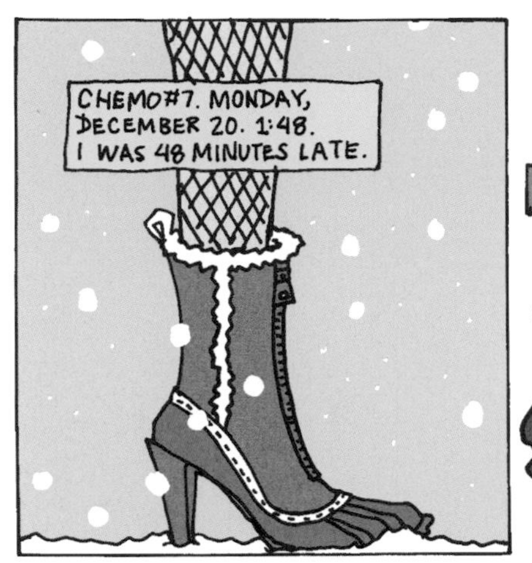
CHEMO#7. MONDAY,
DECEMBER 20. 1:48.
I WAS 48 MINUTES LATE.

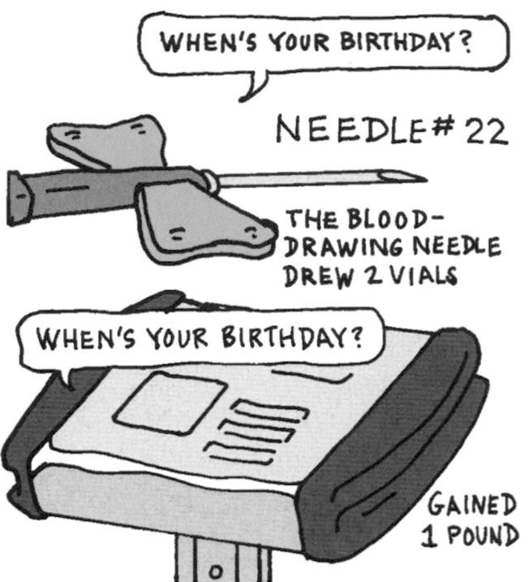
WHEN'S YOUR BIRTHDAY?
NEEDLE# 22
THE BLOOD-
DRAWING NEEDLE
DREW 2 VIALS
WHEN'S YOUR BIRTHDAY?
GAINED
1 POUND

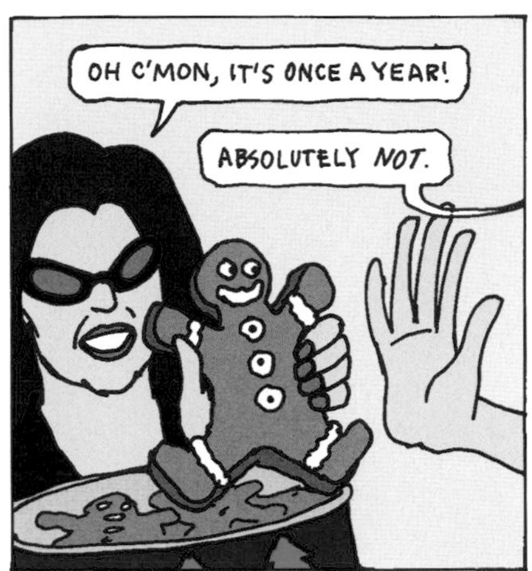
OH C'MON, IT'S ONCE A YEAR!
ABSOLUTELY *NOT*.

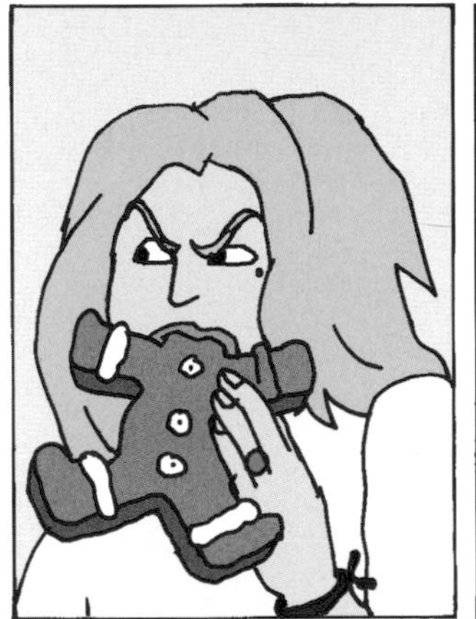

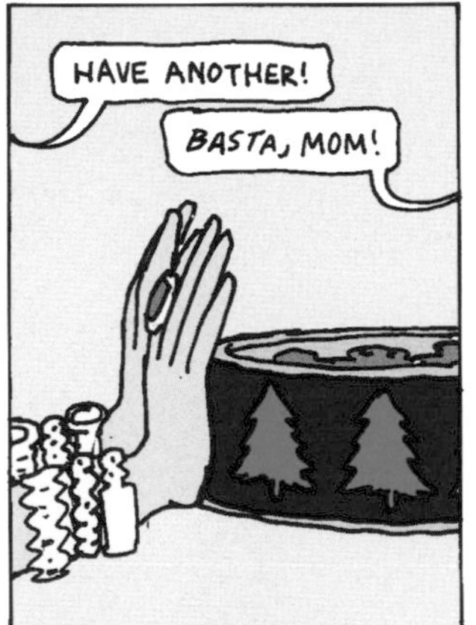
HAVE ANOTHER!
BASTA, MOM!

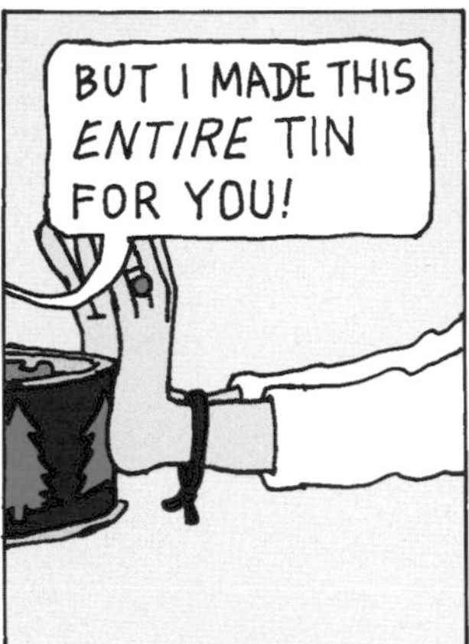
BUT I MADE THIS
ENTIRE TIN
FOR YOU!

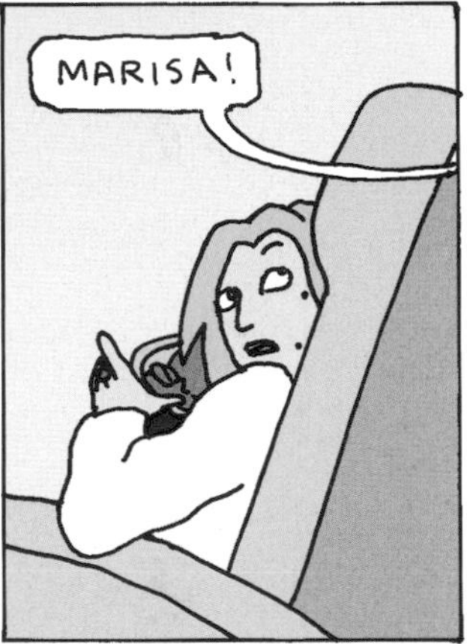
MARISA!

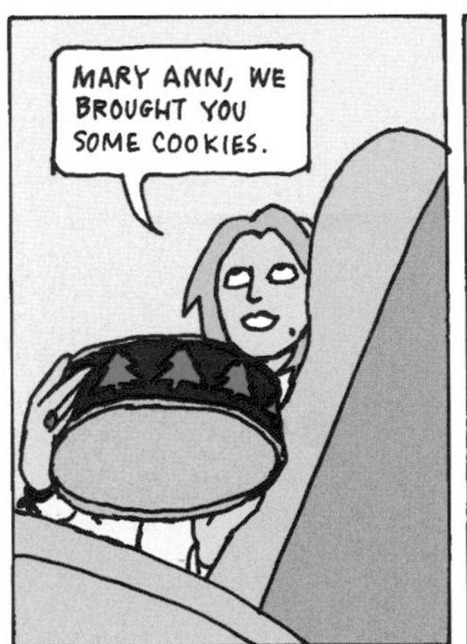
MARY ANN, WE
BROUGHT YOU
SOME COOKIES.

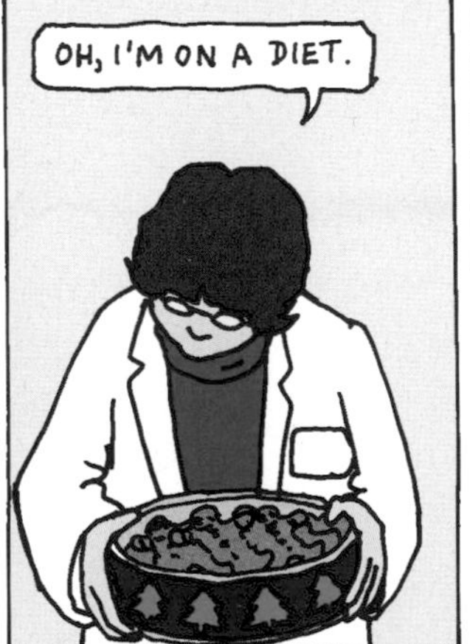
OH, I'M ON A DIET.

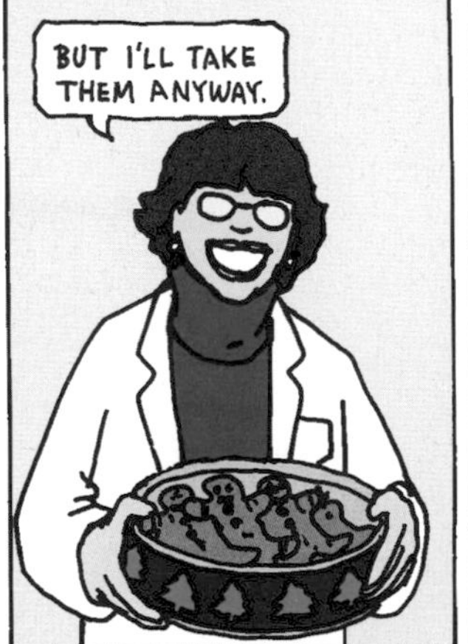
BUT I'LL TAKE
THEM ANYWAY.

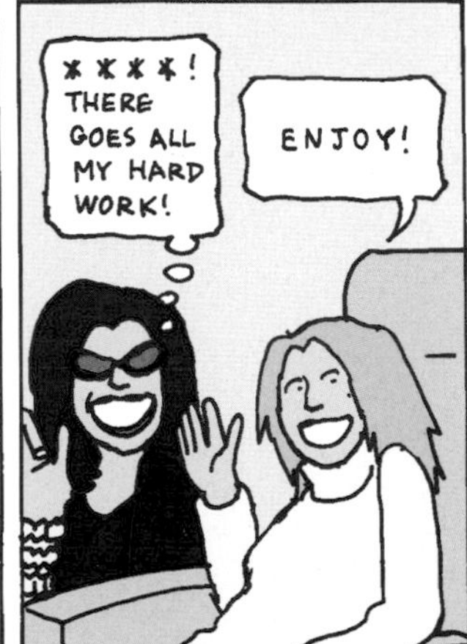
* * * * !
THERE
GOES ALL
MY HARD
WORK!
ENJOY!

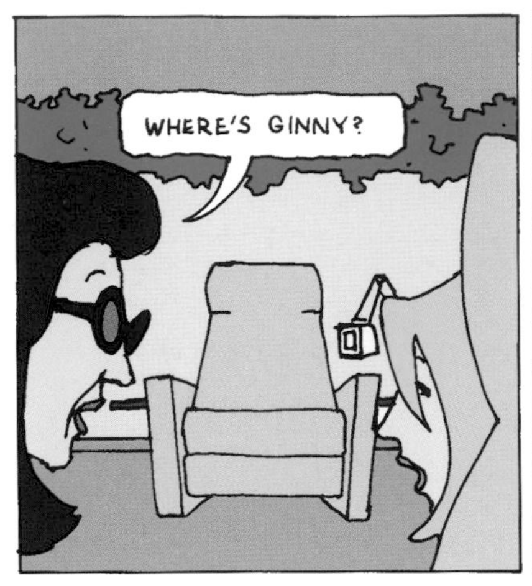

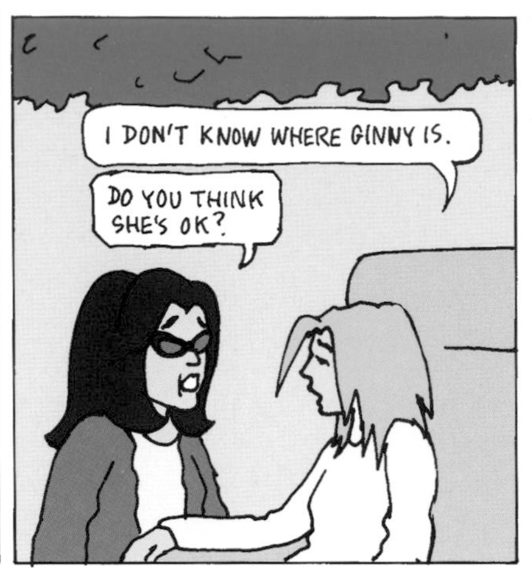

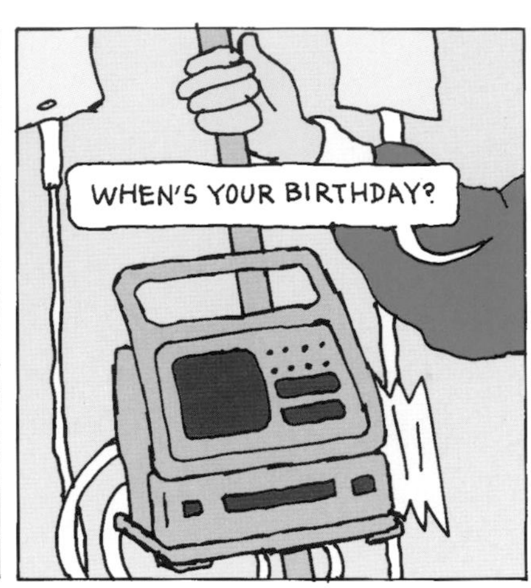

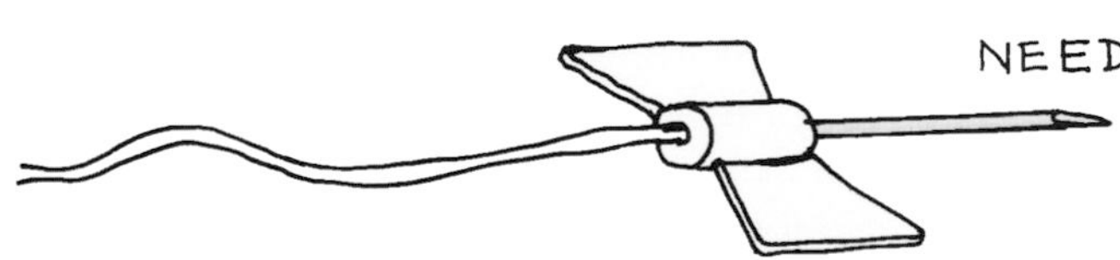

NEEDLE #23

THE CHEMO IV (#7 OF 8)

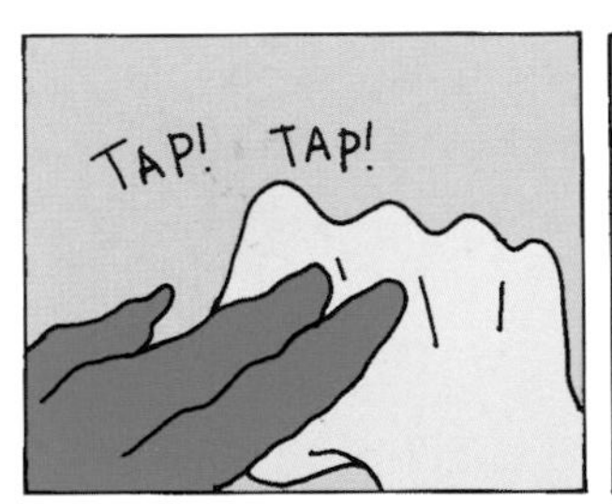

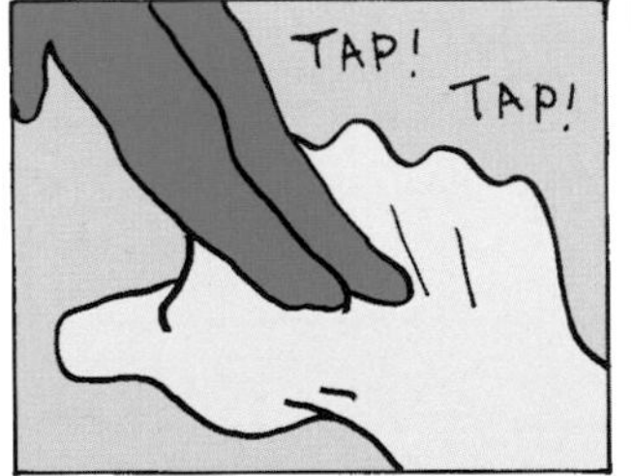

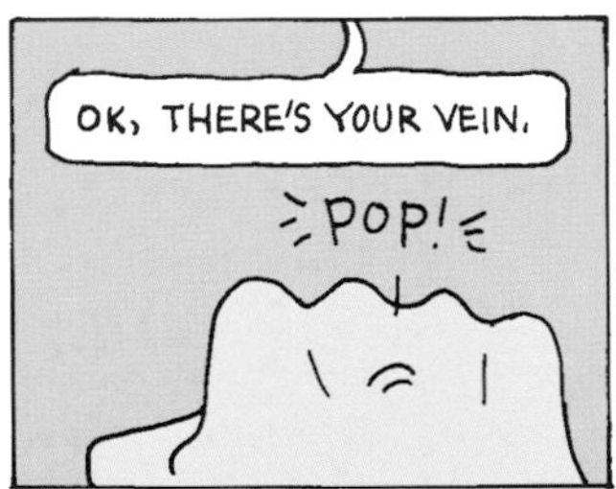

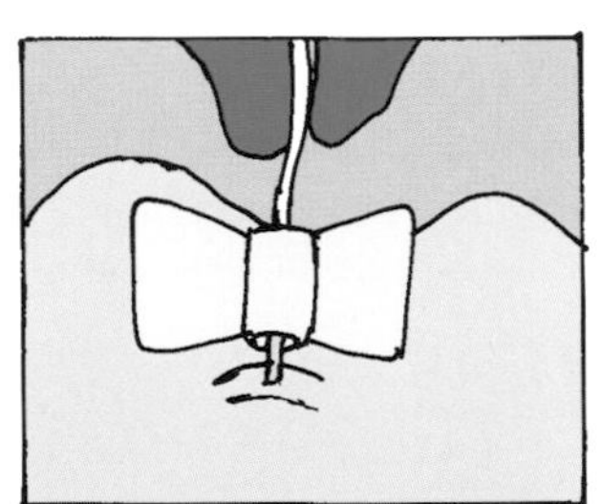

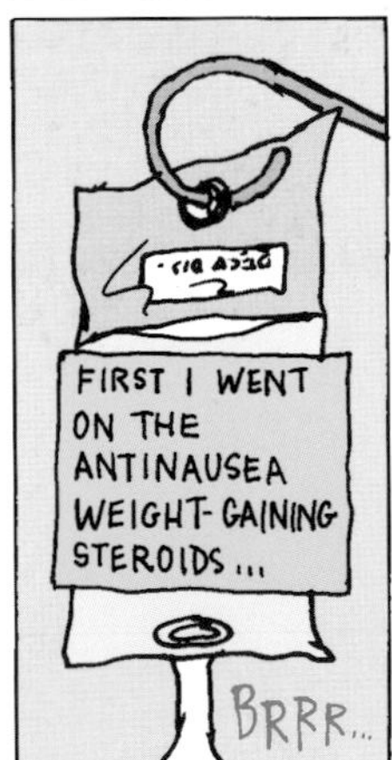

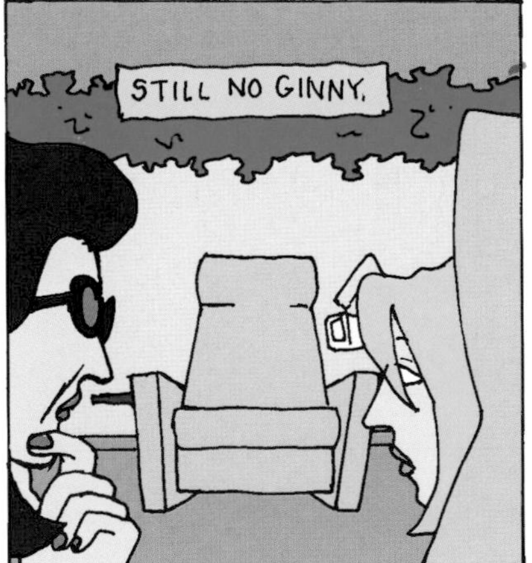

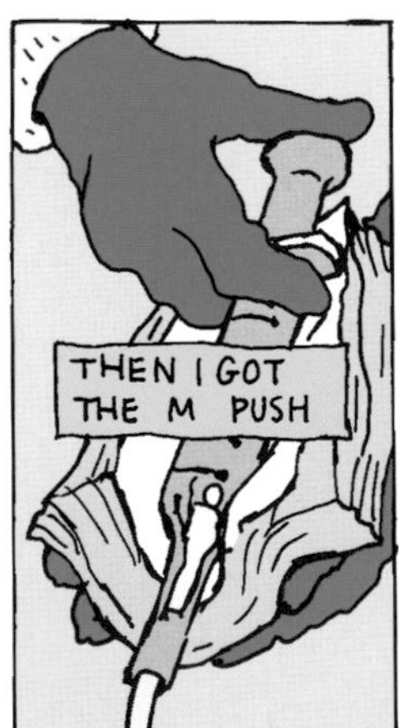

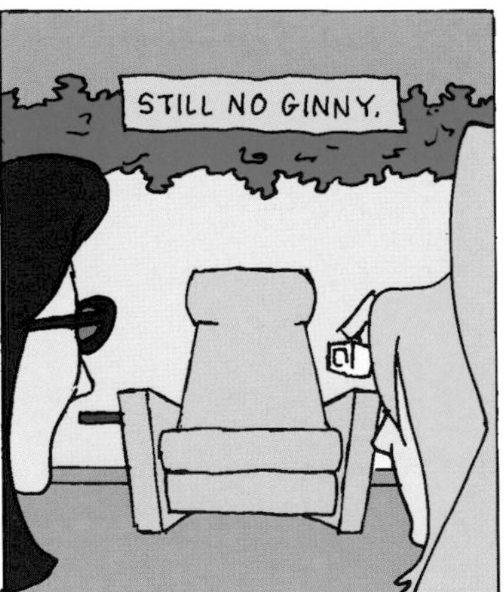

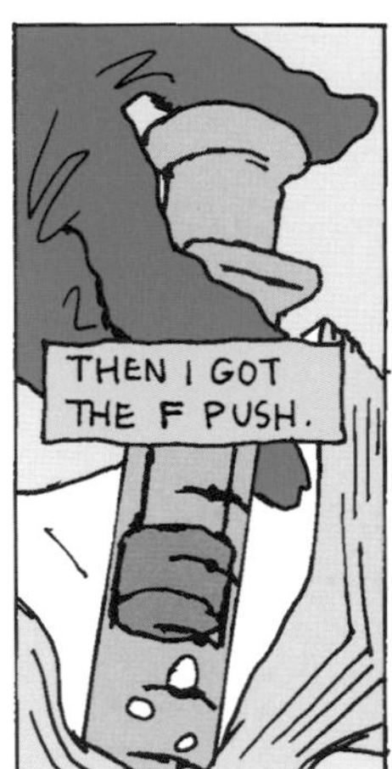
THEN I GOT THE F PUSH.

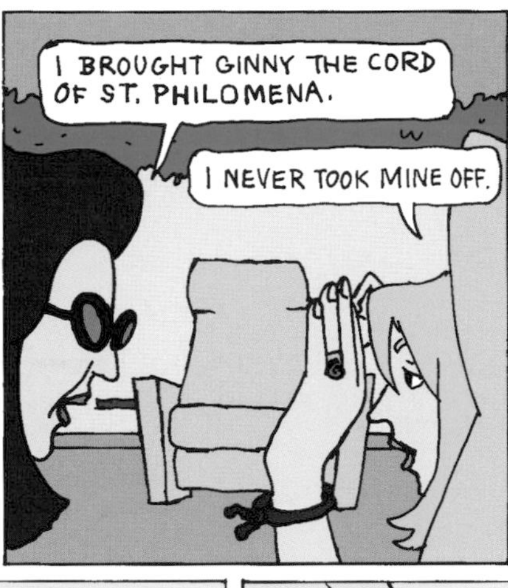
I BROUGHT GINNY THE CORD OF ST. PHILOMENA.
I NEVER TOOK MINE OFF.

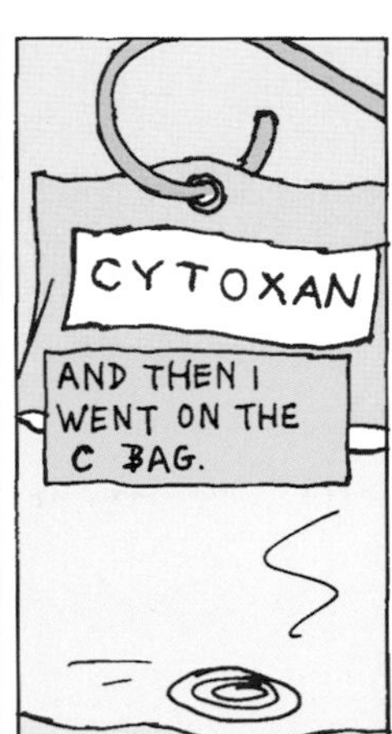
CYTOXAN
AND THEN I WENT ON THE C BAG.

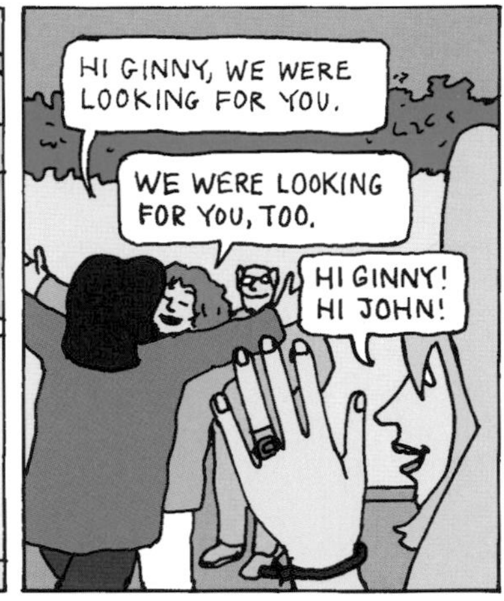
HI GINNY, WE WERE LOOKING FOR YOU.
WE WERE LOOKING FOR YOU, TOO.
HI GINNY! HI JOHN!

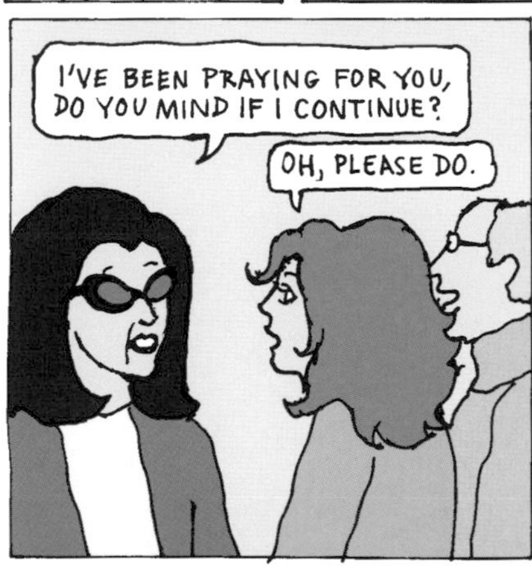
I'VE BEEN PRAYING FOR YOU, DO YOU MIND IF I CONTINUE?
OH, PLEASE DO.

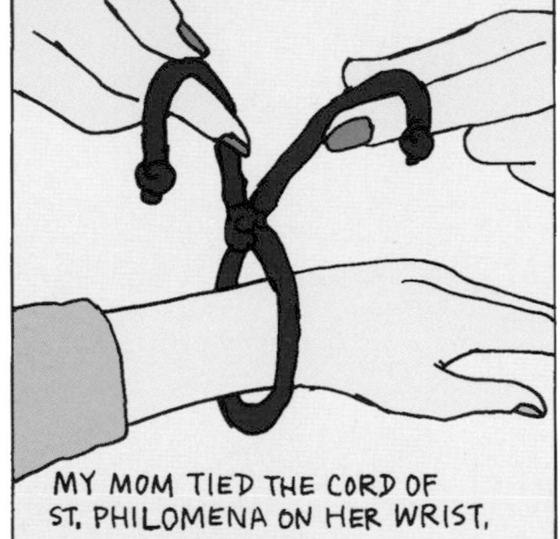
MY MOM TIED THE CORD OF ST. PHILOMENA ON HER WRIST.

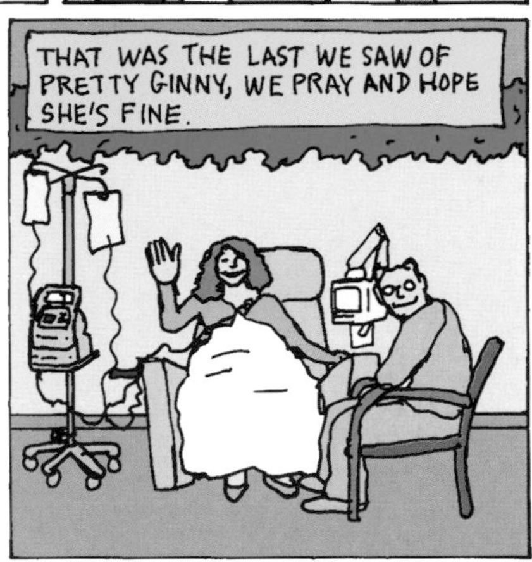
THAT WAS THE LAST WE SAW OF PRETTY GINNY, WE PRAY AND HOPE SHE'S FINE.

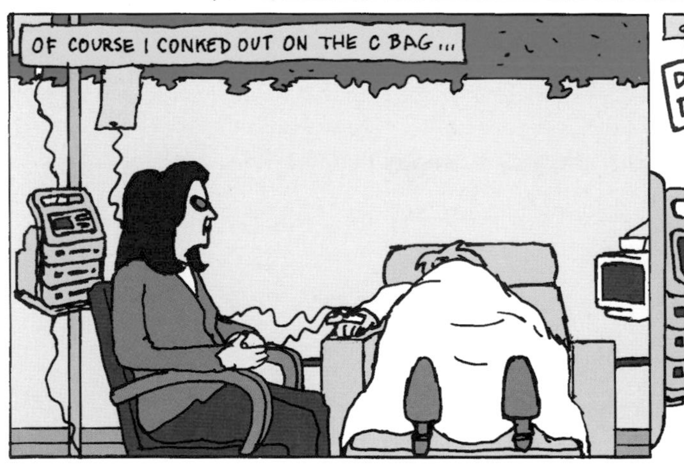
OF COURSE I CONKED OUT ON THE C BAG...

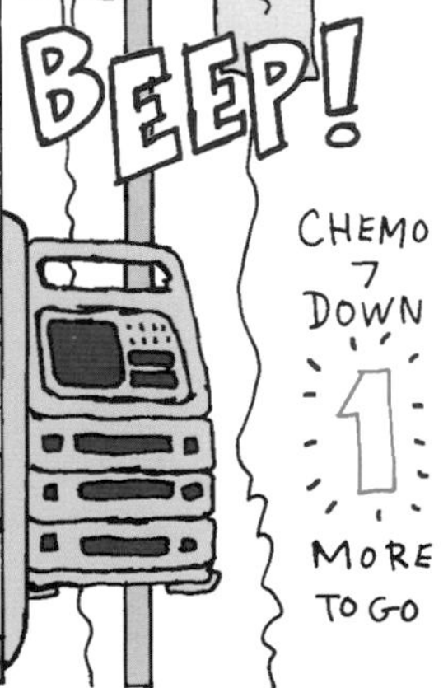
BEEP!
CHEMO
7
DOWN
1
MORE
TO GO

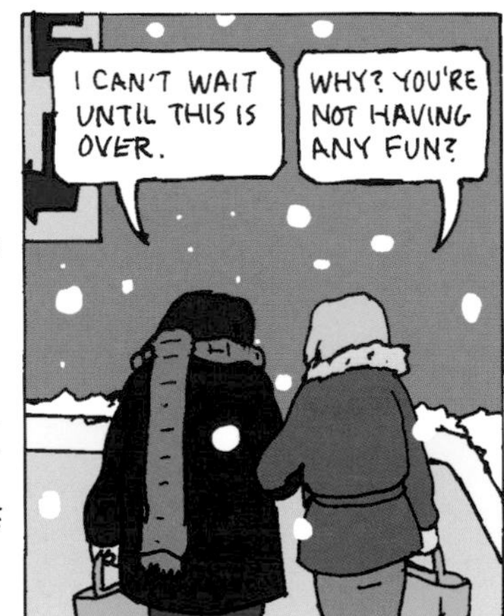
I CAN'T WAIT UNTIL THIS IS OVER.
WHY? YOU'RE NOT HAVING ANY FUN?

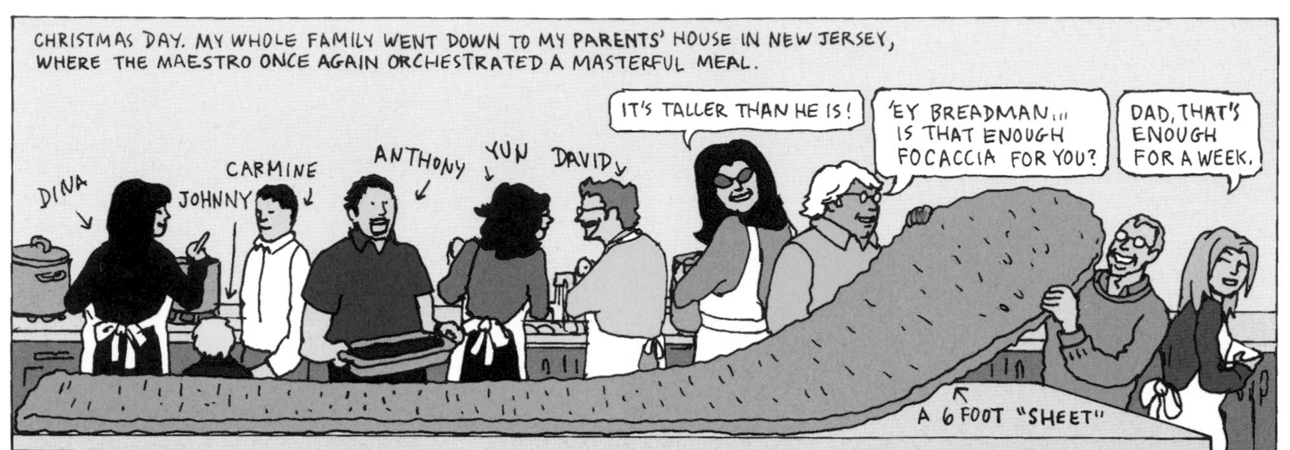
CHRISTMAS DAY. MY WHOLE FAMILY WENT DOWN TO MY PARENTS' HOUSE IN NEW JERSEY, WHERE THE MAESTRO ONCE AGAIN ORCHESTRATED A MASTERFUL MEAL.
IT'S TALLER THAN HE IS!
'EY BREADMAN... IS THAT ENOUGH FOCACCIA FOR YOU?
DAD, THAT'S ENOUGH FOR A WEEK.
DINA
JOHNNY
CARMINE
ANTHONY
YUN
DAVID
A 6 FOOT "SHEET"

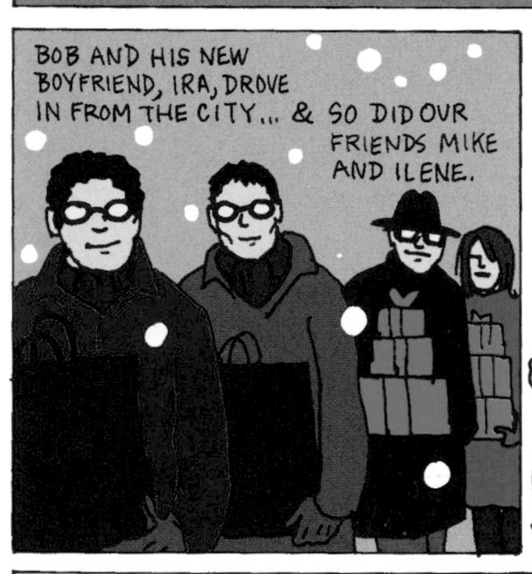
BOB AND HIS NEW BOYFRIEND, IRA, DROVE IN FROM THE CITY... & SO DID OUR FRIENDS MIKE AND ILENE.

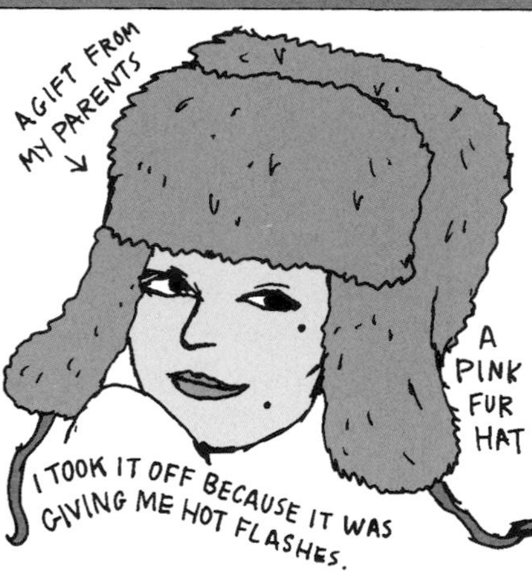
A GIFT FROM MY PARENTS
A PINK FUR HAT
I TOOK IT OFF BECAUSE IT WAS GIVING ME HOT FLASHES.

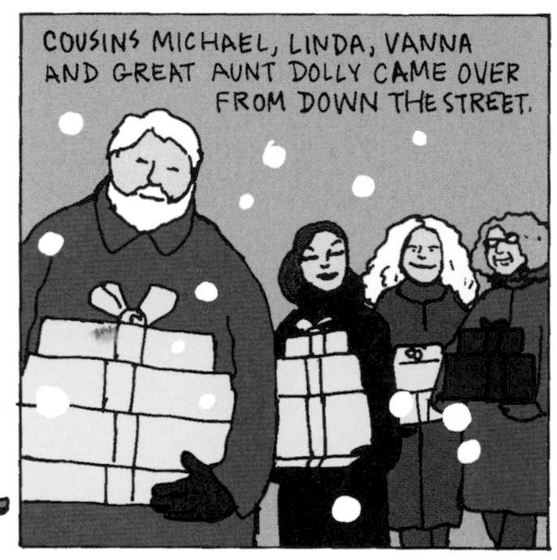
COUSINS MICHAEL, LINDA, VANNA AND GREAT AUNT DOLLY CAME OVER FROM DOWN THE STREET.

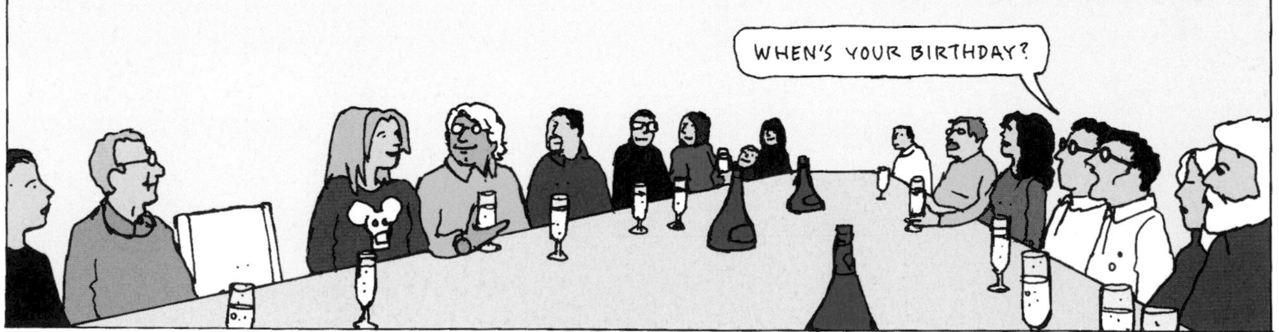
AFTER A SPECTACULAR FEAST OF FOIE GRAS ON FIG BREAD, OYSTERS, A SALAD OF RADICCHIO DI TREVISO, PUNTARELLE, FRESH SCALLOPS ON THE HALF SHELL, GRAPE TOMATOES AND LANGOUSTINES, LASAGNA, BRAISED ARTICHOKES AND PRIME RIB OF BEEF... IT WAS TIME FOR A CELEBRATION. THIS WASN'T JUST CHRISTMAS...
WHEN'S YOUR BIRTHDAY?

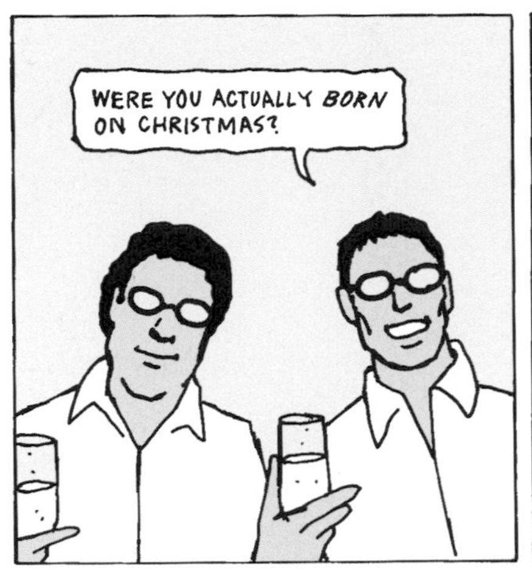
WERE YOU ACTUALLY *BORN* ON CHRISTMAS?

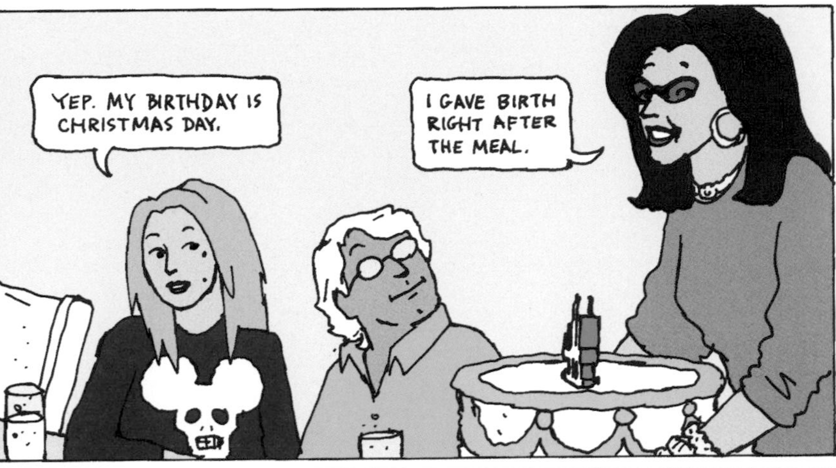
YEP. MY BIRTHDAY IS CHRISTMAS DAY.
I GAVE BIRTH RIGHT AFTER THE MEAL.

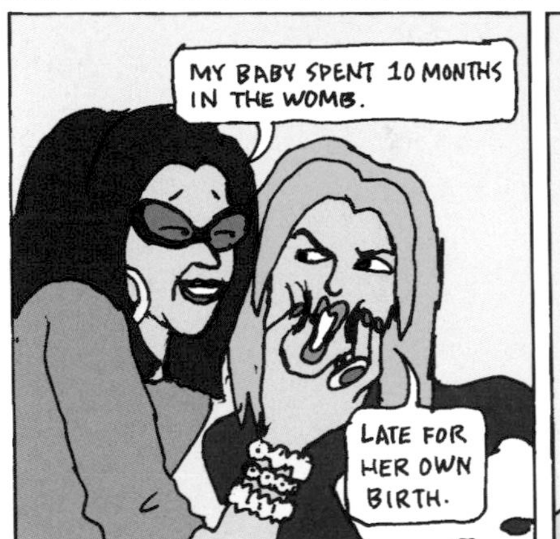
MY BABY SPENT 10 MONTHS IN THE WOMB.
LATE FOR HER OWN BIRTH.

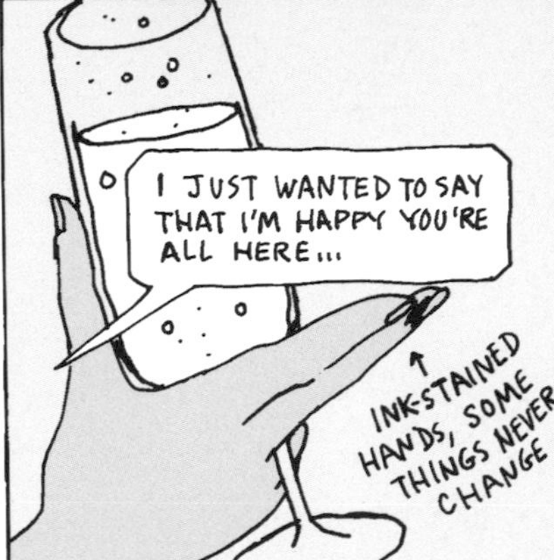
I JUST WANTED TO SAY THAT I'M HAPPY YOU'RE ALL HERE...
INK-STAINED HANDS, SOME THINGS NEVER CHANGE

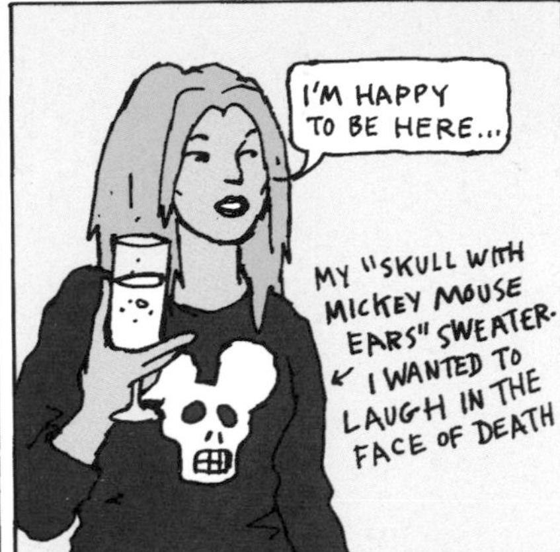
I'M HAPPY TO BE HERE...
MY "SKULL WITH MICKEY MOUSE EARS" SWEATER. I WANTED TO LAUGH IN THE FACE OF DEATH

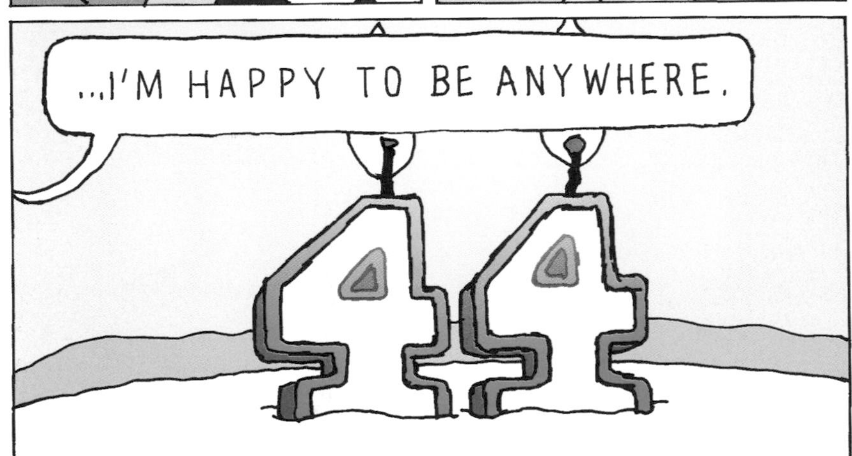
...I'M HAPPY TO BE ANYWHERE.

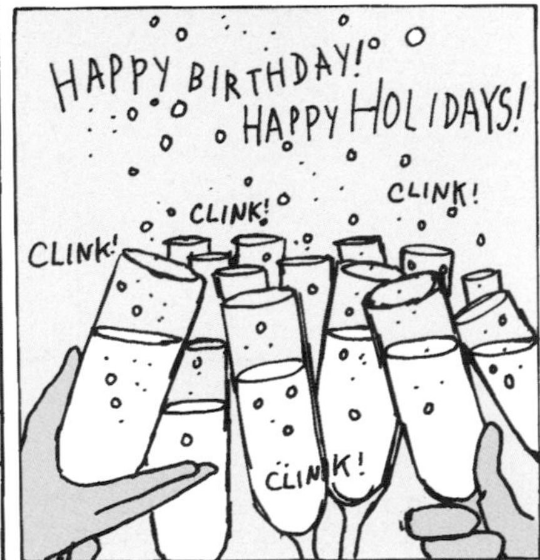
HAPPY BIRTHDAY!
HAPPY HOLIDAYS!
CLINK!
CLINK!
CLINK!
CLINK!

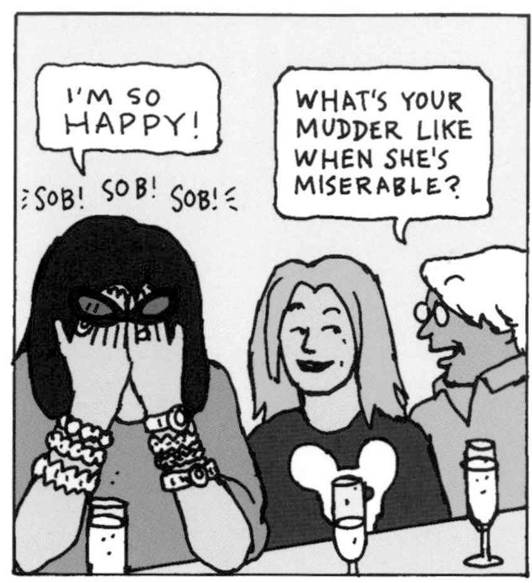
I'M SO HAPPY!
SOB! SOB! SOB!
WHAT'S YOUR MUDDER LIKE WHEN SHE'S MISERABLE?

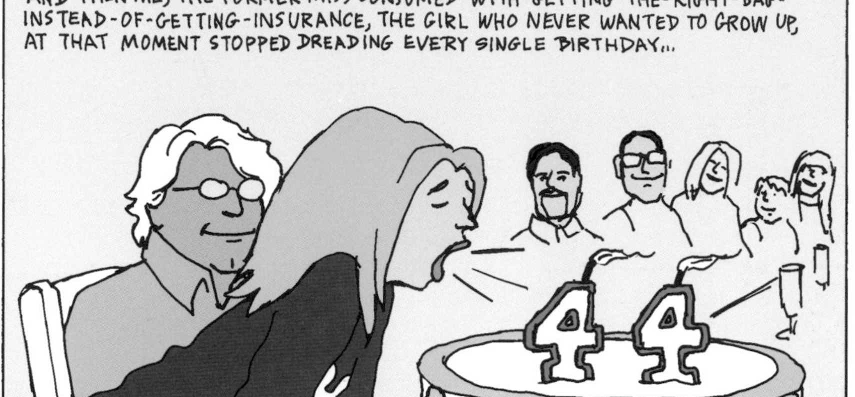
AND THEN ME, THE FORMER MISS CONSUMED-WITH-GETTING-THE-RIGHT-BAG-INSTEAD-OF-GETTING-INSURANCE, THE GIRL WHO NEVER WANTED TO GROW UP, AT THAT MOMENT STOPPED DREADING EVERY SINGLE BIRTHDAY...
44

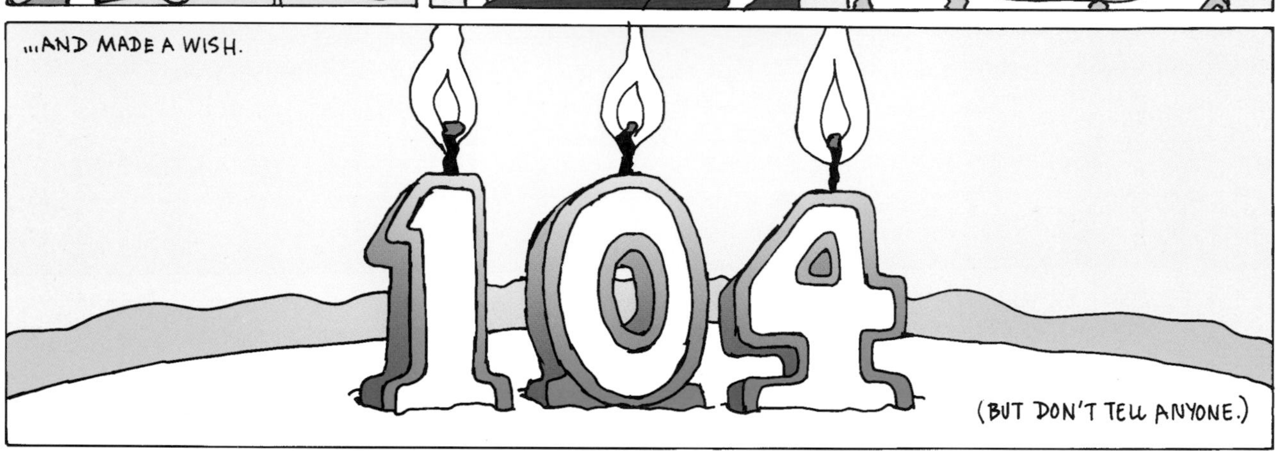
...AND MADE A WISH.
104
(BUT DON'T TELL ANYONE.)

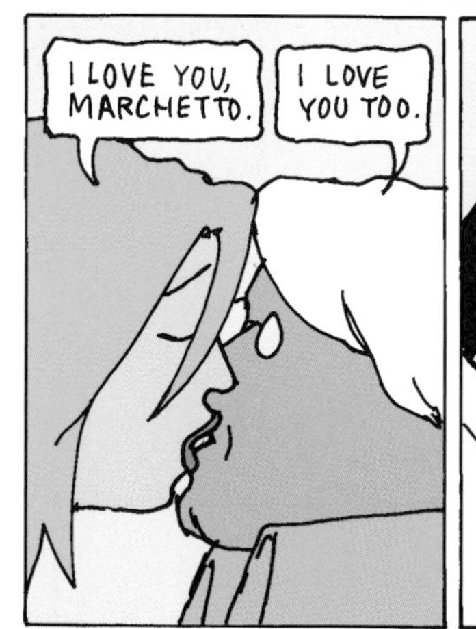
I LOVE YOU, MARCHETTO.
I LOVE YOU TOO.

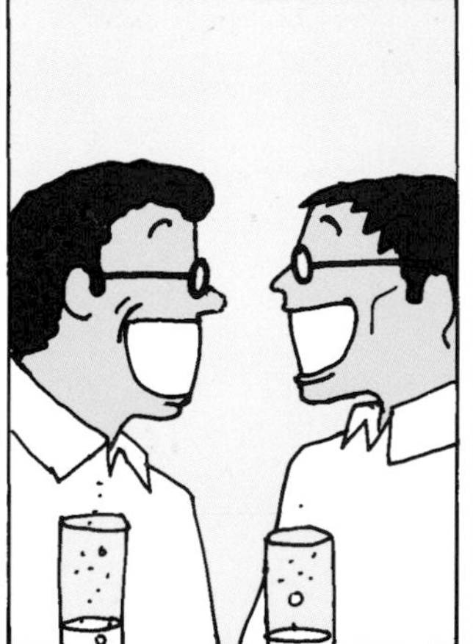

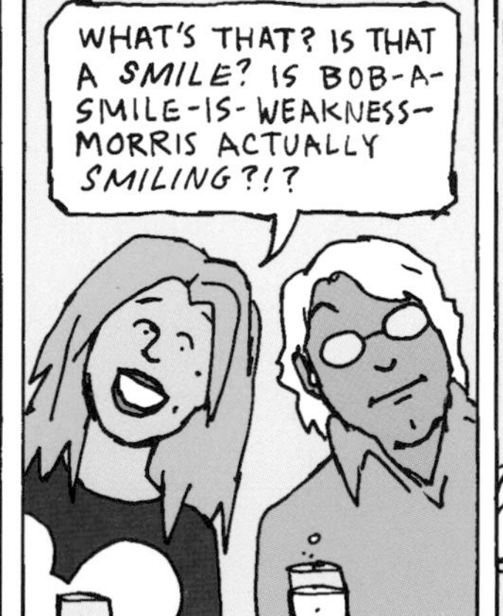
WHAT'S THAT? IS THAT A *SMILE*? IS BOB-A-SMILE-IS-WEAKNESS-MORRIS ACTUALLY *SMILING*?!?

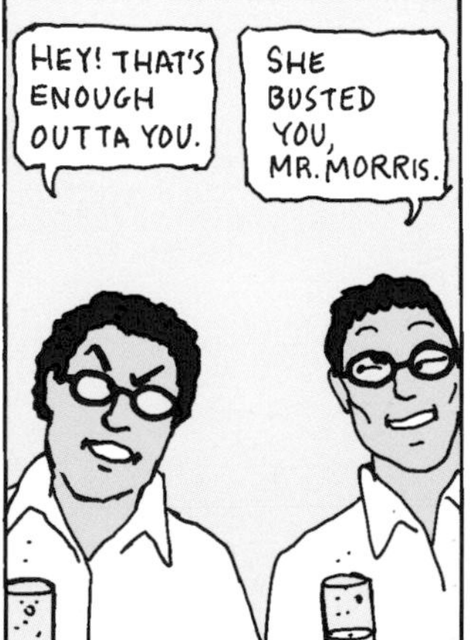
HEY! THAT'S ENOUGH OUTTA YOU.
SHE BUSTED YOU, MR. MORRIS.

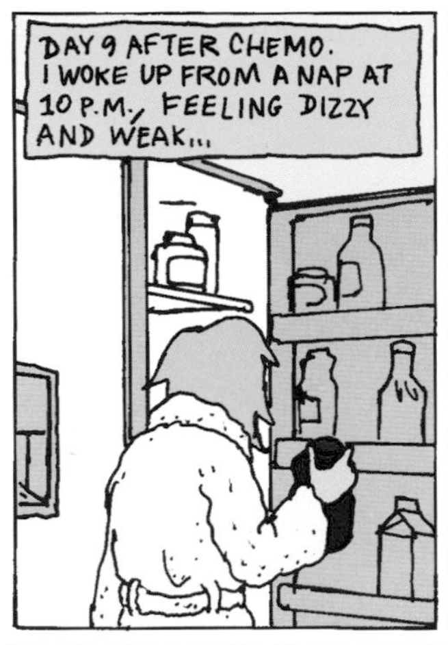
DAY 9 AFTER CHEMO. I WOKE UP FROM A NAP AT 10 P.M., FEELING DIZZY AND WEAK...

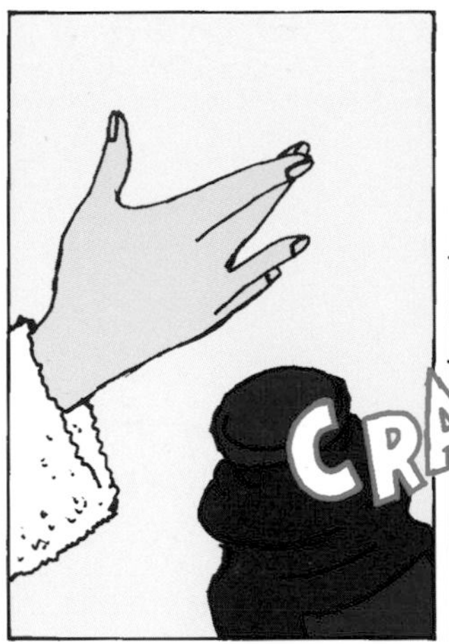
CRASH!

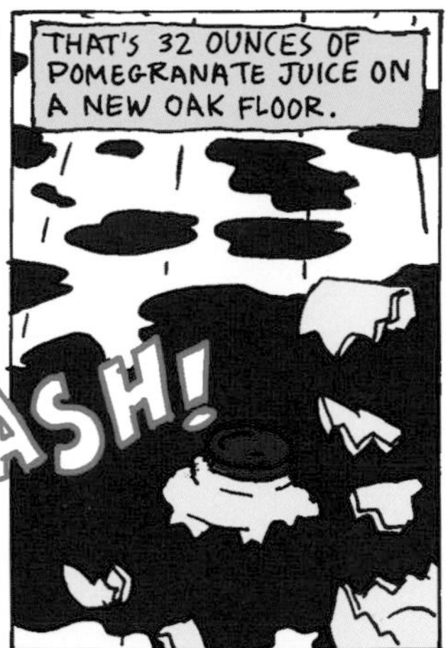
THAT'S 32 OUNCES OF POMEGRANATE JUICE ON A NEW OAK FLOOR.

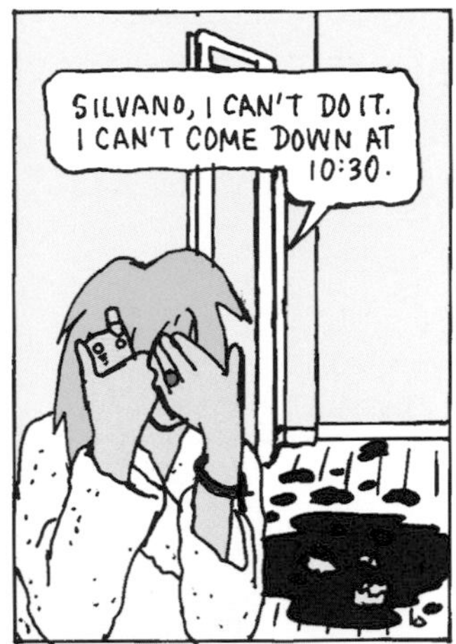
SILVANO, I CAN'T DO IT. I CAN'T COME DOWN AT 10:30.

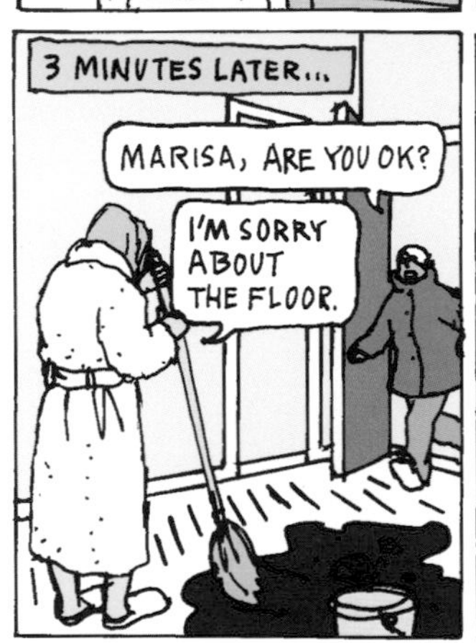
3 MINUTES LATER...
MARISA, ARE YOU OK?
I'M SORRY ABOUT THE FLOOR.

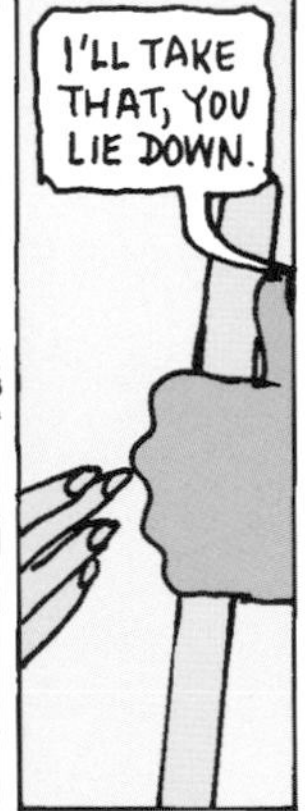
I'LL TAKE THAT, YOU LIE DOWN.

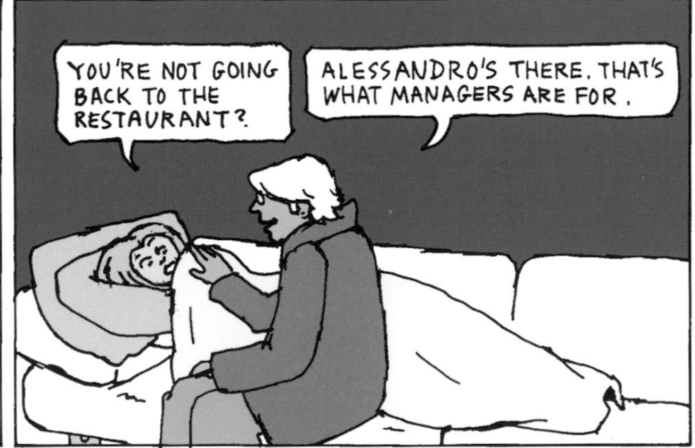
YOU'RE NOT GOING BACK TO THE RESTAURANT?
ALESSANDRO'S THERE. THAT'S WHAT MANAGERS ARE FOR.

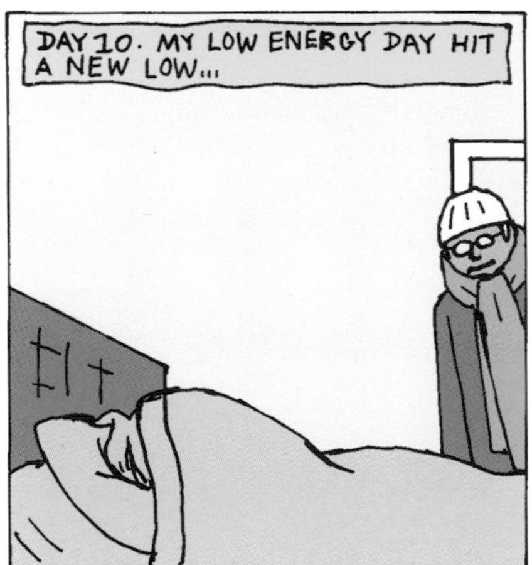
DAY 10. MY LOW ENERGY DAY HIT A NEW LOW...

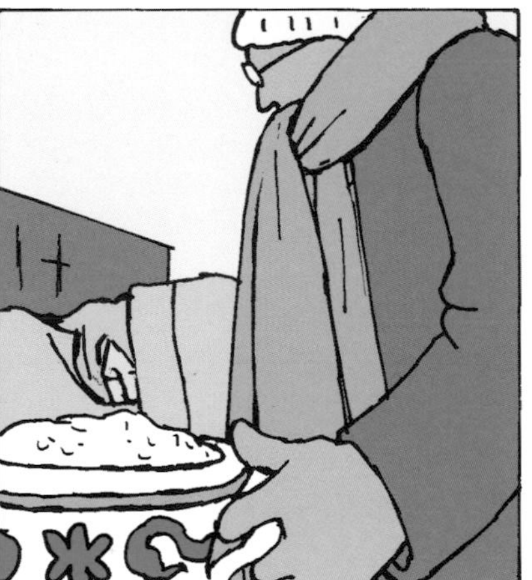

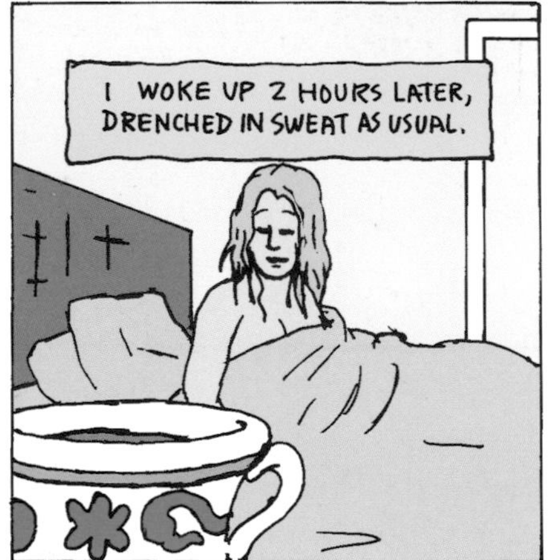
I WOKE UP 2 HOURS LATER, DRENCHED IN SWEAT AS USUAL.

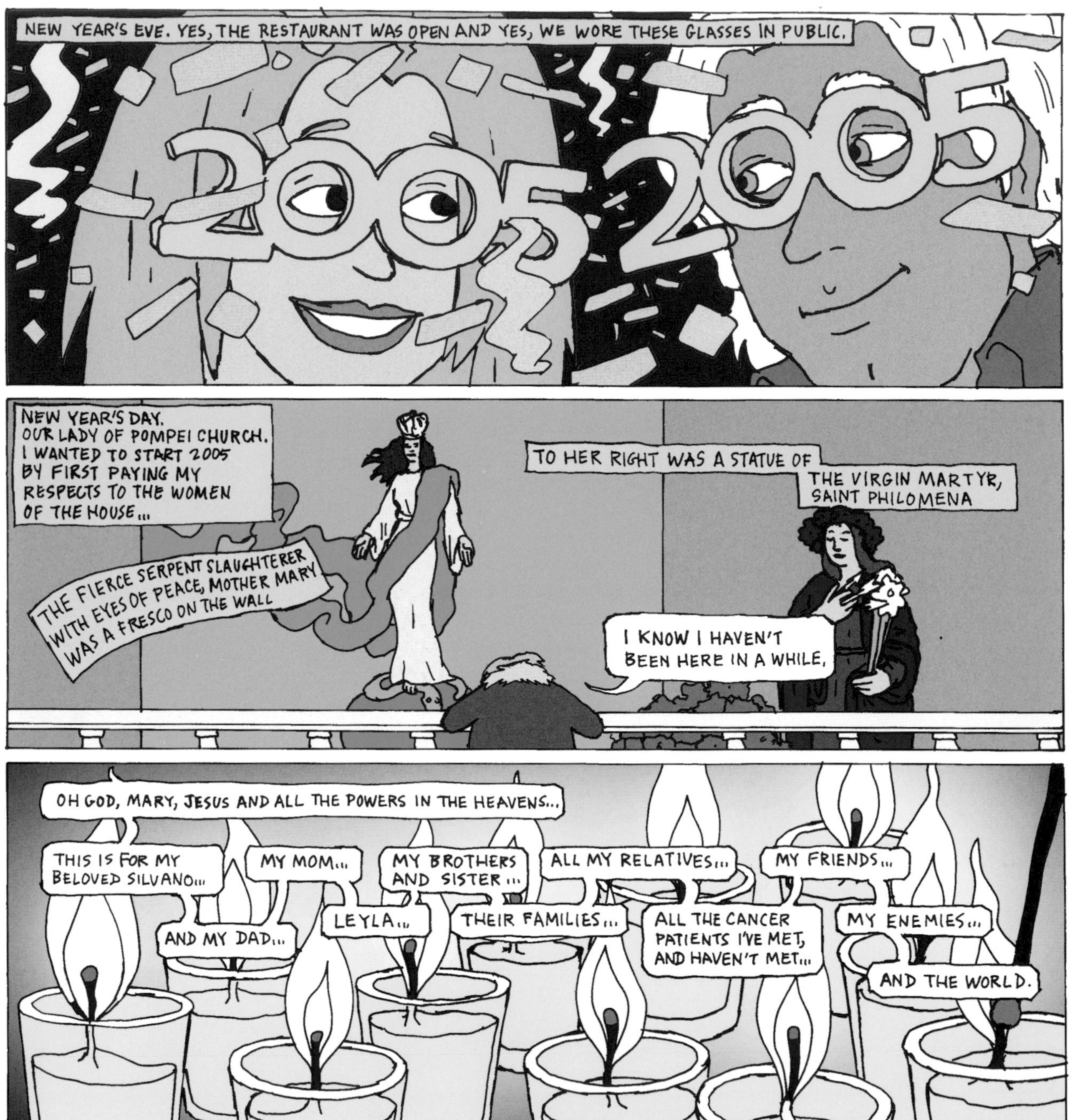
NEW YEAR'S EVE. YES, THE RESTAURANT WAS OPEN AND YES, WE WORE THESE GLASSES IN PUBLIC.
2005
2005
NEW YEAR'S DAY. OUR LADY OF POMPEI CHURCH. I WANTED TO START 2005 BY FIRST PAYING MY RESPECTS TO THE WOMEN OF THE HOUSE...
THE FIERCE SERPENT SLAUGHTERER WITH EYES OF PEACE, MOTHER MARY WAS A FRESCO ON THE WALL
TO HER RIGHT WAS A STATUE OF
THE VIRGIN MARTYR, SAINT PHILOMENA
I KNOW I HAVEN'T BEEN HERE IN A WHILE.
OH GOD, MARY, JESUS AND ALL THE POWERS IN THE HEAVENS...
THIS IS FOR MY BELOVED SILVANO...
AND MY DAD...
MY MOM...
LEYLA...
MY BROTHERS AND SISTER...
THEIR FAMILIES...
ALL MY RELATIVES...
ALL THE CANCER PATIENTS I'VE MET, AND HAVEN'T MET...
MY FRIENDS...
MY ENEMIES...
AND THE WORLD.

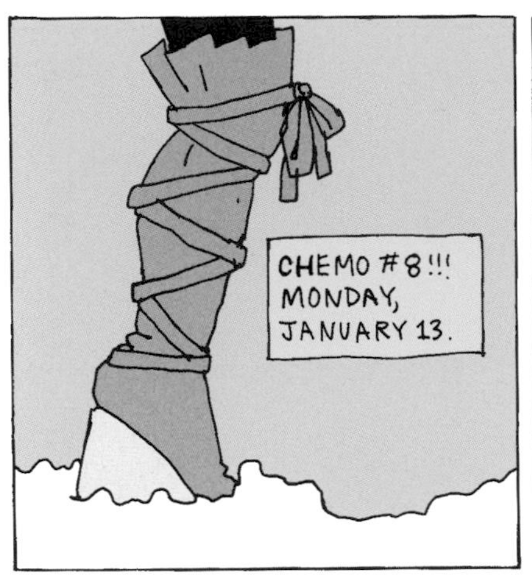
CHEMO #8!!!
MONDAY,
JANUARY 13.

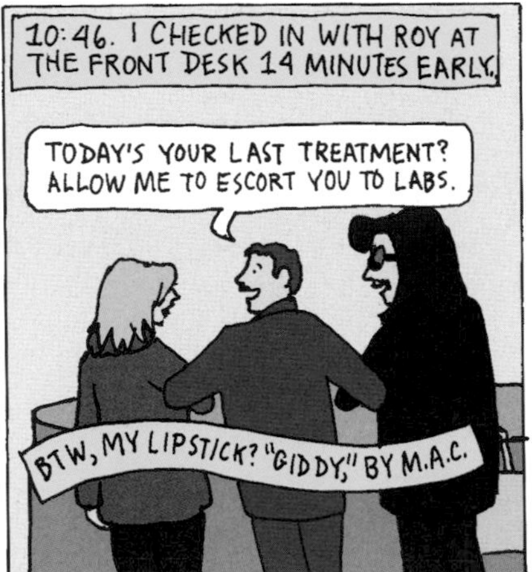
10:46. I CHECKED IN WITH ROY AT THE FRONT DESK 14 MINUTES EARLY.
TODAY'S YOUR LAST TREATMENT? ALLOW ME TO ESCORT YOU TO LABS.
BTW, MY LIPSTICK? "GIDDY," BY M.A.C.

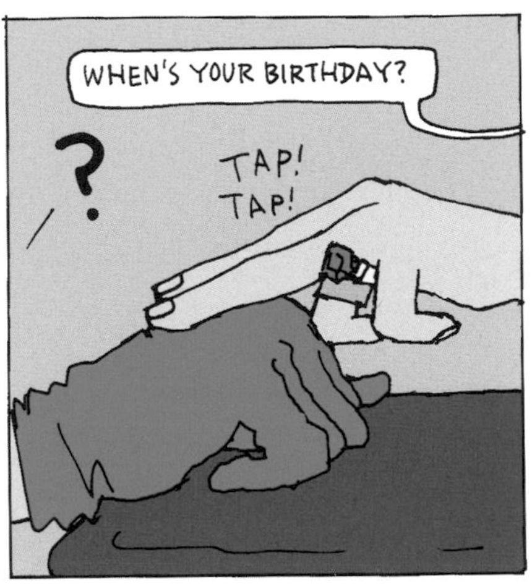
WHEN'S YOUR BIRTHDAY?
?
TAP!
TAP!

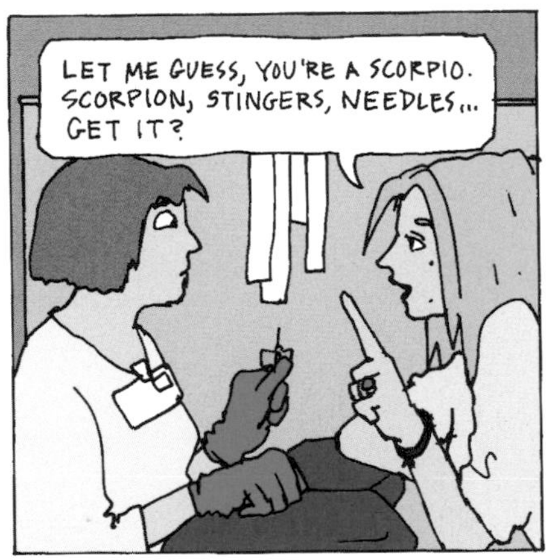
LET ME GUESS, YOU'RE A SCORPIO. SCORPION, STINGERS, NEEDLES... GET IT?

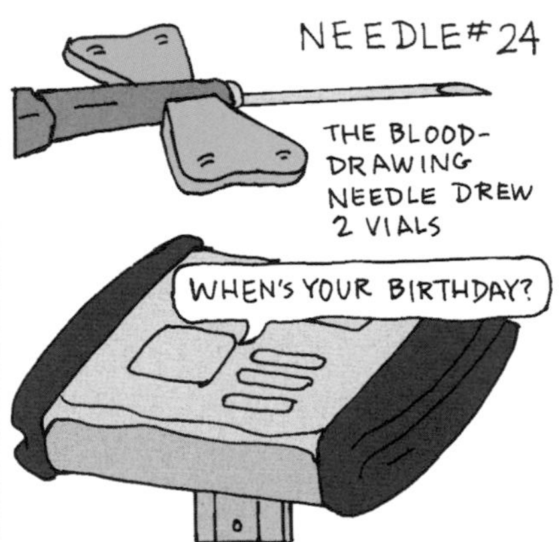
NEEDLE #24
THE BLOOD-DRAWING NEEDLE DREW 2 VIALS
WHEN'S YOUR BIRTHDAY?

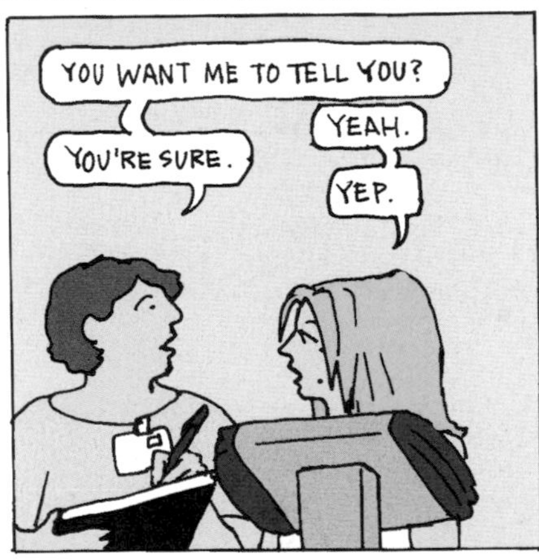
YOU WANT ME TO TELL YOU?
YEAH.
YOU'RE SURE.
YEP.

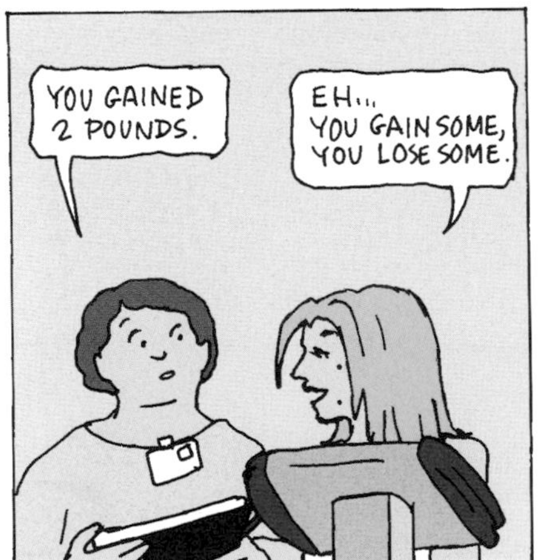
YOU GAINED 2 POUNDS.
EH... YOU GAIN SOME, YOU LOSE SOME.

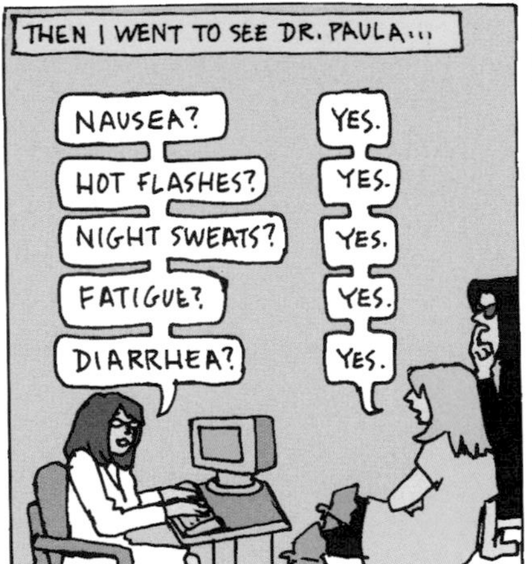
THEN I WENT TO SEE DR. PAULA...
NAUSEA?
YES.
HOT FLASHES?
YES.
NIGHT SWEATS?
YES.
FATIGUE?
YES.
DIARRHEA?
YES.

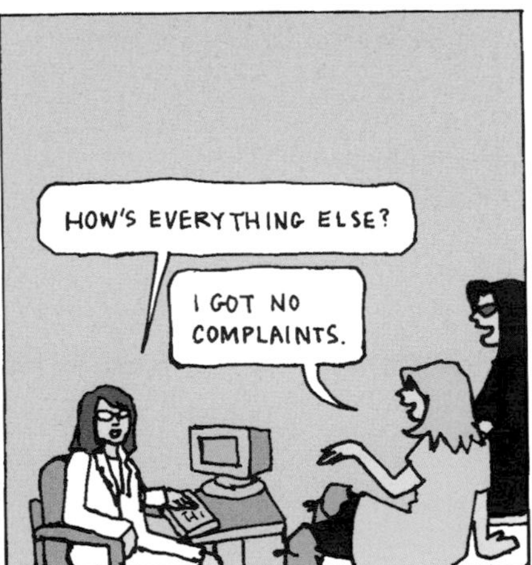
HOW'S EVERYTHING ELSE?
I GOT NO COMPLAINTS.

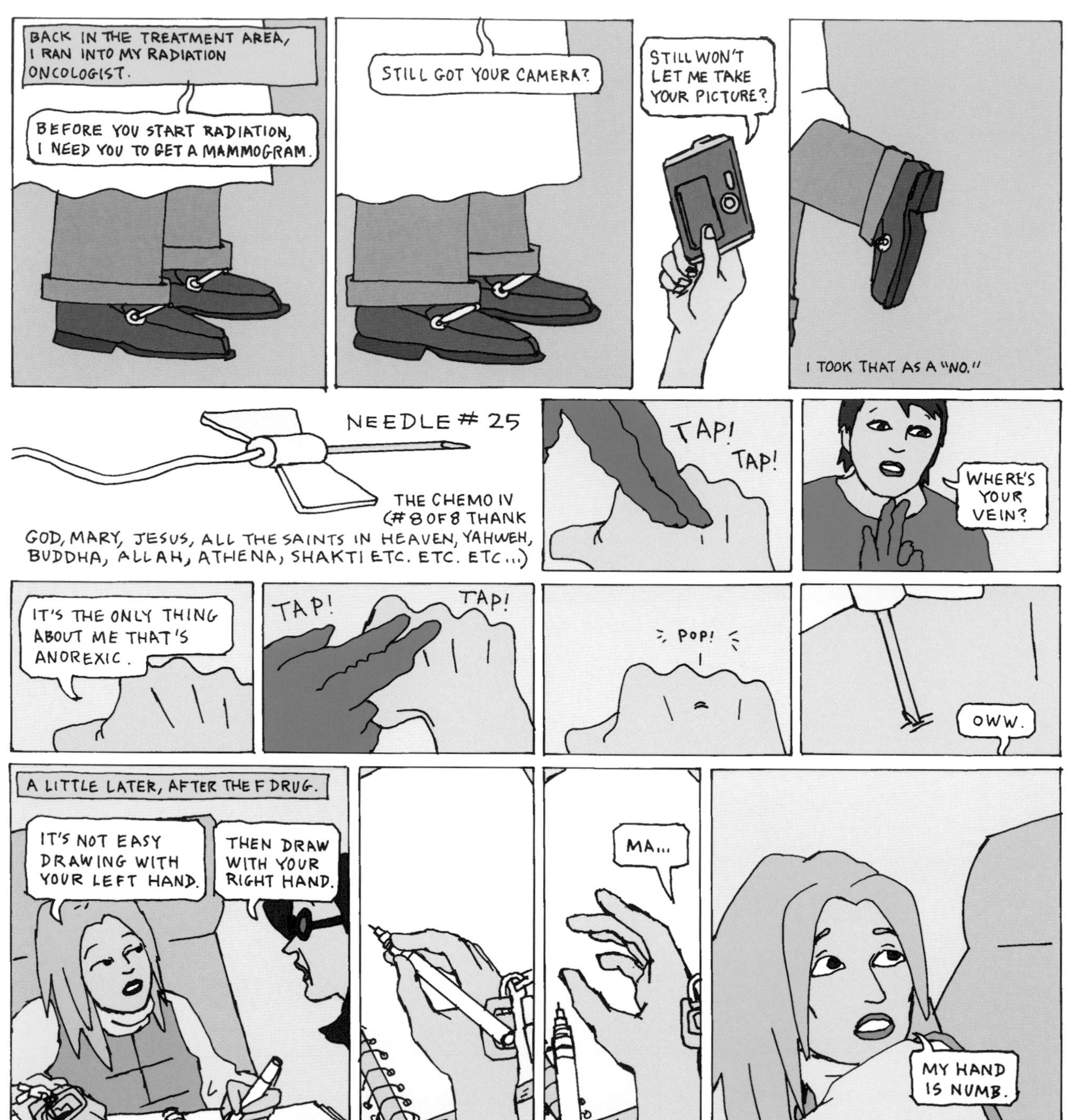
BACK IN THE TREATMENT AREA, I RAN INTO MY RADIATION ONCOLOGIST.
BEFORE YOU START RADIATION, I NEED YOU TO GET A MAMMOGRAM.
STILL GOT YOUR CAMERA?
STILL WON'T LET ME TAKE YOUR PICTURE?
I TOOK THAT AS A "NO."
NEEDLE # 25
THE CHEMO IV (# 8 OF 8 THANK GOD, MARY, JESUS, ALL THE SAINTS IN HEAVEN, YAHWEH, BUDDHA, ALLAH, ATHENA, SHAKTI ETC. ETC. ETC...)
TAP! TAP!
WHERE'S YOUR VEIN?
IT'S THE ONLY THING ABOUT ME THAT'S ANOREXIC.
TAP! TAP!
POP!
OWW.
A LITTLE LATER, AFTER THE F DRUG.
IT'S NOT EASY DRAWING WITH YOUR LEFT HAND.
THEN DRAW WITH YOUR RIGHT HAND.
MA...
MY HAND IS NUMB.

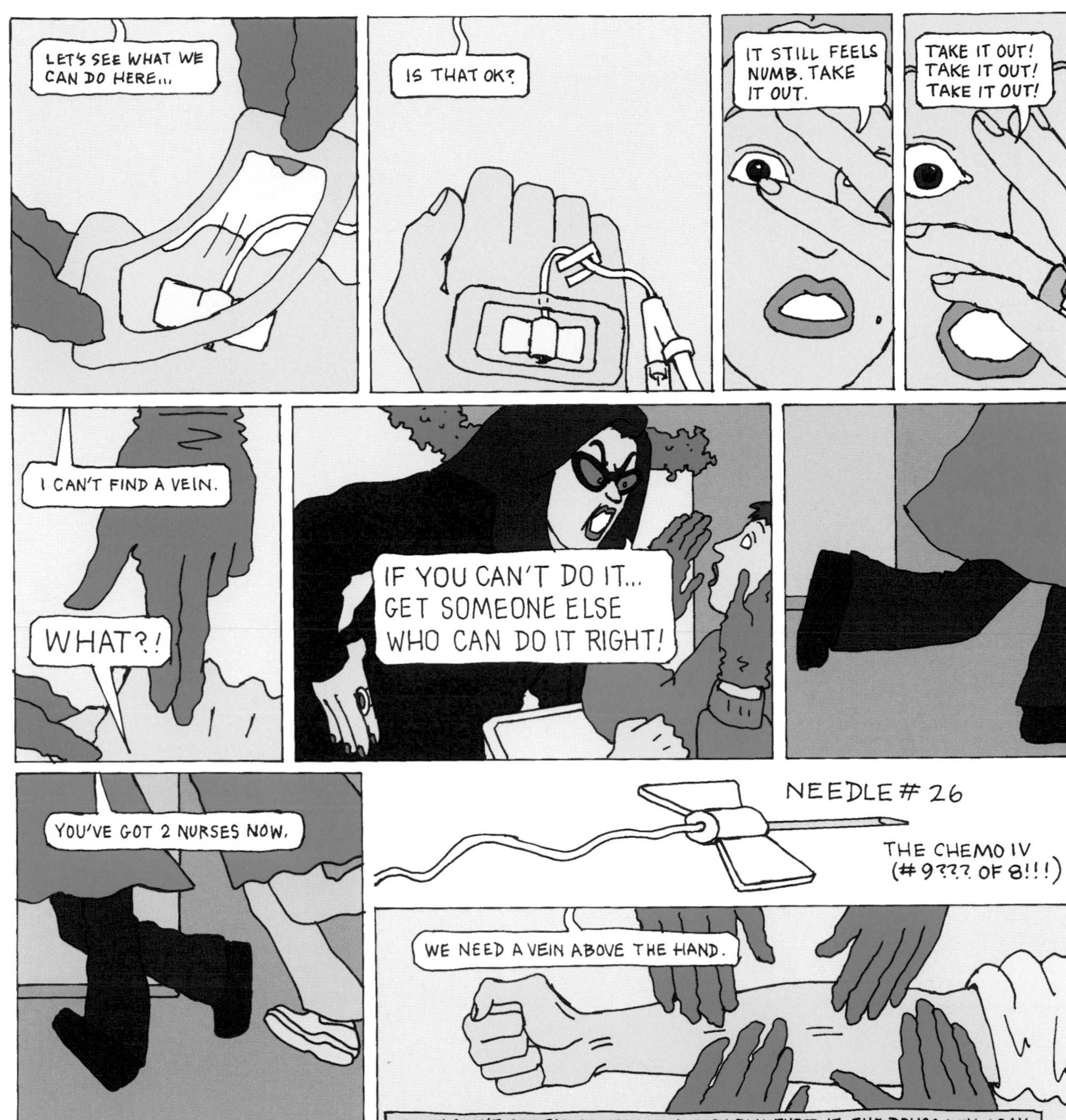
LET'S SEE WHAT WE CAN DO HERE...
IS THAT OK?
IT STILL FEELS NUMB. TAKE IT OUT.
TAKE IT OUT! TAKE IT OUT! TAKE IT OUT!
I CAN'T FIND A VEIN.
WHAT?!
IF YOU CAN'T DO IT... GET SOMEONE ELSE WHO CAN DO IT RIGHT!
YOU'VE GOT 2 NURSES NOW.
NEEDLE # 26
THE CHEMO IV (#9??? OF 8!!!)
WE NEED A VEIN ABOVE THE HAND.
THEY CAN'T GO BELOW A VEIN ONCE THEY PUNCTURED IT. THE DRUGS WILL LEAK.

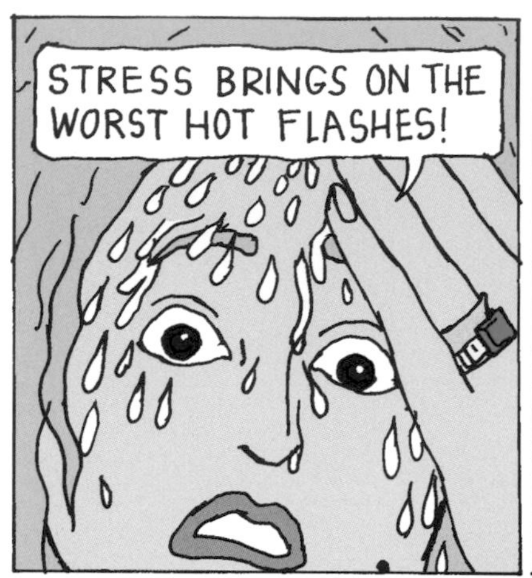
STRESS BRINGS ON THE WORST HOT FLASHES!

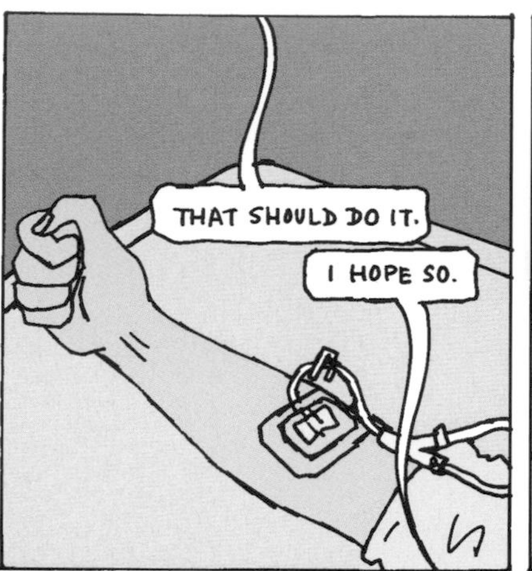
THAT SHOULD DO IT.
I HOPE SO.

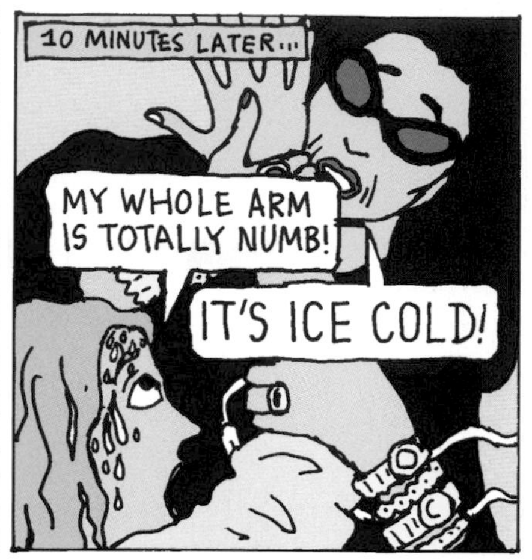
10 MINUTES LATER...
MY WHOLE ARM IS TOTALLY NUMB!
IT'S ICE COLD!

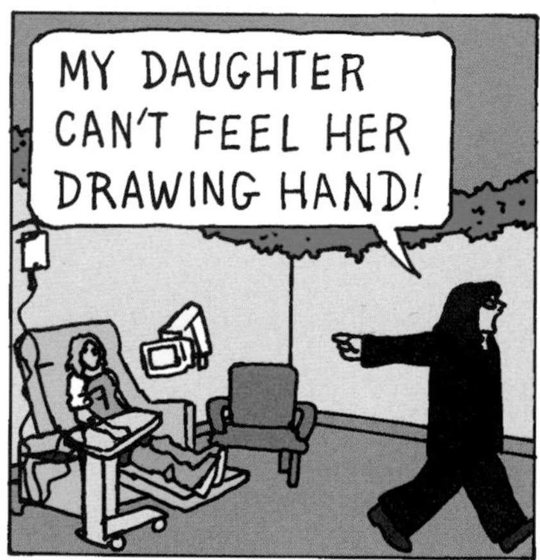
MY DAUGHTER CAN'T FEEL HER DRAWING HAND!

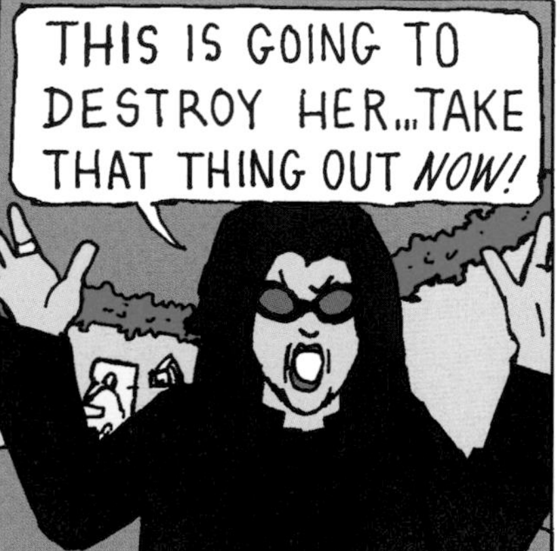
THIS IS GOING TO DESTROY HER...TAKE THAT THING OUT NOW!

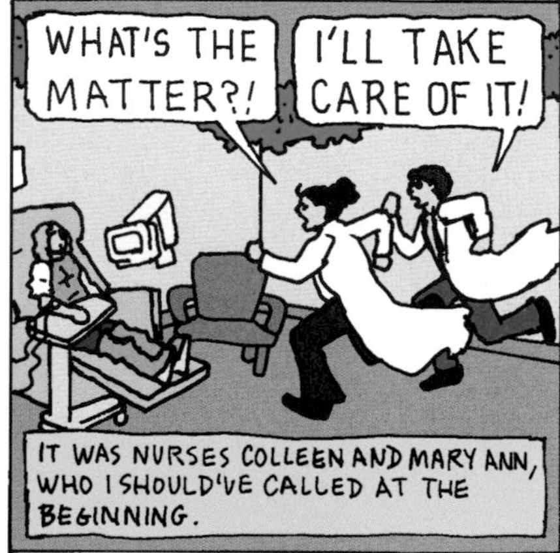
WHAT'S THE MATTER?!
I'LL TAKE CARE OF IT!
IT WAS NURSES COLLEEN AND MARY ANN, WHO I SHOULD'VE CALLED AT THE BEGINNING.

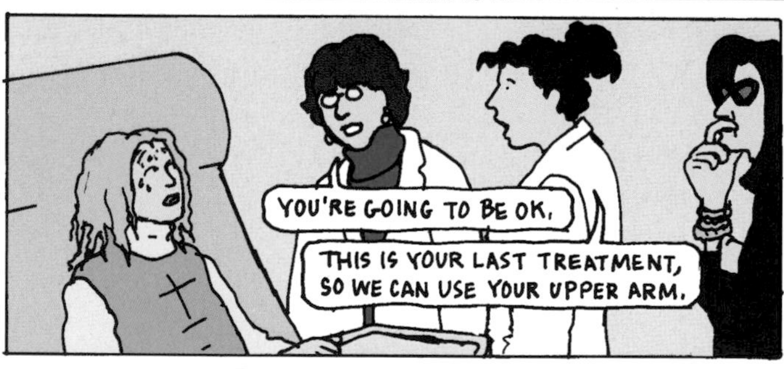
YOU'RE GOING TO BE OK.
THIS IS YOUR LAST TREATMENT, SO WE CAN USE YOUR UPPER ARM.

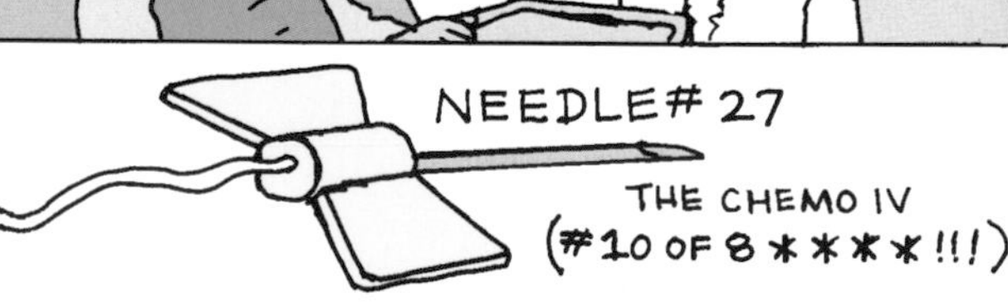
NEEDLE # 27
THE CHEMO IV
(#10 OF 8 **** !!!)

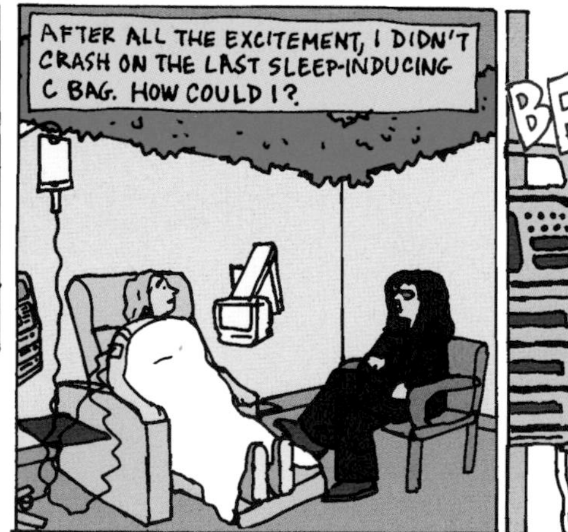
AFTER ALL THE EXCITEMENT, I DIDN'T CRASH ON THE LAST SLEEP-INDUCING C BAG. HOW COULD I?
BEEP!
CHEMO #8 DONE. FINITO. TUTTO BASTA!

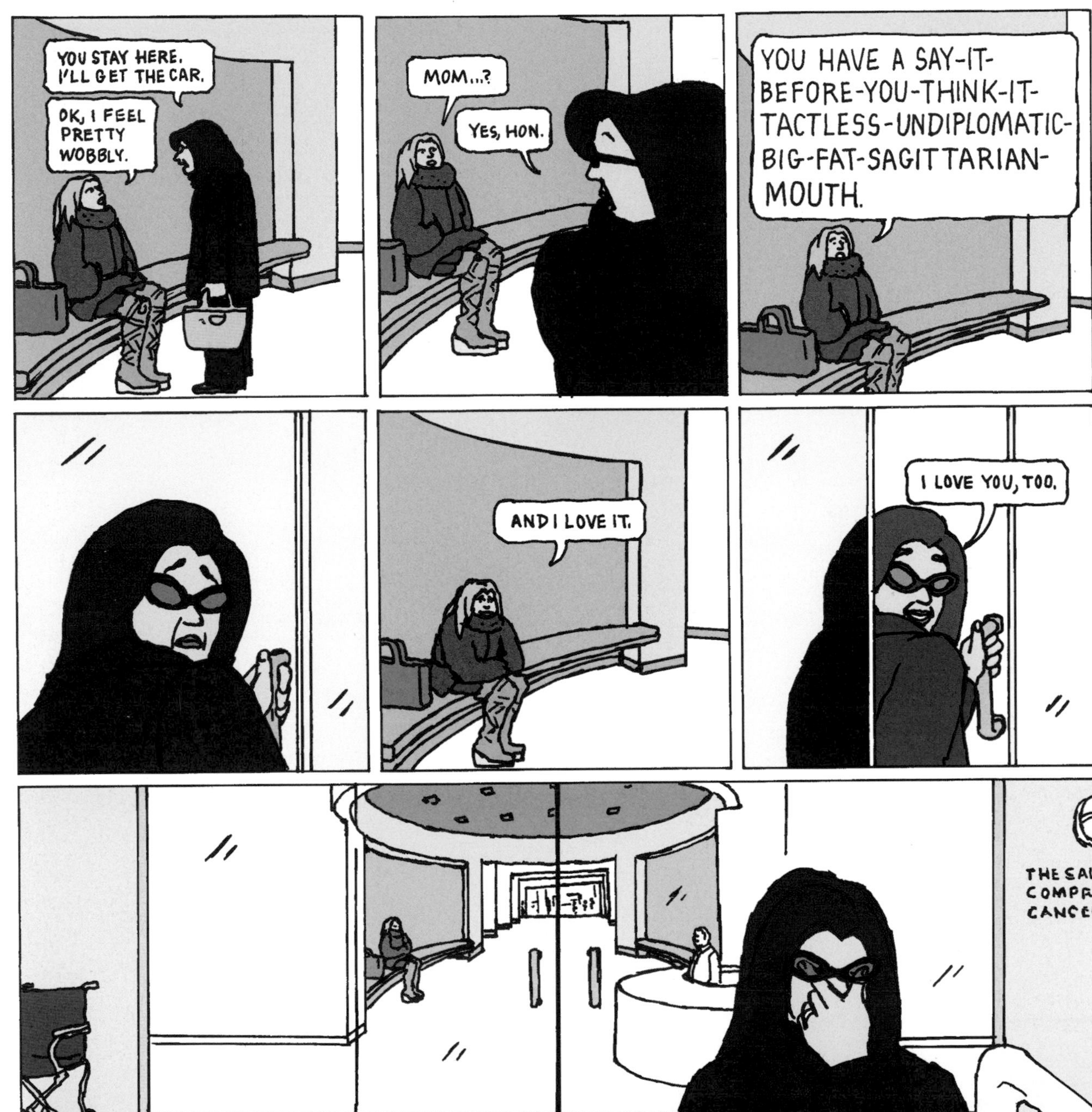
YOU STAY HERE. I'LL GET THE CAR.
OK, I FEEL PRETTY WOBBLY.
MOM...?
YES, HON.
YOU HAVE A SAY-IT-BEFORE-YOU-THINK-IT-TACTLESS-UNDIPLOMATIC-BIG-FAT-SAGITTARIAN-MOUTH.
AND I LOVE IT.
I LOVE YOU, TOO.

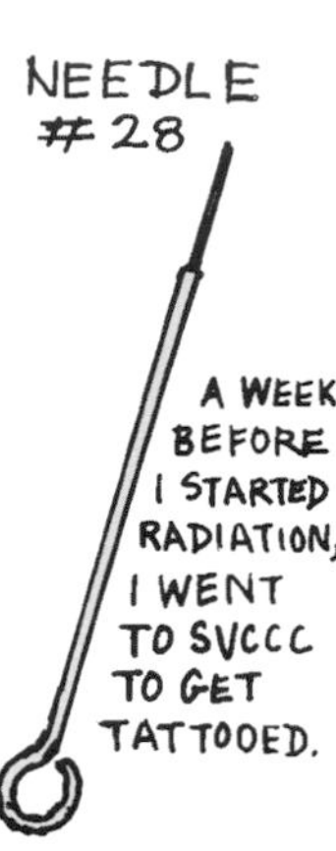
NEEDLE #28
A WEEK BEFORE I STARTED RADIATION, I WENT TO SVCCC TO GET TATTOOED.

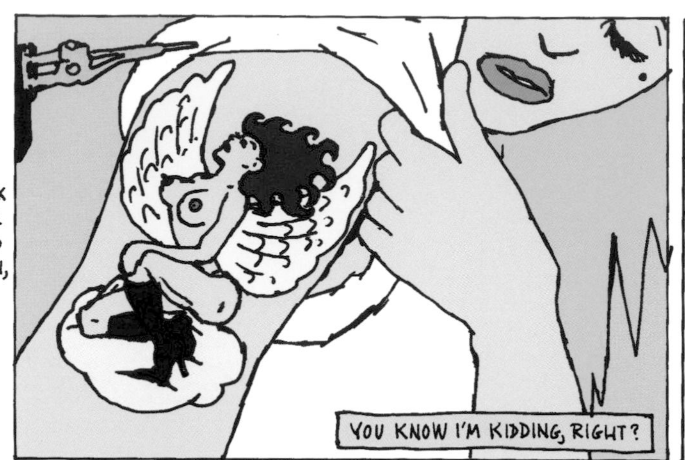
YOU KNOW I'M KIDDING, RIGHT?

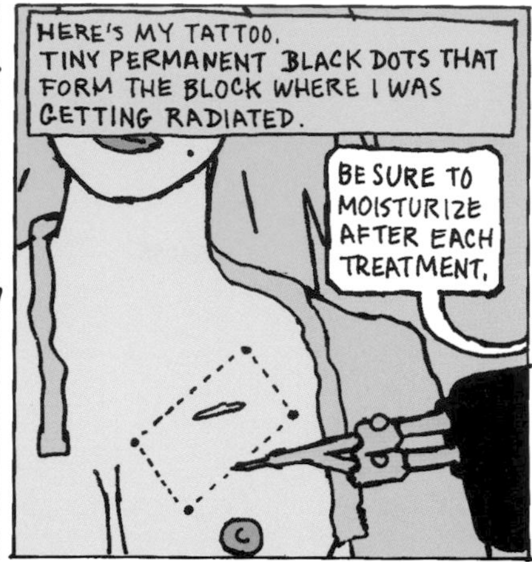
HERE'S MY TATTOO. TINY PERMANENT BLACK DOTS THAT FORM THE BLOCK WHERE I WAS GETTING RADIATED.
BE SURE TO MOISTURIZE AFTER EACH TREATMENT.

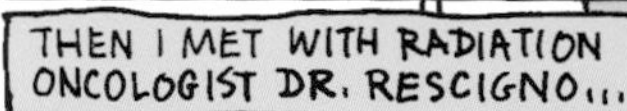
THEN I MET WITH RADIATION ONCOLOGIST DR. RESCIGNO...
THERE COULD STILL BE SOME LINGERING CANCER CELLS IN THE BREAST TISSUE THAT ARE TOO SMALL TO BE DETECTED. WE GIVE RADIATION TO PREVENT RECURRENCE IN THE BREAST, JUST TO BE SAFE.

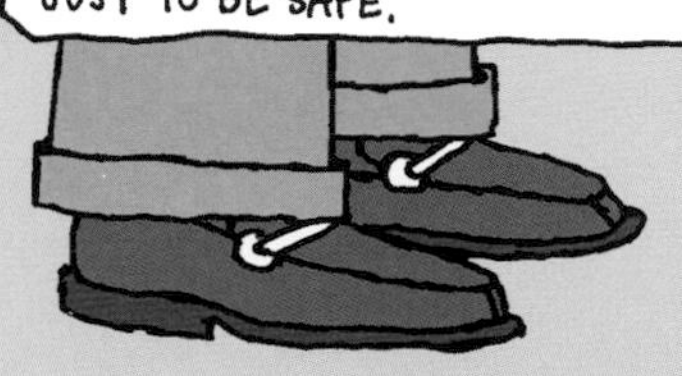

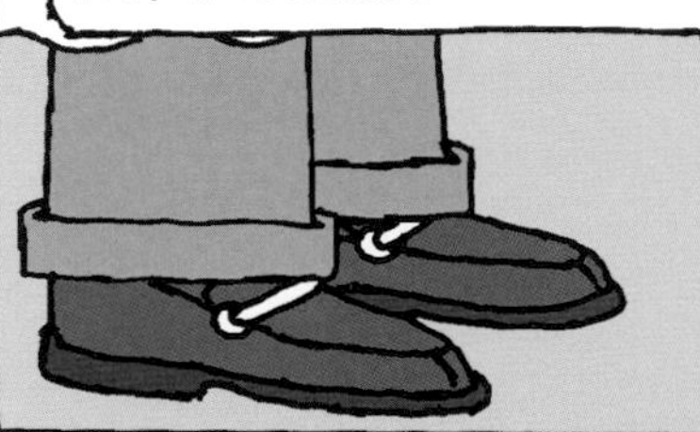
SO, YOU'LL BE STARTING NEXT WEEK. 33 TREATMENTS, 5 DAYS A WEEK MONDAY THROUGH FRIDAY FOR 6½ WEEKS. ANY QUESTIONS?
YEP. I'M DOING FINAL ART ON MY *GLAMOUR* PIECE. ARE YOU SURE YOU DON'T WANT TO BE IN IT?

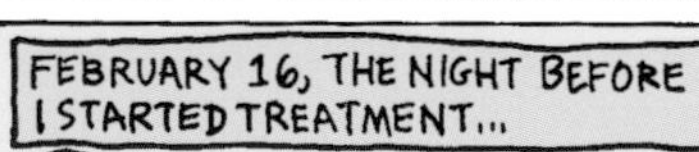
FEBRUARY 16, THE NIGHT BEFORE I STARTED TREATMENT...

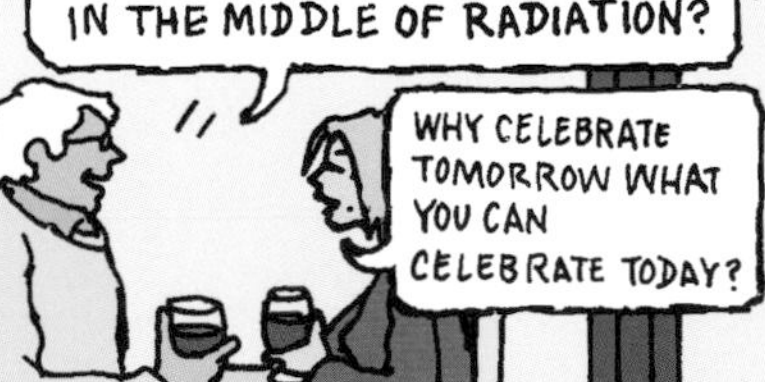
GOD' NEWS, BABY! I GOT THE CAR SHOWROOM! WE'RE 'AVING OUR WEDDING PARTY MARCH 9. BUT DO YOU REALLY WANT TO DO IT IN THE MIDDLE OF RADIATION?
WHY CELEBRATE TOMORROW WHAT YOU CAN CELEBRATE TODAY?

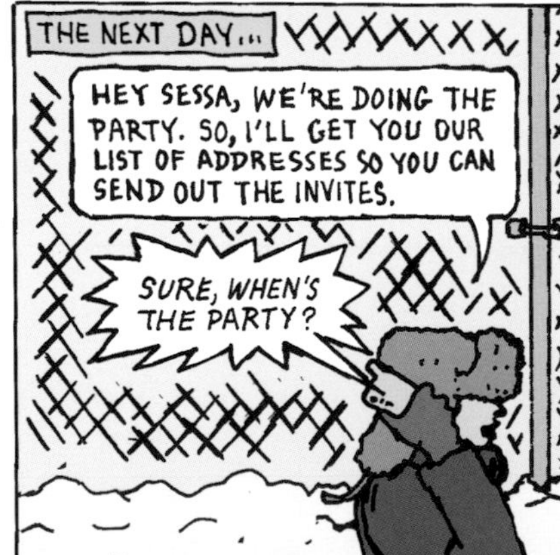
THE NEXT DAY...
HEY SESSA, WE'RE DOING THE PARTY. SO, I'LL GET YOU OUR LIST OF ADDRESSES SO YOU CAN SEND OUT THE INVITES.
SURE, WHEN'S THE PARTY?

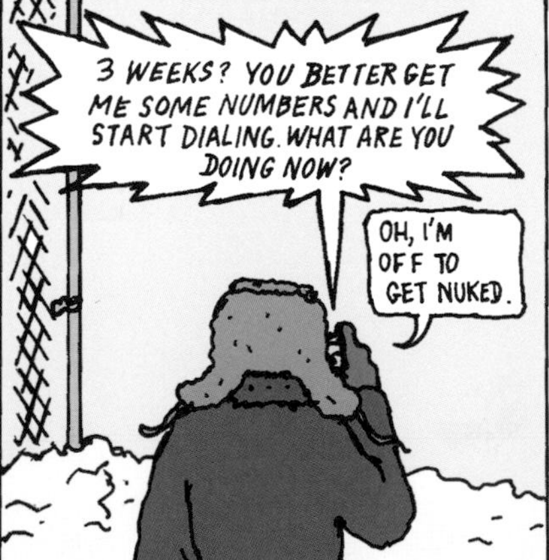
3 WEEKS? YOU BETTER GET ME SOME NUMBERS AND I'LL START DIALING. WHAT ARE YOU DOING NOW?
OH, I'M OFF TO GET NUKED.

AND NOW, IT'S TIME
TO ENTER A NEW PHASE
OF TREATMENT,
YOU KNOW...
"JUST TO BE SAFE"...

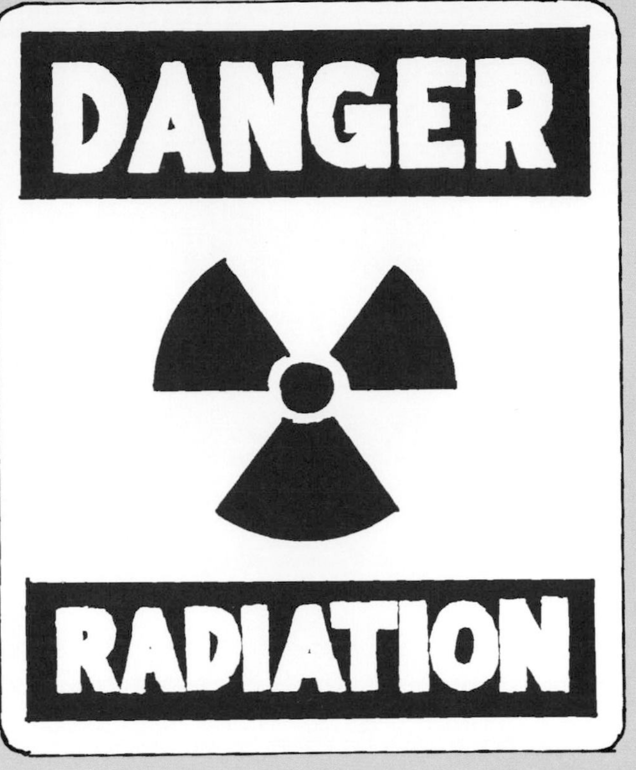

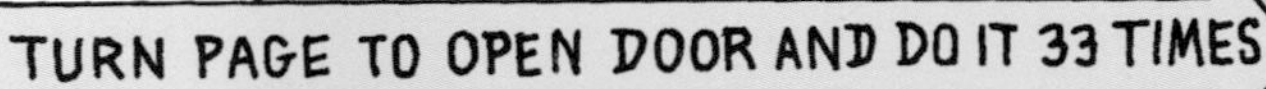

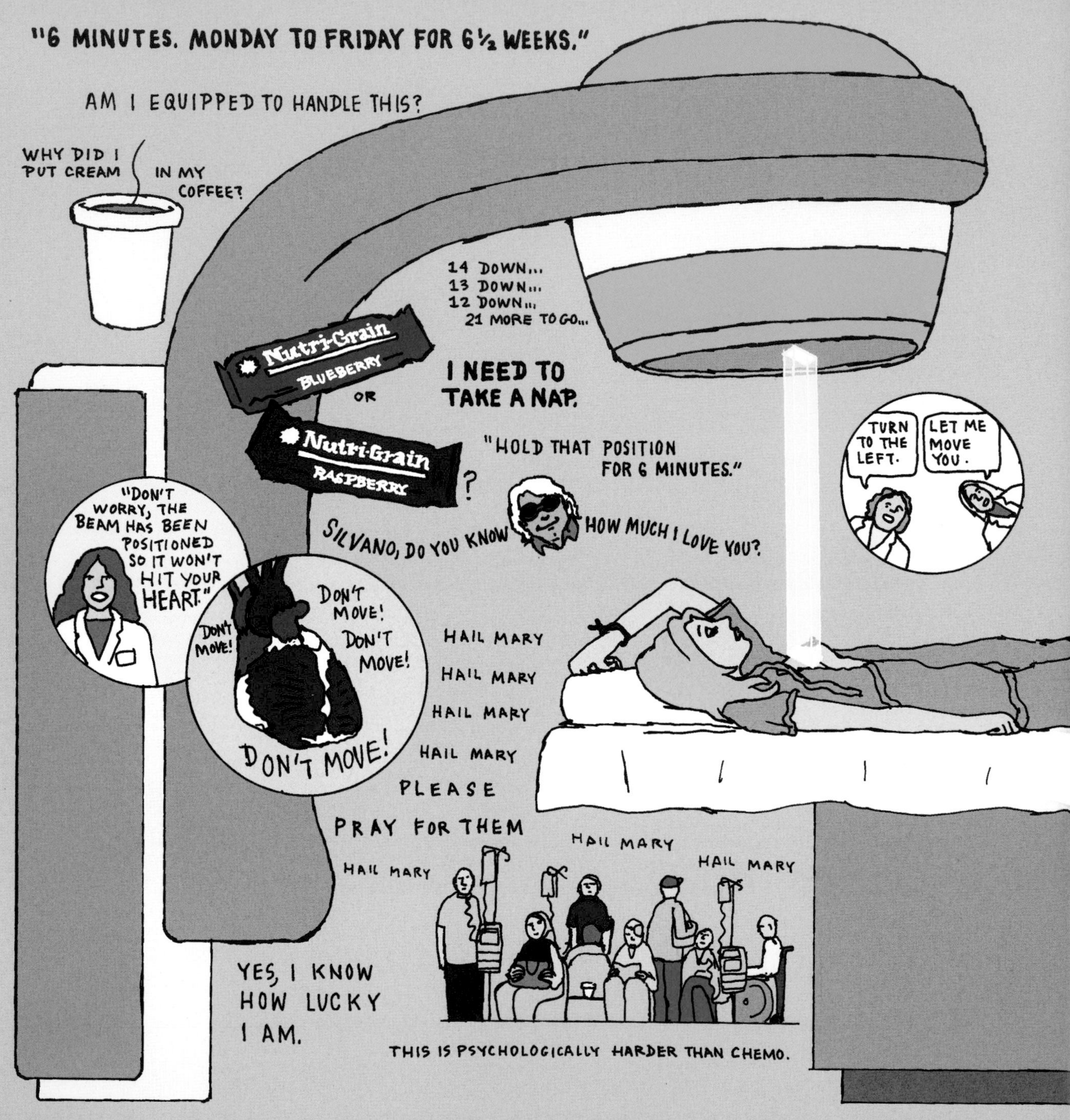
"6 MINUTES. MONDAY TO FRIDAY FOR 6½ WEEKS."
AM I EQUIPPED TO HANDLE THIS?
WHY DID I PUT CREAM IN MY COFFEE?
14 DOWN...
13 DOWN...
12 DOWN...
21 MORE TO GO...
Nutri-Grain
BLUEBERRY
OR
Nutri-Grain
RASPBERRY
?
I NEED TO TAKE A NAP.
"HOLD THAT POSITION FOR 6 MINUTES."
TURN TO THE LEFT.
LET ME MOVE YOU.
SILVANO, DO YOU KNOW HOW MUCH I LOVE YOU?
"DON'T WORRY, THE BEAM HAS BEEN POSITIONED SO IT WON'T HIT YOUR HEART."
DON'T MOVE!
DON'T MOVE!
DON'T MOVE!
DON'T MOVE!
HAIL MARY
HAIL MARY
HAIL MARY
HAIL MARY
PLEASE
PRAY FOR THEM
HAIL MARY
HAIL MARY
HAIL MARY
YES, I KNOW HOW LUCKY I AM.
THIS IS PSYCHOLOGICALLY HARDER THAN CHEMO.

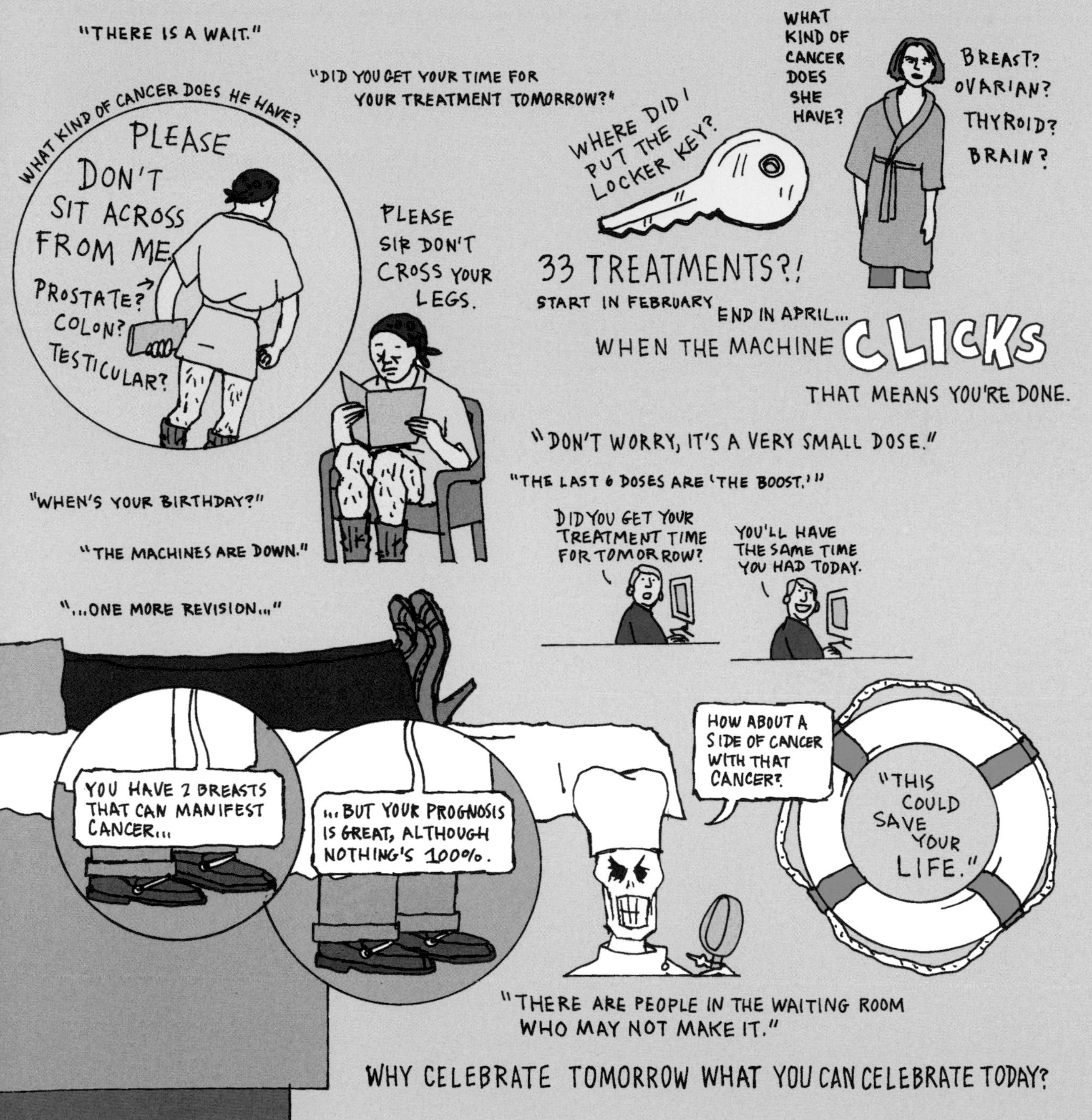

"THERE IS A WAIT."
"DID YOU GET YOUR TIME FOR YOUR TREATMENT TOMORROW?"
WHAT KIND OF CANCER DOES HE HAVE?
PLEASE DON'T SIT ACROSS FROM ME.
PROSTATE?
COLON?
TESTICULAR?
PLEASE SIR DON'T CROSS YOUR LEGS.
WHERE DID I PUT THE LOCKER KEY?
WHAT KIND OF CANCER DOES SHE HAVE?
BREAST?
OVARIAN?
THYROID?
BRAIN?
33 TREATMENTS?!
START IN FEBRUARY
END IN APRIL...
WHEN THE MACHINE CLICKS
THAT MEANS YOU'RE DONE.
"DON'T WORRY, IT'S A VERY SMALL DOSE."
"THE LAST 6 DOSES ARE 'THE BOOST.'"
"WHEN'S YOUR BIRTHDAY?"
"THE MACHINES ARE DOWN."
DID YOU GET YOUR TREATMENT TIME FOR TOMORROW?
YOU'LL HAVE THE SAME TIME YOU HAD TODAY.
"...ONE MORE REVISION..."
YOU HAVE 2 BREASTS THAT CAN MANIFEST CANCER...
...BUT YOUR PROGNOSIS IS GREAT, ALTHOUGH NOTHING'S 100%.
HOW ABOUT A SIDE OF CANCER WITH THAT CANCER?
"THIS COULD SAVE YOUR LIFE."
"THERE ARE PEOPLE IN THE WAITING ROOM WHO MAY NOT MAKE IT."
WHY CELEBRATE TOMORROW WHAT YOU CAN CELEBRATE TODAY?

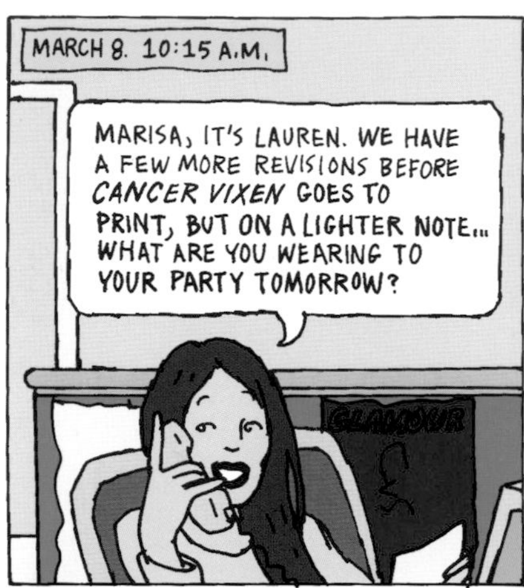
MARCH 8. 10:15 A.M.
MARISA, IT'S LAUREN. WE HAVE A FEW MORE REVISIONS BEFORE CANCER VIXEN GOES TO PRINT, BUT ON A LIGHTER NOTE... WHAT ARE YOU WEARING TO YOUR PARTY TOMORROW?
GLAMOUR

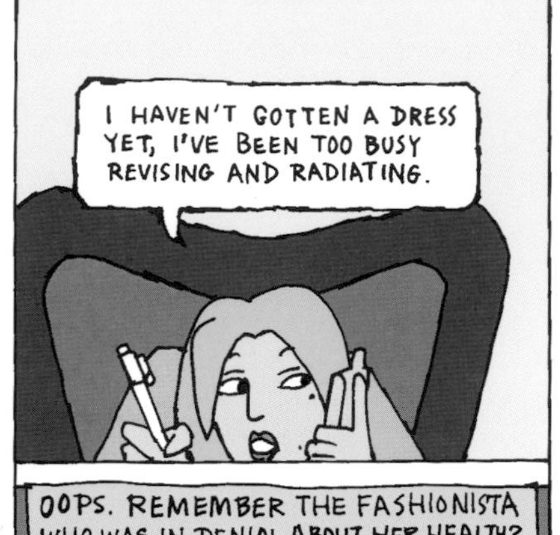
I HAVEN'T GOTTEN A DRESS YET, I'VE BEEN TOO BUSY REVISING AND RADIATING.
OOPS. REMEMBER THE FASHIONISTA WHO WAS IN DENIAL ABOUT HER HEALTH?

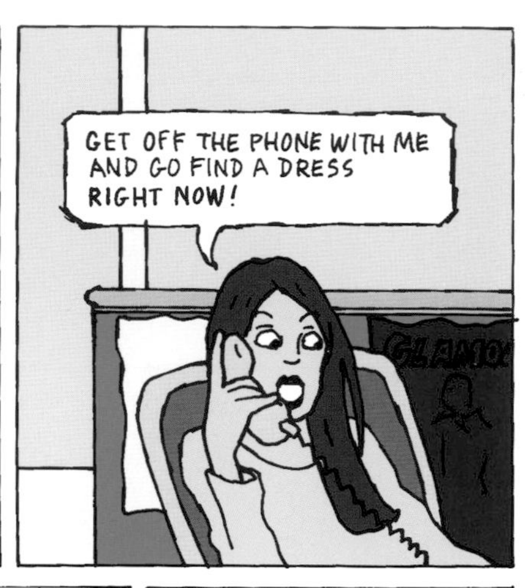
GET OFF THE PHONE WITH ME AND GO FIND A DRESS RIGHT NOW!

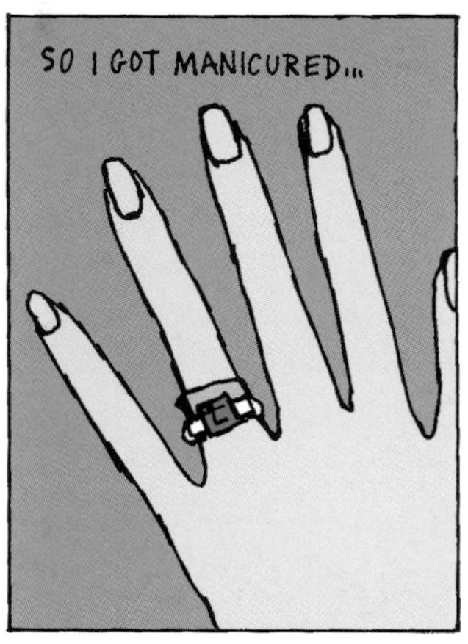
SO I GOT MANICURED...

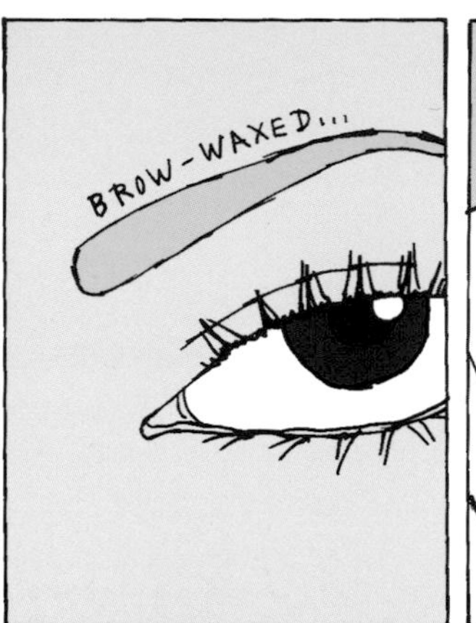
BROW-WAXED...

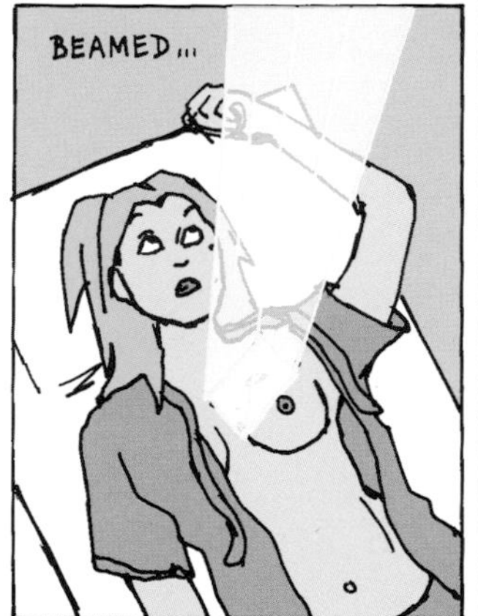
BEAMED...

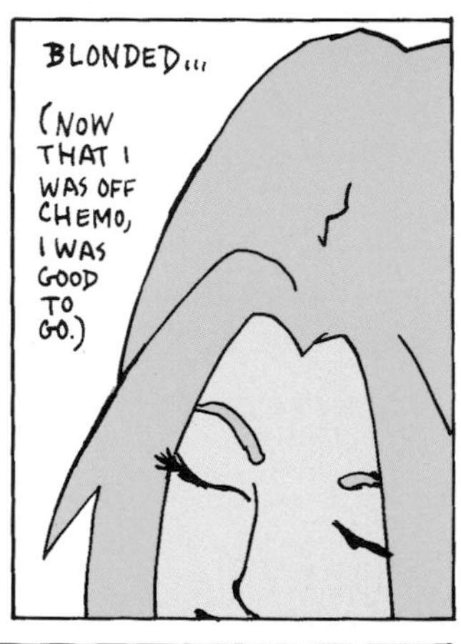
BLONDED...
(NOW THAT I WAS OFF CHEMO, I WAS GOOD TO GO.)

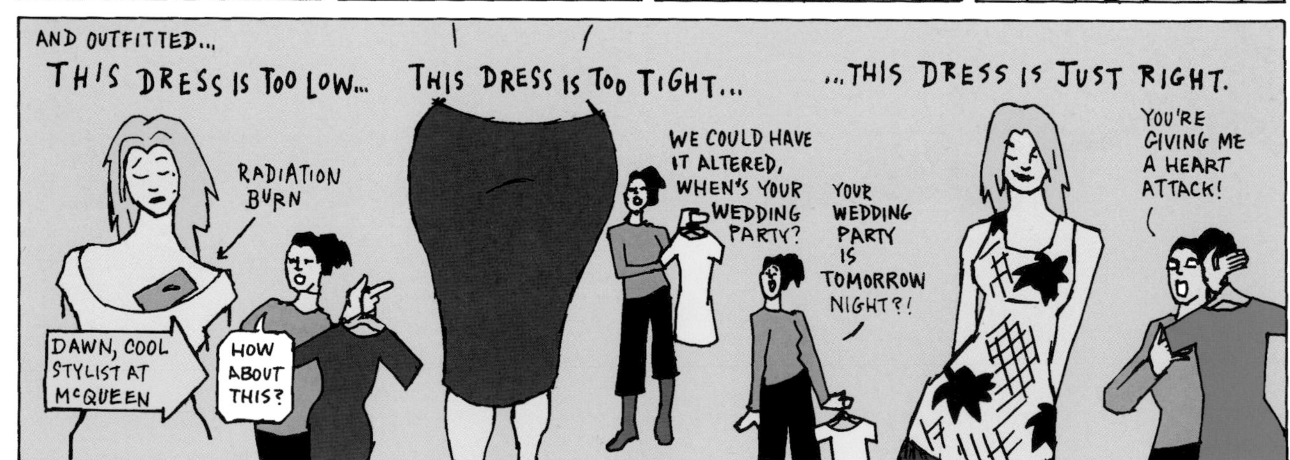
AND OUTFITTED...
THIS DRESS IS TOO LOW...
RADIATION BURN
DAWN, COOL STYLIST AT McQUEEN
HOW ABOUT THIS?
THIS DRESS IS TOO TIGHT...
WE COULD HAVE IT ALTERED, WHEN'S YOUR WEDDING PARTY?
YOUR WEDDING PARTY IS TOMORROW NIGHT?!
...THIS DRESS IS JUST RIGHT.
YOU'RE GIVING ME A HEART ATTACK!

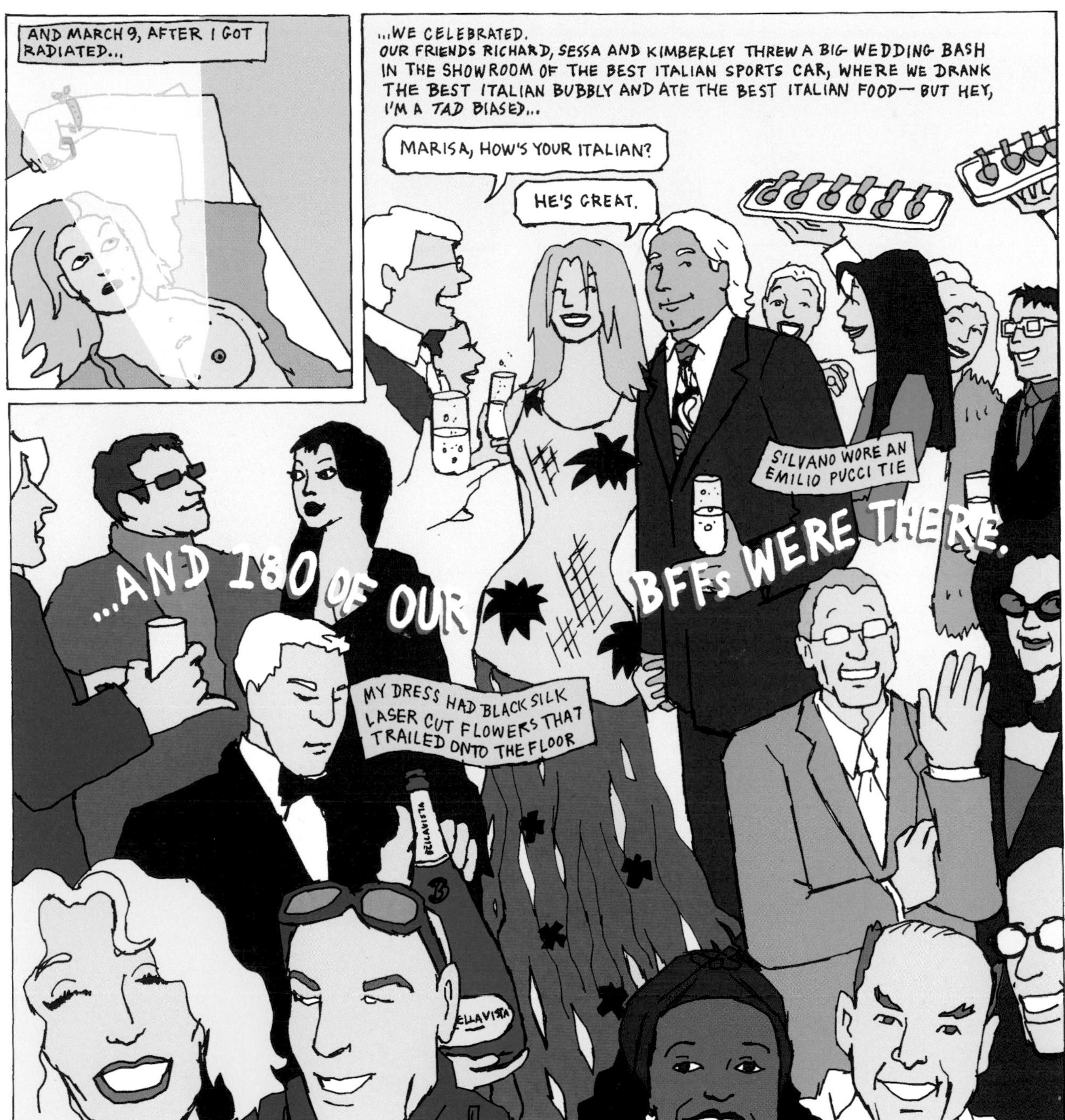
AND MARCH 9, AFTER I GOT RADIATED...
...WE CELEBRATED.
OUR FRIENDS RICHARD, SESSA AND KIMBERLEY THREW A BIG WEDDING BASH IN THE SHOWROOM OF THE BEST ITALIAN SPORTS CAR, WHERE WE DRANK THE BEST ITALIAN BUBBLY AND ATE THE BEST ITALIAN FOOD—BUT HEY, I'M A *TAD* BIASED...
MARISA, HOW'S YOUR ITALIAN?
HE'S GREAT.
SILVANO WORE AN EMILIO PUCCI TIE
...AND 180 OF OUR BFFs WERE THERE.
MY DRESS HAD BLACK SILK LASER CUT FLOWERS THAT TRAILED ONTO THE FLOOR
BELLAVISTA
BELLAVISTA

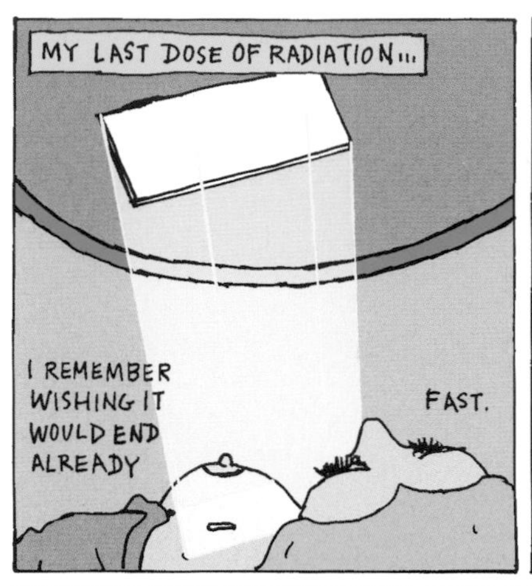
MY LAST DOSE OF RADIATION...
I REMEMBER WISHING IT WOULD END ALREADY
FAST.

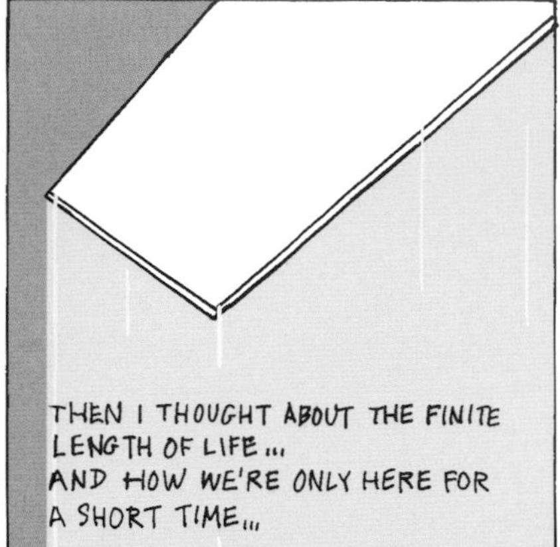
THEN I THOUGHT ABOUT THE FINITE LENGTH OF LIFE...
AND HOW WE'RE ONLY HERE FOR A SHORT TIME...

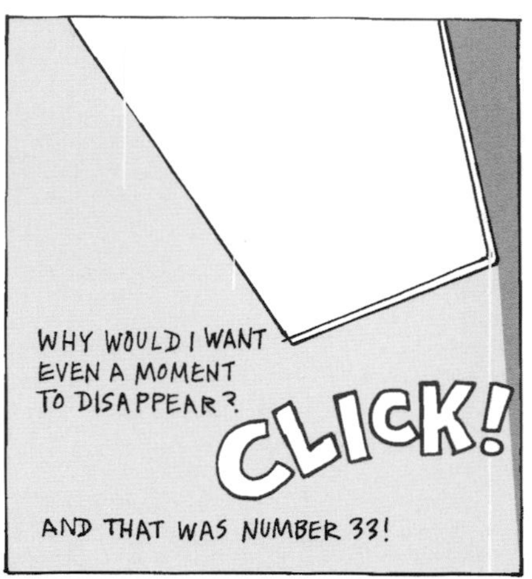
WHY WOULD I WANT EVEN A MOMENT TO DISAPPEAR?
CLICK!
AND THAT WAS NUMBER 33!

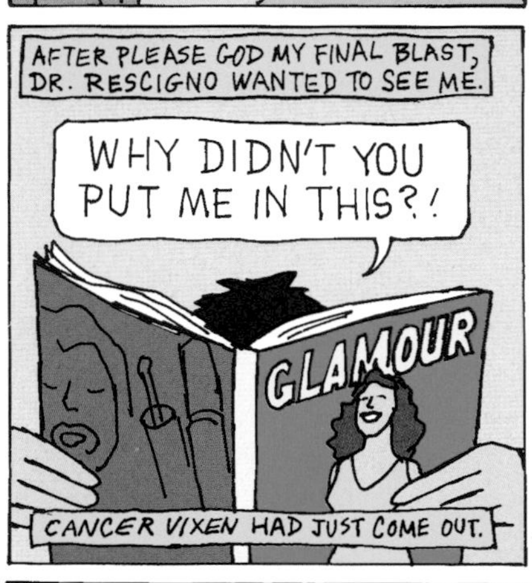
AFTER PLEASE GOD MY FINAL BLAST, DR. RESCIGNO WANTED TO SEE ME.
WHY DIDN'T YOU PUT ME IN THIS?!
GLAMOUR
CANCER VIXEN HAD JUST COME OUT.

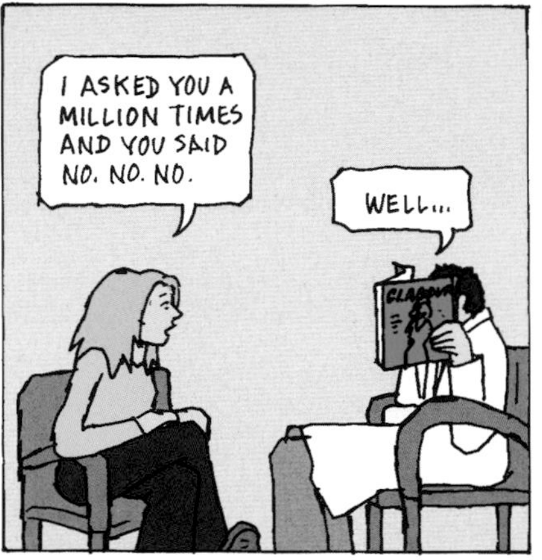
I ASKED YOU A MILLION TIMES AND YOU SAID NO. NO. NO.
WELL...

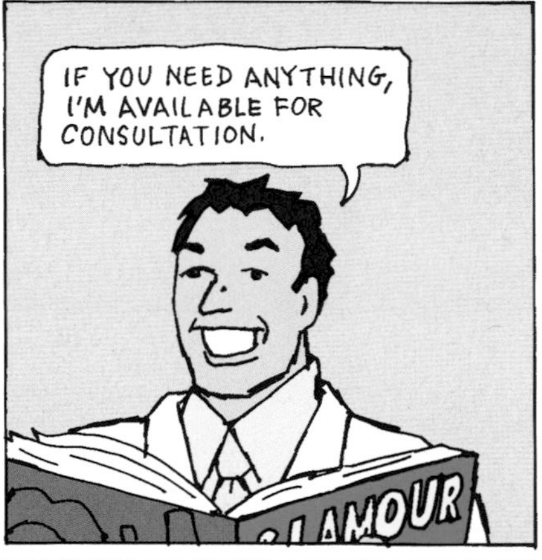
IF YOU NEED ANYTHING, I'M AVAILABLE FOR CONSULTATION.

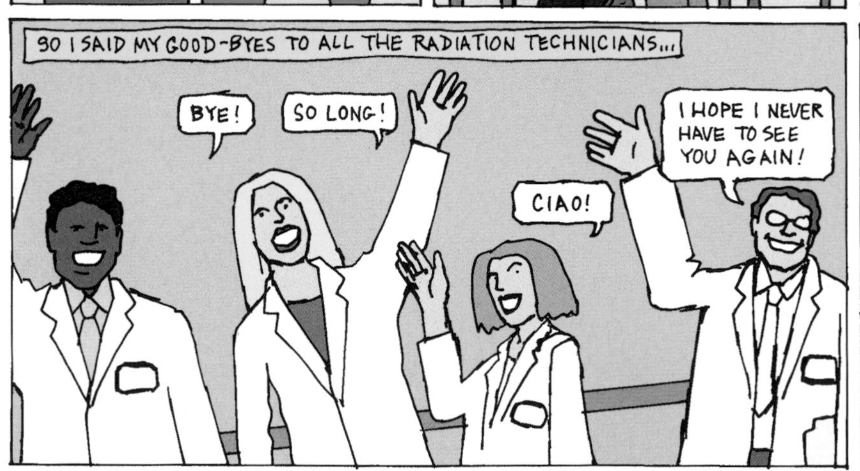
SO I SAID MY GOOD-BYES TO ALL THE RADIATION TECHNICIANS...
BYE!
SO LONG!
CIAO!
I HOPE I NEVER HAVE TO SEE YOU AGAIN!

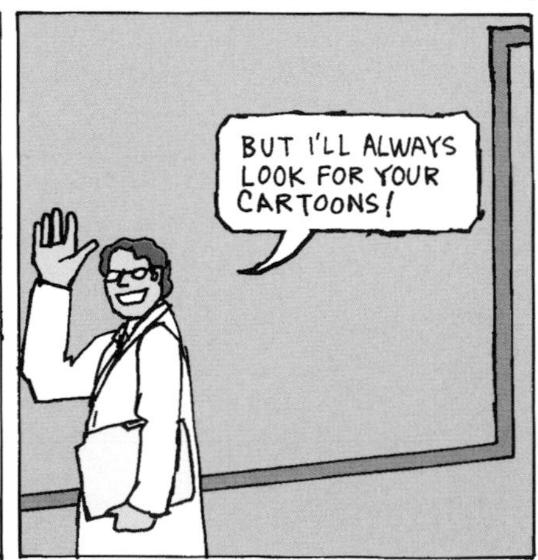
BUT I'LL ALWAYS LOOK FOR YOUR CARTOONS!

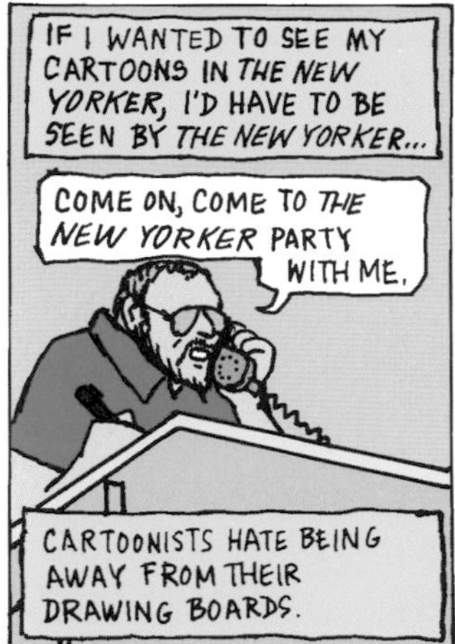
IF I WANTED TO SEE MY CARTOONS IN THE NEW YORKER, I'D HAVE TO BE SEEN BY THE NEW YORKER...
COME ON, COME TO THE NEW YORKER PARTY WITH ME.
CARTOONISTS HATE BEING AWAY FROM THEIR DRAWING BOARDS.

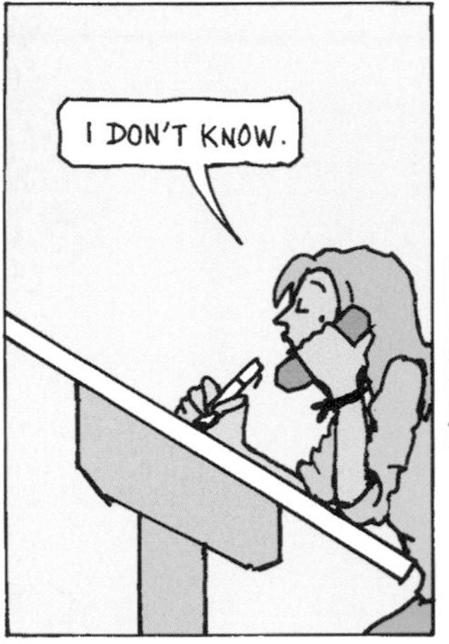
I DON'T KNOW.

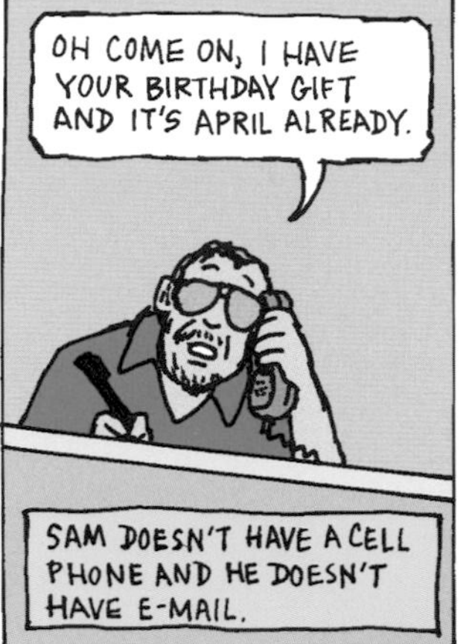
OH COME ON, I HAVE YOUR BIRTHDAY GIFT AND IT'S APRIL ALREADY.
SAM DOESN'T HAVE A CELL PHONE AND HE DOESN'T HAVE E-MAIL.

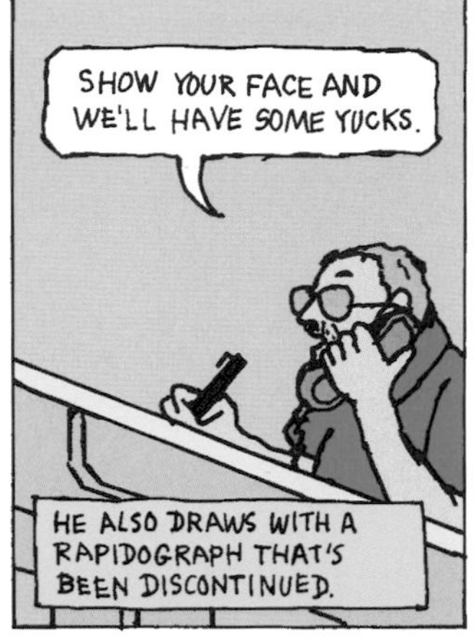
SHOW YOUR FACE AND WE'LL HAVE SOME YUCKS.
HE ALSO DRAWS WITH A RAPIDOGRAPH THAT'S BEEN DISCONTINUED.

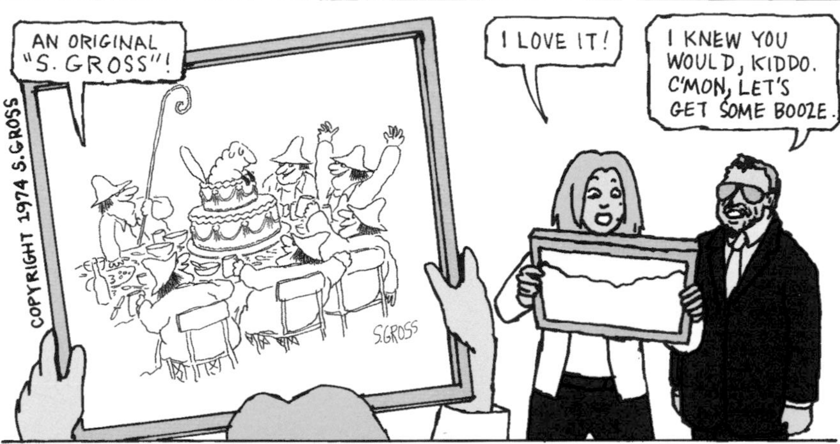
AN ORIGINAL "S. GROSS"!
COPYRIGHT 1974 S. GROSS
S. GROSS
I LOVE IT!
I KNEW YOU WOULD, KIDDO. C'MON, LET'S GET SOME BOOZE.

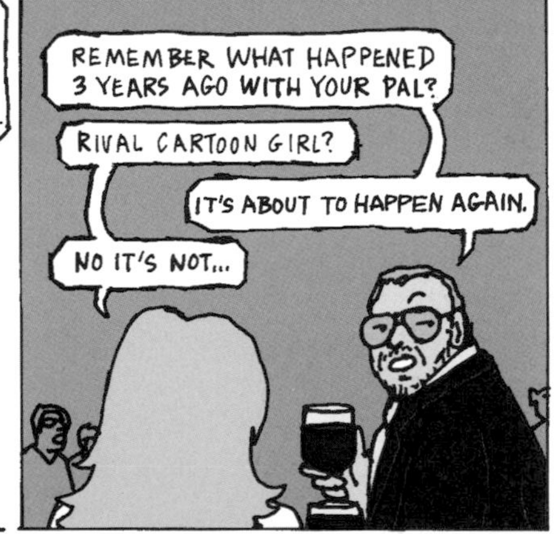
REMEMBER WHAT HAPPENED 3 YEARS AGO WITH YOUR PAL?
RIVAL CARTOON GIRL?
IT'S ABOUT TO HAPPEN AGAIN.
NO IT'S NOT...

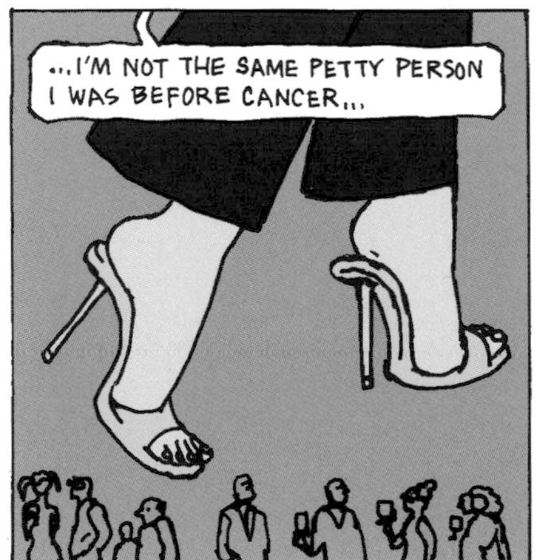
...I'M NOT THE SAME PETTY PERSON I WAS BEFORE CANCER...

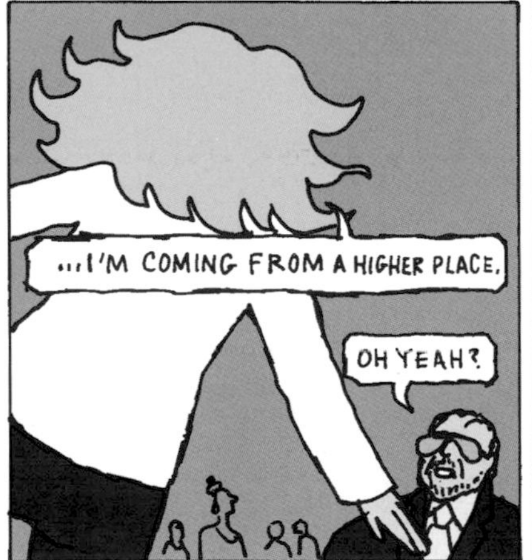
...I'M COMING FROM A HIGHER PLACE.
OH YEAH?

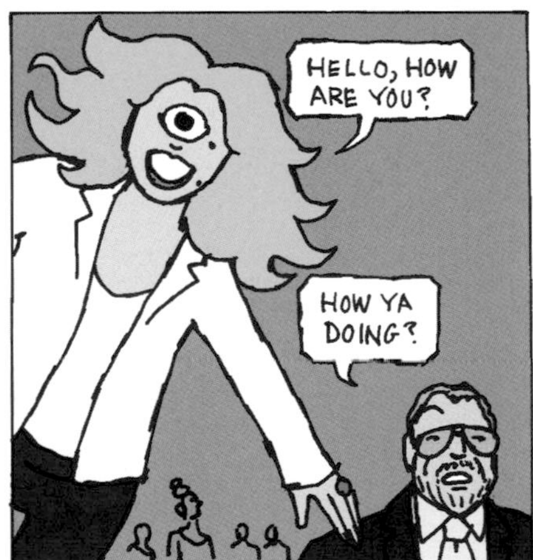
HELLO, HOW ARE YOU?
HOW YA DOING?

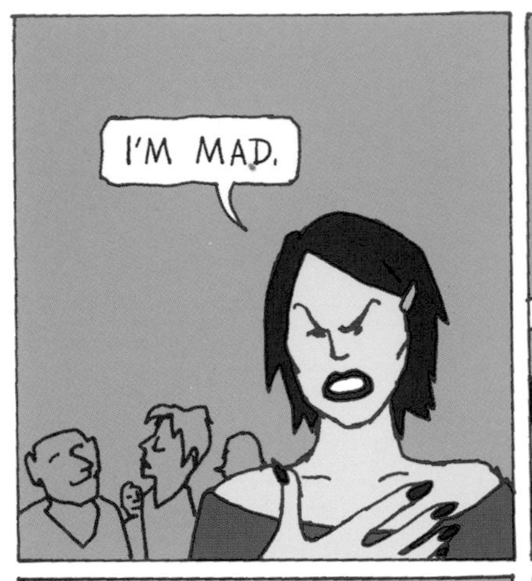
I'M MAD.

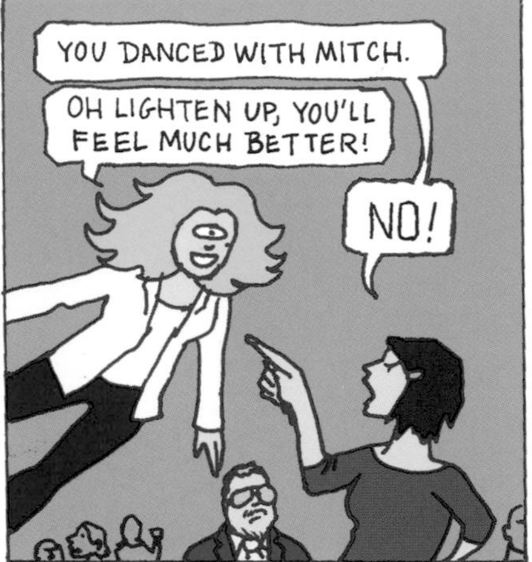
YOU DANCED WITH MITCH.
OH LIGHTEN UP, YOU'LL FEEL MUCH BETTER!
NO!

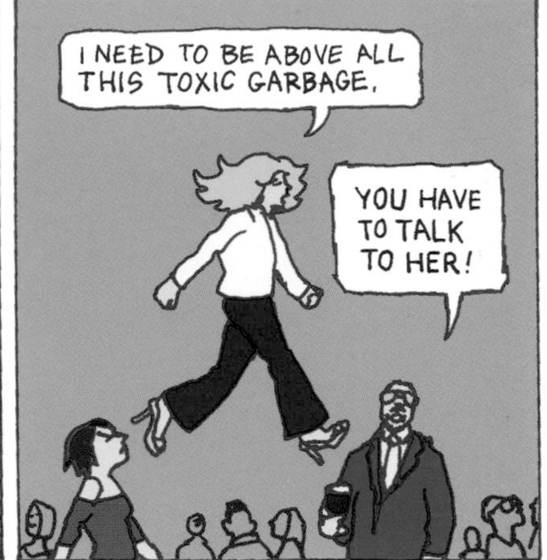
I NEED TO BE ABOVE ALL THIS TOXIC GARBAGE.
YOU HAVE TO TALK TO HER!

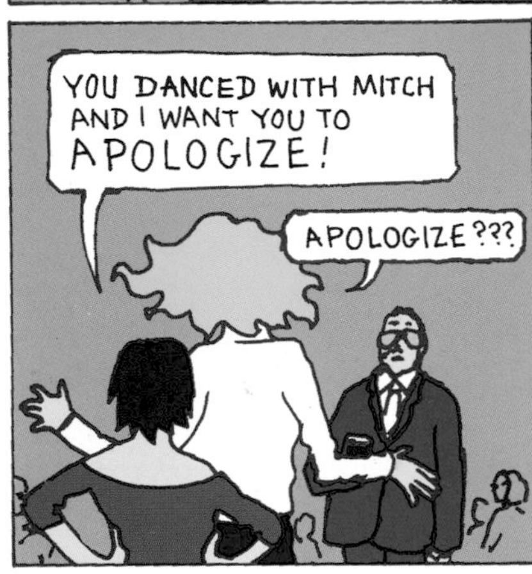
YOU DANCED WITH MITCH AND I WANT YOU TO APOLOGIZE!
APOLOGIZE???

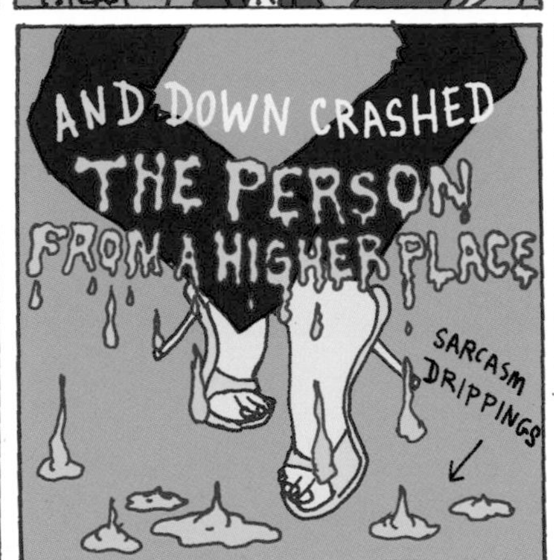
AND DOWN CRASHED THE PERSON FROM A HIGHER PLACE
SARCASM DRIPPINGS

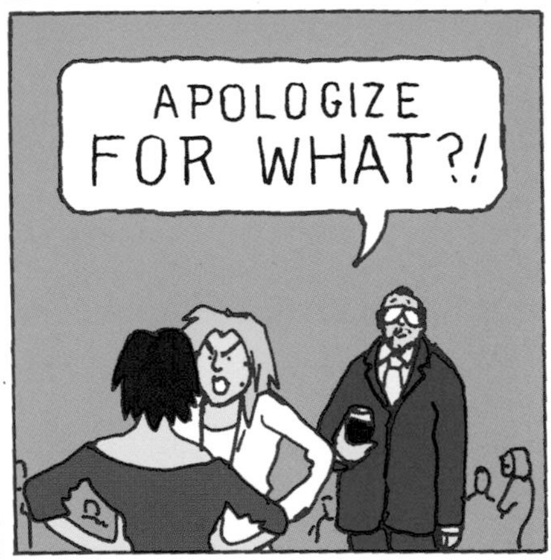
APOLOGIZE FOR WHAT?!

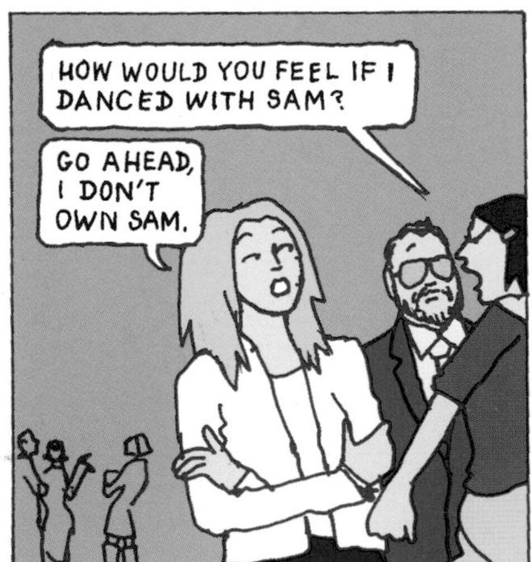
HOW WOULD YOU FEEL IF I DANCED WITH SAM?
GO AHEAD, I DON'T OWN SAM.

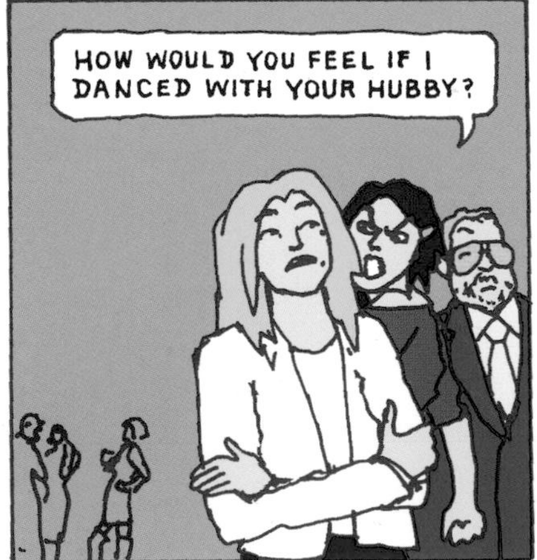
HOW WOULD YOU FEEL IF I DANCED WITH YOUR HUBBY?

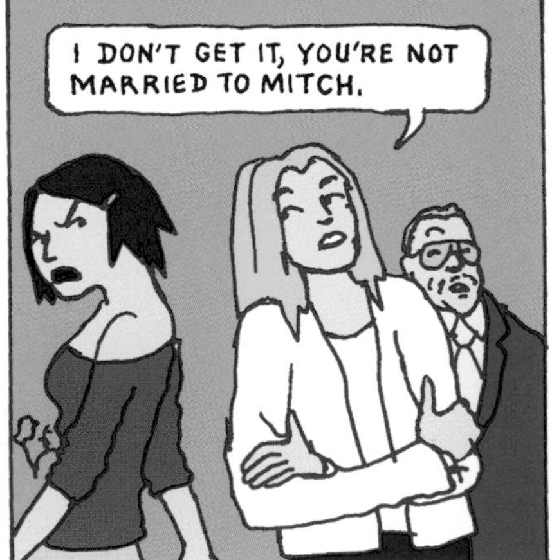
I DON'T GET IT, YOU'RE NOT MARRIED TO MITCH.

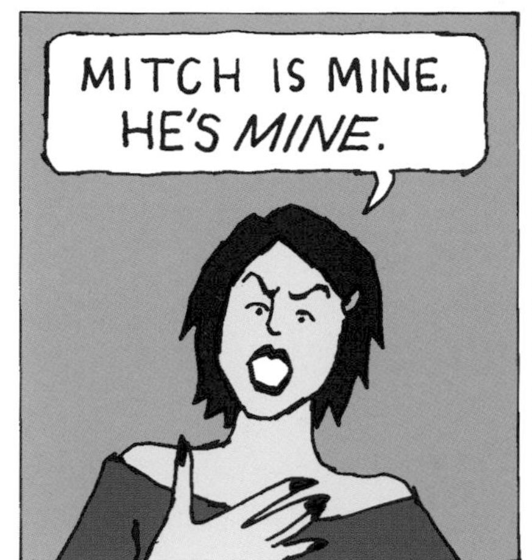

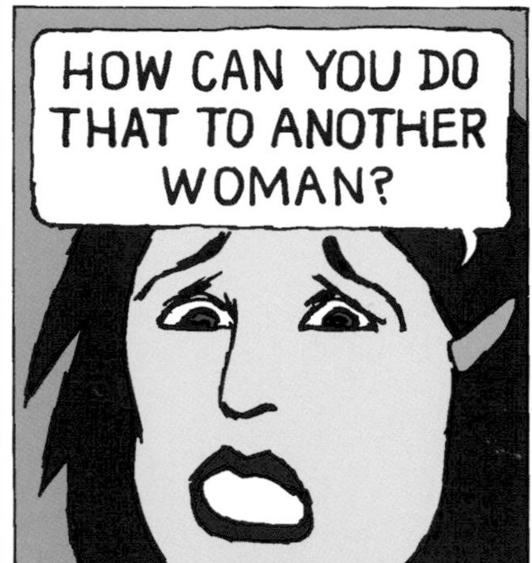

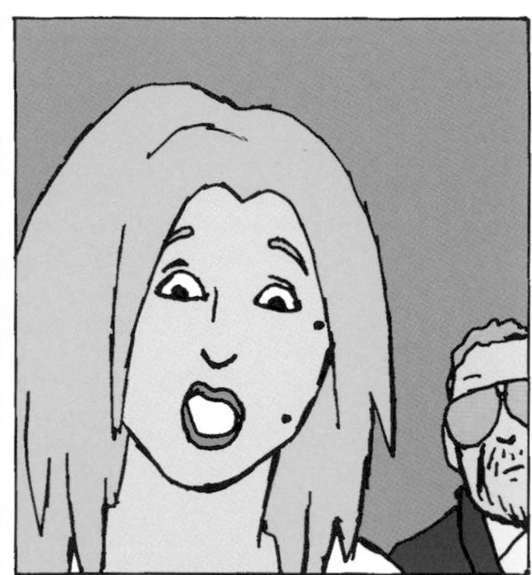

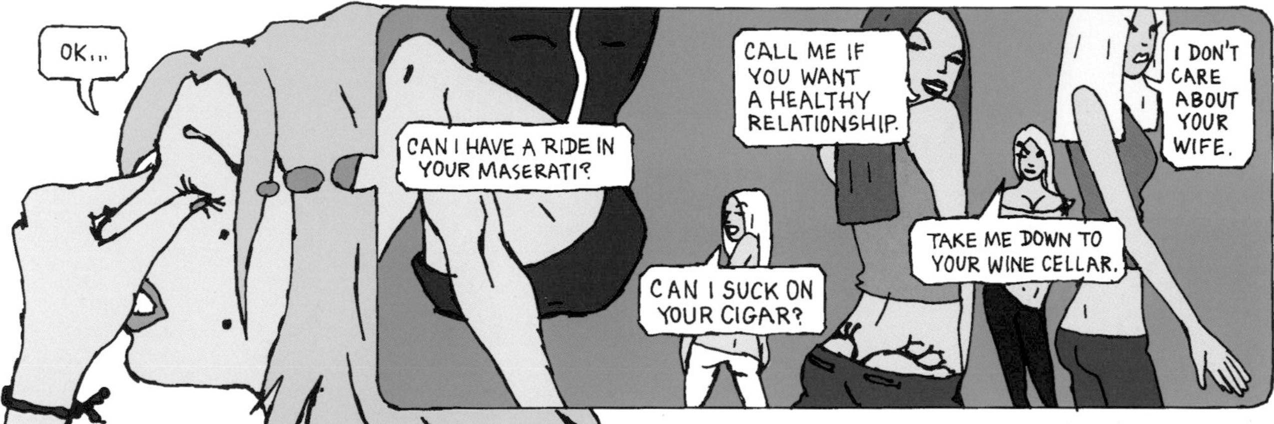

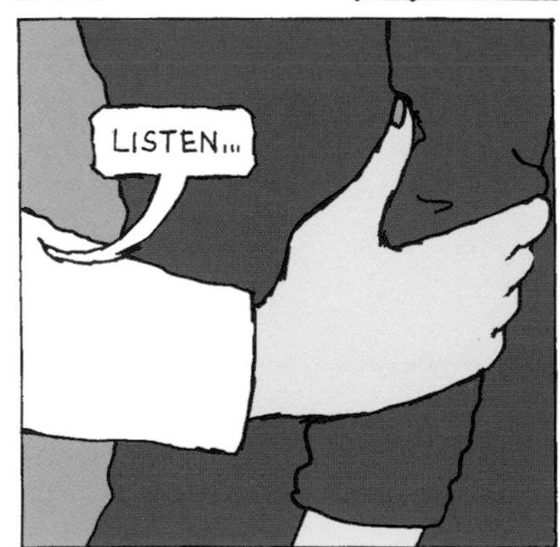

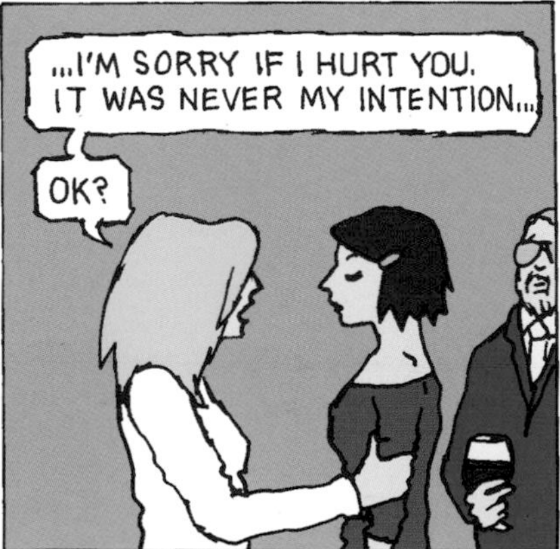

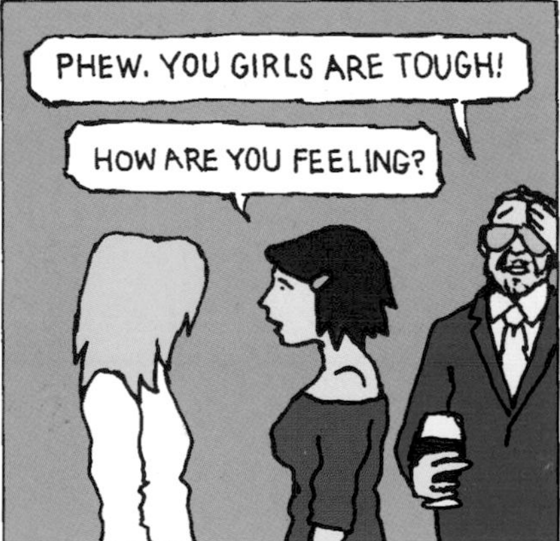

IF I COULD FORGIVE HER, AND SHE COULD FORGIVE ME, MAYBE THERE WAS HOPE IN THE WORLD?

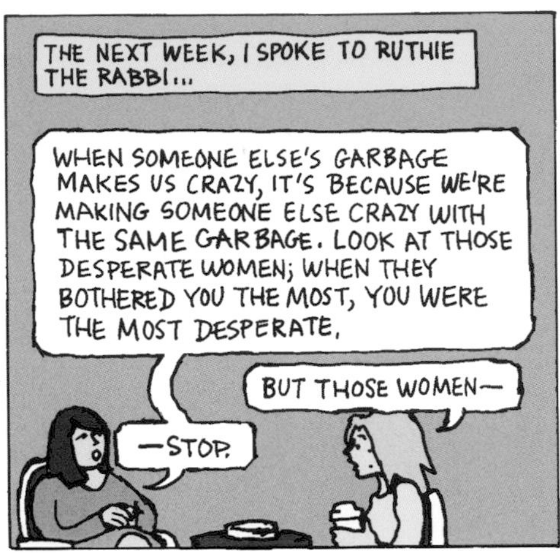
THE NEXT WEEK, I SPOKE TO RUTHIE THE RABBI...
WHEN SOMEONE ELSE'S GARBAGE MAKES US CRAZY, IT'S BECAUSE WE'RE MAKING SOMEONE ELSE CRAZY WITH THE SAME GARBAGE. LOOK AT THOSE DESPERATE WOMEN; WHEN THEY BOTHERED YOU THE MOST, YOU WERE THE MOST DESPERATE.
BUT THOSE WOMEN—
—STOP.

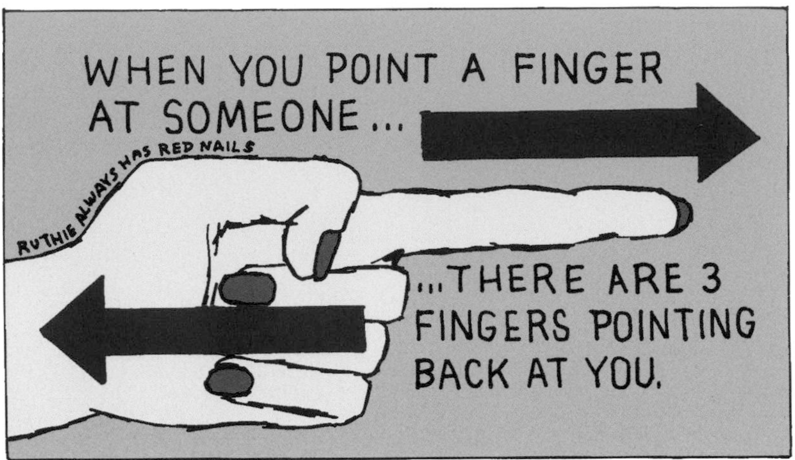
WHEN YOU POINT A FINGER AT SOMEONE...
RUTHIE ALWAYS HAS RED NAILS
...THERE ARE 3 FINGERS POINTING BACK AT YOU.

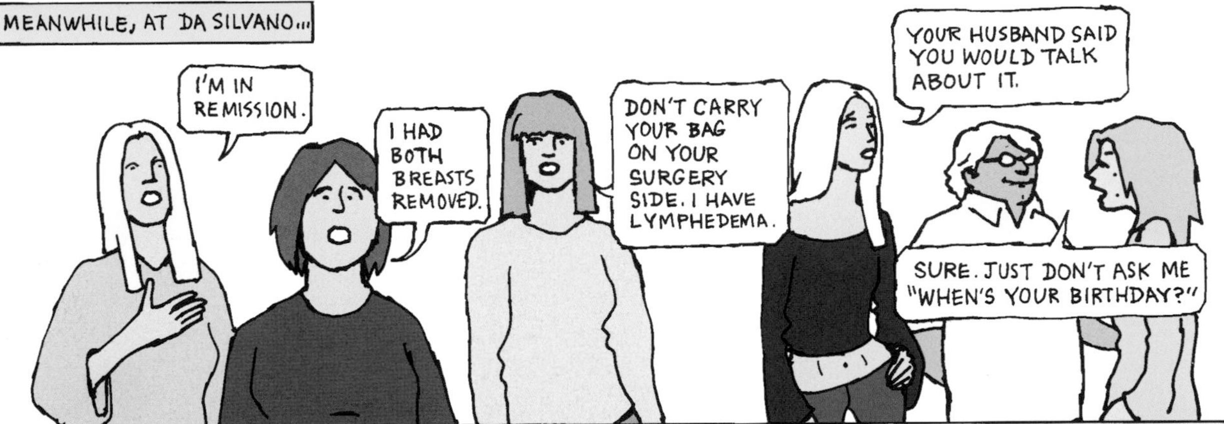
MEANWHILE, AT DA SILVANO...
I'M IN REMISSION.
I HAD BOTH BREASTS REMOVED.
DON'T CARRY YOUR BAG ON YOUR SURGERY SIDE. I HAVE LYMPHEDEMA.
YOUR HUSBAND SAID YOU WOULD TALK ABOUT IT.
SURE. JUST DON'T ASK ME "WHEN'S YOUR BIRTHDAY?"

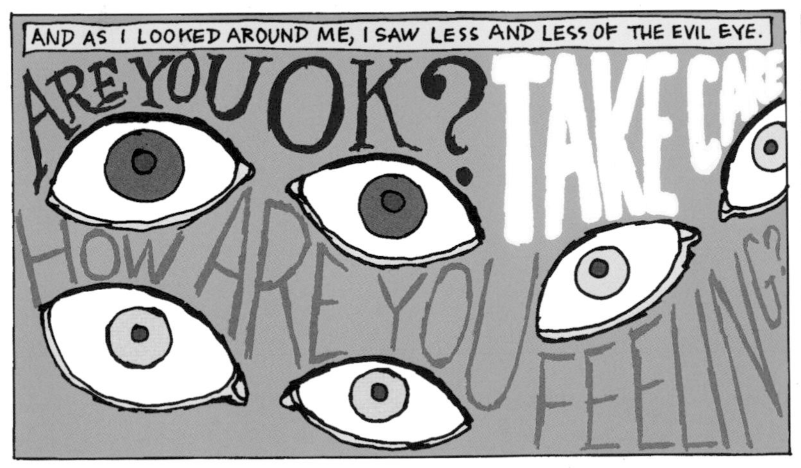
AND AS I LOOKED AROUND ME, I SAW LESS AND LESS OF THE EVIL EYE.
ARE YOU OK?
TAKE CARE
HOW ARE YOU FEELING?

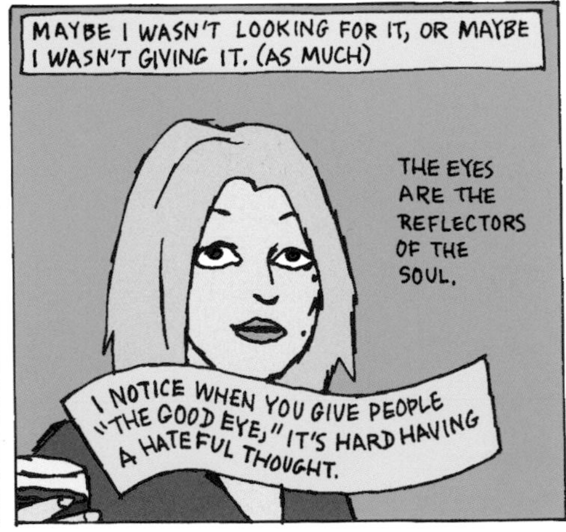
MAYBE I WASN'T LOOKING FOR IT, OR MAYBE I WASN'T GIVING IT. (AS MUCH)
THE EYES ARE THE REFLECTORS OF THE SOUL.
I NOTICE WHEN YOU GIVE PEOPLE "THE GOOD EYE," IT'S HARD HAVING A HATEFUL THOUGHT.

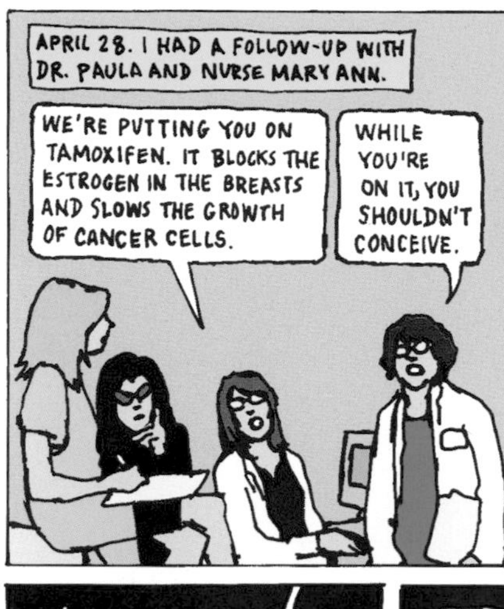
APRIL 28. I HAD A FOLLOW-UP WITH DR. PAULA AND NURSE MARY ANN.
WE'RE PUTTING YOU ON TAMOXIFEN. IT BLOCKS THE ESTROGEN IN THE BREASTS AND SLOWS THE GROWTH OF CANCER CELLS.
WHILE YOU'RE ON IT, YOU SHOULDN'T CONCEIVE.
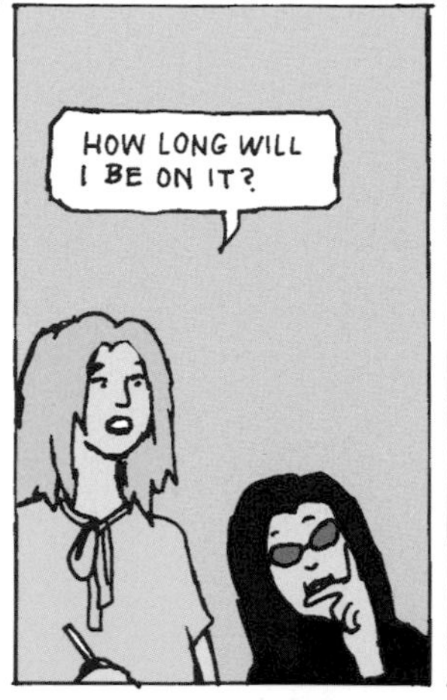
HOW LONG WILL I BE ON IT?
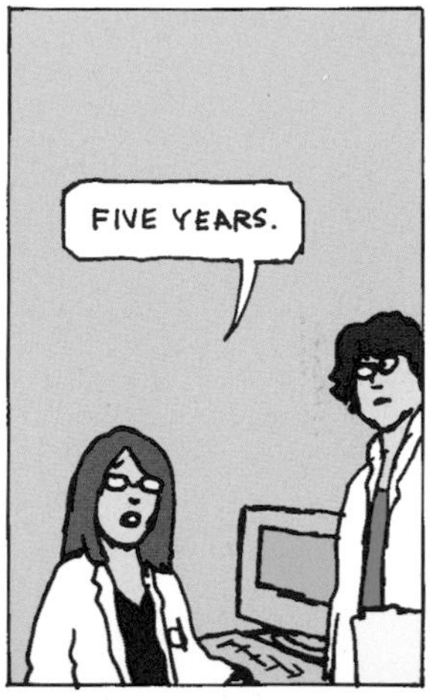
FIVE YEARS.
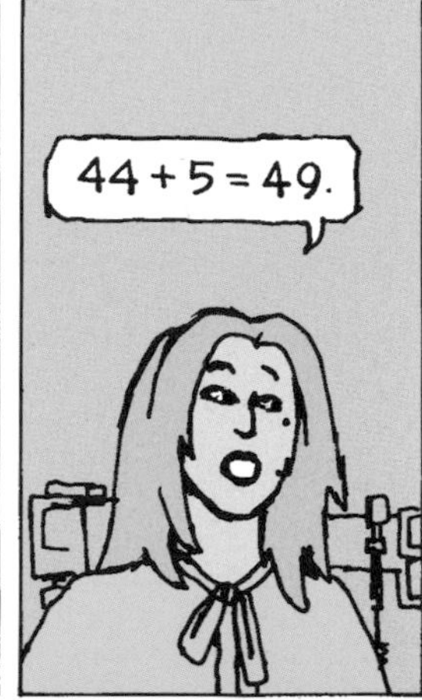
44 + 5 = 49.
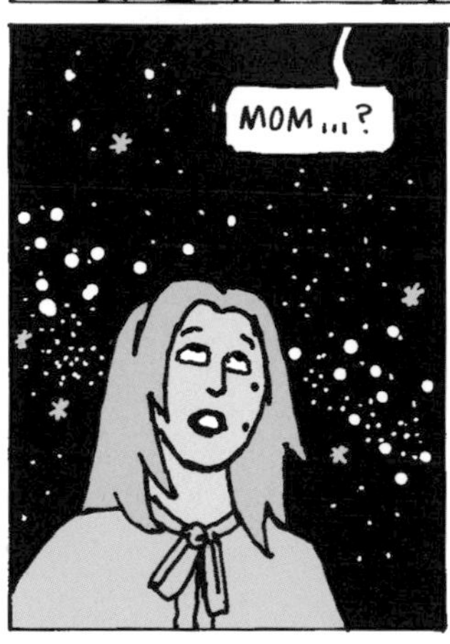
MOM...?
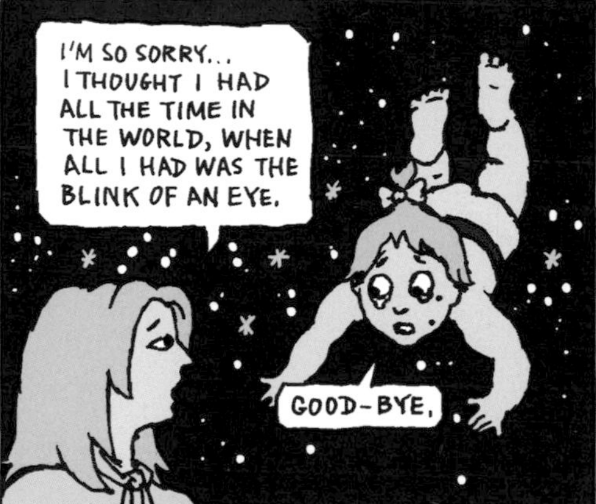
I'M SO SORRY... I THOUGHT I HAD ALL THE TIME IN THE WORLD, WHEN ALL I HAD WAS THE BLINK OF AN EYE.
GOOD-BYE.
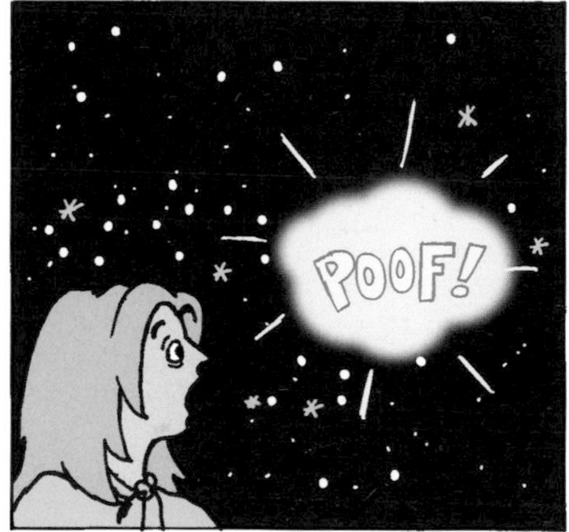
POOF!
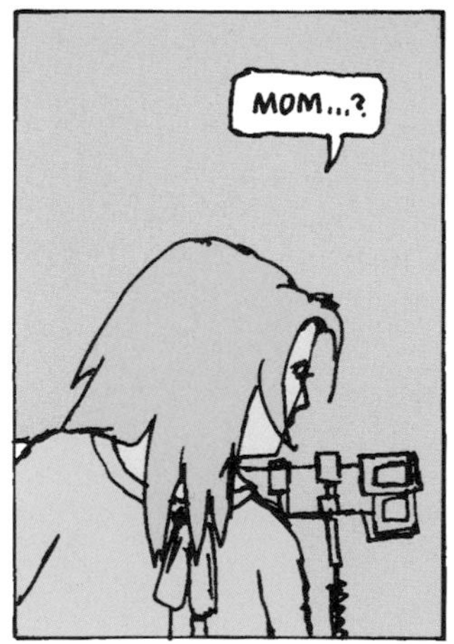
MOM...?
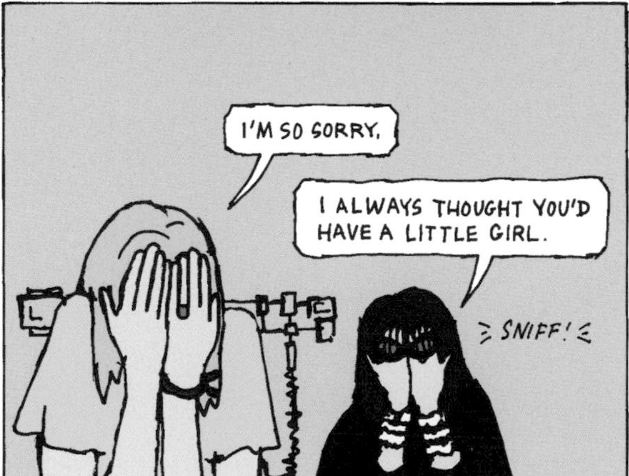
I'M SO SORRY.
I ALWAYS THOUGHT YOU'D HAVE A LITTLE GIRL.
SNIFF!
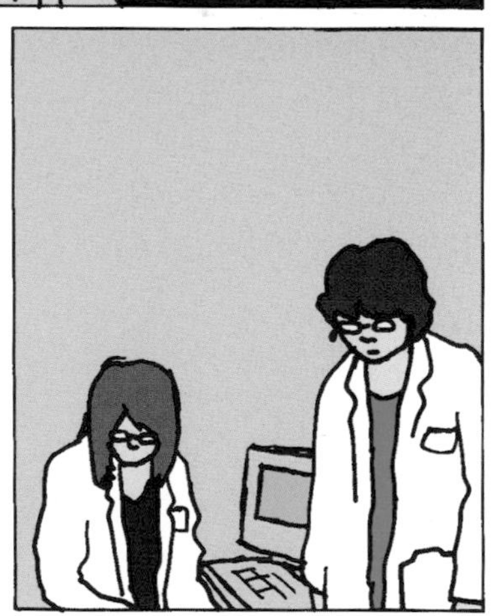

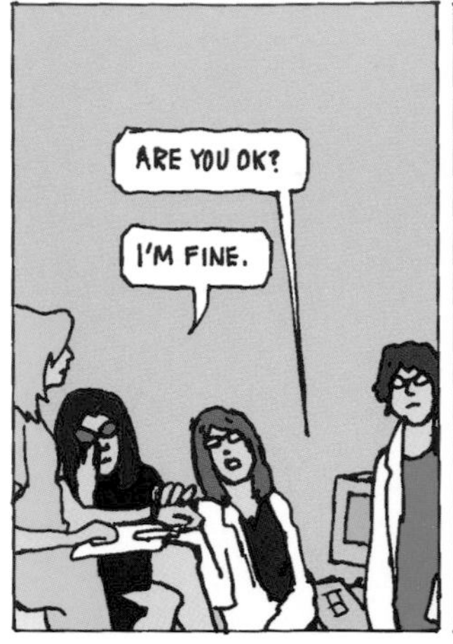

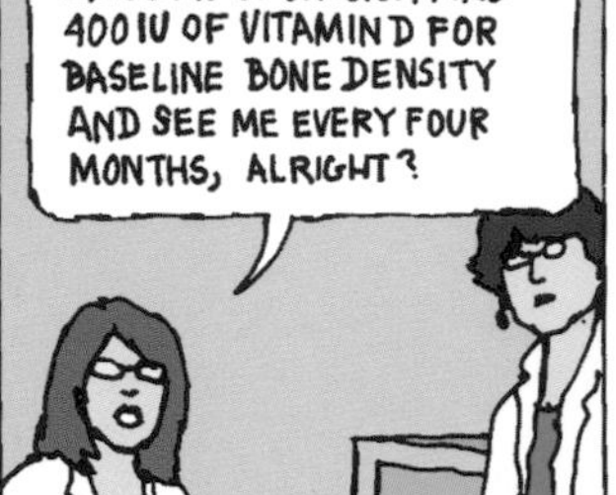

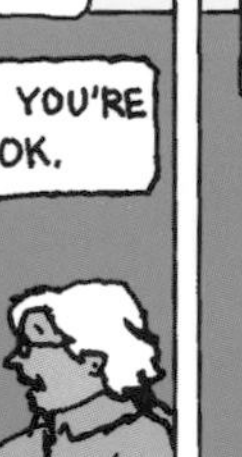

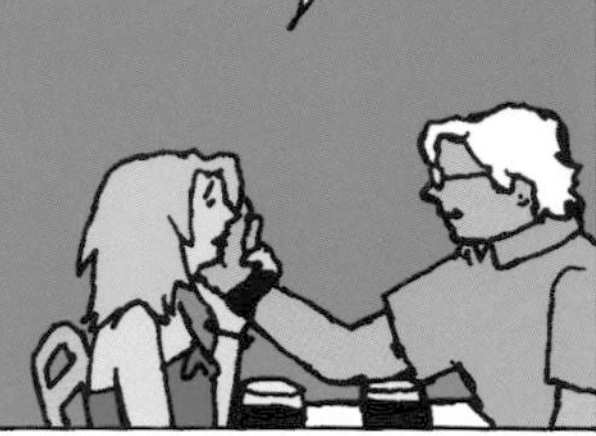

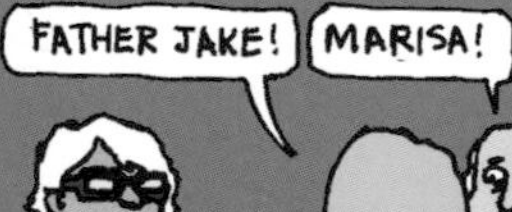

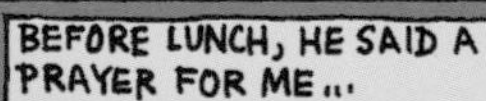

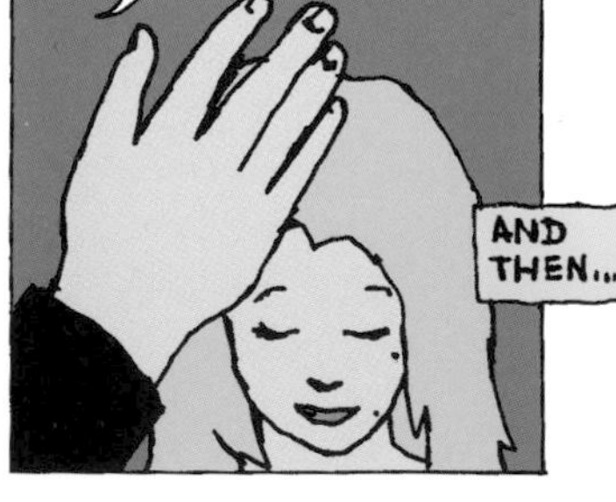

FOLD

BEATVS · IACOBVS · VENETVS

Dear Blessed Iacobus,

During your lifetime you received the sick and the suffering with great tenderness, and you comforted them with words and performed miracles that helped them overcome their pain.
Listen to my prayer, and in your goodness, please help me.
I am trying to be patient in adversity, and I pray to be protected from this cancer, for which people for hundreds of years have prayed to you and invoked your special protection.

Blessed Iacobus, pray for me.

TRANSLATED BY FATHER JAKE

FOLD

FATHER JACOBS GAVE ME THIS HOLY CARD. BLESSED IACOBUS WAS BORN IN VENICE IN 1231, WHERE HIS RELICS ARE CONSERVED IN THE BASILICA OF SAINTS JOHN AND PAUL. HE IS PRAYED TO FOR HELP TO CURE CANCER. FATHER JAKE HAS WITNESSED 4 DRAMATIC MIRACLES.

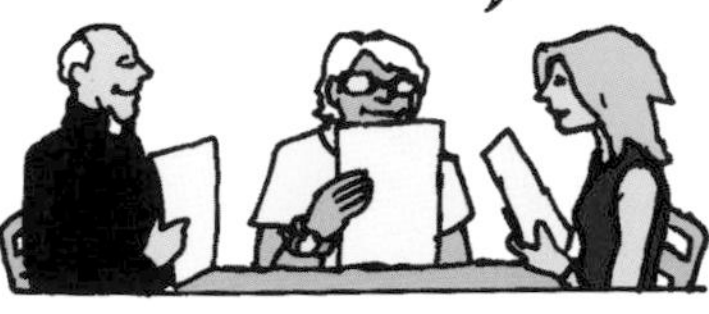

AND HOW AM I TODAY?

I ONLY THINK POSITIVE THOUGHTS!
I FORGIVE ALL MY ENEMIES!
WHAT ENEMIES?! I LOVE EVERYONE!
I GO TO EACH CHECKUP WITH COMPLETE JOY AND ABANDON!
PETTY THINGS DON'T BOTHER ME!
I DON'T HAVE A CARE IN THE WORLD!
I'M ONLY GOING TO CREATE PEACE AND LOVE IN MY LIFE AND JUST HAVE A FEAR-FREE, BLISSFUL EXISTENCE FOR THE REST OF MY DAYS!

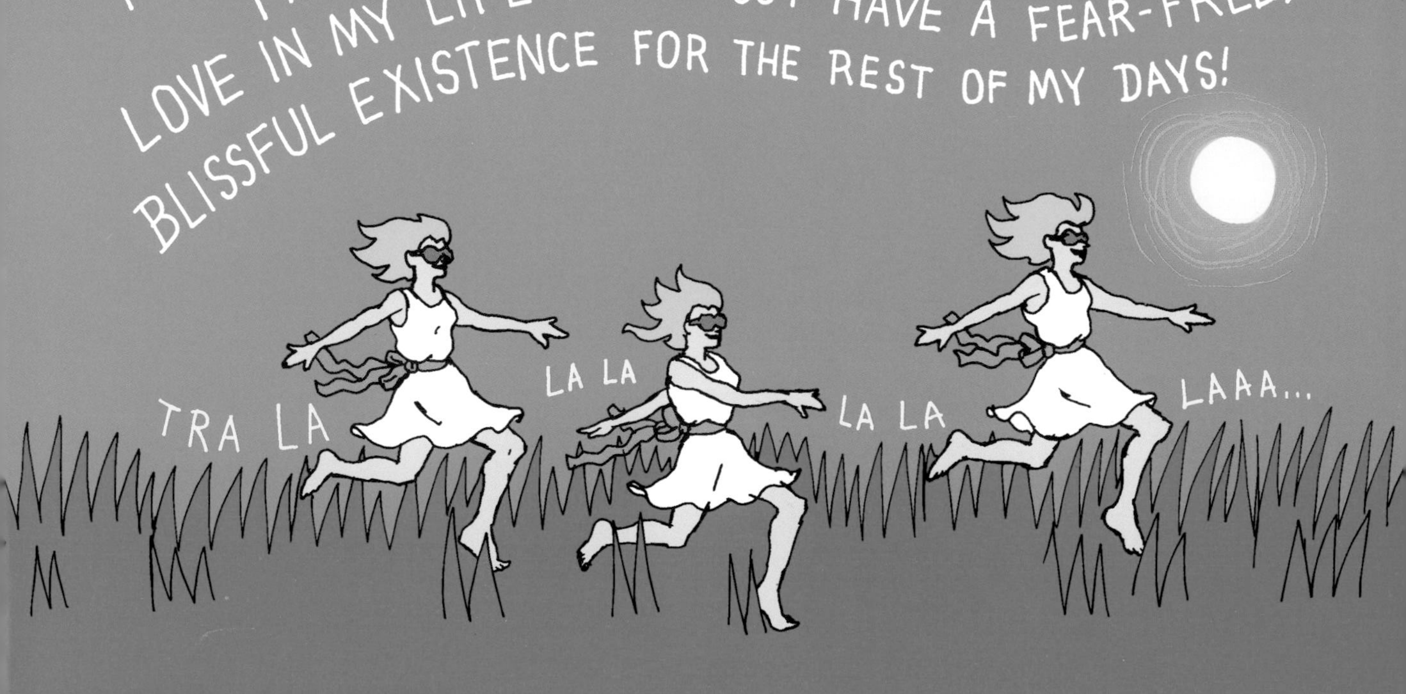

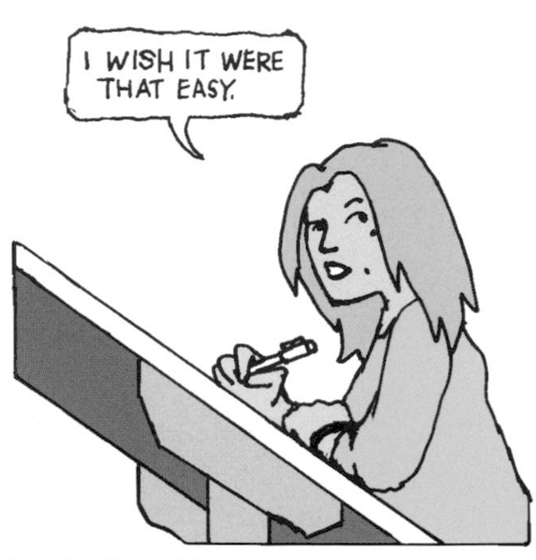
I WISH IT WERE THAT EASY.

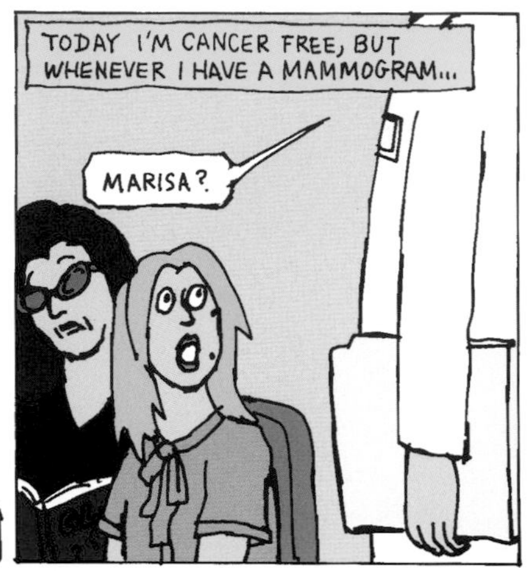
TODAY I'M CANCER FREE, BUT WHENEVER I HAVE A MAMMOGRAM...
MARISA?

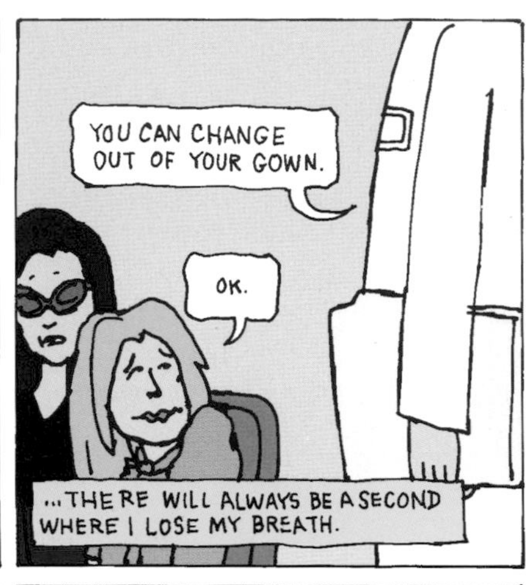
YOU CAN CHANGE OUT OF YOUR GOWN.
OK.
...THERE WILL ALWAYS BE A SECOND WHERE I LOSE MY BREATH.

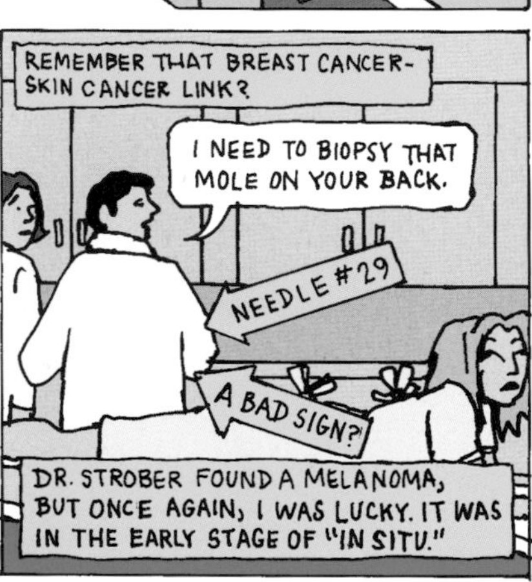
REMEMBER THAT BREAST CANCER-SKIN CANCER LINK?
I NEED TO BIOPSY THAT MOLE ON YOUR BACK.
NEEDLE #29
A BAD SIGN?
DR. STROBER FOUND A MELANOMA, BUT ONCE AGAIN, I WAS LUCKY. IT WAS IN THE EARLY STAGE OF "IN SITU."

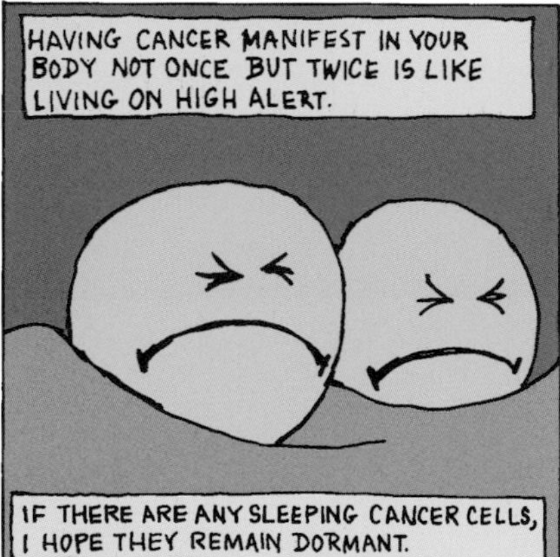
HAVING CANCER MANIFEST IN YOUR BODY NOT ONCE BUT TWICE IS LIKE LIVING ON HIGH ALERT.
IF THERE ARE ANY SLEEPING CANCER CELLS, I HOPE THEY REMAIN DORMANT.

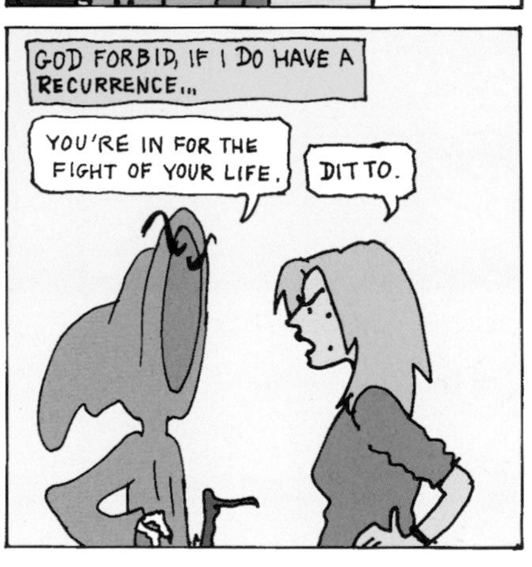
GOD FORBID, IF I DO HAVE A RECURRENCE...
YOU'RE IN FOR THE FIGHT OF YOUR LIFE.
DITTO.

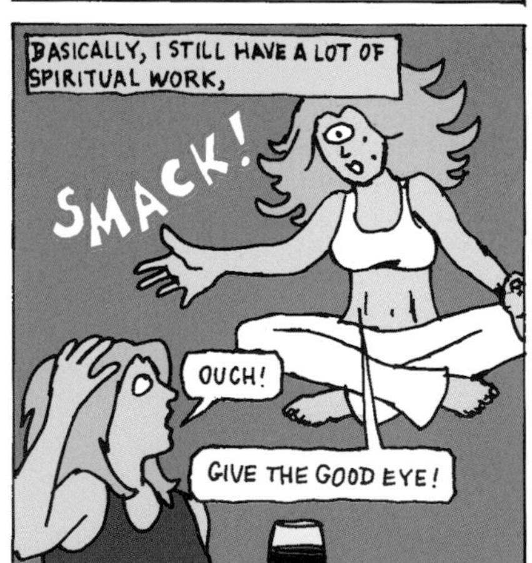
BASICALLY, I STILL HAVE A LOT OF SPIRITUAL WORK,
SMACK!
OUCH!
GIVE THE GOOD EYE!

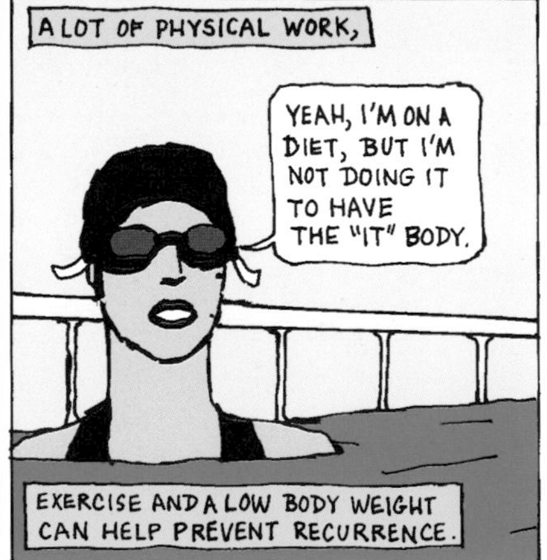
A LOT OF PHYSICAL WORK,
YEAH, I'M ON A DIET, BUT I'M NOT DOING IT TO HAVE THE "IT" BODY.
EXERCISE AND A LOW BODY WEIGHT CAN HELP PREVENT RECURRENCE.

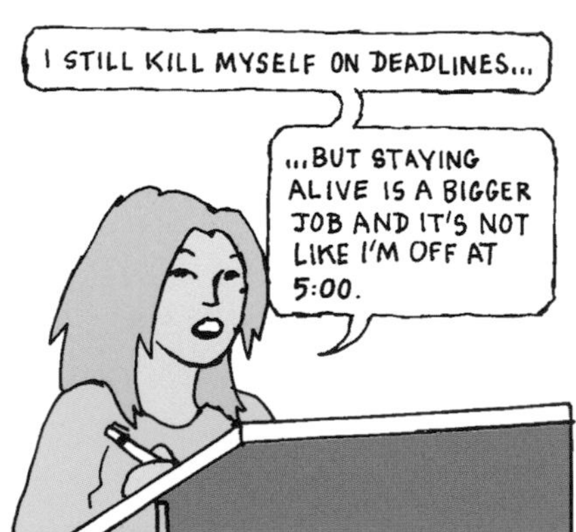
AND A LOT OF EMOTIONAL WORK TO DO.
I STILL KILL MYSELF ON DEADLINES...
...BUT STAYING ALIVE IS A BIGGER JOB AND IT'S NOT LIKE I'M OFF AT 5:00.

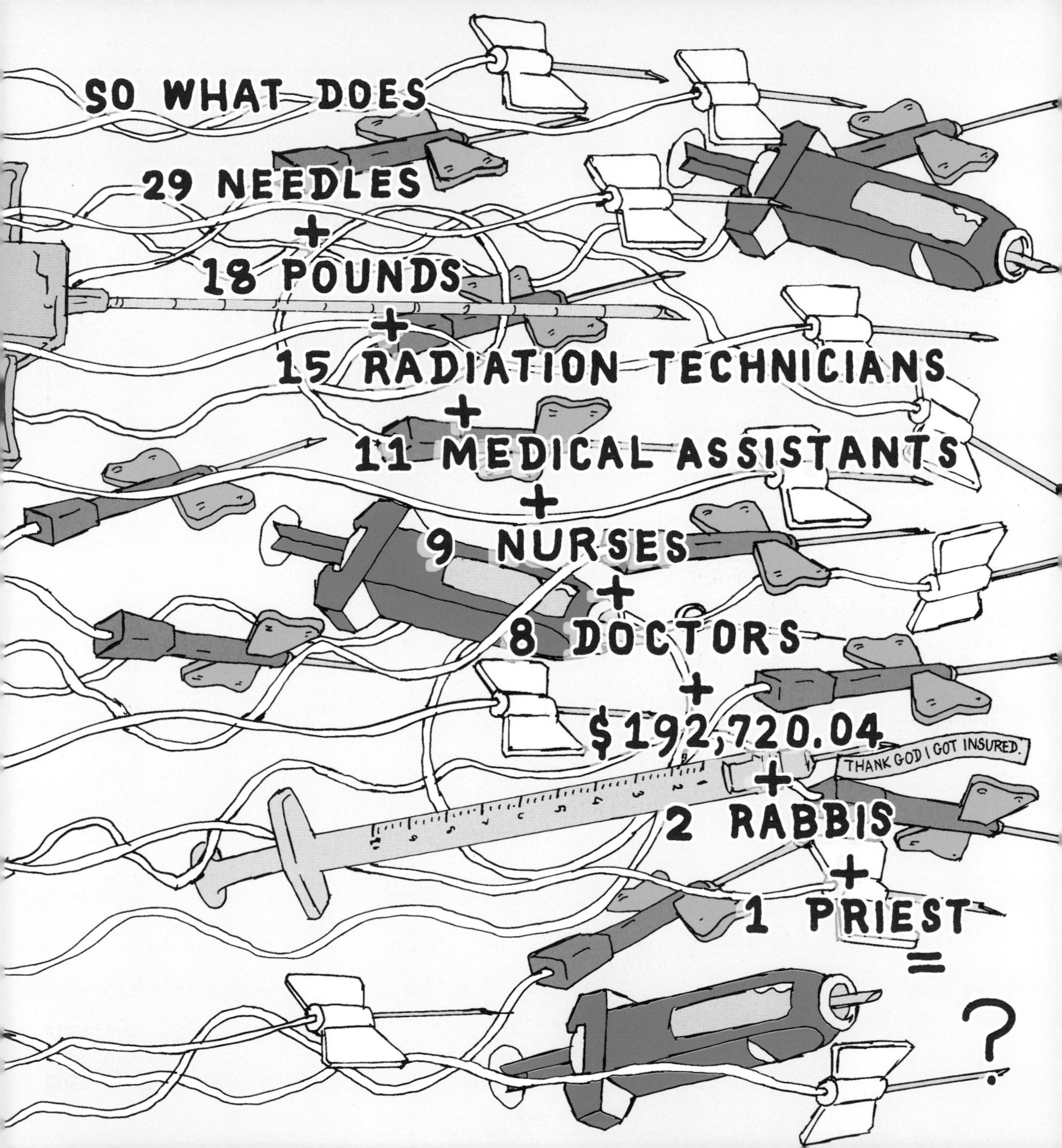
SO WHAT DOES
29 NEEDLES
+
18 POUNDS
+
15 RADIATION TECHNICIANS
+
11 MEDICAL ASSISTANTS
+
9 NURSES
+
8 DOCTORS
+
$192,720.04
THANK GOD I GOT INSURED.
+
2 RABBIS
+
1 PRIEST
=
?

ANSWER:

IT ADDS UP TO AN EXPERIENCE

THAT HAS CHANGED ME FOREVER...

READY TO GO? LET'S PACK UP THE CAR.
WE SHOULD LEAVE NOW, BEFORE IT STARTS TO POUR.

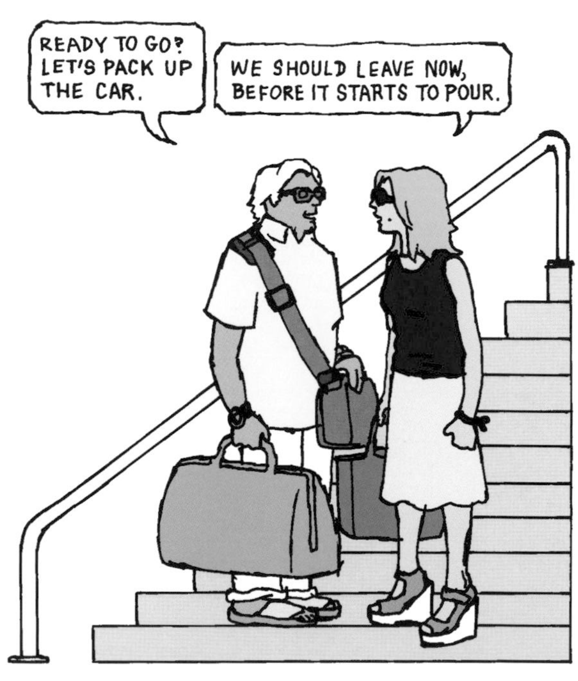

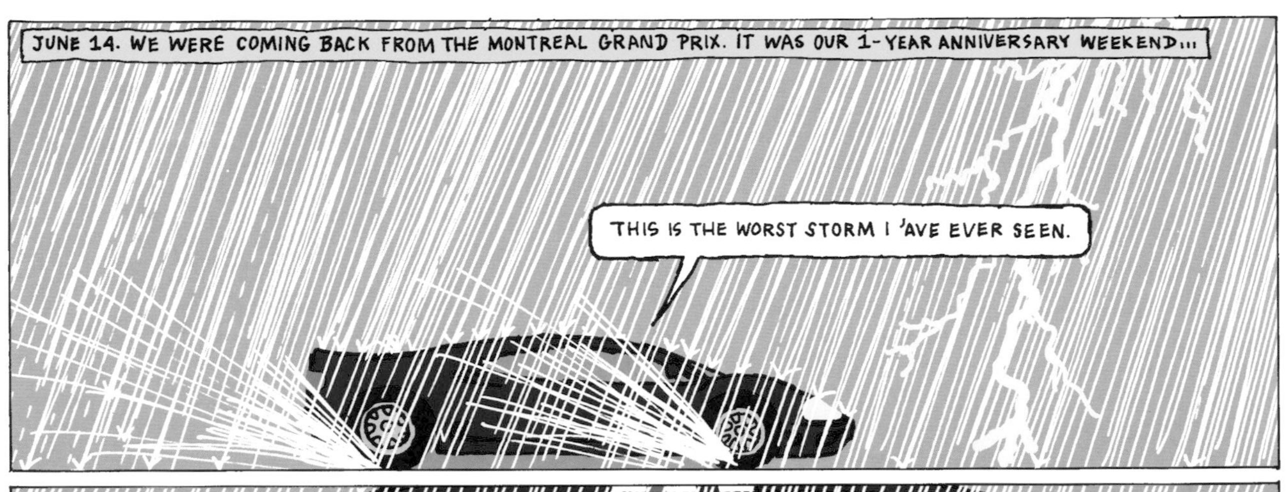
JUNE 14. WE WERE COMING BACK FROM THE MONTREAL GRAND PRIX. IT WAS OUR 1-YEAR ANNIVERSARY WEEKEND...
THIS IS THE WORST STORM I 'AVE EVER SEEN.

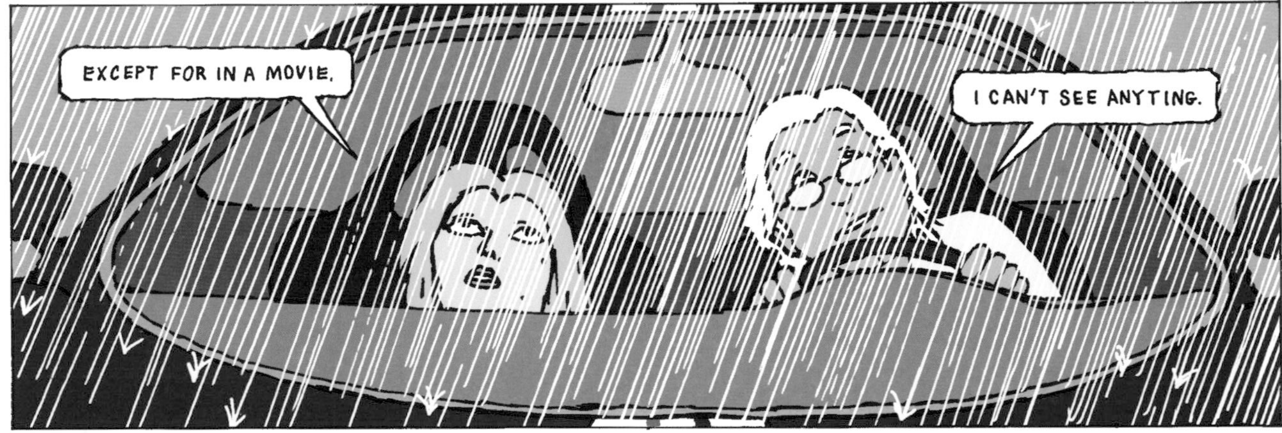
EXCEPT FOR IN A MOVIE.
I CAN'T SEE ANYTING.

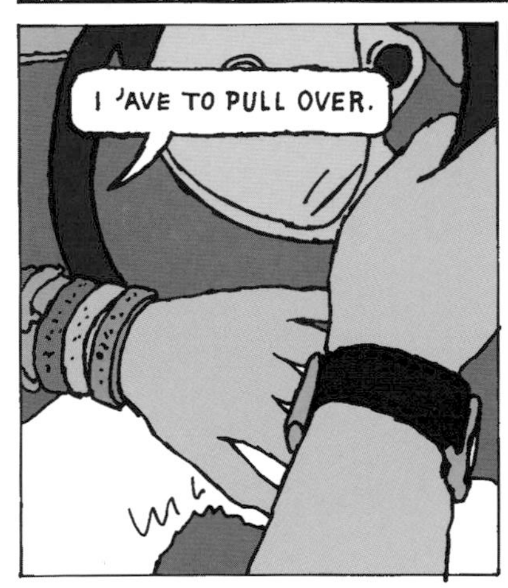
I 'AVE TO PULL OVER.

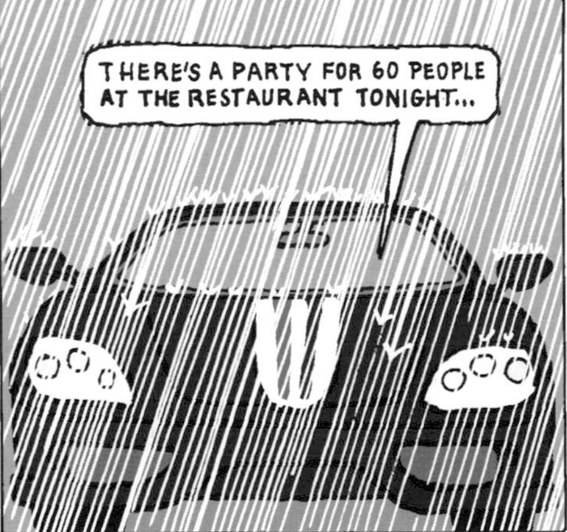
THERE'S A PARTY FOR 60 PEOPLE AT THE RESTAURANT TONIGHT...

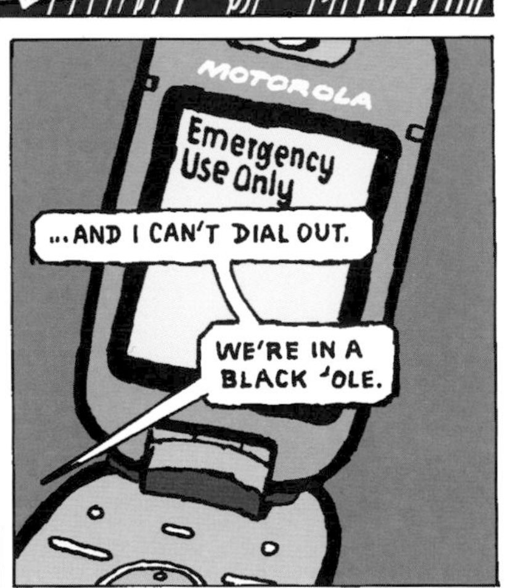
MOTOROLA
Emergency Use Only
...AND I CAN'T DIAL OUT.
WE'RE IN A BLACK 'OLE.

I'M SO MAD ABOUT THIS WEATHER.
DON'T BE...WE WOULDN'T HAVE SEEN SUCH SPECTACULAR LIGHTNING, OR WITNESSED THAT MAJESTIC FOG.

MAYBE YOU'RE RIGHT, MARISA.

SHOULD WE TRY TO GO?
SLOWLY...

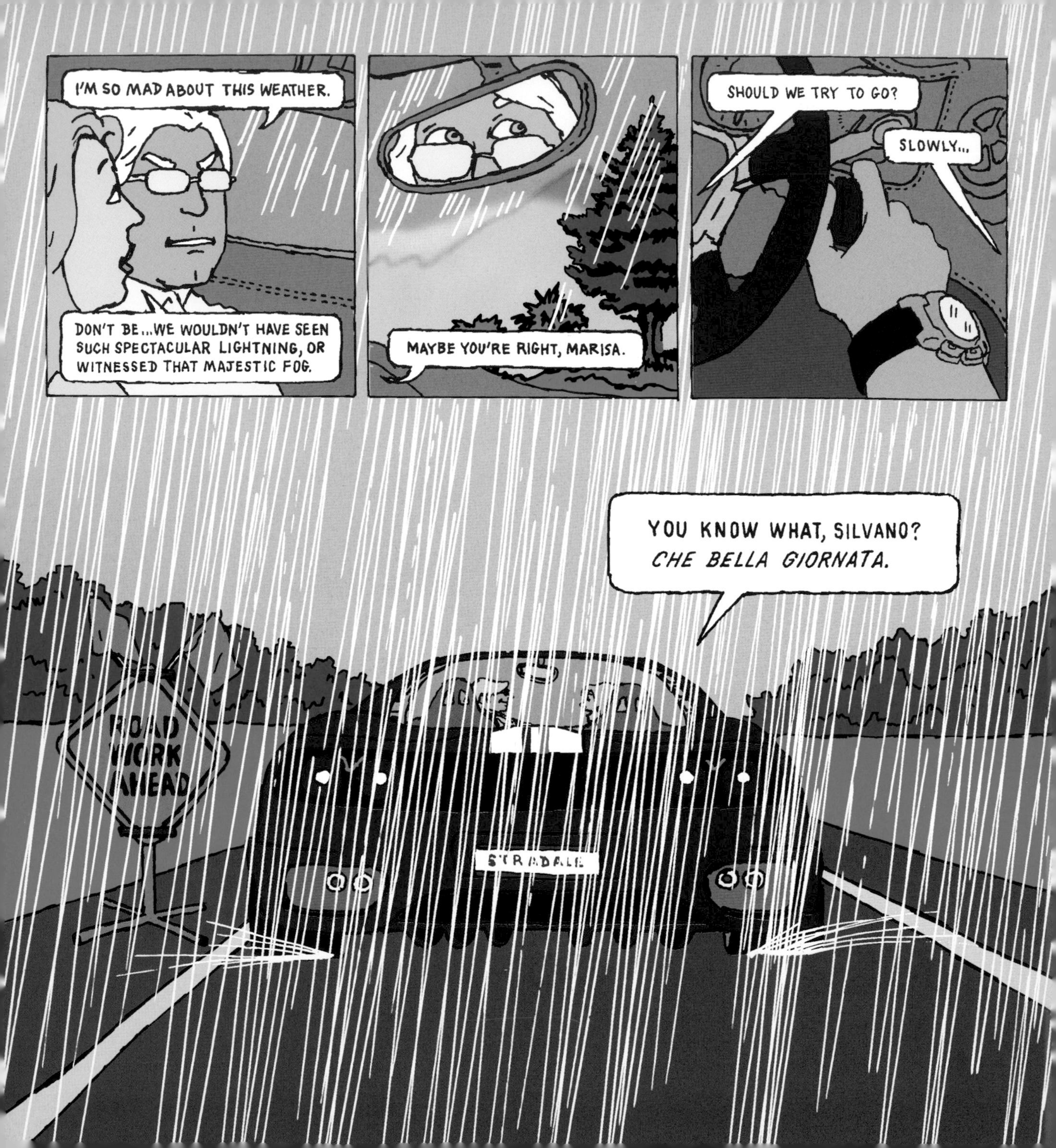

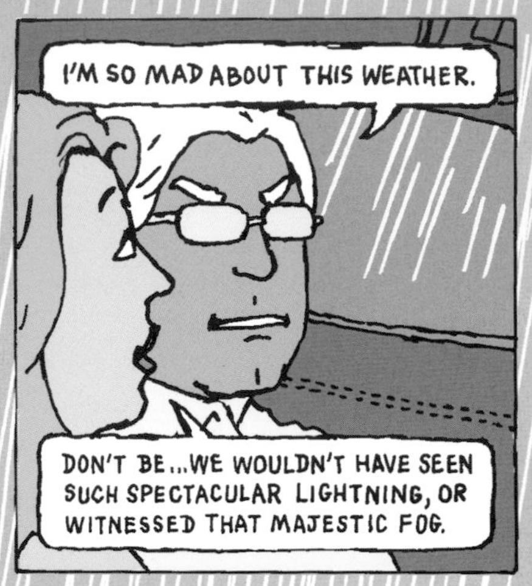

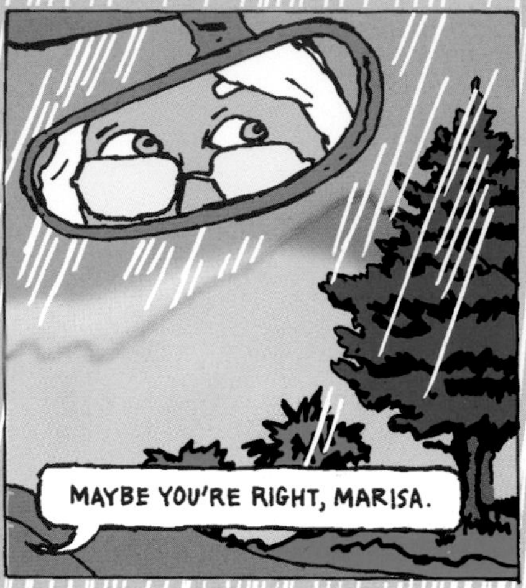

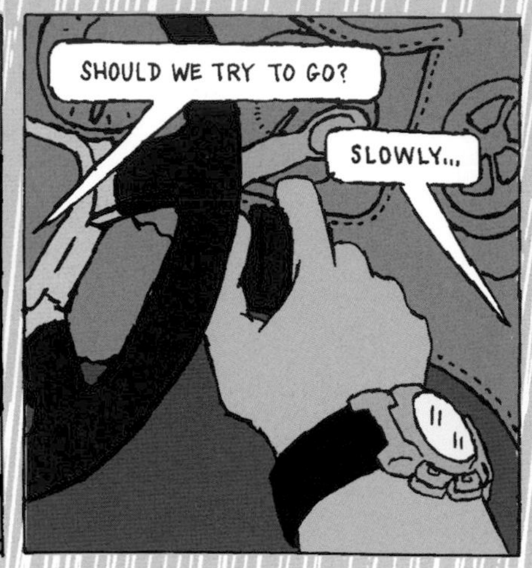

YOU KNOW WHAT, SILVANO? *CHE BELLA GIORNATA.*

ROAD WORK AHEAD

STRADALE

THANK YOU TO MY SUPPORT GROUP OF FAMILY AND FRIENDS.

THIS BOOK WOULD NOT EXIST WITHOUT THE CONTINUAL ENCOURAGEMENT OF CINDI LEIVE AND LAUREN SMITH BRODY OF *GLAMOUR*; MY AGENT, ELIZABETH SHEINKMAN; MY EDITOR/SISTER ROBIN DESSER, DIANA TEJERINA, ANDY HUGHES, PAUL BOGAARDS AND SONNY MEHTA OF KNOPF; AND CRAIG GERING AND SALLY WILLCOX AT CAA.

I WOULD ALSO LIKE TO ACKNOWLEDGE THOSE WHO WILL BATTLE, WHO ARE BATTLING, AND WHO HAVE BATTLED NOT JUST BREAST CANCER, BUT ALL CANCERS.

I PRAY FOR A CURE, AND LOOK FORWARD TO THE DAY WE ARE ALL CANCER-FREE.

IN MEMORY OF JIM MARSHALL AND LORNA CLARKE.

A NOTE ABOUT THE AUTHOR

MARISA ACOCELLA MARCHETTO LIVES IN NEW YORK CITY AND IS A CARTOONIST FOR *THE NEW YORKER* AND *GLAMOUR*. HER WORK HAS APPEARED IN *THE NEW YORK TIMES* AND *MODERN BRIDE*, AMONG OTHER PUBLICATIONS. SHE IS ALSO THE AUTHOR OF *JUST WHO THE HELL IS SHE, ANYWAY?*

GRATEFUL THANKS FOR THE SUPERB COLOR WORK BY JASON ZAMAJTUK AND DENNIS BICKSLER AND THE TEAM AT NORTH MARKET STREET GRAPHICS.